# Emery's
# Elements of Medical Genetics

Commissioning Editor: Alex Stibbe
Project Development Manager: Duncan Fraser
Project Manager: The Partnership Publishing Solutions, Aoibhe O'Shea
Illustration Manager: Mick Ruddy
Design Manager: Andy Chapman
Illustrator: Robert Britton, Antbits Illustration

TWELFTH EDITION

# Emery's Elements of Medical Genetics

Peter D. Turnpenny, BSc, MB, ChB, FRCP, FRCPCH
Consultant Clinical Geneticist
Royal Devon and Exeter Hospital
&
Honorary Senior Clinical Lecturer, Peninsula Medical School
Exeter, UK

Sian Ellard, BSc, PhD, MRCPath
Consultant Clinical Molecular Geneticist
Royal Devon and Exeter Hospital
&
Senior Lecturer, Peninsula Medical School
Exeter, UK

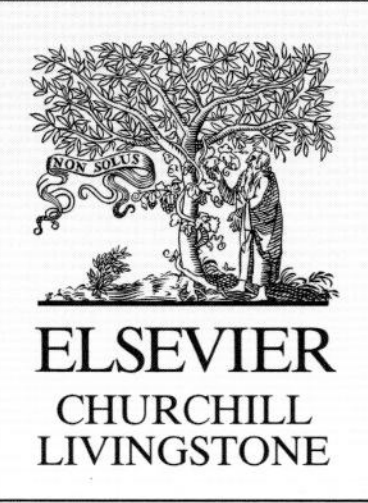


ELSEVIER
CHURCHILL
LIVINGSTONE

EDINBURGH LONDON NEW YORK OXFORD PHILADELPHIA ST LOUIS SYDNEY TORONTO 2005

ELSEVIER
CHURCHILL
LIVINGSTONE

An imprint of Elsevier Ltd



First edition 1968
Second edition 1971
Third edition 1974
Fourth edition 1975
Fifth edition 1979
Sixth edition 1983
Seventh edition 1988
Eighth edition 1992
Ninth edition 1995
Tenth edition 1998
Eleventh edition 2001
This edition 2005

ISBN 0-443-10045-4

**British Library Cataloguing in Publication Data**
A catalogue record for this book is available from the British Library

**Library of Congress Cataloging in Publication Data**
A catalog record for this book is available from the Library of Congress

**Notice**
Medical knowledge is constantly changing. Standard safety precautions must be followed, but as new research and clinical experience broaden our knowledge, changes in treatment and drug therapy may become necessary or appropriate. Readers are advised to check the most current product information provided by the manufacturer of each drug to be administered to verify the recommended dose, the method and duration of administration, and contraindications. It is the responsibility of the practitioner, relying on experience and knowledge of the patient, to determine dosages and the best treatment for each individual patient. Neither the Publisher nor the author assumes any liability for any injury and/or damage to persons or property arising from this publication.
**The Publisher**

Printed in China
Last digit is print number: 9 8 7 6 5 4 3 2 1

The publisher's policy is to use **paper manufactured from sustainable forests**

# Contents



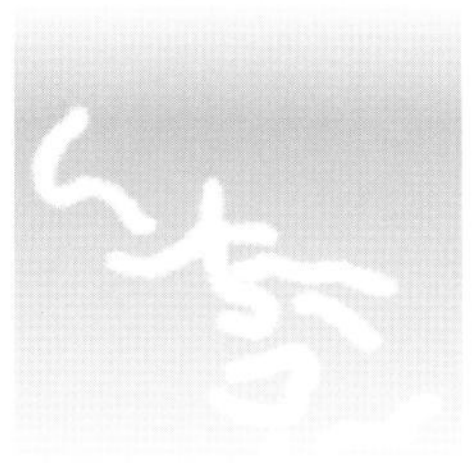

SECTION

# A PRINCIPLES OF HUMAN GENETICS

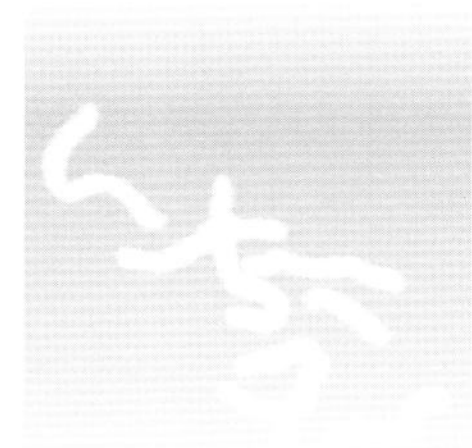

SECTION

# B GENETICS IN MEDICINE

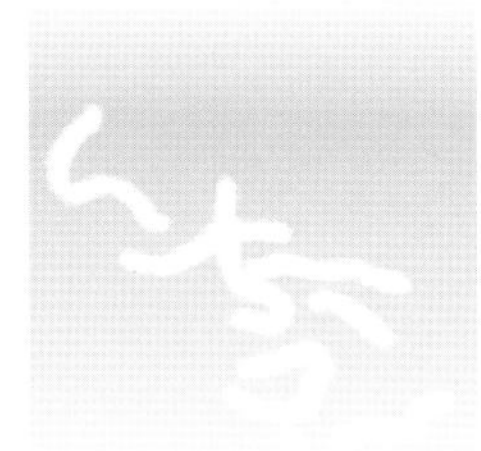

SECTION

# C CLINICAL GENETICS

# Preface

*"A man ought to read just as inclination leads him; for what he reads as a task will do him little good."*

Dr Samuel Johnson

Advances and breakthroughs in genetic science are continually in the news, attracting great interest because of the potential, not only for diagnosing and eventually treating disease, but also for what we learn about humankind through these advances. In addition, almost every new breakthrough raises a fresh ethical, social, and moral debate about the uses to which genetic science will be put. Increasingly, today's medical graduates must be equipped to integrate genetic knowledge and science appropriately into all areas of medicine in order to deliver a dimension of practice and patient care that has hitherto largely been the domain of a small breed of specialists.

In this 12th edition of *Emery's Elements of Medical Genetics* we have sought to provide a comprehensive basic text for medical undergraduates, as well as for specialists experienced in their own fields, who seek a work of reference through which they can swim in calm waters, rather than one in whose rapids they will quickly drown. This is not our work alone: we are building on the dedicated erstwhile efforts of our friends and colleagues – Alan Emery, Bob Mueller and Ian Young – to whom we are indebted. In the short time available to us we have tried to bring the text up to date from the 11th edition. In so doing we have rearranged the structure of the book to reflect some changing emphases in medical genetics and, significantly, added the dimension of self-assessment, which is completely new.

We hope this text proves to be a friendly companion both for those who require familiarity with medical genetics, as well as for those who wish to make it their career, as similar texts once did for us.

PDT, SE
Exeter, UK
June, 2004

# Acknowledgements

Many of our patients were approached for consent to publish their pictures for the first time; not a single one refused, thus making the task of assembling fresh images very much easier than it might have been. In this task, PDT is very grateful to the Graphix Department of the Royal Devon & Exeter Hospital, and Debbie Bristow for secretarial help. We thank our families for tolerating long evenings and weekends, characterized by less than optimal communication whilst the task was at hand.

# Dedication

To our fathers –
sources of encouragement and support
who would have been proud of this work.

SECTION

# A

# PRINCIPLES OF HUMAN GENETICS

CHAPTER 1

# The history and impact of genetics in medicine

*"It's just a little trick, but there is a long story connected with it which it would take too long to tell".*
Gregor Mendel, in conversation with C W Eichling

*"It has not escaped our notice that the specific pairing we have postulated immediately suggests a possible copying mechanism for the genetic material."*
Watson & Crick (April 1953)

Presenting historical truth is at least as challenging as the pursuit of scientific truth and our view of man's endeavours down the ages is heavily biased in favor of winners – those who have conquered on military, political or, indeed, scientific battlefields. The history of genetics in relation to medicine is one of breathtaking discovery from which patients and families already benefit hugely but in today's world success will be measured by continuing progress in the treatment and prevention of disease.

## GREGOR MENDEL AND THE LAWS OF INHERITANCE

### EARLY BEGINNINGS

Developments in genetics during the twentieth century have been truly spectacular. In 1900 Mendel's principles were awaiting rediscovery, chromosomes were barely visible, and the science of molecular genetics did not exist. By contrast, at the time of writing in the year 2003, over 14 000 single-gene disorders or traits have been identified, chromosomes can be analyzed to a very high level of sophistication, and the draft sequence of the entire human genome has been reported.

This revolution in scientific knowledge and expertise has led to the realization that genetics is an area of major importance in almost every medical discipline. Recent discoveries impinge not just on rare and esoteric 'small-print' diseases, but also on many of the common acquired disorders of adult life, such as cardiovascular disease, psychiatric illness and cancer. Consequently genetics is now widely accepted as being at the forefront of medical science and has become an important and integral component of the undergraduate medical curriculum.

In order to put the exciting development and growth of genetic science into context we start with a brief overview of some of the most notable milestones in the history of medical genetics. The importance of understanding its role in medicine is then illustrated by reviewing the overall impact of genetic factors in causing disease; finally, new developments of major importance are discussed.

It is not known very precisely when homo sapiens first appeared on this planet, but according to current scientific consensus it may have been anything from 50 000 to 200 000 years ago. It is reasonable to suppose that man's first thinking ancestors were as curious as ourselves about matters of inheritance and, just as today, they would have experienced the birth of babies with all manner of physical defects. Engravings in Chaldea in Babylonia (now Iraq) dating back at least 6000 years show pedigrees documenting the transmission of certain characteristics of the mane in horses. However, any early attempts to unravel the mysteries of genetics would have been severely hampered by a total lack of knowledge and understanding of basic processes such as conception and reproduction.

Early Greek philosophers and physicians such as Aristotle and Hippocrates concluded, with typical masculine modesty, that important human characteristics were determined by semen, utilizing menstrual blood as a culture medium and the uterus as an incubator. Semen was thought to be produced by the whole body; hence baldheaded fathers would beget baldheaded sons. These ideas prevailed until the seventeenth century, when Dutch scientists such as Leeuwenhoek and de Graaf recognized the existence of sperm and ova, thus explaining how the female could also transmit characteristics to her offspring.

The blossoming of the scientific revolution in the eighteenth and nineteenth centuries saw a revival of interest in heredity by both scientists and physicians among whom two particular names stand out. Pierre de Maupertuis, a French naturalist, studied hereditary traits such as extra digits (polydactyly) and lack of pigmentation (albinism), and showed from pedigree studies that these two conditions were inherited in different ways. Joseph

Adams (1756–1818), a British doctor, also recognized that different mechanisms of inheritance existed and published *A Treatise on the Supposed Hereditary Properties of Diseases*, which was intended as a basis for genetic counseling.

Our present understanding of human genetics owes much to the work of the Austrian monk Gregor Mendel (1822–84, Fig.1.1) who, in 1865, presented the results of his breeding experiments on garden peas to the Natural History Society of Brünn in Bohemia (now Brno in the Czech Republic). Shortly afterwards Mendel's observations were published by this association in the Transactions of the Society, where they remained largely unnoticed until 1900, some 16 years after his death, when their importance was first recognized. In essence Mendel's work can be considered as the discovery of genes and how they are inherited. The term gene was first coined in 1909 by a Danish botanist, Johannsen, and was derived from the term pangen introduced by De Vries. This term was itself a derivative of the word pangenesis coined by Darwin in 1868. In acknowledgement of Mendel's enormous contribution the term *Mendelian* is now applied both to the different patterns of inheritance shown by single gene characteristics and to disorders found to be the result of defects in a single gene.

In his breeding experiments Mendel studied contrasting characters in the garden pea, using for each experiment varieties that differed in only one characteristic. For example, he noted that when strains that were bred for a feature such as tallness were crossed with plants bred to be short, all the offspring in the first *filial* or F1 generation were tall. If plants in this F1 generation were interbred, then this led to both tall and short plants in a ratio of three to one (Fig. 1.2). Those characteristics that were manifest in the F1 hybrids were referred to as *dominant*, whereas those that reappeared in the F2 generation were described as being *recessive*. On reanalysis it has been suggested that Mendel's results were 'too good to be true', in that the segregation ratios he derived were suspiciously closer to the value of 3:1 than the laws of statistics would predict. One possible explanation is that he may have published only those results that best agreed with his preconceived single-gene hypothesis. Whatever the truth of the matter, events have shown that Mendel's interpretation of his results was entirely correct.

Mendel's proposal was that the plant characteristics being studied were each controlled by a pair of factors, one of which was inherited from each parent. The pure-bred plants, with two identical genes, used in the initial cross would now be referred to as *homozygous*. The hybrid F1 plants, each of which has one gene for tallness and one for shortness, would be referred to as *heterozygous*. The genes responsible for these contrasting characteristics are referred to as *allelomorphs*, or *alleles* for short.

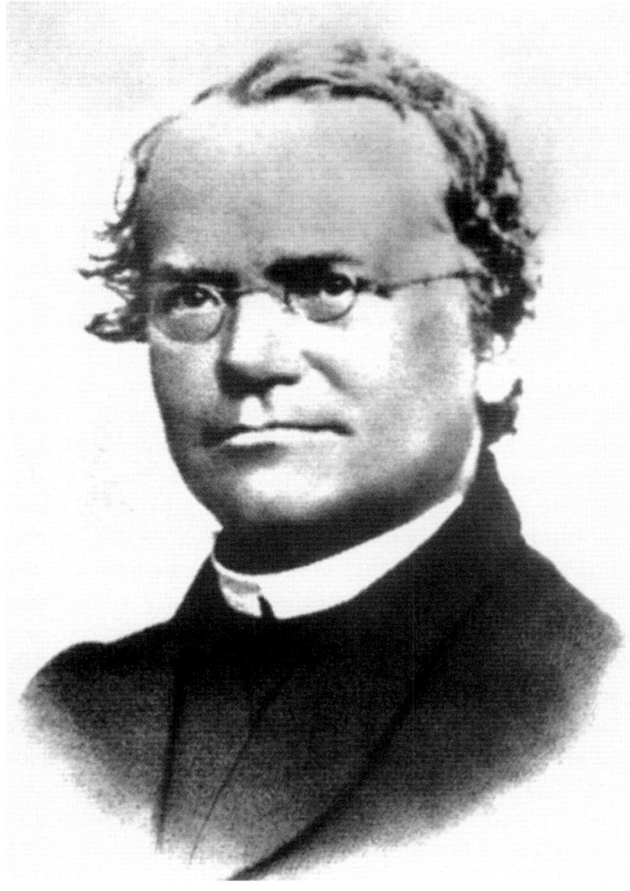

Fig. 1.1
Gregor Mendel. (Reproduced with permission from BMJ Books)

**First filial cross**

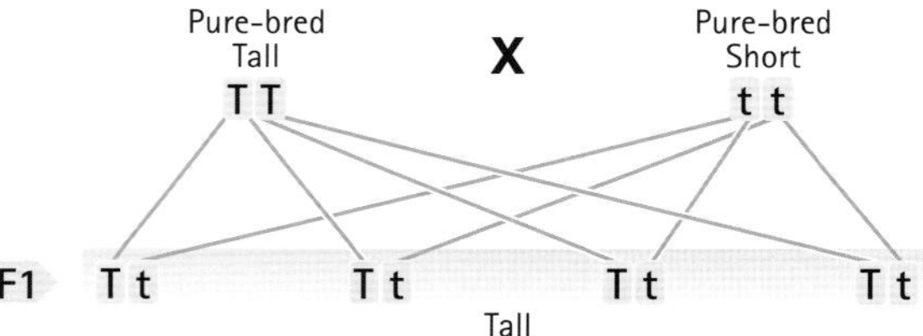


**Second filial cross**

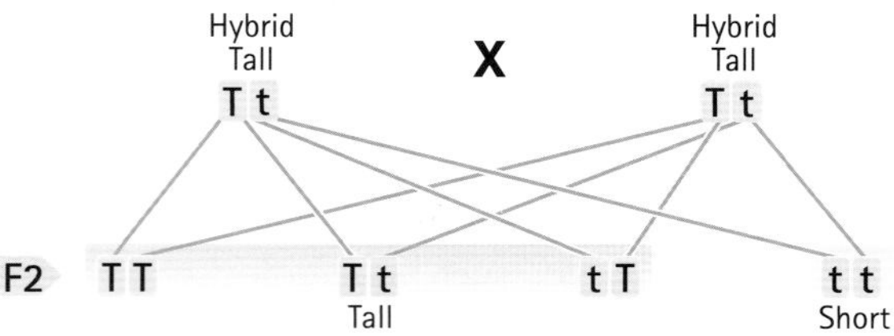


Fig. 1.2
An illustration of one of Mendel's breeding experiments and how he correctly interpreted the results

An alternative method for determining *genotypes* in offspring involves the construction of what is known as a Punnett's square (Fig. 1.3). This will be utilized further in Chapter 7 when considering how genes segregate in large populations.

On the basis of Mendel's plant experiments, three main principles were established. These are known as the laws of uniformity, segregation and independent assortment.

## THE LAW OF UNIFORMITY

The *law of uniformity* refers to the fact that when two homozygotes with different alleles are crossed, all the offspring in the F1 generation are identical and heterozygous. In other words, the characteristics do not blend, as had been believed previously, and can reappear in later generations.

## THE LAW OF SEGREGATION

The *law of segregation* refers to the observation that each individual possesses two genes for a particular characteristic, only one of which can be transmitted at any one time. Rare exceptions to this rule can occur when two allelic genes fail to separate because of chromosome non-disjunction at the first meiotic division (p. 44).

## THE LAW OF INDEPENDENT ASSORTMENT

The *law of independent assortment* refers to the fact that members of different gene pairs segregate to offspring independently of one another. In reality, this is not always true, as genes that are close together on the same chromosome tend to be inherited together, i.e. they are 'linked' (p. 131). There are a number of other ways by which the laws of Mendelian inheritance are breached but, overall, they remain foundational to our understanding of the science.

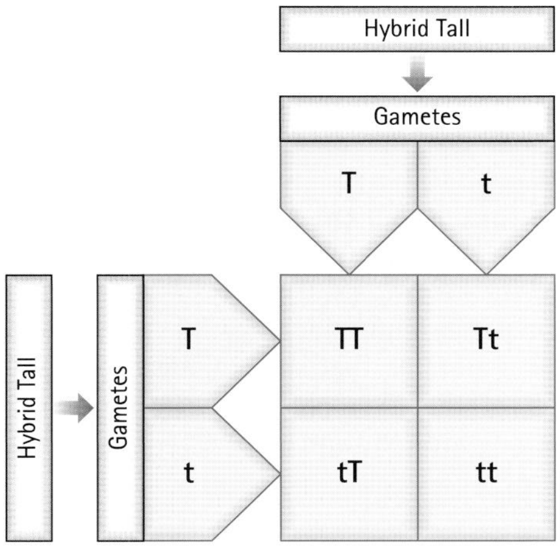

Hybrid Tall

Gametes

| | T | t |
|---|---|---|
| **T** | TT | Tt |
| **t** | tT | tt |

Hybrid Tall → Gametes

Fig. 1.3
A Punnett's square showing the different ways in which genes can segregate and combine in the second filial cross from Figure 1.2. Construction of a Punnett's square provides a simple method for showing the possible gamete combinations in different matings

## THE CHROMOSOMAL BASIS OF INHERITANCE

As interest in Mendelian inheritance grew, there was much speculation as to how it actually occurred. At that time it was also known that each cell contains a nucleus within which there are several thread-like structures known as *chromosomes*, so called because of their affinity for certain stains (*chroma* = color, *soma* = body). In 1903, Walter Sutton, an American medical student, and Theodor Boveri, a German biologist, independently proposed that chromosomes carry the hereditary factors, or genes. These suggestions were prompted by the realization that the behaviour of chromosomes at cell division could provide an explanation for how genes could segregate (Fig. 1.4).

When the connection between Mendelian inheritance and chromosomes was first made, it was thought that the normal chromosome number in humans was 48; the correct number of 46 was not established until 1956, 3 years after the correct structure of DNA was proposed. Within a few years it was shown that some disorders in humans could be caused by loss or gain of a whole chromosome as well as an abnormality in a single gene. Chromosome disorders are discussed at length in Chapter 18. Some chromosome abnormalities, such as translocations, can run in families (p. 49), and are sometimes said to be segregating in a Mendelian fashion.

# DNA AS THE BASIS OF INHERITANCE

Whilst James Watson and Francis Crick are justifiably credited with discovering the structure of DNA in 1953, they were only attracted to working on it because its key role as the genetic material was established in the 1940s. Formerly many believed that hereditary characteristics were transmitted by proteins, until it was appreciated that their molecular structure was far too cumbersome. Nucleic acids were in fact discovered in 1849. In 1928 Fred Griffith was working on two strains of *streptococcus* and realized that characteristics of one strain could be conferred on the other by something that he called the *transforming principle*. In 1944, at the Rockefeller Institute in New York, Oswald Avery, Maclyn McCarty and Colin MacLeod identified DNA as the genetic material whilst working on the *pneumococcus*. Even then, many in the scientific community were skeptical; DNA was only a simple molecule with lots of repetition of four nucleic

A 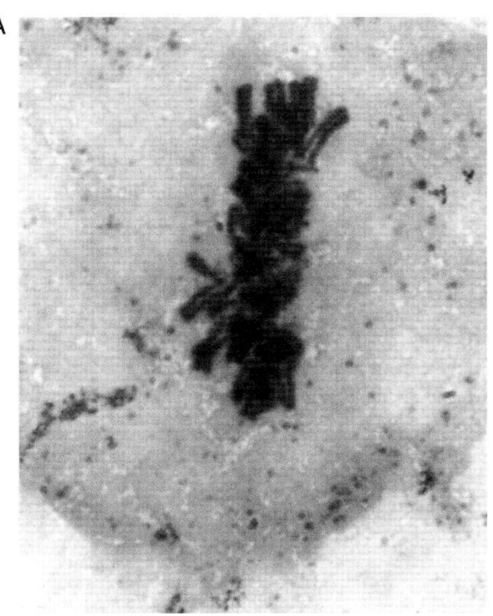
B 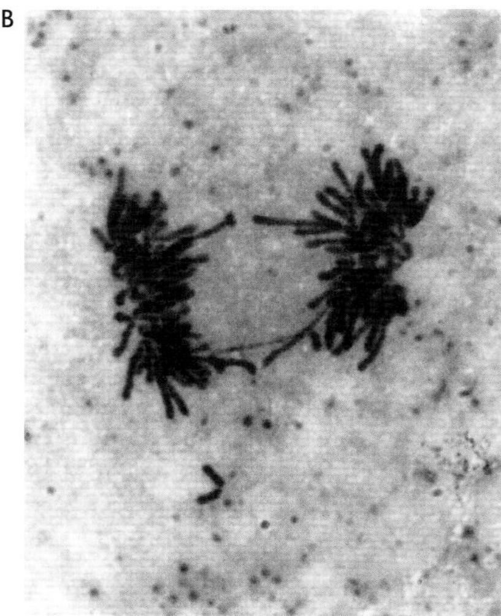
C 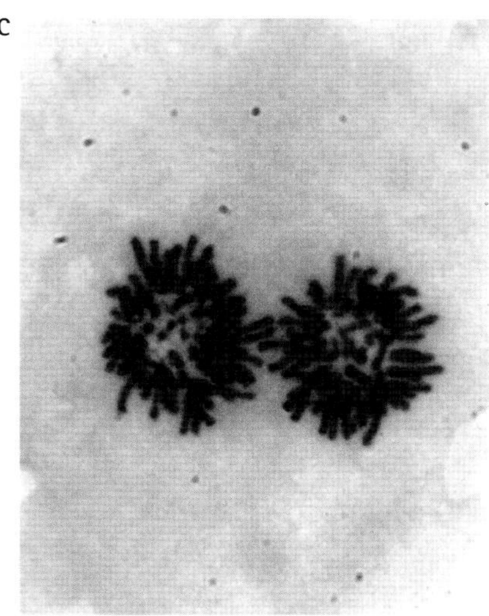

Fig. 1.4
Shows chromosomes dividing into two daughter cells at different stages of cell division. A = metaphase; B = anaphase; C = telophase. The behaviour of chromosomes in cell division (mitosis) is described at length in Chapter 3. (Photographs courtesy of Dr K Ocraft, City Hospital, Nottingham)

acids – very boring! The genius of Watson and Crick, at Cambridge, was to hit on a structure for DNA that would explain the very fact of biological reproduction, and their elegant double helix has stood the test of time. Crucial to their discovery was the X-ray crystallography work of Maurice Wilkins and Rosalind Franklin at King's College, London.

The relationship between the sequence of bases in DNA and the sequence of amino acids in protein, i.e. the *genetic code*, was unravelled in some very elegant biochemical experiments in the 1960s. Thus it became possible to predict the base change in DNA that led to the amino acid change in the protein. However, direct confirmation of that prediction had to wait until DNA sequencing methods became available after the advent of recombinant DNA techniques. Interestingly, however, the first genetic trait to be characterized at the molecular level had already been identified in 1957 by laborious sequencing of the purified proteins. This was sickle-cell anemia, in which the mutation affects the amino-acid sequence of the blood protein hemoglobin.

## THE FRUIT FLY

Before returning to historical developments in human genetics, it is worth a brief diversion to consider the merits of this unlikely creature that has proved to be of great value in genetic research. The fruit fly, *Drosophila* possesses several distinct advantages for the study of genetics. These are as follows:

1. It can be bred easily in a laboratory.
2. It reproduces rapidly and prolifically at a rate of 20–25 generations per annum.
3. It has a number of easily recognized characteristics, such as *curly wings* and a *yellow body*, which show Mendelian inheritance.
4. *Drosophila melanogaster*, the species most frequently studied, has only four pairs of chromosomes, each of which has a distinct appearance so that they can be identified easily.
5. The chromosomes in the salivary glands of *Drosophila* larvae are among the largest known in nature, being at least 100 times bigger than those in other body cells.

In view of these unique properties, fruit flies were used extensively in early breeding experiments. Today their study is still proving of great value in fields such as developmental biology, where knowledge of gene homology throughout the animal kingdom has enabled scientists to identify families of genes that are very important in human embryogenesis (Ch. 6). When considering major scientific achievements in the history of genetics it is notable that sequencing of the 180 million base pairs of the *Drosophila melanogaster* genome was completed towards the end of 1999.

## THE ORIGINS OF MEDICAL GENETICS

Mention has already been made of the pioneering studies of far-sighted individuals such as Pierre de Maupertuis and Joseph Adams, whose curiosity was aroused by familial conditions such as polydactyly and albinism. Others, such as John Dalton of atomic theory fame, observed that some conditions, notably color blindness and hemophilia, show what is now referred to as sex- or X-linked inheritance, and to this day color blindness is still sometimes referred to as daltonism. Inevitably, these founders of human and medical genetics could only speculate as to the nature of the mechanisms underlying their observations.

In 1900 Mendel's work resurfaced. His papers were quoted almost simultaneously by three European botanists – De Vries (Holland), Correns (Germany) and Von Tschermak (Austria) – and this marked the real beginning of medical genetics, providing an enormous impetus for the study of inherited disease. Credit for the first recognition of a single gene trait is shared by William Bateson and Archibald Garrod, who together proposed that alkaptonuria was a rare recessive disorder. In this relatively benign condition urine turns dark on standing or on exposure to alkali because of an inability on the part of the patient to metabolize homogentisic acid (p. 165). Young children show skin discoloration in the napkin (diaper) area and affected adults are prone to develop arthritis in large joints. Realizing that this was an inherited disorder involving a chemical process, Garrod coined the term inborn error of metabolism. Several hundred such disorders have now been identified, giving rise to the field of study known as biochemical genetics (Ch. 11). The history of alkaptonuria neatly straddles almost the entire twentieth century, starting with Garrod's original observations of recessive inheritance in 1902 and culminating in cloning of the relevant gene on chromosome 3 in 1996.

During the course of the twentieth century it gradually became clear that hereditary factors are implicated in many conditions and that different genetic mechanisms are involved. Traditionally, hereditary conditions have been considered under the headings of *single gene*, *chromosomal* and *multifactorial*. Increasingly, it is becoming clear that the interplay of different genes (polygenic inheritance) is important in disease and a further category – *acquired* somatic genetic disease – should also be included.

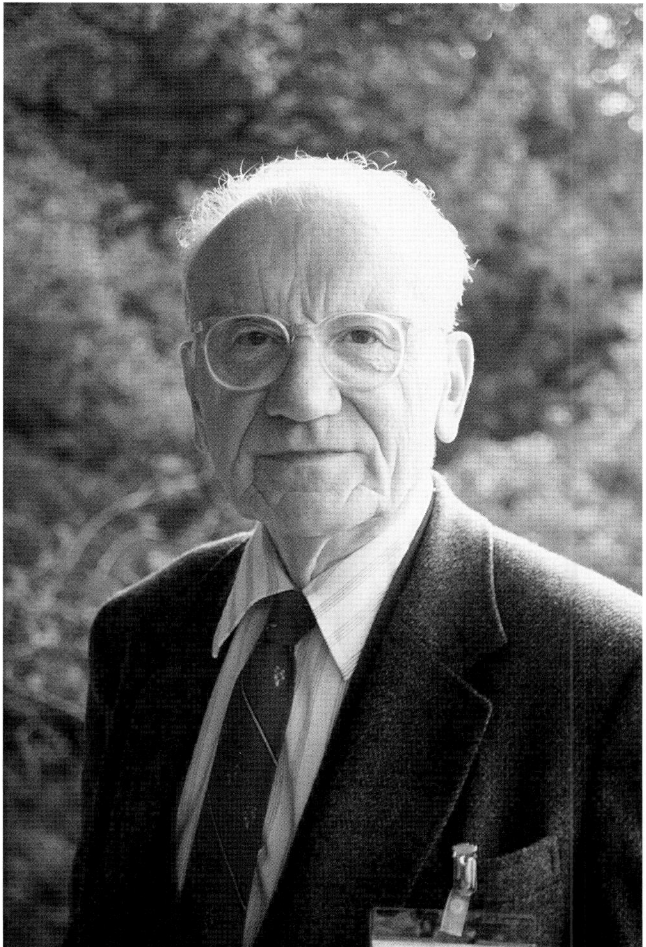

Fig. 1.5
Victor McKusick in 1994, whose studies and catalogs have been so important to medical genetics.

## SINGLE-GENE DISORDERS

In addition to alkaptonuria, Garrod suggested that albinism and cystinuria could also show recessive inheritance. Soon other examples followed, leading to an explosion in knowledge and disease delineation. By 1966 almost 1500 single-gene disorders or traits had been identified, prompting the publication by an American physician, Victor McKusick (Fig. 1.5), of a catalog of all known single-gene conditions. By 1998 when the twelfth edition of this catalog was published, it contained over 8500 entries (Fig. 1.6). The growth of 'McKusick's Catalog' has been exponential and it is now accessible via the Internet as *Online Mendelian Inheritance in Man* (OMIM) (see Appendix). By late 2003 OMIM contained a total of 14830 entries with 11031 established gene loci and 8784 gene map loci (fewer than the established gene loci because many genes are associated with more than one phenotype).

## CHROMOSOME ABNORMALITIES

Improved techniques for studying chromosomes led to the demonstration in 1959 that the presence of an additional number 21 chromosome (*trisomy 21*) results in Down syndrome. Other similar discoveries followed rapidly. The identification of chromosome abnormalities

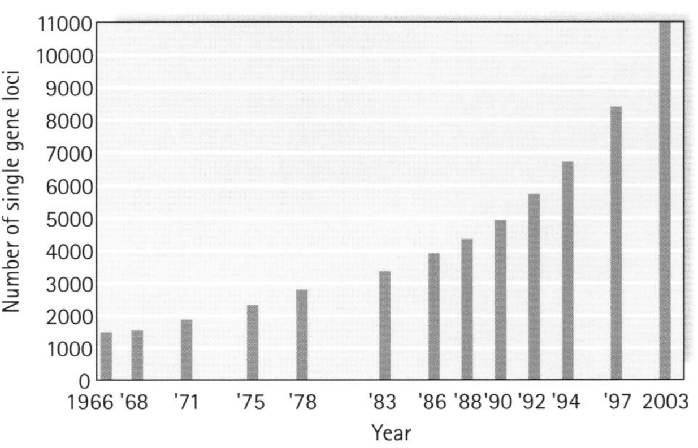


**Fig. 1.6**
Histogram showing the rapid increase in recognition of conditions and characteristics (traits) showing single gene inheritance. (Adapted from McKusick 1998 and OMIM – see Appendix.)

was further aided by the development of banding techniques in 1970 (p. 33). These enabled reliable identification of individual chromosomes and helped confirm that loss or gain of even a very small segment of a chromosome can have devastating effects on human development (Ch. 18).

Most recently it has been shown that several rare conditions featuring learning difficulties and abnormal physical features are due to loss of such a tiny amount of chromosome material that no abnormality can be detected using even the most high-powered light microscope. These conditions are referred to as microdeletion syndromes (p. 274) and are diagnosed using a technique known as FISH (*fluorescent in-situ hybridization*), which combines conventional chromosome analysis (*cytogenetics*) with much newer DNA diagnostic technology (*molecular genetics*) (p. 35).

## MULTIFACTORIAL DISORDERS

Francis Galton, a cousin of Charles Darwin, had a longstanding interest in human characteristics such as stature, physique and intelligence. Much of his research was based on the study of identical twins, in whom it was realized that differences in these parameters must largely be the result of environmental influences. Galton introduced to genetics the concept of the *regression coefficient* as a means of estimating the degree of resemblance between various relatives. This concept was later extended to incorporate Mendel's discovery of genes, to try to explain how parameters such as height and skin color could be determined by the interaction of many genes, each exerting a small additive effect. This is in contrast to single-gene characteristics in which the action of one gene is exerted independently, i.e. in a non-additive fashion.

This model of *quantitative inheritance* is now widely accepted and has been adapted to explain the pattern of inheritance observed for many relatively common conditions (Ch. 9). These include congenital malformations such as cleft lip and palate, and late-onset conditions such as hypertension, diabetes mellitus and Alzheimer disease. The prevailing view is that genes at several loci interact to generate a susceptibility to the effects of adverse environmental trigger factors. Recent research has confirmed that many genes are involved in most of these adult-onset disorders, although progress in identifying specific susceptibility loci has been disappointingly slow. It has also emerged that in some conditions, such as type I diabetes mellitus, different genes can exert major or minor effects in determining susceptibility (p. 145). Overall, multifactorial/polygenic conditions are now known to make a very major contribution to chronic illness in adult life (Ch. 15).

## ACQUIRED SOMATIC GENETIC DISEASE

Not all genetic errors are present from conception. Many billions of cell divisions (mitoses) occur in the course of an average human lifetime. During each *mitosis* there is an opportunity for both single-gene mutations to occur, because of DNA copy errors, and for numerical chromosome abnormalities to arise as a result of errors in chromosome separation. Accumulating somatic mutations and chromosome abnormalities are now known to play a major role in causing cancer (Ch. 14), and they probably also explain the rising incidence with age of many other serious illnesses, as well as the aging process itself. It is, therefore, necessary to appreciate that not all disease with a genetic basis is hereditary.

Before considering the impact of hereditary disease it is necessary to introduce a few definitions.

### Incidence

*Incidence* refers to the rate at which new cases occur. Thus, if the birth incidence of a particular condition equals 1 in 1000, then on average 1 in every 1000 newborn infants is affected.

### Prevalence

This refers to the proportion of a population affected at any one time. The prevalence of a genetic disease will usually be less than its birth incidence, either because life expectancy is reduced or because the condition shows a delayed age of onset.

### Frequency

*Frequency* is a general term that lacks scientific specificity, although the word is often taken as being synonymous with incidence when calculating gene 'frequencies' (Ch. 8).

### Congenital

*Congenital* means that a condition is present at birth. Thus, cleft palate represents an example of a congenital malformation. Not all genetic disorders are congenital in terms of age of onset (for example, Huntington disease), nor are all congenital abnormalities genetic in origin (e.g. fetal disruptions, as discussed in Ch. 16).

## THE IMPACT OF GENETIC DISEASE

During the twentieth century improvements in all areas of medicine, most notably public health and therapeutics, resulted in changing patterns of disease, with increasing recognition of the role of genetic factors in causing illness at all ages. For some parameters, such as perinatal mortality, the actual numbers of cases with exclusively genetic causes have probably remained constant but their *relative* contribution to overall figures has increased as other causes, such as infection, have declined. For other conditions, such as the chronic diseases of adult life, the overall contribution of genetics has almost certainly increased as greater life expectancy has provided more opportunity for adverse genetic and environmental interaction to manifest itself, for example in coronary heart disease and diabetes mellitus.

An indication of the incidence of genetic disorders and their impact on health at all ages can be gauged from the following observations.

### *Spontaneous miscarriages*

A chromosome abnormality is present in 40–50% of all recognized first-trimester pregnancy loss. Approximately 1 in 6 of all pregnancies results in spontaneous miscarriage, thus around 5–7% of all recognized conceptions are chromosomally abnormal (p. 290). This figure would be much higher if unrecognized pregnancies could also be included and it is likely that a significant proportion of miscarriages with normal chromosomes do in fact have catastrophic submicroscopic genetic errors.

### *Newborn infants*

Of all neonates, 2–3% have at least one major congenital abnormality, at least 50% of which are caused exclusively or partially by genetic factors (Ch. 16). The incidences of chromosome abnormalities and single-gene disorders in neonates are approximately $\frac{1}{200}$ and $\frac{1}{100}$ respectively.

### *Childhood*

Genetic disorders account for 50% of all childhood blindness, 50% of all childhood deafness and 50% of all cases of severe learning difficulty. In developed countries genetic disorders and congenital malformations together also account for 30% of all childhood hospital admissions and 40–50% of all childhood deaths.

### *Adult life*

Approximately 1% of all malignancy is caused by single-gene inheritance, and between 5% and 10% of common cancers such as breast, colon and ovary have a strong hereditary component. By the age of 25, 5% of the population will have a disorder in which genetic factors play an important role. Taking into account the genetic contribution to cancer and cardiovascular diseases, such as coronary artery occlusion and hypertension, it has been estimated that over 50% of the older adult population in developed countries will have a genetically determined medical problem.

## MAJOR NEW DEVELOPMENTS

The study of genetics and its role in causing human disease is now widely acknowledged as being among the most exciting and influential areas of medical research. Since 1962 when Francis Crick, James Watson and Maurice Wilkins gained acclaim for their elucidation of the structure of DNA, the Nobel Prize for Medicine and/or Physiology has been won on 18 occasions by scientists working in human and molecular genetics or related fields (Table 1.1). These pioneering studies have spawned a thriving molecular technology industry with applications as diverse as the development of genetically modified disease-resistant crops, the use of genetically engineered animals to produce therapeutic drugs, and the possible introduction of DNA-based vaccines for conditions such as malaria.

### THE HUMAN GENOME PROJECT

With DNA technology rapidly progressing, a group of visionary scientists in the USA persuaded Congress in 1988 to fund a coordinated international program to sequence the entire human genome. The program would run from 1990 to 2005 and 3 billion US dollars were initially allocated to the project, including 5% allocated to the study of the ethical and social implications of the new knowledge. The project has been likened to the Apollo moon mission in terms of its complexity, although in practical terms the benefits are likely to be much more tangible. The draft DNA sequence of 3 billion base pairs was successfully completed in 2000 and the complete sequence was announced ahead of schedule in 2003 amid considerable anticipation and excitement. Prior to the

**Table 1.1 Genetic discoveries that have led to the award of the Nobel Prize for Medicine and/or Physiology 1962–2003**

| Year | Prize-winners | Discovery |
|---|---|---|
| 1962 | Francis Crick<br>James Watson<br>Maurice Wilkins | The molecular structure of DNA |
| 1965 | Francois Jacob<br>Jacques Monod<br>André Lwoff | Genetic regulation |
| 1966 | Peyton Rous | Oncogenic viruses |
| 1968 | Robert Holley<br>Gobind Khorana<br>Marshall Nirenberg | Deciphering of the genetic code |
| 1975 | David Baltimore<br>Renato Dulbecco<br>Howard Temin | Interaction between tumor viruses and nuclear DNA |
| 1978 | Werner Arber<br>Daniel Nathans<br>Hamilton Smith | Restriction endonucleases |
| 1980 | Baruj Benacerraf<br>Jean Dausset<br>George Snell | Genetic control of immunological response |
| 1983 | Barbara McClintock | Mobile genes (transposons) |
| 1985 | Michael Brown<br>Joseph Goldstein | Cell receptors in familial hypercholesterolemia |
| 1987 | Susumu Tonegawa | Genetic aspects of antibodies |
| 1989 | Michael Bishop<br>Harold Varmus | Study of oncogenes |
| 1993 | Richard Roberts<br>Phillip Sharp | 'Split genes' |
| 1995 | Edward Lewis<br>Christiane Nüsslein-Volhard<br>Eric Wieschaus | Homeotic and other developmental genes |
| 1997 | Stanley Prusiner | Prions |
| 1999 | Günter Blobel | Protein transport signaling |
| 2000 | Arvid Carlsson<br>Paul Greengard<br>Eric Kandel | Signal transduction in the nervous system |
| 2001 | Leland Hartwell<br>Timothy Hunt<br>Paul Nurse | Regulators of the cell cycle |
| 2002 | Sydney Brenner<br>Robert Horvitz<br>John Sulston | Genetic regulation in development and programmed cell death (apoptosis) |

closing stages of the project it was believed that there might be approximately 100 000 coding genes that provide the blueprint for human life. It has come as a surprise to many that the number is much lower, with current estimates at around 30 000. However, many genes have the capacity to perform multiple functions, which in some cases is challenging traditional concepts of disease classification. The immediate benefits of the sequence data are being realized in research that is leading to better diagnosis and counseling for families with a genetic disease. In the longer term an improved understanding of how genes are expressed will hopefully lead to the development of new strategies for the prevention and treatment of both single-gene and polygenic disorders. Rapid DNA sequencing technologies currently under development will in due course greatly extend the range and ease of genetic testing, though the application has important ethical and social implications.

## GENE THERAPY

Most genetic disease is resistant to conventional treatment so that the prospect of successfully modifying the genetic code in a patient's cells is extremely attractive. Despite major investment and extensive research success in humans has so far been limited to a few very rare immunological disorders. For more common conditions, such as cystic fibrosis, major problems have been encountered, such as targeting the correct cell populations, overcoming the body's natural defense barriers and identifying suitably non-immunogenic vectors. However, the availability of mouse models for genetic disorders such as cystic fibrosis (p. 302) and Duchenne muscular dystrophy (p. 308) has greatly enhanced research opportunities and there is universal optimism that in the short-to-medium term the prospects for successful gene therapy are good (p. 358).

## THE INTERNET

The availability of information in genetics has been greatly enhanced by the development of several excellent online databases, a selection of which are listed in the Appendix. These are updated regularly and provide instant access to a vast amount of contemporary information. For the basic scientist facilities such as the Genome Database and GenBank enable rapid determination of whether a particular gene has been cloned, together with details of its sequence, location and pattern of expression. For the clinician OMIM offers a full account of the important genetic aspects of all Mendelian disorders, together with pertinent clinical details and extensive references. Although it is unlikely that more traditional sources of information, such as this textbook, will become totally obsolete, it is clear that only electronic technology can hope to match the explosive pace of developments in all areas of genetic research.

## FURTHER READING

Baird P A, Anderson T W, Newcombe H B, Lowry R B 1988 Genetic disorders in children and young adults: a population study. Am J Hum Genet 42: 677–693
*A comprehensive study of the incidence of genetic disease in a large Western urban population.*

Dunham I, Shimizu N, Roe B A et al 1999 The DNA sequence of human chromosome 22. Nature 402: 489–495
*The first report of the complete sequencing of a human chromosome.*

Emery A E H 1989 Portraits in medical genetics – Joseph Adams 1756–1818. J Med Genet 26: 116–118
*An account of the life of a London doctor who made remarkable observations about hereditary disease in his patients.*

Garrod A E 1902 The incidence of alkaptonuria: a study in chemical individuality. Lancet ii: 1916–1920
*A landmark paper in which Garrod proposed that alkaptonuria could show Mendelian inheritance and also noted that 'the mating of first cousins gives exactly the conditions most likely to enable a rare, and usually recessive, character to show itself'.*

McKusick V A 1998 Mendelian inheritance in man, 11th edn. Johns Hopkins University Press, Baltimore
*An exhaustive three-volume catalogue of all known conditions and traits showing Mendelian inheritance.*

On-line Mendelian inheritance in man, OMIM (TM). Johns Hopkins University, Baltimore. World Wide Web URL:http://www3.ncbi.nlm.nih.gov/omim/
*Regularly updated online version of Mendelian inheritance in man.*

Orel V 1995 Gregor Mendel: the first geneticist. Oxford University Press, Oxford
*A detailed biography of the life and work of the Moravian monk who was described by his abbot as being 'very diligent in the study of the sciences but much less fitted for work as a parish priest'.*

Ouellette F 1999 Internet resources for the clinical geneticist. Clin Genet 56: 179–185
*A guide to how to access some of the most useful online databases.*

Shapiro R 1991 The human blueprint: the race to unlock the secrets of our genetic script. St Martin's Press, New York

Watson J 1968 The Double Helix. Atheneum, New York.
*The story of the discovery of the structure of DNA, through the eyes of Watson himself.*

## ELEMENTS

1. A characteristic manifest in a hybrid (heterozygote) is dominant. A recessive characteristic is expressed only in an individual with two copies of the gene, i.e. a homozygote.
2. Mendel proposed that each individual has two genes for each characteristic: one is inherited from each parent and one is transmitted to each child. Genes at different loci act and segregate independently.
3. Chromosome separation at cell division facilitates gene segregation.
4. Genetic disorders are present in at least 2% of all neonates, account for 50% of childhood blindness, deafness, learning difficulties and deaths, and affect 5% of the population by the age of 25.
5. Molecular genetics is at the forefront of medical research. The Human Genome Project and the prospect of gene therapy represent major new initiatives that will revolutionize the management and treatment of genetic diseases.

CHAPTER

# 2 The cellular and molecular basis of inheritance

*"There is nothing, Sir, too little for so little a creature as man. It is by studying little things that we attain the great art of having as little misery and as much happiness as possible."*

Samuel Johnson

The hereditary material is present in the nucleus of the cell, while protein synthesis takes place in the cytoplasm. What is the chain of events that leads from the gene to the final product?

This chapter covers basic cellular biology outlining the structure of DNA, the process of DNA replication, the types of DNA sequences, gene structure, the genetic code, the processes of transcription and translation, the various types of mutations, mutagenic agents and DNA repair.

## THE CELL

Within each cell of the body, visible with the light microscope, is the *cytoplasm* and a darkly staining body, the *nucleus*, the latter containing the hereditary material in the form of *chromosomes* (Fig. 2.1). The phospholipid bilayer of the plasma membrane protects the interior of the cell but remains selectively permeable and has integral proteins involved in recognition and signaling between cells. The nucleus has a darkly staining area, the *nucleolus*. The nucleus is surrounded by a membrane, the *nuclear envelope*, which separates it from the cytoplasm but still allows communication through *nuclear pores*.

The cytoplasm contains the *cytosol*, which is semifluid in consistency containing both soluble elements and cytoskeletal structural elements. In addition, in the cytoplasm there is a complex arrangement of very fine, highly convoluted interconnecting channels, the *endoplasmic reticulum*. The endoplasmic reticulum, in association with the *ribosomes*, is involved in the biosynthesis of proteins and lipids. Also situated within the cytoplasm are other even more minute cellular organelles that can only be visualized with an electron microscope. These include the Golgi apparatus, which is responsible for the secretion of cellular products, the *mitochondria*, which are involved in energy production through the oxidative phosphorylation metabolic *pathways* (p. 178), and the *peroxisomes* (p. 177) and the *lysozomes*, both of which are involved in the degradation and disposal of cellular waste material and toxic molecules.

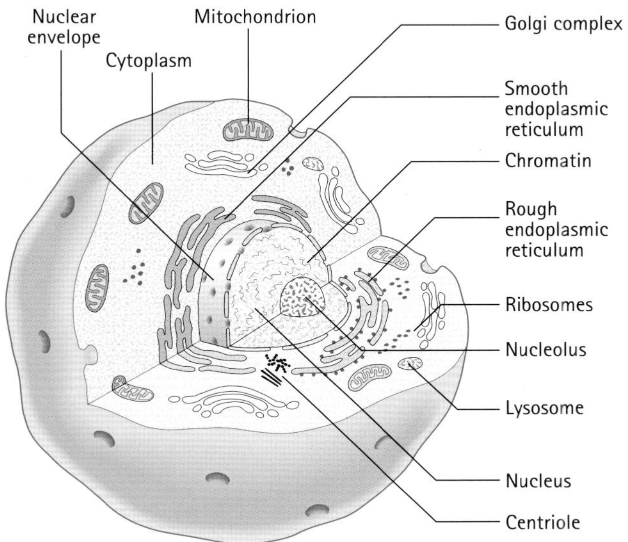


**Fig. 2.1**
Diagrammatic representation of an animal cell.

## DNA: THE HEREDITARY MATERIAL

### COMPOSITION

Nucleic acid is composed of a long polymer of individual molecules called *nucleotides*. Each nucleotide is composed of a nitrogenous base, a sugar molecule and a phosphate molecule. The nitrogenous bases fall into two types, *purines* and *pyrimidines*. The purines include adenine and guanine; the pyrimidines include cytosine, thymine and uracil.

There are two different types of nucleic acid, *ribonucleic acid* (RNA), which contains the five carbon sugar ribose, and *deoxyribonucleic acid* (DNA), in which the hydroxyl group at the 2′ position of the ribose sugar is replaced by a hydrogen, i.e. an oxygen molecule is lost, hence deoxy. DNA and RNA both contain the purine bases adenine and guanine and the pyrimidine cytosine, but thymine occurs only in DNA and uracil is only found in RNA.

RNA is present in the cytoplasm and in particularly high concentrations in the nucleolus of the nucleus. DNA, on the other hand, is found mainly in the chromosomes.

## STRUCTURE

For genes to be composed of DNA it is necessary that the latter should have a structure sufficiently versatile to account for the great variety of different genes and yet, at the same time, be able to reproduce itself in such a manner that an identical replica is formed at each cell division. In 1953, Watson and Crick, based on X-ray diffraction studies by themselves and others, proposed a structure for the DNA molecule which fulfilled all the essential requirements. They suggested that the DNA molecule is composed of two chains of nucleotides arranged in a double helix. The backbone of each chain is formed by phosphodiester bonds between the 3′ and 5′ carbons of adjacent sugars, the two chains being held together by hydrogen bonds between the nitrogenous bases which point in towards the centre of the helix. Each DNA chain has a polarity determined by the orientation of the sugar-phosphate backbone. The chain end terminated by the 5′ carbon atom of the sugar molecule is referred to as the 5′ end, and the end terminated by the 3′ carbon atom is called the 3′ end. In the DNA duplex the 5′ end of one strand is opposite the 3′ end of the other, i.e. they have opposite orientations and are said to be *antiparallel*.

The arrangement of the bases in the DNA molecule is not random: a purine in one chain always pairs with a pyrimidine in the other chain, with specific pairing of the base pairs: guanine in one chain always pairs with cytosine in the other chain and adenine always pairs with thymine, i.e. this base pairing forms complementary strands (Fig. 2.2). For their work Watson and Crick, along with Maurice Wilkins, were awarded the Nobel Prize for Medicine or Physiology in 1962 (p. 10).

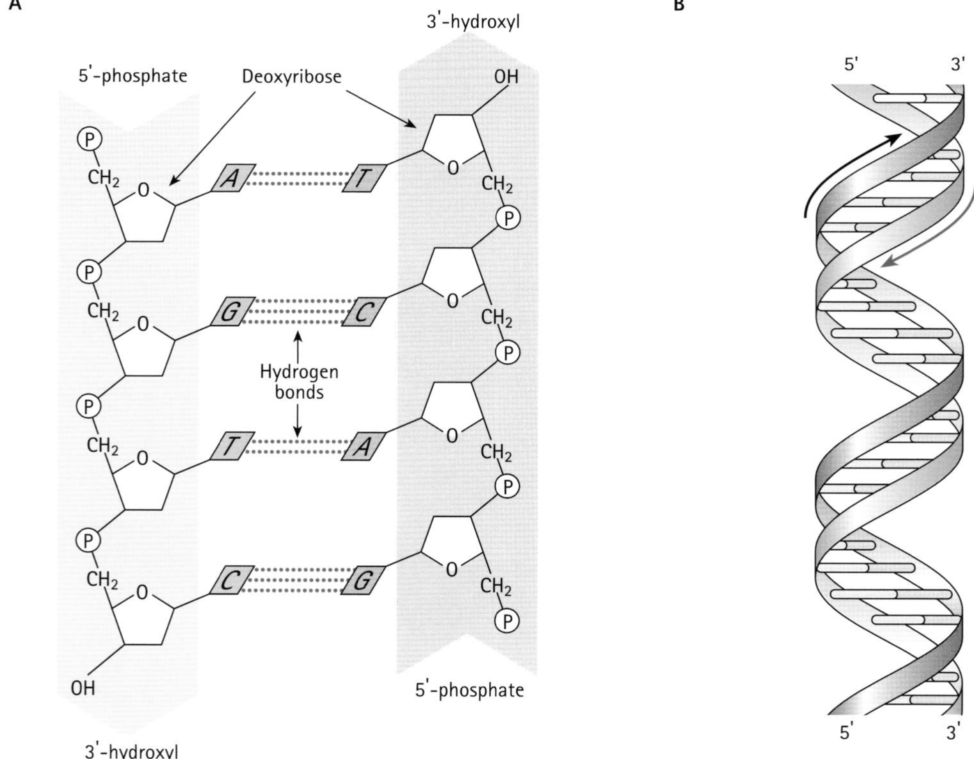


**Fig. 2.2**
DNA double helix. (A) Sugar-phosphate backbone and nucleotide pairing of the DNA double helix (P = phosphate; A = adenine; T = thymine; G = guanine; C = cytosine). (B) Representation of the DNA double helix.

## REPLICATION

The process of *DNA replication* provides an answer to the question of how genetic information is transmitted from one generation to the next. During nuclear division the two strands of the DNA double helix separate through the action of enzyme DNA helicase, each DNA strand directing the synthesis of a complementary DNA strand through specific base pairing, resulting in two daughter DNA duplexes that are identical to the original parent molecule. In this way, when cells divide, the genetic information is conserved and transmitted unchanged to each daughter cell. The process of DNA replication is termed *semiconservative*, as only one strand of each resultant daughter molecule is newly synthesized.

DNA replication, through the action of the enzyme DNA polymerase, takes place at multiple points known as *origins of replication*, forming bifurcated Y-shaped structures known as *replication forks*. The synthesis of both complementary antiparallel DNA strands occurs in the 5′ to 3′ direction. One strand, known as the *leading strand*, is synthesized as a continuous process. The other strand, known as the *lagging strand*, is synthesized in pieces called Okazaki fragments, which are then joined together as a continuous strand by the enzyme DNA ligase (Fig. 2.3A).

DNA replication progresses in both directions from these points of origin, forming bubble-shaped structures, or *replication bubbles* (Fig. 2.3B). Neighbouring replication origins are approximately 50–300 kb apart and occur in clusters or *replication units* of 20–80 origins of replication. DNA replication in individual replication units takes place at different times in the S phase of the cell cycle (p. 30), adjacent replication units fusing until all the DNA is copied, forming two complete identical daughter molecules.

## CHROMOSOME STRUCTURE

The idea that each chromosome is composed of a single DNA double helix is an oversimplification. A chromosome is very much wider than the diameter of a DNA double helix. In addition, the amount of DNA in the nucleus of each cell in humans means that the total length of DNA contained in the chromosomes, if fully extended, would be several meters long! In fact, the total length of the human chromosome complement is less than half a millimeter.

The packaging of DNA into chromosomes involves several orders of DNA coiling and folding. In addition to the primary coiling of the DNA double helix, there is secondary coiling around spherical *histone* 'beads', forming what are called *nucleosomes*. There is a tertiary coiling of the nucleosomes to form the *chromatin fibres* that form long loops on a scaffold of non-histone acidic proteins, which are further wound in a tight coil to make up the chromosome as visualized under the light microscope (Fig. 2.4), the whole structure making up the so-called *solenoid* model of chromosome structure.

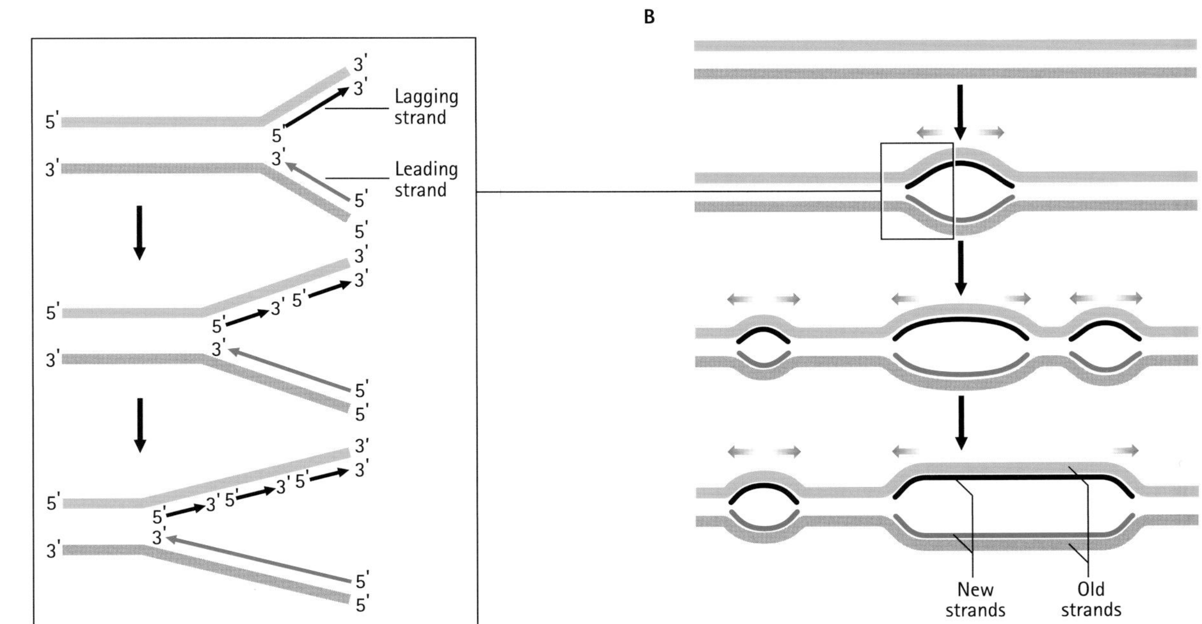


Fig. 2.3
DNA replication. (A) Detailed diagram of DNA replication at the site of origin in the replication fork showing asymmetric strand synthesis with the continuous synthesis of the leading strand and the discontinuous synthesis of the lagging strand with ligation of the Okazaki fragments.
(B) Multiple points of origin and semiconservative mode of DNA replication.

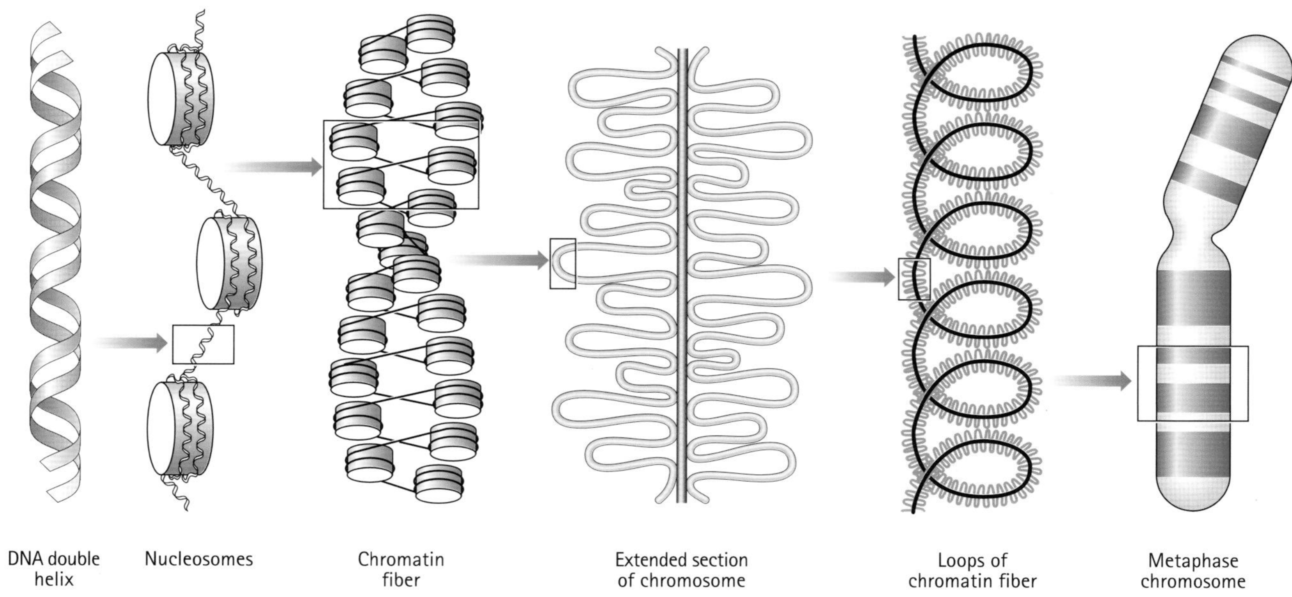


Fig. 2.4
Simplified diagram of proposed solenoid model of DNA coiling which leads to the visible structure of the chromosome.

## TYPES OF DNA SEQUENCES

DNA, if denatured, will reassociate as a duplex at a rate that is dependent on the proportion of unique and repeat sequences present, the latter occurring more rapidly. Analysis of the results of the kinetics of the reassociation of human DNA have shown that approximately 60–70% of the human *genome* consists of single or low copy number DNA sequences. The remainder of the genome, some 30–40%, consists of either moderately or highly *repetitive* DNA sequences that are not transcribed. This latter portion consists of mainly satellite DNA and interspersed DNA sequences (Table 2.1).

**Table 2.1 Types of DNA sequence**

**Nuclear (~3 × $10^9$ bp)**
- Genes (~30 000)
  - Unique single copy
  - Multigene families
    - Classic gene families
    - Gene superfamilies
- Extragenic DNA (unique/low copy number or moderate/highly repetitive)
  - Tandem repeat
    - Satellite
    - Minisatellite
      - Telomeric
      - Hypervariable
    - Microsatellite
  - Interspersed
    - Short interspersed nuclear elements
    - Long interspersed nuclear elements

**Mitochondrial (16.6 kb, 37 genes)**
- Two rRNA genes
- 22 tRNA genes

## NUCLEAR GENES

It is estimated that there are approximately 30 000 genes in the nuclear genome. The distribution of these genes varies greatly between chromosomal regions. For example, heterochromatic and centromeric (p. 32) regions are mostly non-coding, with the highest gene density observed in sub-telomeric regions (p. 32). Chromosomes 19 and 22 are gene rich, whereas 4 and 18 are relatively gene poor. The size of genes also shows great variability: from small genes with single exons to genes with up to 79 exons (e.g. dystophin, which occupies 2.5 Mb of the genome).

### Unique single-copy genes

Most human genes are unique single-copy genes coding for polypeptides that are involved in or carry out a variety of cellular functions. These include enzymes, hormones, receptors, and structural and regulatory proteins.

### Multigene families

Many genes have similar functions, having arisen through gene duplication events with subsequent evolutionary divergence making up what are known as *multigene families*. Some are found physically close together in clusters, e.g. the α- and β-globin gene clusters on chromosomes 16 and

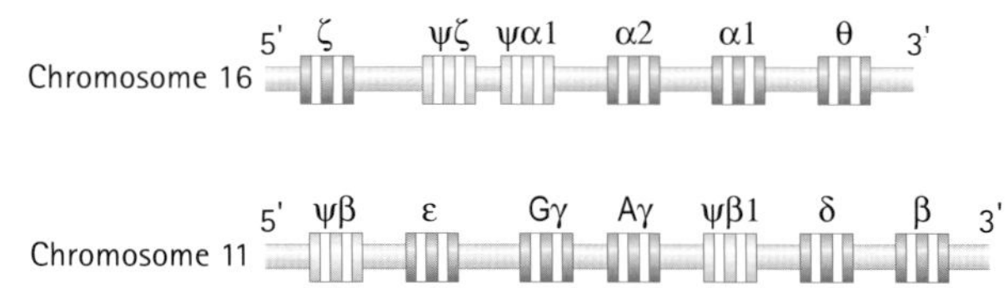


Fig. 2.5
Representation of the α- and β-globin regions on chromosomes 16 and 11.

11 (Fig. 2.5), whereas others are widely dispersed throughout the genome occurring on different chromosomes, e.g. the *HOX* homeobox gene family (p. 87).

Multigene families can be split into two types, *classic gene families* that show a high degree of sequence homology and *gene superfamilies* that have limited sequence homology but are functionally related, having similar structural domains.

### Classic gene families

Examples of classic gene families include the numerous copies of genes coding for the various ribosomal RNAs, which are clustered as tandem arrays at the nucleolar organizing regions on the short arms of the five acrocentric chromosomes (p. 32), and the different transfer RNA (p. 20) gene families, which are dispersed in numerous clusters throughout the human genome.

### Gene superfamilies

Examples of gene superfamilies include the HLA genes on chromosome 6 (p. 193) and the T-cell receptor genes, which have structural homology with the immunoglobulin (Ig) genes (p. 193). It is believed that these are almost certainly derived from duplication of a precursor gene, with subsequent evolutionary divergence forming the Ig superfamily.

### Gene structure

The original concept of a gene as a continuous sequence of DNA coding for a protein was turned on its head in the early 1980s by detailed analysis of the structure of the human β-globin gene. It was revealed that the gene was much longer than necessary to code for the β-globin protein, containing non-coding intervening sequences or introns, which separate the coding sequences or exons (Fig. 2.6). It appears to be the exception for genes in humans to consist of uninterrupted coding sequences. The number and size of introns in various genes in humans are extremely variable, although there is a general trend that the larger the gene, the greater the number and size of the exons. Individual introns can be far larger than the coding sequences and some have been found to contain coding sequences for other genes, i.e. genes occurring within genes (p. 300). Genes in humans do not usually overlap, being separated from each other by an average of 30 kb, although some of the genes in the HLA complex (p. 194) have been shown to be overlapping.

### Pseudogenes

Particularly fascinating is the occurrence of genes that closely resemble known structural genes but which, in general, are not functionally expressed: so-called *pseudogenes* (p. 151). These are thought to have arisen in two main ways, either by genes undergoing duplication events that are rendered silent through the acquisition of mutations in coding or regulatory elements, or as the result of the insertion of complementary DNA sequences, produced by the action of the enzyme *reverse transcriptase* on a naturally occurring mRNA transcript, which lack the promoter sequences necessary for expression.

## EXTRAGENIC DNA

The estimated 30 000 unique single-copy genes in humans represent less than 2% of the genome encoding proteins. The remainder of the human genome is made up of repetitive DNA sequences that are predominantly transcriptionally inactive. It has been described as *junk* DNA, but some regions show evolutionary conservation and may play a role in the regulation of gene expression.

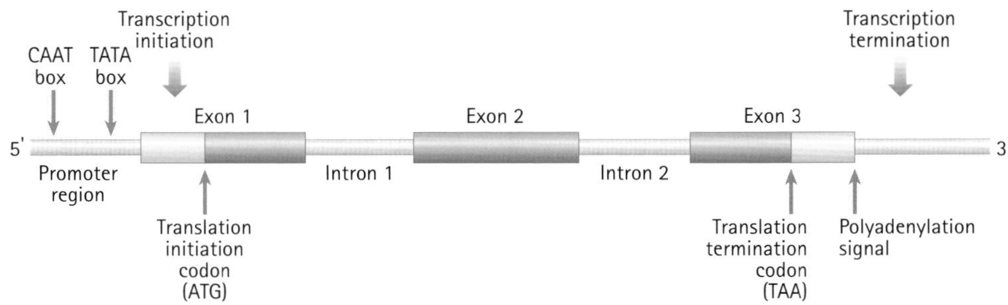


Fig. 2.6
Representation of a typical human structural gene.

## Tandemly repeated DNA sequences

*Tandemly repeated DNA sequences* consist of blocks of tandem repeats of non-coding DNA that can be either highly dispersed or restricted in their location in the genome. Tandemly repeated DNA sequences can be divided into three subgroups: satellite, minisatellite and microsatellite DNA.

### *Satellite DNA*

*Satellite DNA* accounts for approximately 10–15% of the repetitive DNA sequences of the human genome and consists of very large series of simple or moderately complex short tandemly repeated DNA sequences that are transcriptionally inactive and are clustered around the centromeres of certain chromosomes. This class of DNA sequences can be separated on density-gradient centrifugation as a shoulder, or 'satellite', to the main peak of genomic DNA, and has therefore been referred to as satellite DNA.

### *Minisatellite DNA*

*Minisatellite DNA* consists of two families of tandemly repeated short DNA sequences, telomeric and hypervariable minisatellite DNA sequences, that are transcriptionally inactive.

**Telomeric DNA**
The terminal portion of the telomeres of the chromosomes (p. 32) contains 10–15 kb of tandem repeats of a 6 bp DNA sequence known as *telomeric DNA*. The telomeric repeat sequences are necessary for chromosomal integrity in replication and are added to the chromosome by a specialized enzyme known as telomerase (p. 32).

**Hypervariable minisatellite DNA**
*Hypervariable minisatellite* DNA is made up of highly polymorphic DNA sequences consisting of short tandem repeats of a common core sequence, the highly variable number of repeat units in different hypervariable minisatellites forming the basis of DNA fingerprinting used in forensic and paternity testing (p. 70). Although often located near the telomeres, hypervariable minisatellite DNA also occurs at other locations in the chromosomes.

### *Microsatellite DNA*

*Microsatellite DNA* consists of tandem single, di-, tri- and tetranucleotide repeat base pair sequences located throughout the genome. Microsatellite repeats rarely occur within coding sequences but trinucleotide repeats in or near genes are associated with certain inherited disorders (p. 25).

DNA microsatellites are highly polymorphic (p. 71), i.e. the number of CA repeats varies between persons, and can be used in linkage studies in gene mapping (p. 132). This variation in repeat number is thought to arise by incorrect pairing of the tandem repeats of the two complementary DNA strands during DNA replication, or what is known as *slipped strand mispairing*. Duplications or deletions of longer sequences of tandemly repeated DNA are thought to arise through unequal cross-over of non-allelic DNA sequences on chromatids of homologous chromosomes or sister chromatids (p. 32).

## Highly repeated interspersed repetitive DNA sequences

Approximately one-third of the human genome is made up of two main classes of short and long repetitive DNA sequences that are interspersed throughout the genome.

### *Short interspersed nuclear elements*

About 5% of the human genome consists of some 750 000 copies of *short interspersed nuclear elements* or *SINEs*. The most common are DNA sequences of approximately 300 bp that have sequence similarity to a signal recognition particle involved in protein synthesis. They are called *Alu repeats* because they contain an *AluI* restriction enzyme recognition site.

### *Long interspersed nuclear elements*

About 5% of the DNA of the human genome is made up of *long interspersed nuclear elements* or *LINEs*. The most commonly occurring LINE, known as LINE-1 or an L1 element, consists of over 100 000 copies of a DNA sequence of up to 6000 bp that encodes a reverse transcriptase.

The function of these interspersed repeat sequences is not clear at present. Members of the *Alu* repeat family are flanked by short direct repeat sequences and therefore resemble unstable DNA sequences called transposable elements or *transposons*. Transposons, originally identified in maize by Barbara McClintock (p. 10), move spontaneously throughout the genome from one chromosome location to another and appear to be ubiquitous in the plant and animal kingdoms. It is postulated that *Alu* repeats could promote unequal recombination, which could lead to pathogenic mutations (p. 23) or provide selective advantage in evolution by gene duplication. Both *Alu* and LINE-1 repeat elements have been implicated as a cause of mutation in inherited human disease.

## MITOCHONDRIAL DNA

In addition to nuclear DNA, the several thousand mitochondria of each cell possess their own 16.6 kb

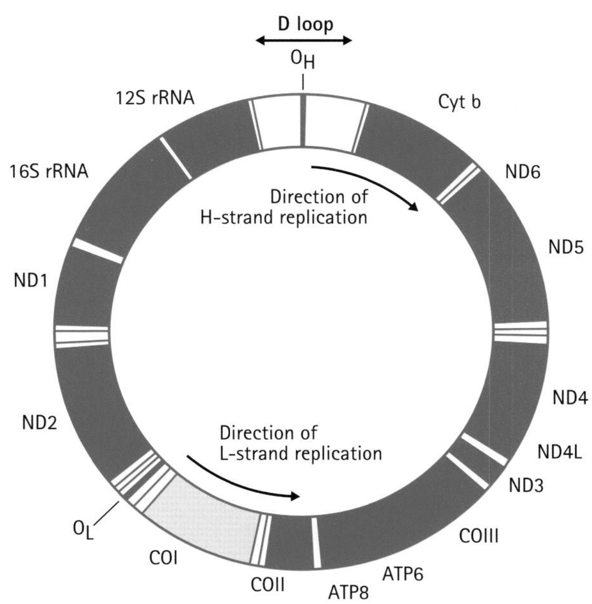


**Fig 2.7**
The human mitochondrial genome.

circular double-stranded DNA, *mitochondrial DNA* or mtDNA (Fig. 2.7). The mitochondrial DNA genome is very compact, containing little repetitive DNA, and codes for 37 genes which include two types of ribosomal RNA, 22 transfer RNAs (p. 20) and 13 protein subunits for enzymes, such as cytochrome b and cytochrome oxidase, which are involved in the energy-producing oxidative phosphorylation pathways. The genetic code of the mtDNA differs slightly from that of nuclear DNA.

The mitochondria of the fertilized zygote are inherited almost exclusively from the oocyte, leading to the maternal pattern of inheritance of mitochondrially inherited disorders (p. 120).

## TRANSCRIPTION

The process whereby genetic information is transmitted from DNA to RNA is called *transcription*. The information stored in the genetic code is transmitted from the DNA of a gene to *messenger RNA* or mRNA. Every base in the mRNA molecule is complementary to a corresponding base in the DNA of the gene but with uracil replacing thymine in mRNA. mRNA is single stranded, being synthesized by the enzyme RNA polymerase that adds the appropriate complementary ribonucleotide to the 3′ end of the RNA chain.

In any particular gene only one DNA strand of the double helix acts as the so-called *template strand*. The transcribed mRNA molecule is a copy of the complementary strand or what is called the *sense strand* of the DNA double helix. The template strand is sometimes called the *antisense strand*. The particular strand of the DNA double helix used for RNA synthesis appears to differ throughout different regions of the genome.

## RNA PROCESSING

Before the primary mRNA molecule leaves the nucleus it undergoes a number of modifications, or what is known as *RNA processing*. This involves splicing, capping and polyadenylation.

### mRNA splicing

After transcription, the non-coding introns in the primary mRNA are excised, and the non-contiguous coding exons are spliced together to form a shorter mature mRNA before its transportation to the ribosomes in the cytoplasm for translation. The process is known as *mRNA splicing* (Fig. 2.8). The boundary between the introns and exons consists of a 5′ donor GT dinucleotide and a 3′ acceptor AG dinucleotide. These, along with surrounding short splicing consensus sequences, another intronic sequence known as the splicing branch site, small nuclear RNA molecules and associated proteins, are necessary for the splicing process.

### 5′ capping

Shortly after transcription the nascent mRNA is modified by the addition of a methylated guanine nucleotide to the 5′ end of the molecule by an unusual 5′ to 5′ phosphodiester bond, the so-called *5′ cap*. The 5′ cap is thought to facilitate transport of the mRNA to the cytoplasm and attachment to the ribosomes, as well as to protect the RNA transcript from degradation by endogenous cellular exonucleases.

### Polyadenylation

The cleavage of the 3′ end of the mRNA molecule from the DNA involves the addition of approximately 200 adenylate residues, the so-called *poly(A) tail*, after cleavage of the RNA transcript at a site downstream from a specific six-nucleotide sequence. The addition of the poly(A) tail is thought to facilitate transport of the mRNA to the cytoplasm and translation.

## TRANSLATION

*Translation* is the transmission of the genetic information from mRNA to protein. Newly processed mRNA is transported from the nucleus to the cytoplasm, where it becomes associated with the *ribosomes* which are the site of protein synthesis. Ribosomes are made up of two different sized subunits which consist of four different

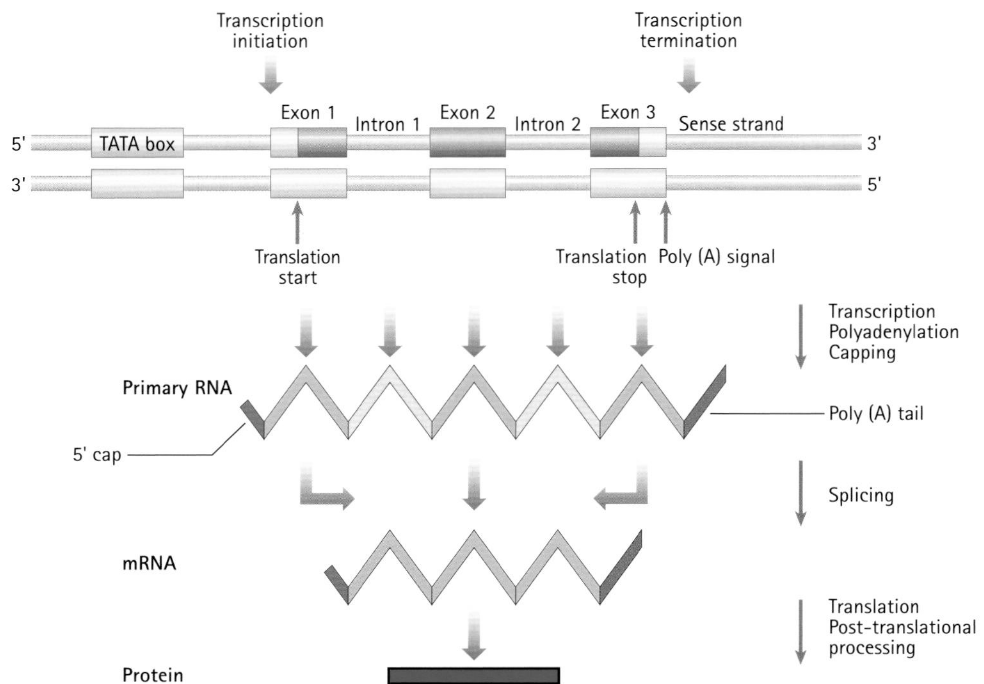


**Fig. 2.8**
Transcription, post-transcriptional processing, translation and post-translational processing.

types of *ribosomal RNA* (rRNA) molecules, and a large number of ribosomal specific proteins. Groups of ribosomes associated with the same molecule of mRNA are referred to as *polyribosomes* or *polysomes*. In the ribosomes the mRNA forms the template for producing the specific sequence of amino acids of a particular *polypepetide*.

## TRANSFER RNA

In the cytoplasm there is another form of RNA called *transfer RNA* or tRNA. The incorporation of amino acids into a *polypeptide* chain requires the amino acids to be covalently bound by reacting with ATP to the specific tRNA molecule by the activity of the enzyme aminoacyl tRNA synthetase. The ribosome, with its associated rRNAs, moves along the mRNA, the amino acids linking up by the formation of peptide bonds through the action of the enzyme peptidyl transferase to form a polypeptide chain (Fig. 2.9).

## POST-TRANSLATIONAL MODIFICATION

Many proteins, before they attain their normal structure or functional activity, undergo *post-translational modification* that can include chemical modification of amino acid side-chains (e.g. hydroxylation, methylation etc.), the addition of carbohydrate or lipid moieties (e.g. glycosylation), or proteolytic cleavage of polypeptides (e.g. the conversion of proinsulin to insulin).

This post-translational modification, along with certain short amino acid sequences known as *localization sequences* in the newly synthesized proteins, results in transport to specific cellular locations, e.g. the nucleus, or their secretion.

# THE GENETIC CODE

Twenty different amino acids are found in proteins and, as DNA is composed of four different nitrogenous bases, then obviously a single base cannot specify one amino acid. If two bases were to specify one amino acid, there would only be $4^2$ or 16 possible combinations. If, however, three bases specified one amino acid then the possible number of combinations of the four bases would be $4^3$ or 64. This is more than enough to account for all the 20 known amino acids and is known as the genetic code.

## TRIPLET CODONS

The triplet of nucleotide bases in the mRNA that codes for a particular amino acid is called a *codon*. Each triplet codon in sequence codes for a specific amino acid in sequence and so the genetic code is non-overlapping. The order of the triplet codons in a gene is known as the translational *reading frame*. However, some amino acids are coded for by more than one triplet and so the code is

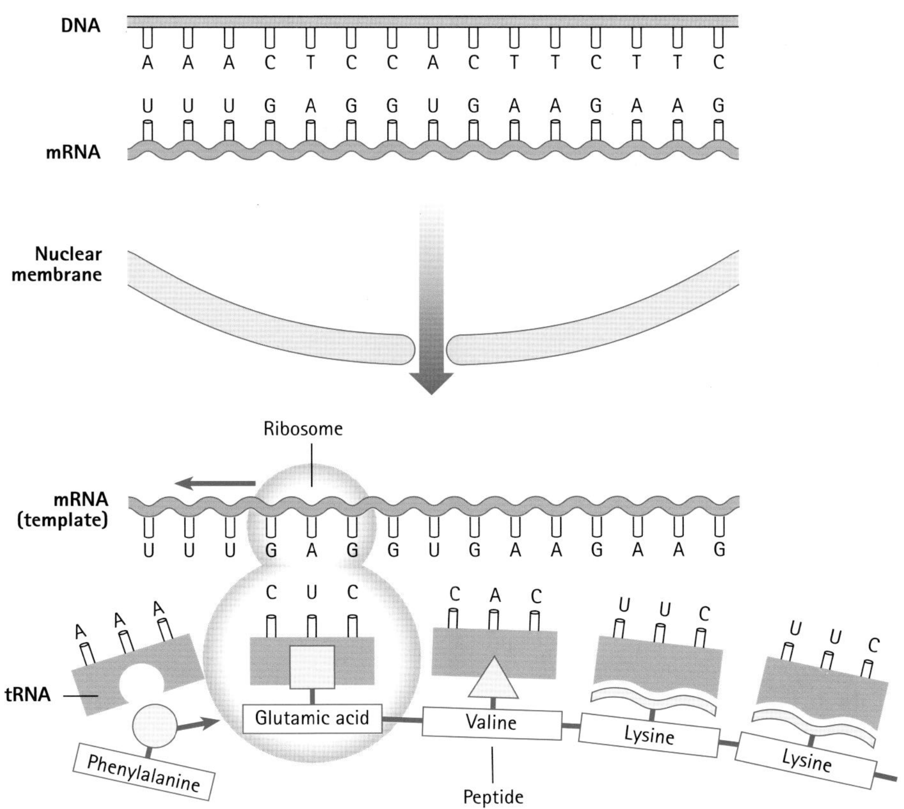


Fig. 2.9
Representation of the way in which genetic information is translated into protein.

said to be *degenerate* (Table 2.2). Each tRNA species for a particular amino acid has a specific trinucleotide sequence called the *anticodon*, which is complementary to the codon of the mRNA. Although there are 64 codons, there are only 30 cytoplasmic tRNAs, the anticodons of a number of the tRNAs recognizing codons that differ at the position of the third base, with guanine being able to pair with uracil as well as cytosine. Termination of translation of the mRNA is signaled by the presence of one of the three *stop* or *termination codons*.

The genetic code of mtDNA differs from that of the nuclear genome. Eight of the 22 tRNAs are able to recognize codons that differ only at the third base of the codon, 14 can recognize pairs of codons that are identical at the first two bases, with either a purine or pyrimidine for the third base, the other four codons acting as stop codons (Table 2.2).

## REGULATION OF GENE EXPRESSION

Many cellular processes, and therefore the genes that are expressed, are common to all cells, for example ribosomal, chromosomal and cytoskeleton proteins, constituting what are called the *housekeeping* genes. Some cells express large quantities of a specific protein in certain tissues or at specific times in development, e.g. hemoglobin in red blood cells (p. 149). This differential control of gene expression can occur at a variety of stages.

### CONTROL OF TRANSCRIPTION

The control of transcription can be affected permanently or reversibly by a variety of factors, both environmental (e.g. hormones) and genetic (cell signaling). This occurs through a number of different mechanisms which include signaling molecules that bind to regulatory sequences in the DNA known as *response elements*, intracellular receptors known as *hormone nuclear receptors*, and receptors for specific ligands on the cell surface involved in the process of *signal transduction*.

All these mechanisms affect transcription through the binding of transcription factors to short specific DNA promoter elements that are located within 200 bp 5′ or *upstream* of most eukaryotic genes in the so-called *promoter region* that leads to activation of RNA polymerase (Fig. 2.10). This includes the TATA (or Hogness), the GC

**Table 2.2 The genetic code of the nuclear and mitochondrial genomes (Differences in mitochondrial genetic code are in *italics*.)**

| | 2nd base | | | | |
|---|---|---|---|---|---|
| **1st base** | **U** | **C** | **A** | **G** | **3rd base** |
| U | Phenylalanine | Serine | Tyrosine | Cysteine | U |
| | Phenylalanine | Serine | Tyrosine | Cysteine | C |
| | Leucine | Serine | Stop | Stop (*Tryptophan*) | A |
| | Leucine | Serine | Stop | Tryptophan | G |
| C | Leucine | Proline | Histidine | Arginine | U |
| | Leucine | Proline | Histidine | Arginine | C |
| | Leucine | Proline | Glutamine | Arginine | A |
| | Leucine | Proline | Glutamine | Arginine | G |
| A | Isoleucine | Threonine | Asparagine | Serine | U |
| | Isoleucine | Threonine | Asparagine | Serine | C |
| | Isoleucine (*Methionine*) | Threonine | Lysine | Arginine (*Stop*) | A |
| | Methionine | Threonine | Lysine | Arginine (*Stop*) | G |
| G | Valine | Alanine | Aspartic acid | Glycine | U |
| | Valine | Alanine | Aspartic acid | Glycine | C |
| | Valine | Alanine | Glutamic acid | Glycine | A |
| | Valine | Alanine | Glutamic acid | Glycine | G |

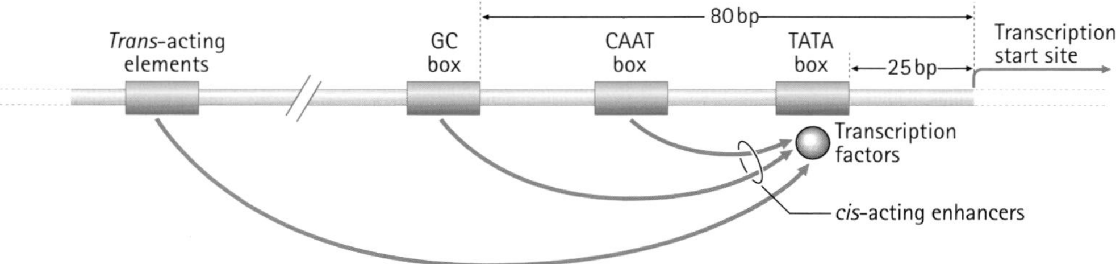


Fig. 2.10
Diagrammatic representation of the factors regulating gene expression.

(or GGGCGGG *consensus sequence*) and the CAAT boxes. The TATA box, which is about 25 bp upstream of the transcription start site, is involved in the initiation of transcription at a basal constitutive level and mutations in it can lead to alteration of the transcription start site. The GC box, which is about 80 bp upstream, and the CAAT box increase the basal level of transriptional activity of the TATA box.

The regulatory elements in the promoter region are said to be *cis-acting*, that is, they only affect the expression of the adjacent gene on the same DNA duplex, while the transcription factors are said to be *trans-acting*, acting on both copies of a gene on each chromosome being synthesized from genes that are located at a distance. DNA sequences that increase transcriptional activity, such as the GC and CAAT boxes, are known as *enhancers*. There are also negative regulatory elements or *silencers* that inhibit transcription. In addition, there are short sequences of DNA, usually 500 bp to 3 kb in size, which are known as *boundary elements*, that block or inhibit the influence of regulatory elements of adjacent genes.

## TRANSCRIPTION FACTORS

An increasing number of genes are being identified that encode proteins involved in the regulation of gene expression. They have DNA-binding activity to short nucleotide sequences, usually mediated through α helical protein motifs, and are known as *transcription factors*. These gene regulatory proteins have a transcriptional activation domain and one of four main types of DNA-binding domains. The most common type of gene regulatory protein are the *helix-turn-helix proteins*, so named because they are made up of two α helices connected by a short chain of amino acids that make up the 'turn'. Perhaps not surprisingly, structural analysis of the homeodomain sequence of the homeotic genes (p. 87) has revealed that they contain a helix-turn-helix motif. Analysis of other gene-regulatory proteins has shown them to contain one of three other types of DNA-binding motif that include the *zinc finger*, *leucine zipper* or *helix-loop-helix* motifs, so named as a result of specific structural features.

## POST-TRANSCRIPTIONAL CONTROL OF GENE EXPRESSION

Regulation of expression of most genes occurs at the level of transcription but can also occur at the levels of RNA processing, RNA transport, mRNA degradation and translation. For example, the G to A variant at position 20210 in the 3′ untranslated region of the prothrombin gene increases the stability of the mRNA transcript, resulting in higher plasma prothrombin levels.

## ALTERNATIVE SPLICING

Many human genes undergo *alternative splicing* and therefore encode more than one protein. Some genes have more than one promoter, and these *alternative* promoters may result in tissue-specific isoforms. Alternative splicing of exons is also seen with individual exons present in only some isoforms. The extent of alternative splicing in humans may be inferred from the finding that the human genome includes only about 30 000 genes, far fewer than the original prediction of over 100 000.

# RNA-DIRECTED DNA SYNTHESIS

The process of the transfer of the genetic information from DNA to RNA to protein has been called the central dogma. It was initially believed that genetic information was only transferred from DNA to RNA and thence translated into protein. However, there is evidence from the study of certain types of virus – retroviruses – that genetic information can occasionally flow in the reverse direction, i.e. from RNA to DNA (p. 205). This is referred to as *RNA-directed DNA synthesis*. It has been suggested that regions of DNA in normal cells serve as templates for the synthesis of RNA, which in turn then acts as a template for the synthesis of DNA that later becomes integrated into the nuclear DNA of other cells. Homology between human and retroviral oncogene sequences could reflect this process (p. 205), which could be an important therapeutic approach for the treatment of inherited disease in humans.

# MUTATIONS

A *mutation* is defined as a heritable alteration or change in the genetic material. Mutations drive evolution but can also be pathogenic. Mutations can arise through exposure to mutagenic agents (p. 27), but the vast majority occur spontaneously through errors in DNA replication and repair. Sequence variants with no obvious effect upon phenotype may be termed polymorphisms.

*Somatic* mutations may cause adult-onset disease such as cancer but cannot be transmitted to offspring. A mutation in *gonadal tissue* or a *gamete* can be transmitted to future generations unless it affects fertility or survival into adulthood. It is estimated that each individual carries up to six lethal or semilethal recessive mutant alleles that in the homozygous state would have very serious effects. These are conservative estimates and the actual figure could be many times greater. Harmful alleles of all kinds constitute the so-called genetic load of the population.

There are also rare examples of 'back mutation' in patients with recessive disorders. For example, reversion of inherited deleterious mutations has been demonstrated in phenotypically normal cells present in a small number of patients with Fanconi anemia.

## TYPES OF MUTATION

Mutations can range from single base substitutions, through insertions and deletions of single or multiple bases to loss or gain of entire chromosomes (see Table 2.3). A standard nomenclature to describe mutations (see Table 2.4) has been agreed although it is not universally used! Examples of chromosome abnormalities are discussed in Chapter 3.

### Substitutions

A *substitution* is the replacement of a single nucleotide by another. These are the most common type of mutation. If the substitution involves replacement by the same type of nucleotide, i.e. a pyrimidine for a pyrimidine (C for T or vice versa) or a purine for a purine (A for G or vice versa), this is termed a *transition*. Substitution of a pyrimidine by a purine or vice versa is termed a *transversion*. Transitions occur more frequently than transversions. This may be due to the relatively high frequency of C to T transitions, which is likely to be the result of the nucleotides cytosine and guanine occurring together, or what are known as CpG dinucleotides (p represents the phosphate) frequently being methylated in genomic DNA with spontaneous deamination of methylcytosine converting them to thymine. CpG dinucleotides have been termed 'hot spots' for mutation.

### Deletions

A *deletion* involves the loss of one or more nucleotides. If it occurs in coding sequences and involves one, two or more nucleotides that are not a multiple of three, it will disrupt the reading frame (p. 18). Larger deletions may result in partial or whole gene deletions and may arise through unequal crossover between repeat sequences (e.g. HNPP, p. 298).

**Table 2.3 The main classes, groups and types of mutation and effects on protein product**

| Class | Group | Type | Effect on protein product |
|---|---|---|---|
| Substitution | Synonymous | *Silent | Same amino acid |
| | Non-synonymous | *Missense | Altered amino acid – may affect protein function or stability |
| | | *Nonsense | Stop codon – loss of function or expression due to degradation of mRNA |
| | | Splice site | Aberrant splicing – exon skipping or intron retention |
| | | Promoter | Altered gene expression |
| Deletion | Multiple of 3 (codon) | | In-frame deletion of one or more amino acid(s) – may affect protein function or stability |
| | Not multiple of 3 | Frameshift | Likely to result in premature termination with loss of function or expression |
| | Large deletion | Partial gene deletion | May result in premature termination with loss function or expression |
| | | Whole gene deletion | Loss of expression |
| Insertion | Multiple of 3 (codon) | | In-frame insertion of one or more amino acid(s) – may affect protein function or stability |
| | Not multiple of 3 | Frameshift | Likely to result in premature termination with loss of function or expression |
| | Large insertion | Partial gene duplication | May result in premature termination with loss of function or expression |
| | | Whole gene duplication | May have an effect due to increased gene dosage |
| | Expansion of trinucleotide repeat | Dynamic mutation | Altered gene expression or altered protein stability/function |

*Some have been shown to cause aberrant splicing

**Table 2.4 Mutation nomenclature: examples of *CFTR* gene mutations. (Mutations can be designated according to the genomic or cDNA [mRNA] sequence and are prefixed by g. or c., respectively. The first base of the start codon [ATG] is c.1. However, for historical reasons this is not always the case and the first base of the *CFTR* cDNA is actually nucleotide 133.)**

| Type of mutation | Designation | Description | Consequence |
|---|---|---|---|
| Missense | c.482G>A | R117H | Arginine to histidine |
| Nonsense | c.1756G>T | G542X | Glycine to Stop |
| Splicing | c.621+1G>T | | Splice donor site mutation |
| Deletion (1bp) | c.1078delT | | Frameshift mutation |
| Deletion (3bp) | c. 1652–1654delTCT | ΔF508 | In-frame deletion of phenylalanine |
| Insertion | c.3905^3906insT | | Frameshift mutation |

## Insertions

An *insertion* involves the addition of one or more nucleotides into a gene. Again, if an insertion occurs in a coding sequence and involves one, two or more nucleotides that are not a multiple of three, it will disrupt the reading frame (p. 20). Large insertions can also result from unequal crossover (e.g. HMSN type 1a, p. 297) or the insertion of transposable elements (p. 18).

In 1991, expansion of trinucleotide repeat sequences was identified as a mutational mechanism. A number of single-gene disorders have subsequently been shown to be associated with triplet repeat expansions (Table 2.5). These are described as *dynamic* mutations because the repeat sequence becomes more unstable as it expands in size. The mechanism by which amplification or expansion of the triplet repeat sequence occurs is not clear at present. Triplet repeats below a certain length for each disorder are faithfully transmitted in mitosis and meiosis. Above a certain repeat number for each disorder they are more likely to be transmitted unstably, usually with an increase or decrease in repeat number. A variety of possible explanations have been offered as to how the increase in triplet repeat number occurs. These include unequal cross-over or unequal sister chromatid exchange (pp. 44, 288) in non-replicating DNA, and slipped strand mispairing and polymerase slippage in replicating DNA.

Triplet repeat expansions usually take place over a number of generations within a family, providing an

**Table 2.5 Examples of diseases arising from triplet repeat expansion**

| Disease | Repeat sequence | Normal range (repeats) | Pathogenic range (repeats) | Repeat location |
|---|---|---|---|---|
| Huntington disease (HD) | CAG | 9–35 | 36–100 | Coding |
| Myotonic dystrophy type 1 (DM1) | CTG | 5–35 | 50–4000 | 3′ UTR |
| Myotonic dystrophy type 2 (DM2) | CCTG | <25 | 75–11 000 | Intronic |
| Fragile X site A (FRAXA) | CGG | 10–50 | 200–2000 | 5′ UTR |
| Kennedy disease (SBMA) | CAG | 13–30 | 40–62 | Coding |
| Spino-cerebellar ataxia 1 (SCA1) | CAG | 6–38 | 39–80 | Coding |
| Spino-cerebellar ataxia 2 (SCA2) | CAG | 16–30 | 36–52 | Coding |
| Machado–Joseph disease (MJD, SCA3) | CAG | 14–40 | 60–>85 | Coding |
| Spinocerebellar ataxia 6 (SCA6) | CAG | 5–20 | 21–28 | Coding |
| Spinocerebellar ataxia 7 (SCA7) | CAG | 7–19 | 37–220 | Coding |
| Spinocerebellar ataxia 8 (SCA8) | CTG | 16–37 | 100–>500 | 3′ UTR |
| Dentatorubral-pallidoluysian atrophy (DRPLA) | CAG | 7–23 | 49–>75 | Coding |
| Friedreich ataxia (FA) | GAA | 8–33 | 100–900 | Intronic |
| Fragile X site E (FRAXE) | CCG | 6–25 | >200 | Promoter |
| Oculopharyngeal muscular dystrophy | GCG | 6 | 8–13 | Coding |

UTR: untranslated region.

explanation for some unusual aspects of patterns of inheritance as well as possibly being the basis of the previously unexplained phenomenon of anticipation (p. 116).

The exact mechanisms by which triplet repeat expansions cause disease are not known. Unstable trinucleotide repeats may be within coding or non-coding regions of genes and hence vary in their pathogenic mechanisms. Expansion of the CAG repeat in the coding region of the HD gene and some *SCA* genes results in a protein with an elongated polyglutamine tract that forms toxic aggregates within certain cells. In Fragile X the repeat expansion in the 5′ UTR results in methylation of promoter sequences and lack of expression of the FMR1 protein.

The spectrum of repeat expansion mutations has recently been extended by the finding of a dodecamer repeat expansion upstream from the cystatin B gene that causes progressive myoclonus epilepsy (EPM1), and a tetranucleotide repeat expansion in intron 1 of the *ZNF9* gene which causes a second type of myotonic dystrophy (PROMM).

## STRUCTURAL EFFECTS OF MUTATIONS ON THE PROTEIN

Mutations can also be subdivided into two main groups according to the effect on the polypeptide sequence of the encoded protein, being either synonymous or non-synonymous.

### Synonymous/silent mutations

If a mutation does not alter the polypeptide product of the gene, this is termed a *synonymous* or *silent mutation*. A single base pair substitution, particularly if it occurs in the third position of a codon because of the degeneracy of the genetic code, will often result in another triplet that codes for the same amino acid with no alteration in the properties of the resulting protein.

### Non-synonymous mutations

If a mutation leads to an alteration in the encoded polypeptide, it is known as a *non-synonymous mutation*. Non-synonymous mutations are observed to occur less frequently than synonymous mutations. Synonymous mutations will be selectively neutral, whereas alteration of the amino acid sequence of the protein product of a gene is likely to result in abnormal function that is usually associated with disease or lethality that has an obvious selective disadvantage.

Non-synonymous mutations can occur in one of three main ways.

#### *Missense*

A single base pair substitution can result in coding for a different amino acid and the synthesis of an altered protein, a so-called *missense* mutation. If the mutation codes for an amino acid that is chemically dissimilar, e.g.

a different charge, the structure of the protein will be altered. This is termed a *non-conservative* substitution and can lead to a gross reduction, or even a complete loss, of biological activity. Single base pair mutations can lead to qualitative rather than quantitative changes in the function of a protein, such that it retains its normal biological activity (e.g. enzyme activity) but differs in characteristics such as its mobility on electrophoresis, its pH optimum, or its stability so that it is more rapidly broken down in vivo. Many of the abnormal hemoglobins (p. 152) are the result of missense mutations.

Some single base pair substitutions, although resulting in the replacement by a different amino acid if it is chemically similar, will often have no functional effect. These are termed *conservative* substitutions.

#### *Nonsense*

A substitution that leads to the generation of one of the stop codons (Table 2.2) will result in premature termination of translation of a peptide chain or what is termed a *nonsense* mutation. In most cases the shortened chain is unlikely to retain normal biological activity, particularly if the termination codon results in the loss of an important functional domain(s) of the protein. Messenger RNA transcripts containing premature termination codons are frequently degraded by a process known as *nonsense-mediated decay*. This is a form of RNA surveillance that is believed to have evolved to protect the body from the possible consequences of truncated proteins interfering with normal function.

#### *Frameshift*

If a mutation involves the insertion or deletion of nucleotides that are not a multiple of three, it will disrupt the reading frame and constitute what is known as a *frameshift* mutation. The amino acid sequence of the protein subsequent to the mutation bears no resemblance to the normal sequence and may have an adverse effect upon its function. Most frameshift mutations result in a premature stop codon downstream to the mutation. This may lead to expression of a truncated protein, unless the mRNA is degraded by nonsense-mediated decay.

## MUTATIONS IN NON-CODING DNA

In general, mutations in non-coding DNA are less likely to have a phenotypic effect. Exceptions include mutations in promoter sequences or other regulatory regions that affect the level of gene expression.

### Splicing mutations

Mutations of the highly conserved splice donor (GT) and splice acceptor (AG) sites (p. 19) usually result in aberrant splicing. This can result in the loss of coding sequence (exon skipping) or retention of intronic sequence, and may lead to frameshift mutations. *Cryptic splice* sites are sequences similar to conserved splice sites that may be mutated with similar consequences. The spectrum of splicing mutations has recently been extended with the observation that base substitutions resulting in apparent silent, missense and nonsense mutations can cause aberrant splicing through mutation of *exon splicing enhancer* sequences. These purine-rich sequences are required for the correct splicing of exons with weak splice site consensus sequences.

## FUNCTIONAL EFFECTS OF MUTATIONS ON THE PROTEIN

Mutations exert their phenotypic effect in one of two ways, through either loss or gain of function.

### Loss-of-function

*Loss-of-function* mutations can result in either reduced activity or complete loss of the gene product. The former can be the result of either reduced activity or of decreased stability of the gene product and is known as a *hypomorph*, the latter being known as a *null allele* or *amorph*. Loss-of-function mutations in the heterozygous state would, at worst, be associated with half normal levels of the protein product. Loss-of-function mutations involving enzymes will usually be inherited in an autosomal or X-linked recessive manner, because the catalytic activity of the product of the normal allele is more than adequate to carry out the reactions of most metabolic pathways.

#### *Haploinsufficiency*

Loss-of-function mutations in the heterozygous state in which half normal levels of the gene product result in phenotypic effects are termed *haploinsufficiency mutations*. The phenotypic manifestations sensitive to gene dosage are a result of mutations occurring in genes that code for either receptors, or more rarely enzymes, the functions of which are rate limiting, e.g. familial hypercholesterolemia (p. 170) and acute intermittent porphyria (p. 175).

There are a number of autosomal dominant disorders where the mutational basis of the functional abnormality is the result of haploinsufficiency, in which, not surprisingly, homozygous mutations result in more severe phenotypic effects, e.g. angioneurotic edema (p. 195) and familial hypercholesterolemia (p. 170).

### Gain-of-function mutations

*Gain-of-function* mutations, as the name suggests, result in either increased levels of gene expression or the development of a new function(s) of the gene product. Increased expression levels due to activating point mutations or increased gene dosage are responsible for one type of Charcot–Marie–Tooth disease, hereditary motor and sensory neuropathy type I (p. 277). The expanded triplet repeat mutations in the Huntington gene cause qualitative changes in the gene product, which result in its aggregation in the central nervous system leading to the classic clinical features of the disorder (p. 293).

Mutations that alter the timing or tissue specificity of the expression of a gene can also be considered to be gain-of-function mutations. Examples include the chromosomal rearrangements that result in the combination of sequences from two different genes seen with specific tumors (p. 206). The novel function of the resulting chimeric gene causes the neoplastic process.

Gain-of-function mutations are dominantly inherited and the rare instances of gain-of-function mutations occurring in the homozygous state are associated with a much more severe phenotype, which is often a prenatally lethal disorder, e.g. homozygous achondroplasia (p. 92) or Waardenburg syndrome type I (p. 90).

#### Dominant-negative mutations

A *dominant-negative* mutation is one in which a mutant gene in the heterozygous state results in the loss of protein activity/function, as a consequence of the mutant gene product interfering with the function of the normal gene product of the corresponding allele. Dominant-negative mutations are particularly common in proteins that are dimers or multimers, e.g. structural proteins such as the collagens, mutations in which can lead to osteogeneis imperfecta (p. 117).

### GENOTYPE–PHENOTYPE CORRELATION

Many genetic disorders are well recognized as being very variable in the severity of involvement (p. 108) or in the particular features a person with the disorder will manifest (p. 108). Developments in molecular genetics increasingly allow identification of the mutational basis of the specific features that occur in a person with a particular inherited disease, or what is known as the phenotype. This has resulted in attempts to correlate the presence of a particular mutation, which is often called the genotype, with the specific features seen in a person with an inherited disorder, this being referred to as *genotype–phenotype correlation*. This can be important in the management of a patient. One example includes the association of mutations in the *BRCA1* gene with the risk of developing ovarian cancer as well as breast cancer (p. 217). Particularly striking examples are mutations in the receptor tyrosine kinase gene *RET* which, depending on their location, can lead to four different syndromes that differ in the functional mechanism and clinical phenotype. Loss-of-function nonsense mutations lead to lack of migration of neural crest-derived cells to form the ganglia of the myenteric plexus of the large bowel, leading to Hirschsprung disease, while gain-of-function missense mutations result in familial medullary thyroid carcinoma or one of the two types of multiple endocrine neoplasia type 2 (pp. 92, 95). Mutations in the *LMNA* gene are associated with an even broader spectrum of disease (p. 107).

## MUTATIONS AND MUTAGENESIS

Naturally occurring mutations are referred to as *spontaneous mutations* and are thought to arise through chance errors in chromosomal division or DNA replication. Environmental agents that cause mutations are known as mutagens.

### MUTAGENS

These include natural or artificial ionizing radiation and chemical or physical mutagens.

#### Ionizing radiation

*Ionizing radiation* includes electromagnetic waves of very short wavelength (X-rays and $\gamma$ rays), and high-energy particles ($\alpha$ particles, $\beta$ particles and neutrons). X-rays, $\gamma$ rays and neutrons have great penetrating power, but $\alpha$ particles can penetrate soft tissues to a depth of only a fraction of a millimeter and $\beta$ particles only up to a few millimeters.

##### *Measures of radiation*

The amount of radiation received by irradiated tissues is often referred to as the 'dose', which is measured in terms of the *radiation absorbed dose* or *rad*. The rad is a measure of the amount of any ionizing radiation that is actually absorbed by the tissues, 1 rad being equivalent to 100 ergs of energy absorbed per gram of tissue. The biological effects of ionizing radiation depend on the volume of tissue exposed. In humans, irradiation of the whole body with a dose of 300–500 rads is usually fatal, but as much as 10 000 rads can be given to a small volume of tissue in the treatment of malignant tumors without serious effects.

Humans can be exposed to a mixture of radiation, and the rem (r*oentgen* e*quivalent for* m*an*) is a convenient unit as it is a measure of any radiation in terms of X-rays. A rem of radiation is that absorbed dose that produces in a given tissue the same biological effect as 1 rad of X-rays.

Expressing doses of radiation in terms of rems permits us to compare the amounts of different types of radiation to which humans are exposed. A millirem (mrem) is one-thousandth of a rem. 100 rem is equivalent to 1 *sievert* (Sv), and 100 rad is equivalent to 1 gray (Gy) in SI units. For all practical purposes, sieverts and grays are approximately equal. In this discussion sieverts and millisieverts (mSv) will be used as the units of measure.

### Dosimetry

*Dosimetry* is the measurement of radiation. The dose of radiation is expressed in relation to the amount received by the gonads because it is the effects of radiation on germ cells rather than somatic cells that are important as far as transmission of mutations to future progeny is concerned. The *gonad dose* of radiation is often expressed as the amount received in 30 years. This period of time has been chosen because it corresponds roughly to the generation time in humans.

### Sources of radiation

The various sources and average annual doses of the different types of natural and artificial ionizing radiation are listed in Table 2.6. Natural sources of radiation include cosmic rays, external radiation from radioactive materials in certain rocks, and internal radiation from radioactive materials in tissues. Artificial sources include diagnostic and therapeutic radiology, occupational exposure and fallout from nuclear explosions.

The average gonad dose of ionizing radiation from radioactive fallout resulting from the testing of nuclear weapons is less than that from any of the sources of background radiation. However, the possibility of serious accidents involving nuclear reactors, as occurred at Three Mile Island in the United States in 1979 and at Chernobyl in the Soviet Union in 1986 with widespread effects, always must be borne in mind.

**Table 2.6 Approximate average doses of ionizing radiation from various sources to the gonads of the general population**

| Source of radiation | Average dose per year (mSv) | Average dose per 30 years (mSv) |
|---|---|---|
| **Natural** | | |
| Cosmic radiation | 0.25 | 7.5 |
| External $\gamma$ radiation* | 1.50 | 45.0 |
| Internal $\gamma$ radiation | 0.30 | 9.0 |
| **Artificial** | | |
| Medical radiology | 0.30 | 9.0 |
| Radioactive fallout | 0.01 | 0.3 |
| Occupational and miscellaneous | 0.04 | 1.2 |
| **Total** | **2.40** | **72.0** |

*Including radon in dwelling.
(Data from Clarke R H, Southwood T R E 1989 Risks from ionizing radiation. Nature 338: 197–198)

### Genetic effects

Experiments with animals and plants have shown that the number of mutations produced by irradiation is proportional to the dose: the larger the dose the more mutations produced. It is believed that there is no threshold below which irradiation has no effect – even the smallest dose of radiation can result in a mutation. The genetic effects of ionizing radiation are also cumulative, so that each time a person is exposed to radiation the dose received has to be added to the amount of radiation already received. The total number of radiation-induced mutations is directly proportional to the total gonad dose.

### Permissible dose

The hazard from mutations induced in humans by radiation is not so much to ourselves as to our descendants. Unfortunately, in humans there is no easy way to demonstrate genetic damage caused by mutagens. Nevertheless, the International Commission of Radiological Protection (ICRP), working in close liaison with various agencies of the United Nations (WHO, UNESCO, IAEA etc.), has been mainly responsible for defining what is referred to as the maximum permissible dose of radiation. This is an arbitrary safety limit and is probably very much less than that which would cause any significant effect on the frequency of harmful mutations within the population. It has been recommended that occupational exposure should not exceed 50 mSv in a year. However, there is currently much controversy over exactly what the permissible dose should be and some countries, such as the USA, set the upper limit significantly lower than many others. In the UK the National Radiological Protection Board advises that occupational exposure should not in fact exceed 15 mSv in a year. To put this into perspective, 1mSv is roughly 50 times the dose received in a single chest X-ray and 100 times the dose incurred in flying from the UK to Spain in a jet aircraft!

There is no doubting the potential dangers, both somatic and genetic, of exposure to ionizing radiation. In the case of medical radiology the dose of radiation resulting from a particular procedure has to be weighed against the ultimate beneficial effect to the patient. In the case of occupational exposure to radiation, the answer lies in defining the risks and introducing and enforcing adequate legislation. With regard to the dangers from fallout from nuclear accidents and explosions the solution would seem obvious.

### Chemical mutagens

In humans, chemical mutagenesis may be more important than radiation in producing genetic damage. Experiments have shown that certain chemicals, such as mustard gas, formaldehyde, benzene, some basic dyes and food additives, are mutagenic in animals. Exposure to environmental chemicals may result in the formation of DNA adducts, chromosome breaks or aneuploidy. Consequently all new pharmaceutical products are subject to a battery of mutagenicity tests which include both *in vitro* and *in vivo* studies in animals.

## DNA REPAIR

The occurrence of mutations in DNA, if left unrepaired, would have serious consequences for both the individual and subsequent generations. The stability of DNA is dependent upon continuous *DNA repair* by a number of different mechanisms (Table 2.7). Some types of DNA damage can be repaired directly. Examples include the dealkylation of $O^6$-alkyl guanine or the removal of thymine dimers by photoreactivation in bacteria. The majority of DNA repair mechanisms involve cleavage of the DNA strand by an endonuclease, removal of the damaged region by an exonuclease, insertion of new bases by the enzyme DNA polymerase, and sealing of the break by DNA ligase.

*Nucleotide excision repair* (NER) removes thymine dimers and large chemical adducts. It is a complex process involving over 30 proteins which remove fragments of approximately 30 nucleotides. Mutations in at least eight of the genes encoding these proteins can cause Xeroderma pigmentosum (p. 288), which is characterized by extreme sensitivity to UV light and a high frequency of skin cancer. A different set of repair enzymes is utilized to excise single abnormal bases (*base excision repair* or BER), with mutations in the gene encoding the DNA glycosylase MYH having recently been shown to cause an autosomal recessive form of colorectal cancer (p. 216).

Naturally occurring reactive oxygen species and ionizing radiation induce breakage of DNA strands. Double-strand breaks result in chromosome breaks that can be lethal if not repaired. *Post-replication repair* is required to correct double-strand breaks and usually involves homologous recombination with a sister DNA molecule. Human genes involved in this pathway include *NBS*, *BLM* and *BRCA1/2* (mutated in Nijmegen breakage syndrome Bloom syndrome p. 287 and hereditary breast cancer p. 217, respectively). Alternatively, the broken ends may be rejoined by non-homologous end-joining which is an error-prone pathway.

*Mismatch repair* (MMR) corrects mismatched bases introduced during DNA replication. Cells defective in MMR have very high mutation rates (up to 1000x higher than normal). Mutations in at least six different MMR genes cause hereditary non-polyposis colorectal cancer (HNPCC, p. 215).

Although DNA repair pathways have evolved to correct DNA damage and hence protect the cell from the deleterious consequences of mutations, some mutations arise from the cell's attempts to tolerate damage. One example is *translesion DNA synthesis*, where the DNA replication machinery bypasses sites of DNA damage, allowing normal DNA replication and gene expression to proceed downstream. Human disease may also be caused by defective cellular response to DNA damage. Cells have complex signaling pathways which allow cell cycle arrest to provide increased time for DNA repair. If the DNA damage is irreparable, the cell may initiate programmed cell death (*apoptosis*). The ATM protein is involved in sensing DNA damage and has been described as the 'guardian of the genome'. Mutations in the *ATM* gene cause ataxia telangiectasia (AT, p. 287), characterized by hypersensitivity to radiation and a high risk of cancer.

**Table 2.7 DNA repair pathways, genes and associated disorders**

| Type of DNA repair | Mechanism | Genes | Disorders |
|---|---|---|---|
| Base excision repair (BER) | Removal of abnormal bases | *MYH* | Colorectal cancer |
| Nucleotide excision repair (NER) | Removal of thymine dimers and large chemical adducts | *XP* genes | Xeroderma pigmentosum |
| Post-replication repair | Removal of double-strand breaks by homologous recombination or non-homologous end-joining | *NBS*<br>*BLM*<br>*BRCA1/2* | Nijmegen breakage syndrome<br>Bloom syndrome<br>Breast cancer |
| Mismatch repair (MMR) | Corrects mismatched bases caused by mistakes in DNA replication | *MSH* and *MLH* genes | Colorectal cancer (HNPCC) |

## FURTHER READING

Alberts B, Bray D, Lewis J et al 1995 Molecular biology of the cell, 3rd edn. Garland, London
*Very accessible, well written and lavishly illustrated comprehensive text of molecular biology with accompanying problems book and CD ROM using multimedia review and self-assessment.*
Alberts B, Bray D, Johnson A et al 1997 Essential cell biology: an introduction to the molecular biology of the cell. Garland, London
*An excellent introductory textbook with full colour illustrations.*
Beir V 1990 Health effects of exposure to low levels of ionizing radiation. National Academy Press, Washington
*The fifth report of the National Research Council's Committee on the Biological Effects of Ionizing Radiation.*
Dawkins R 1989 The selfish gene, 2nd edn. Oxford University Press, Oxford
*An interesting controversial concept.*
Epstein RJ 2003 Human molecular biology: an introduction to the molecular basis of health and disease. Cambridge University Press, Cambridge
*A modern textbook about molecules and their role in human disease.*
Lewin B 2000 Genes VII, 7th edn. Oxford University Press, Oxford
*The seventh edition of this excellent textbook of molecular biology with colour diagrams and figures. Hard to improve upon.*
Lodisch H, Berk A, Zipursky S L et al 1999 Molecular cell biology, 2nd edn. W H Freeman, London
*A revised and updated edition of the first edition, clearly written with excellent diagrams.*
Mettler F A, Moseley R D 1985 Medical effects of ionising radiation. Grune & Stratton, London
*Good overview of all aspects of the medical consequences of ionizing radiation.*
Schull W J, Neel J V 1958 Radiation and the sex ratio in man. Sex ratio among children of survivors of atomic bombings suggests induced sex-linked lethal mutations. Science 228: 434–438
*The original report of possible evidence of the effects of atomic radiation.*
Strachan T, Read A P 2004 Human molecular genetics 3rd edn. Garland Science, London and New York
*An up-to-date, comprehensive textbook of all aspects of molecular and cellular biology as it relates to inherited disease in humans.*
Turner J E 1995 Atoms, radiation and radiation protection. John Wiley, Chichester
*Basis of the physics of radiation, applications and harmful effects.*
Watson J D, Crick F H C 1953 Molecular structure of nucleic acids – a structure for deoxyribose nucleic acid. Nature 171: 737–738
*The concepts in this paper, presented in just over one page, resulted in the authors receiving the Nobel Prize!*
Weaver R F 1998 Molecular biology. WCB/McGraw-Hill, London
*Well written and illustrated textbook covering the breadth of molecular biology.*

## ELEMENTS

1. Genetic information is stored in DNA (deoxyribonucleic acid) as a linear sequence of two types of nucleotide, the purines (adenine [A] and guanine [G]) and the pyrimidines (cytosine [C] and thymine [T]), linked by a sugar-phosphate backbone.

2. A molecule of DNA consists of two antiparallel strands held in a double helix by hydrogen bonds between the complementary G-C and A-T base pairs.

3. DNA replication has multiple sites of origin and is semiconservative, each strand acting as a template for synthesis of a complementary strand.

4. Genes coding for proteins in higher organisms (eukaryotes) consist of coding (exons) and non-coding (introns) sections.

5. Transcription is the synthesis of a single-stranded complementary copy of one strand of a gene that is known as messenger RNA (mRNA). RNA (ribonucleic acid) differs from DNA in containing the sugar ribose and the base uracil instead of thymine.

6. mRNA is processed during transport from the nucleus to the cytoplasm, eliminating the non-coding sections. In the cytoplasm it becomes associated with the ribosomes, where translation, i.e. protein synthesis, occurs.

7. The genetic code is 'universal' and consists of triplets (codons) of nucleotides, each of which codes for an amino acid or termination of peptide chain synthesis. The code is degenerate, i.e. all but two amino acids are specified by more than one codon.

8. The major control of gene expression is at the level of transcription by DNA regulatory sequences in the 5′ flanking promoter region of structural genes in eukaryotes. General and specific transcription factors are also involved in the regulation of genes.

9. Mutations occur both spontaneously and as a result of exposure to mutagenic agents such as ionizing radiation. Mutations are continuously corrected by DNA repair enzymes.

CHAPTER

3

# Chromosomes and cell division

*"Let us not take it for granted that life exists more fully in what is commonly thought big than in what is commonly thought small."*

Virginia Woolf

At the molecular or submicroscopic level DNA can be regarded as the basic template that provides a blueprint for the formation and maintenance of an organism. DNA is packaged into *chromosomes* and at a very simple level these can be considered as being made up of tightly coiled long chains of genes. Unlike DNA, chromosomes can be visualized during cell division using a light microscope, under which they appear as thread-like structures or 'colored bodies'. The word chromosome is derived from the Greek *chroma* (= color) and *soma* (= body).

Chromosomes are the factors that distinguish one species from another and that enable transmission of genetic information from one generation to the next. Their behavior at somatic cell division in *mitosis* provides a means of ensuring that each daughter cell retains its own complete genetic complement. Similarly, their behavior during gamete formation in *meiosis* enables each mature ovum and sperm to contain a unique single set of parental genes. Chromosomes are quite literally the vehicles that facilitate reproduction and the maintenance of a species.

The study of chromosomes and cell division is referred to as *cytogenetics*. Prior to the 1950s it was believed, incorrectly, that each human cell contained 48 chromosomes and that human sex was determined by the number of X chromosomes present at conception. Following the development in 1956 of more reliable techniques for studying human chromosomes it was realized that the correct chromosome number in humans is 46 and that maleness is determined by the presence of a Y chromosome regardless of the number of X chromosomes present in each cell. It was also realized that abnormalities of chromosome number and structure could seriously disrupt normal growth and development.

## HUMAN CHROMOSOMES

### MORPHOLOGY

At the submicroscopic level chromosomes consist of an extremely elaborate complex, made up of supercoils of DNA, which has been likened to the tightly coiled network of wiring seen in a solenoid (p. 15). Under the electron microscope chromosomes can be seen to have a rounded and rather irregular morphology (Fig 3.1). However, most of our knowledge of chromosome structure has been gained using light microscopy. Special stains selectively taken up by DNA have enabled each individual chromosome to be identified. These are best seen during cell division, when the chromosomes are maximally contracted and the constituent genes can no longer be transcribed.

At this time each chromosome can be seen to consist of two identical strands known as *chromatids*, or *sister chromatids*, which are the result of DNA replication having taken place during the S (synthesis) phase of the cell cycle (p. 43). These sister chromatids can be seen to be joined at a primary constriction known as the *centromere*. Centromeres consist of several hundred kilobases of repetitive DNA and are responsible for the movement of chromosomes at cell division. Each centromere divides the chromosome into short and long arms, designated p (= petite) and q ('g' = grande), respectively.

The tip of each chromosome arm is known as the *telomere*. Telomeres play a crucial role in sealing the ends of chromosomes and maintaining their structural integrity. Telomeres have been highly conserved throughout evolution and in humans they consist of many tandem repeats of a TTAGGG sequence. During DNA replication an enzyme known as *telomerase* replaces the 5′ end of the long strand (p. 18), which would otherwise become progressively shorter until a critical length is reached when the cell can no longer divide and thus becomes

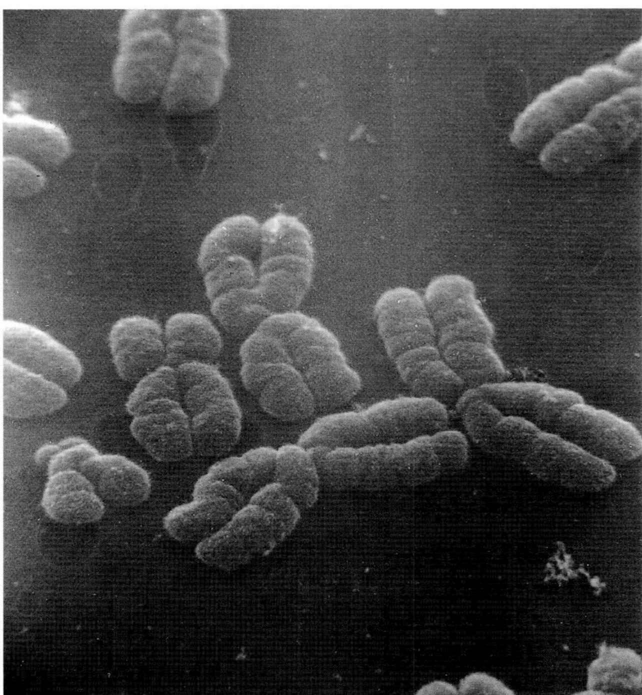

Fig. 3.1
Electron micrograph of human chromosomes showing the centromeres and well-defined chromatids. (Courtesy of Dr Christine Harrison. Reproduced from Cytogenetics and Cell Genetics 1983, 35: 21–27 with permission of the publisher, S Karger A G, Basel.)

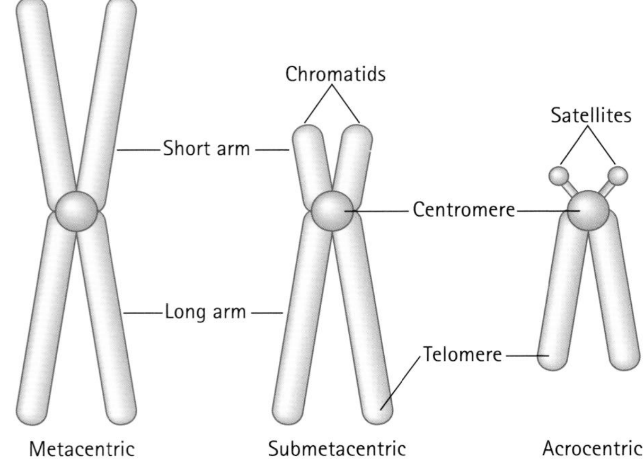


Fig. 3.2
Morphologically chromosomes are divided into metacentric, submetacentric and acrocentric depending on the position of the centromere.

senescent. This is in fact part of the normal cellular aging process, with most cells being unable to undergo more than 50–60 divisions. However, in some tumors increased telomerase activity has been implicated as a cause of abnormally prolonged cell survival.

Morphologically chromosomes are classified according to the position of the centromere. If this is located centrally, the chromosome is *metacentric*, if terminal it is *acrocentric*, and if the centromere is in an intermediate position the chromosome is *submetacentric* (Fig. 3.2). Acrocentric chromosomes sometimes have stalk-like appendages called *satellites* that form the nucleolus of the resting interphase cell and contain multiple repeat copies of the genes for ribosomal RNA.

## CLASSIFICATION

Individual chromosomes differ not only in the position of the centromere but also in their overall length. Based on the three parameters of length, position of the centromere and the presence or absence of satellites, early pioneers of cytogenetics were able to identify most individual chromosomes, or at least subdivide them into groups labelled A–G on the basis of overall morphology (A = 1–3, B = 4–5, C = 6–12 + X, D = 13–15, E = 16–18, F = 19–20, G = 21–22 + Y). In humans the normal cell nucleus contains 46 chromosomes, made up of 22 pairs of *autosomes* and a single pair of sex chromosomes – XX in the female and XY in the male. One member of each of these pairs is derived from each parent. Somatic cells are said to have a *diploid* complement of 46 chromosomes, whereas gametes (i.e. ova and sperm) have a *haploid* complement of 23 chromosomes. Members of a pair of chromosomes are known as *homologs*.

The development of chromosome banding (p. 33) enabled very precise recognition of individual chromosomes and the detection of subtle chromosome abnormalities. This technique also revealed that *chromatin*, the combination of DNA and histone proteins of which chromosomes are made, exists in two main forms. *Euchromatin* stains lightly and consists of genes that are actively expressed. In contrast, *heterochromatin* stains darkly and is made up largely of inactive unexpressed repetitive DNA.

The total number of chromosomes in different organisms varies considerably but is constant for any particular species. Whereas the marmoset and certain monkeys resemble man in having 46 chromosomes, higher primates more closely related to humans, such as the chimpanzee, gorilla and orangutan, have 48 chromosomes. Among these primates the chromosomes of the chimpanzee most closely resemble those of humans. This is consistent with the fact that there is a difference of only 1% between human and chimpanzee DNA. There is general agreement that the human number 2 chromosome is the product of the fusion of two chimpanzee chromosomes, with many other differences between the chromosome complements in the two species being due to paracentric and pericentric inversions (p. 53). These observations have been exploited by molecular biologists to help map and clone genes in humans.

## THE SEX CHROMOSOMES

The X and Y chromosomes are known as the sex chromosomes because of their crucial role in sex determination. The X chromosome was originally labeled as such because of uncertainty as to its function when it was realized that in some insects this chromosome is present in some gametes but not in others. In these insects the male has only one sex chromosome (X), whereas the female has two (XX). In humans, and in most mammals, both the male and the female have two sex chromosomes – XX in the female and XY in the male. The Y chromosome is much smaller than the X and carries only a few genes of functional importance, most notably the testis-determining factor, known as *SRY* (p. 97). Other genes on the Y chromosome are known to be important in maintaining spermatogenesis.

In the female each ovum carries an X chromosome, whereas in the male each sperm carries either an X or a Y chromosome. As there is a roughly equal chance of either an X-bearing sperm or a Y-bearing sperm fertilizing an ovum, the numbers of male and female conceptions are approximately equal (Fig. 3.3). In fact, slightly more male babies are born than females, although during childhood and adult life the sex ratio evens out at 1:1.

The process of sex determination will be considered in detail later (p. 97).

# METHODS OF CHROMOSOME ANALYSIS

It was generally believed that each cell contained 48 chromosomes until 1956, when Tjio and Levan correctly concluded on the basis of their studies that the normal human somatic cell contains only 46 chromosomes. The methods they used, with certain modifications, are now universally employed in cytogenetic laboratories to analyze the chromosome constitution of an individual, which is known as a *karyotype*. This term is also used to describe a photomicrograph of an individual's chromosomes, arranged in a standard manner.

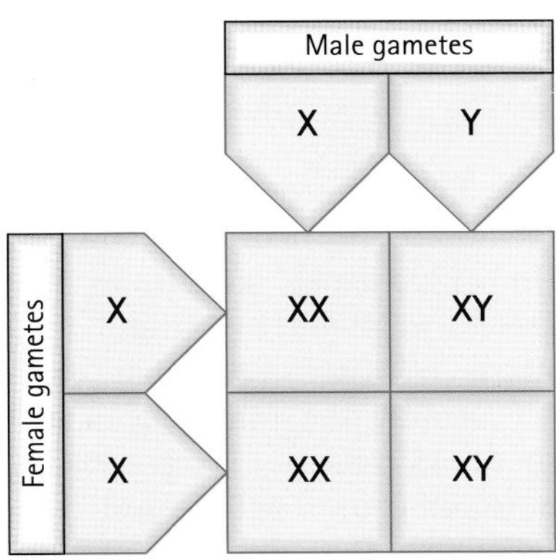


Fig. 3.3
Punnett's square showing sex chromosome combinations for male and female gametes.

## CHROMOSOME PREPARATION

Any tissue with living nucleated cells that undergo division can be used for studying human chromosomes. Most commonly circulating lymphocytes from peripheral blood are used, although samples for chromosomal analysis can be prepared relatively easily using skin, bone marrow, chorionic villi or cells from amniotic fluid (amniocytes).

In the case of peripheral (venous) blood, a sample is added to a small volume of nutrient medium containing phytohemagglutinin, which stimulates T lymphocytes to divide. The cells are cultured under sterile conditions at 37°C for about 3 days, during which they divide, and colchicine is then added to each culture. This drug has the extremely useful property of preventing formation of the spindle, thereby arresting cell division during metaphase, the time when the chromosomes are maximally condensed and therefore most easily visible. Hypotonic saline is then added, which causes the red blood cells to lyze and results in spreading of the chromosomes, which are then fixed, mounted on a slide and stained ready for analysis (Fig. 3.4).

## CHROMOSOME BANDING

Several different staining methods can be utilized to identify individual chromosomes.

### G (giemsa) banding

This is the method most commonly used. The chromosomes are treated with trypsin, which denatures their protein content, and then stained with a DNA-binding dye known as Giemsa, which gives each chromosome a characteristic and reproducible pattern of light and dark bands (Fig. 3.5).

### Q (quinacrine) banding

This gives a banding pattern similar to that obtained with Giemsa, and requires examination of the chromosomes with an ultraviolet fluorescent microscope.

### R (reverse) banding

The chromosomes are heat-denatured before staining with Giemsa, yielding light and dark bands which are the reverse of those obtained using conventional G banding (Fig. 3.6).

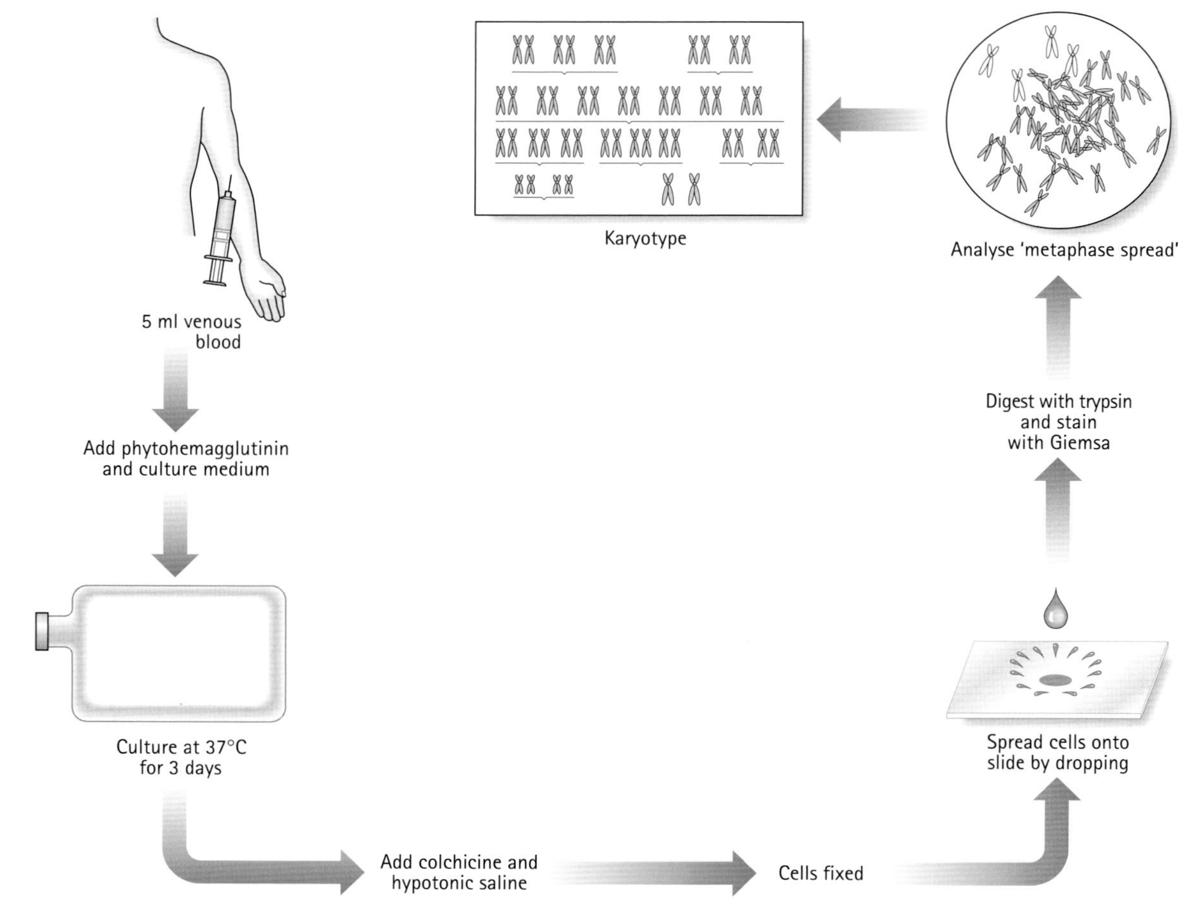


**Fig. 3.4**
Preparation of a karyotype.

### C (centromeric heterochromatin) banding

If the chromosomes are pretreated with acid followed by alkali prior to G banding, the centromeres and other heterochromatic regions containing highly repetitive DNA sequences are preferentially stained.

### High-resolution banding

G banding generally provides high-quality chromosome analysis with approximately 400–500 bands per haploid set. Each of these bands corresponds on average to approximately 6000–8000 kb (i.e. 6–8 megabases) of DNA. High-resolution banding of the chromosomes at an earlier stage of mitosis, such as prophase or prometaphase, provides greater sensitivity with up to 800 bands per haploid set, but is much more demanding technically. This involves first inhibiting cell division with an agent such as methotrexate or thymidine. Folic acid or deoxycytidine is added to the culture medium, which releases the cells into mitosis. Colchicine is then added at a specific time interval, when a higher proportion of cells will be in prometaphase and the chromosomes will not be fully contracted, giving a more detailed banding pattern.

## KARYOTYPE ANALYSIS

The next stage in chromosome analysis involves first counting the number of chromosomes present in a specified number of cells, sometimes referred to as *metaphase spreads*, followed by careful analysis of the banding pattern of each individual chromosome in selected cells. Usually the total chromosome count is determined in 10–15 cells, but if mosaicism is suspected then 30 or more cell counts will be undertaken. Detailed analysis of the banding pattern of the individual chromosomes is carried out on both members of each pair of homologs in approximately 3–5 metaphase spreads, which show high-quality banding.

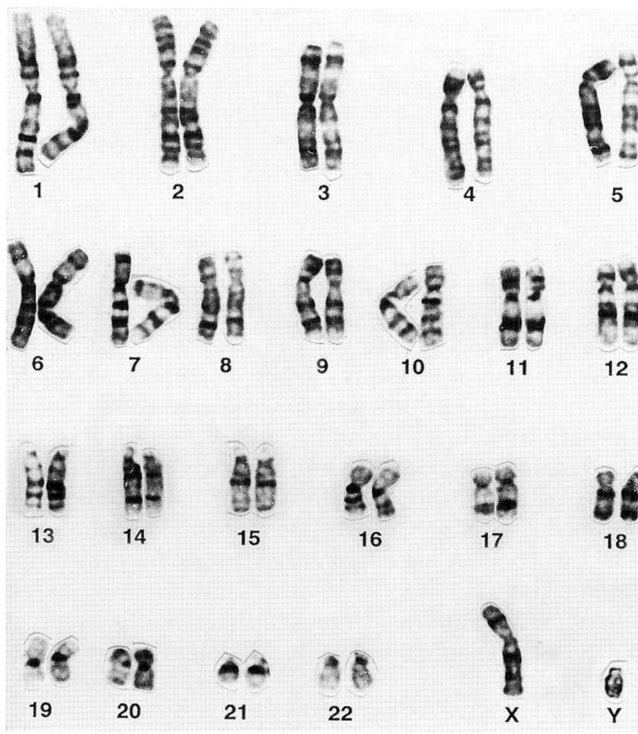


**Fig. 3.5**
A normal G-banded male karyotype.

The banding pattern of each chromosome is specific and can be shown in the form of a stylized ideal karyotype known as an *idiogram* (Fig. 3.7). The cytogeneticist analyses each pair of homologous chromosomes, either while looking down the microscope or, increasingly, on a photograph of the metaphase spread, which can now be produced electronically (Fig. 3.8). Until the advent of banding in 1971, chromosomes could be classified only on the basis of their overall morphology. Now a formally presented karyotype or *karyogram* will show each chromosome pair in descending order of size.

## MOLECULAR CYTOGENETICS

### FLUORESCENT IN-SITU HYBRIDIZATION

This relatively new diagnostic tool combines conventional cytogenetics with molecular genetic technology. It is based on the unique ability of a portion of single-stranded DNA, i.e. a probe (p. 64), to anneal with its complementary target sequence wherever it is located on a metaphase spread. Unlike most other methods used for chromosome analysis, *fluorescent in-situ hybridization* (FISH) can also be used to study chromosomes in cells that are resting between cell division in the interval known as *interphase*.

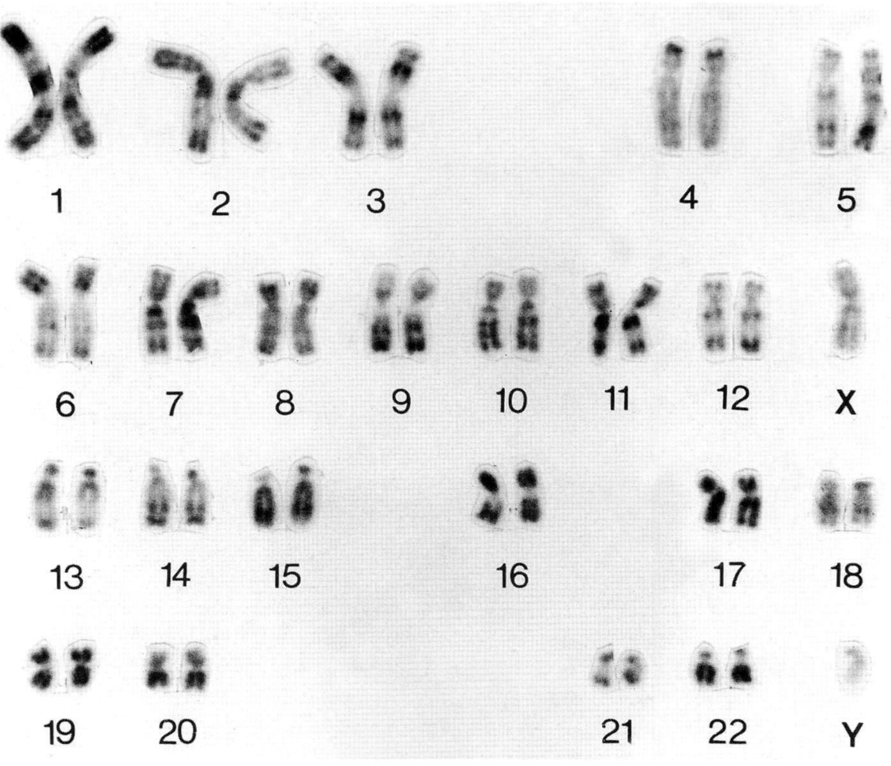


**Fig. 3.6**
A normal R-banded male karyotype.
(Courtesy of H. J. Evans.)

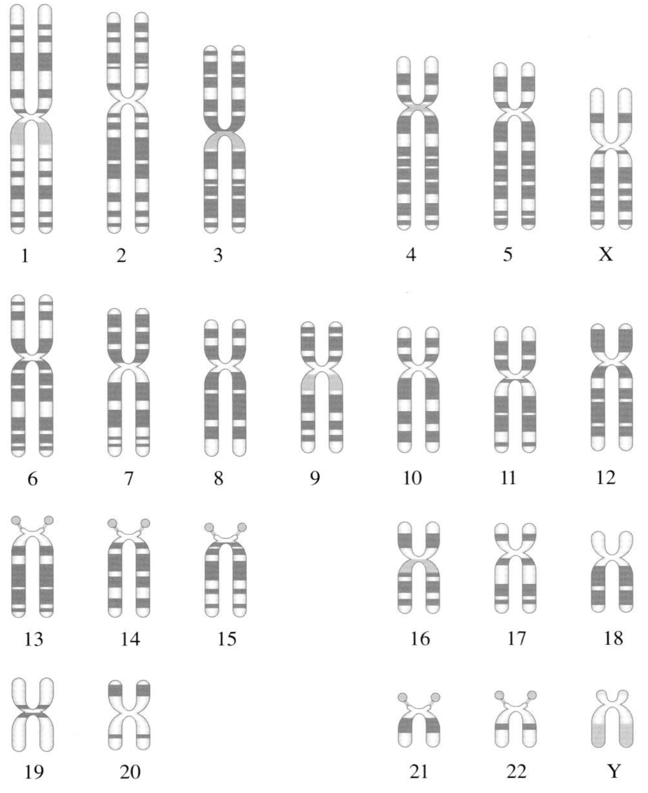


**Fig. 3.7**
An idiogram showing the banding patterns of individual chromosomes as revealed by fluorescent and Giemsa staining.

In this technique the DNA probe is conjugated with modified nucleotides which, after hybridization with the patient sample, allows the region where hybridization has occurred to be visualized using a fluorescent microscope. FISH is now used widely for clinical diagnostic purposes and one major advantage is that results are usually obtained very rapidly with interphase FISH.

## Different types of fish probes

### *Centromeric probes*

These consist of repetitive DNA sequences found in and around the centromere of a specific chromosome. They are suitable for making a rapid diagnosis of one of the common aneuploidy syndromes (trisomies 13, 18, 21 – see p. 271) using non-dividing cells in interphase obtained from a prenatal diagnostic sample of chorionic villi (Fig. 3.9). A set of centromere-specific probes for chromosomes 13, 18, 21, X and Y can be used as an adjunct to provide rapid prenatal diagnosis for some of the more common numerical chromosomal abnormalities (p. 327).

### *Chromosome-specific unique sequence probes*

These are specific for a particular single locus. They are particularly useful for identifying tiny submicroscopic deletions and duplications (Fig. 3.10). The group of disorders referred to as the *microdeletion* syndromes are

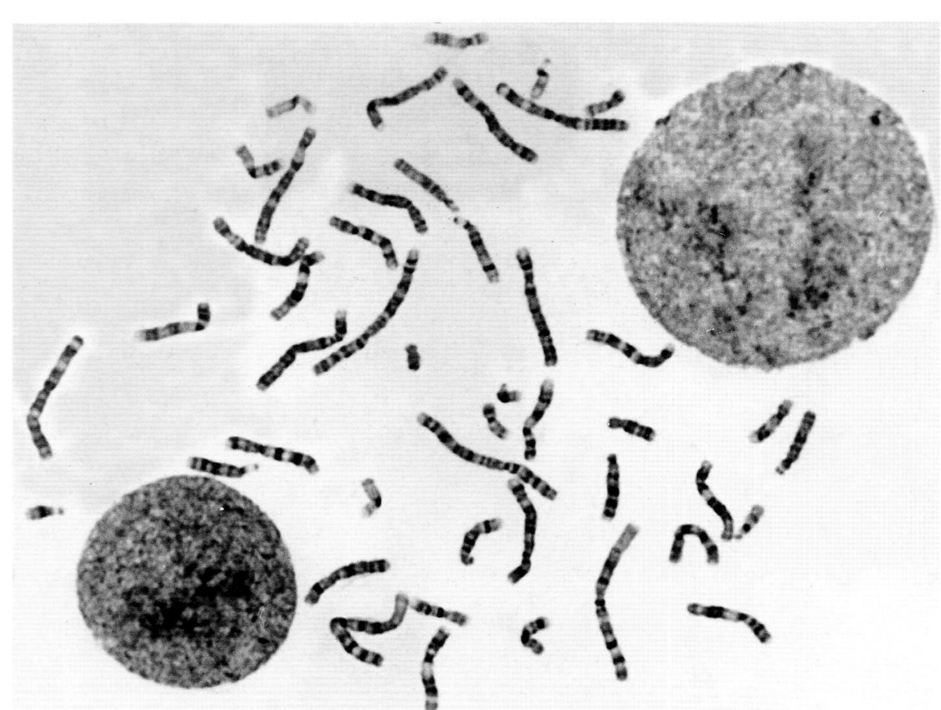

**Fig. 3.8**
A G-banded metaphase spread. (Courtesy of Mr A Wilkinson, Cytogenetics Unit, City Hospital, Nottingham.)

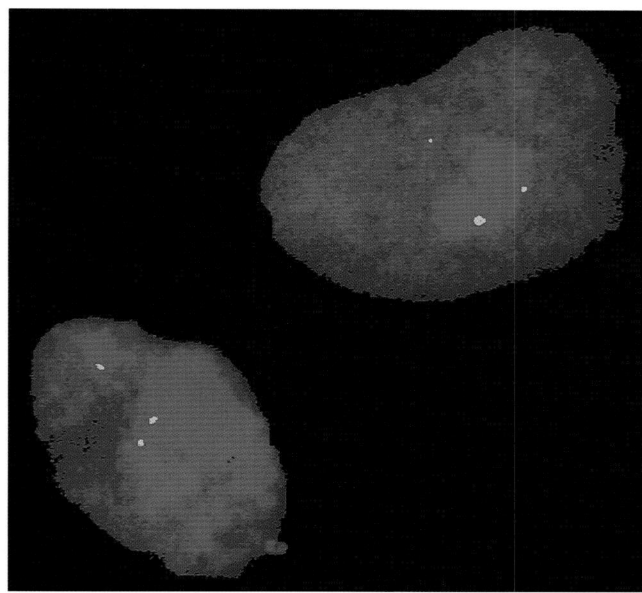

**Fig. 3.9**
Fluorescent in situ hybridization (FISH) of interphase nuclei with a chromosome 21 centromeric probe (CAMBIO) showing three signals consistent with trisomy 21. (Courtesy of Nigel Smith, City Hospital, Nottingham.)

described in Chapter 18. Unique sequence probes are widely used in gene mapping studies (p. 76).

### Telomeric probes

A complete set of telomeric probes has been developed for all 24 chromosomes (i.e. autosomes 1–22 plus X and Y). Using these a method has been devised which enables the simultaneous analysis of the subtelomeric region of every chromosome using only a single microscope slide per patient. This has proved to be a particularly useful technique for identifying tiny 'cryptic' subtelomeric abnormalities, such as deletions and translocations, in a small but significant proportion of children with unexplained mental retardation (p. 280).

### Whole chromosome paint probes

These consist of a cocktail of probes obtained from different parts of a particular chromosome. When this mixture of probes is used together in a single hybridization, the entire relevant chromosome fluoresces, i.e. is 'painted'. Chromosome painting is extremely useful for characterizing complex rearrangements such as subtle translocations (Fig. 3.11) and for identifying the origin of additional chromosome material, such as small supernumerary markers or rings (Fig. 3.12).

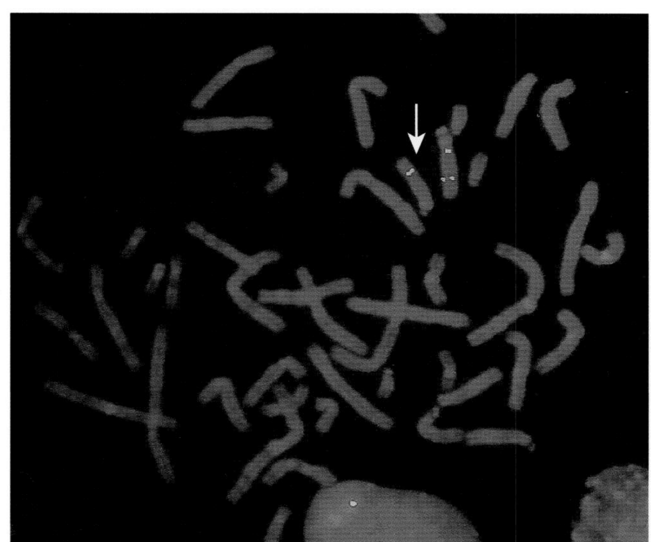

**Fig. 3.10**
Shows FISH demonstration of a microdeletion in one number 15 chromosome in a child with Prader-Willi syndrome using chromosome 15 locus specific probes (ONCOR). The arrow indicates the deleted chromosome, which shows only the signal generated by the chromosome 15 marker probe. (Courtesy of Meg Heath, City Hospital, Nottingham.)

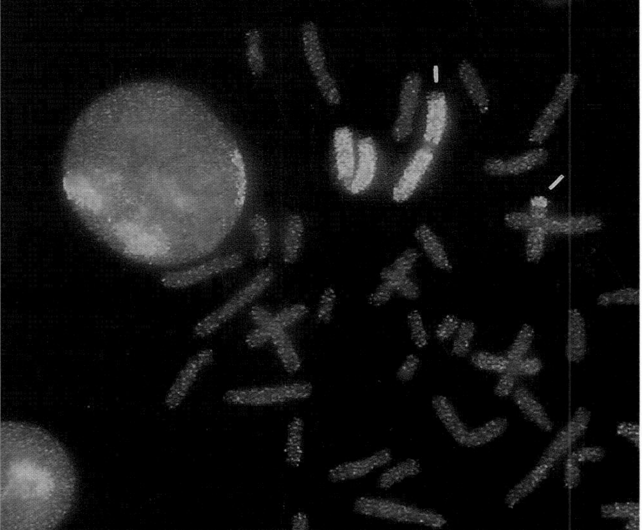

**Fig. 3.11**
Chromosome painting showing a subtle reciprocal translocation involving chromosomes 1 (white) and 9 (purple). The small translocated segments are indicated. (Courtesy of Meg Heath, City Hospital, Nottingham.)

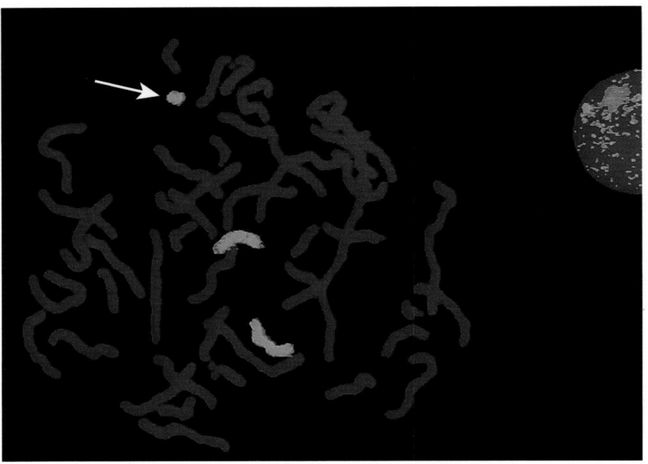

Fig. 3.12
Chromosome painting showing two normal number 17 chromosomes and a small ring 17 chromosome (arrowed) (paint provided by CAMBIO). (Courtesy of Nigel Smith, City Hospital, Nottingham.)

## Reverse painting

In this procedure a portion of unidentified chromosome material, such as a small supernumerary marker or ring, is used as a paint for hybridization to a normal metaphase spread. The unidentified chromosome is obtained using a fluorescent activated cell sorter (see below) and is then amplified using the polymerase chain reaction (p. 62) to prepare the labeled paint. The origin of the unidentified chromosome segment is then revealed by identifying the chromosome(s) to which it hybridizes.

## Multicolor spectral karyotyping (SKY) and multicolor fish (M-FISH)

These latest developments in FISH technology utilize pools of whole human chromosome paint probes to provide a multicolour human karyotype in which each pair of homologous chromosomes can be identified on the basis of its unique color when studied using computer-based image analysis (Fig. 3.13). These

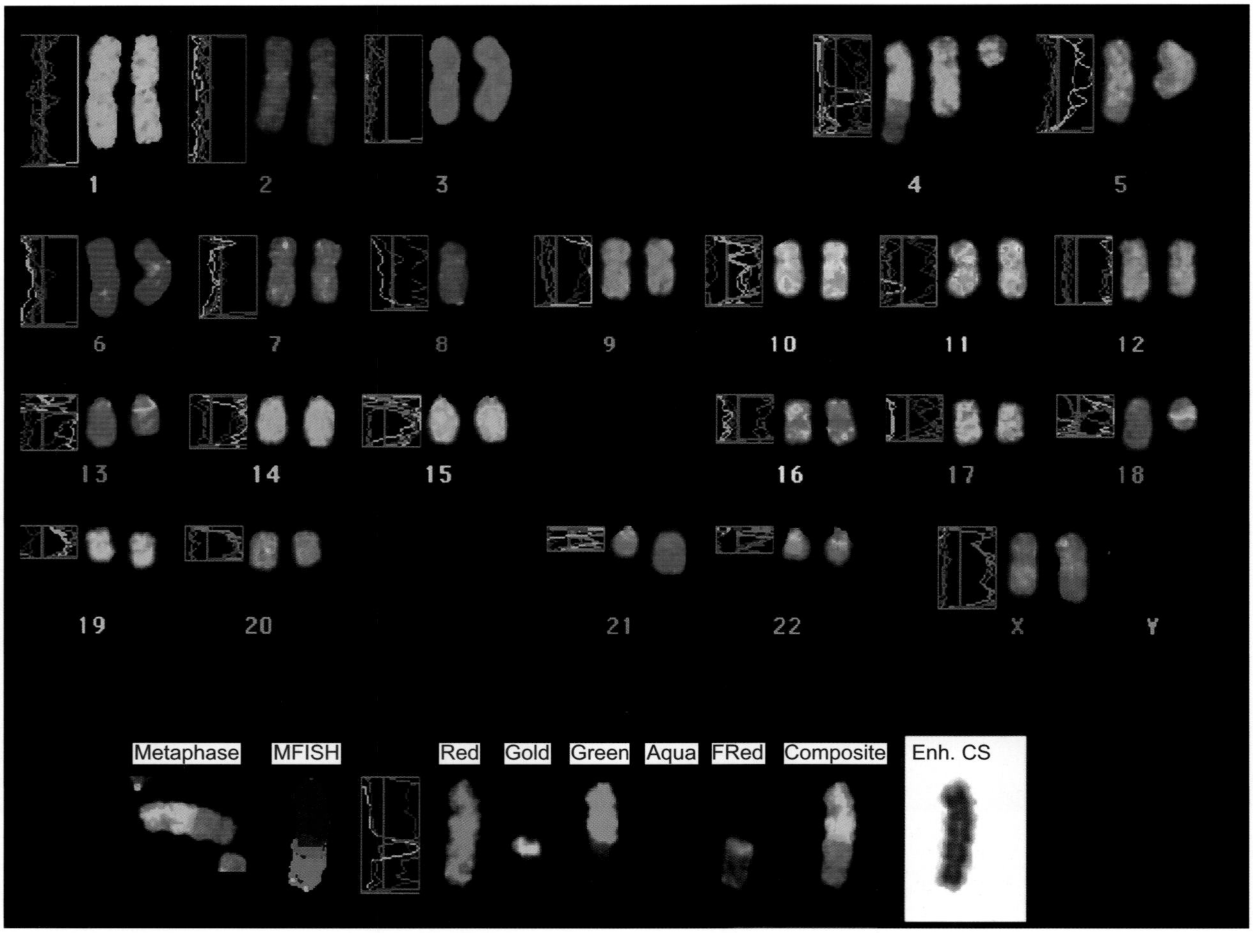

Fig. 3.13
M-FISH showing complex chromosome rearrangement involving chromosomes 4, 8, 13, 18 and 21 as observed in cultured blood lymphocytes. (Courtesy of Dr Rhona Anderson, Radiation and Genome Stability Unit, MRC Harwell, Oxon, UK and Applied Imaging.)

approaches have proved to be extremely useful for detecting subtle chromosome rearrangements, such as deletions and translocations, and for identifying small supernumerary markers and ring chromosomes.

## FLOW CYTOMETRY

Because of their differing size and DNA composition chromosomes bind different amounts of fluorescent dyes, some of which bind specifically to GC ('gene-rich') sequences and others to AT ('gene-poor') sequences. This property of differential binding allows chromosomes to be separated by the process of *flow cytometry* or *fluorescent activated cell sorting* (FACS). This involves staining metaphase chromosomes with a fluorescent DNA-binding dye and then projecting them in a fine jet of droplets across a focused laser beam that excites the chromosomes to fluoresce. The fluorescence intensity is measured by a photomultiplier and the results are analyzed by a computer that draws up a distribution histogram of chromosome size. This is referred to as a *flow karyotype*.

Flow cytometry can be used to analyze an individual's chromosomes, but its clinical application is limited by its expense and by the relatively poor separation achieved for certain chromosomes, most noticeably those in the C group. It finds greater application in separating preparations of single chromosomes for the construction of chromosome-specific DNA libraries and in the manufacture of chromosome paints for FISH.

## COMPARATIVE GENOMIC HYBRIDIZATION

This ingenious modification of reverse painting is widely used in cancer genetics to detect regions of allele loss and gene amplification (p. 210). Tumor or 'test' DNA is labeled with a green paint and control normal DNA is labeled with a red paint. The two samples are mixed and hybridized competitively to normal metaphase chromosomes, and photographed using a fluorescence microscope (Fig. 3.14). If the test sample contains more DNA from a particular chromosome region than the control sample, then that region is identified by an increase in the green to red fluorescence ratio (Fig. 3.15). Similarly a deletion in the test sample is identified by a reduction in the green to red fluorescence ratio.

Metaphase comparative genomic hybridization (CGH) has significantly contributed to our understanding of cancer cytogenetics, particularly for solid tumors where it

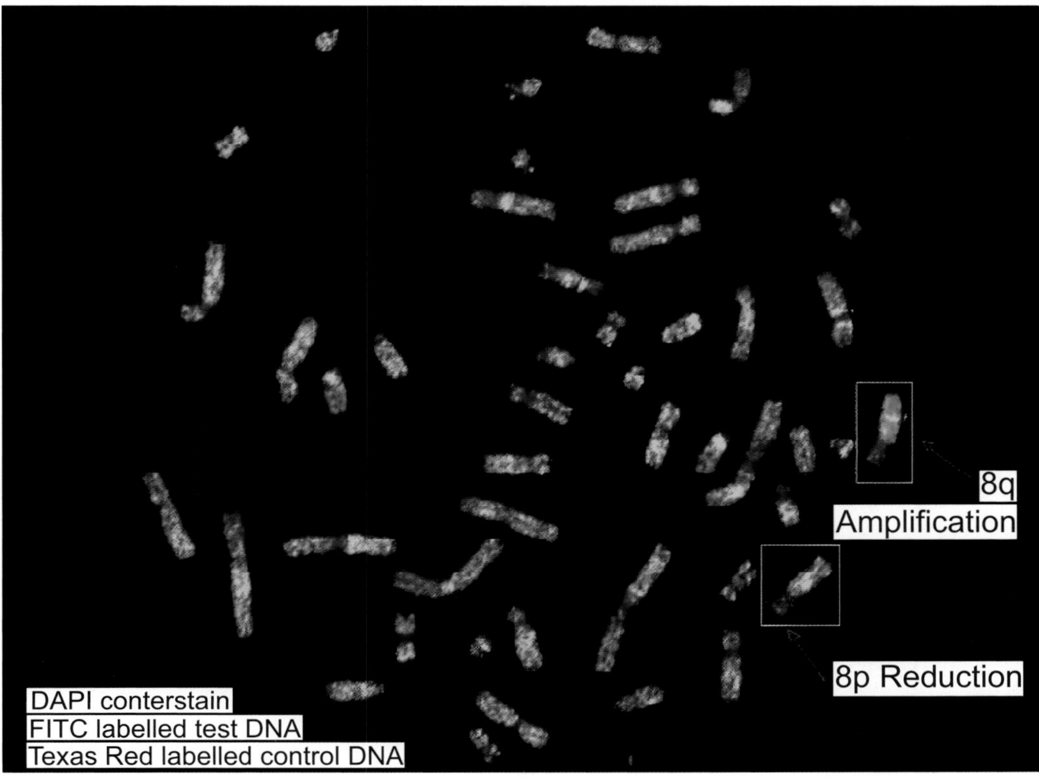


**Fig. 3.14**
Comparative genomic hybridization (CGH) analysis showing areas of gene amplification and reduction (deletion) in tumor DNA. (Courtesy of Dr Peter Lichter, DKFZ, Heidelberg and Applied Imaging.)

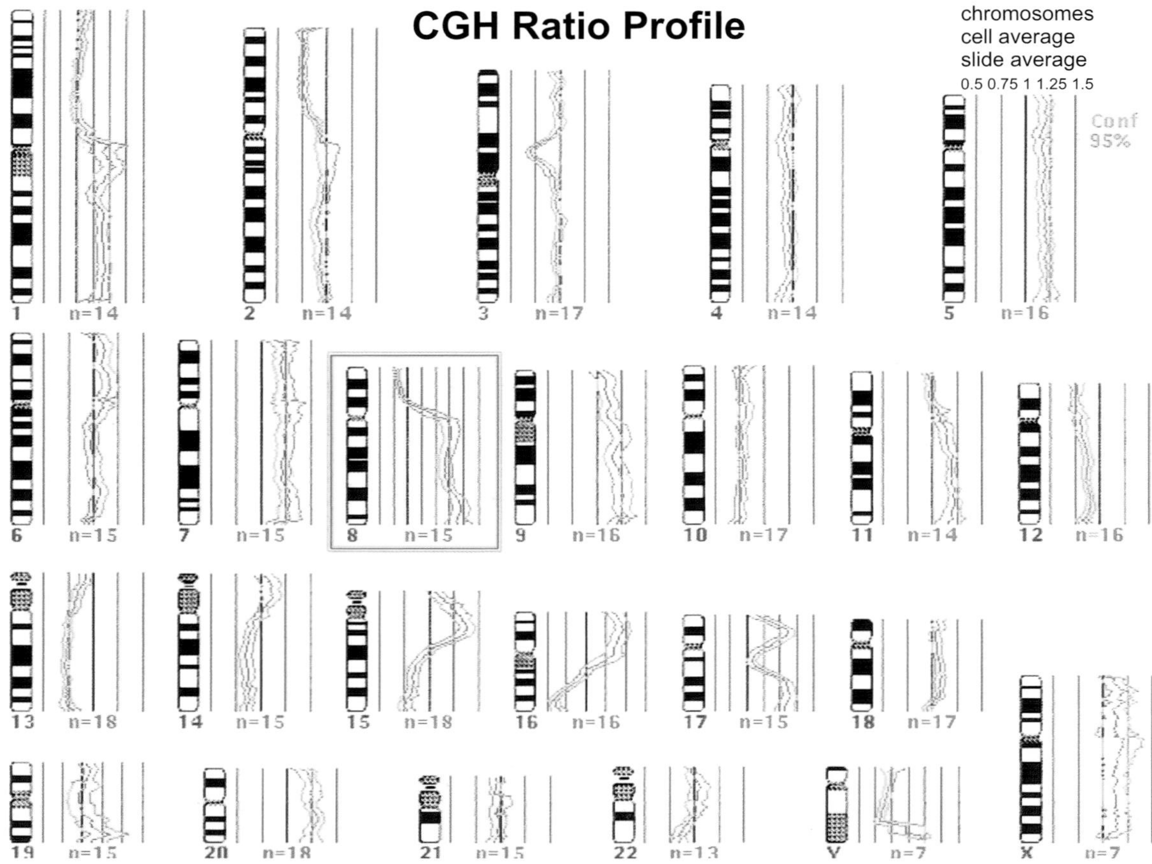


Fig. 3.15
CGH ratio profiles for the CGH analysis shown in Figure 3.14. The vertical lines adjacent to each chromosome show fluorescence ratios of 0.5 to 1.5 between test and control DNA. (Courtesy of Dr Peter Lichter, DKFZ, Heidelberg and Applied Imaging.)

obviates the need for metaphase spreads from tumors. However, its utility is limited by its resolution and technical difficulty. Current limits of resolution are 10 megabases (10 000 000 bases or 10 Mb) for losses and 2 Mb for gains, which provides a starting point for positional cloning (p. 78) but not precise localization of genes involved in tumor development. *Microarray CGH* is likely to supersede metaphase CGH.

## MICROARRAY COMPARATIVE GENOMIC HYBRIDIZATION

This technique involves hybridization of patient and reference DNA (as for metaphase CGH) on to short sequences of DNA bound to glass slides. The DNA target sequences are spotted on to the microscope slides using robotics to create a microarray where each DNA target has a unique location. Following hybridization and washing to remove unbound DNA, the relative levels of fluorescence are measured using computer software. Two types of DNA target have been described: either cDNA or genomic clones (YAC, BAC, PAC or cosmid). For detection of single-copy gains and losses the use of genomic probes is favored, and this is called *array CGH*. Increased uniformity in hybridization and subsequent signal fidelity is achieved because the genomic DNA targets have greater complexity and coverage.

The application of microarray CGH has extended from cancer cytogenetics to the detection of any type of gain/loss, including the detection of subtelomeric deletions in patients with unexplained mental retardation.

A further development is *array painting*, which extends the concept of reverse painting. Flow-sorted chromosomes are used as probes to analyze translocation breakpoints in order to identify the requisite genes.

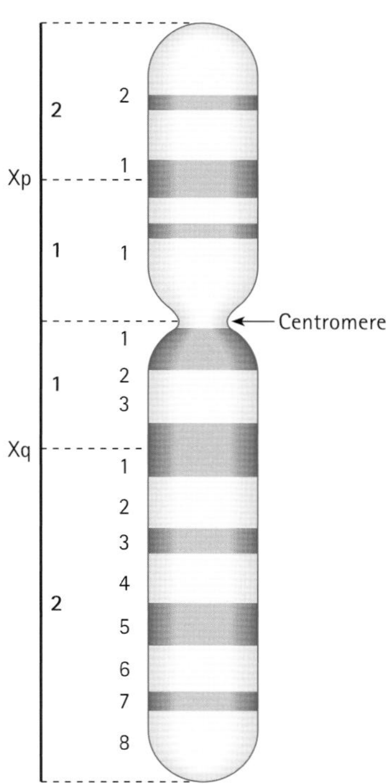


Fig. 3.16
An X chromosome showing the short and long arms each subdivided into regions and bands.

## CHROMOSOME NOMENCLATURE

By convention each chromosome arm is divided into regions and each region is subdivided into bands, numbering always from the centromere outwards (Fig. 3.16). A given point on a chromosome is designated by the chromosome number, the arm (p or q), the region and the band, e.g. 15q12. Sometimes the word region is omitted, so that 15q12 would be referred to simply as band 12 on the long arm of chromosome 15.

A shorthand notation system exists for the description of chromosome abnormalities (Table 3.1). Normal male and female karyotypes are depicted as 46,XY and 46,XX, respectively. A male with Down syndrome as a result of trisomy 21 would be represented as 47,XY,+21, whereas a female with a deletion of the short arm of one number 5 chromosome (*Cri du chat* syndrome, p. 274) would be represented as 46,XX,del(5p). A chromosome report reading 46,XY,t(2;4)(p23;q25) would indicate a male with a reciprocal translocation involving the short arm of chromosome 2 at region 2 band 3 and the long arm of chromosome 4 at region 2 band 5.

This system of karyotype nomenclature has been extended to include the results of FISH studies. For example, a karyotype which reads 46,XX.ish del(15)(q11.2q11.2)(D15S10–) refers to a female with a microdeletion involving 15q11.2 identified by in-situ hybridization analysis using a probe for the D15S10 locus (D15S10 = DNA from chromosome 15 site 10). This individual will have either Prader–Willi or Angelman syndrome, as discussed in Chapter 18.

**Table 3.1 Symbols used in describing a karyotype**

| Term | Explanation |
|---|---|
| p | Short arm |
| q | Long arm |
| cen | Centromere |
| del | Deletion, e.g. 46,XX,del(1)(q21) |
| dup | Duplication, e.g. 46,XY,dup(13)(q14) |
| fra | Fragile site |
| i | Isochromosome, e.g. 46,X,i(Xq) |
| inv | Inversion, e.g. 46XX,inv(9)(p12q12) |
| ish | In situ hybridization |
| r | Ring, e.g. 46,XX,r(21) |
| t | Translocation, e.g. 46,XY,t(2;4)(q21;q21) |
| ter | Terminal or end, i.e. tip of arm, e.g. pter or qter |
| / | Mosaicism, e.g. 46,XY/47,XXY |
| + or – | Sometimes used after a chromosome arm in text to indicate gain or loss of part of that chromosome, e.g. 46,XX,5p– |

## CELL DIVISION

### MITOSIS

At conception the human zygote consists of a single cell. This undergoes rapid division, leading ultimately to the mature human adult consisting of approximately $1 \times 10^{14}$ cells in total. In most organs and tissues, such as bone marrow and skin, cells continue to divide throughout life. This process of somatic cell division, during which the nucleus also divides, is known as *mitosis*. During mitosis each chromosome divides into two daughter chromosomes, one of which segregates into each daughter cell. Consequently the number of chromosomes per nucleus remains unchanged.

Prior to a cell entering mitosis, each chromosome consists of two identical sister chromatids as a result of DNA replication having taken place during the S phase of the cell cycle (p. 43). Mitosis is the process whereby each of these pairs of chromatids separates and disperses into separate daughter cells.

Mitosis is a continuous process that usually lasts 1–2 h, but for descriptive purposes it is convenient to distinguish five distinct stages. These are prophase, prometaphase, metaphase, anaphase and telophase (Fig. 3.17).

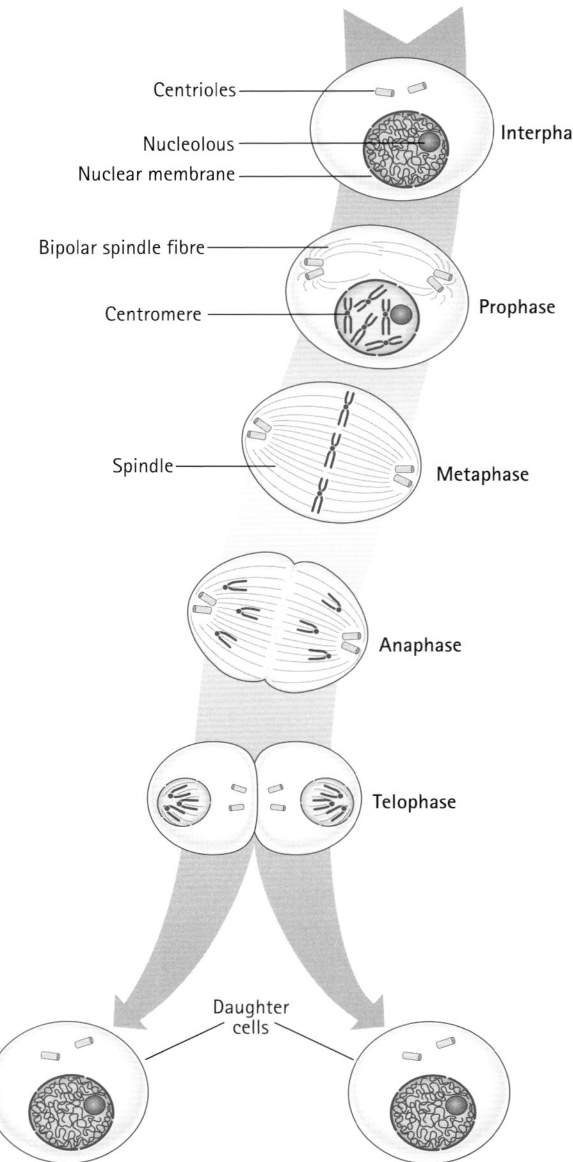


Fig. 3.17
Stages of mitosis.

## Prophase

During the initial stage of *prophase* the chromosomes condense and the mitotic spindle begins to form. Two *centrioles* form in each cell, from which *microtubules* radiate as the centrioles move towards opposite poles of the cell.

## Prometaphase

During *prometaphase* the nuclear membrane begins to disintegrate, allowing the chromosomes to spread around the cell. Each chromosome becomes attached at its centromere to a microtubule of the mitotic spindle.

## Metaphase

In *metaphase* the chromosomes become aligned along the equatorial plane or plate of the cell, where each chromosome is attached to the centriole by a microtubule forming the mature spindle. At this point the chromosomes are maximally contracted and, therefore, most easily visible. Each chromosome resembles the letter X in shape as the chromatids of each chromosome have separated longitudinally but remain attached at the centromere that has not yet undergone division.

## Anaphase

In *anaphase* the centromere of each chromosome divides longitudinally and the two daughter chromatids separate to opposite poles of the cell.

## Telophase

By *telophase* the chromatids, which are now independent chromosomes consisting of a single double helix, have separated completely and the two groups of daughter chromosomes each become enveloped in a new nuclear membrane. The cell cytoplasm also separates (cytokinesis), resulting in the formation of two new daughter cells each of which contains a complete diploid chromosome complement.

# THE CELL CYCLE

The period between successive mitoses is known as the *interphase* of the cell cycle (Fig. 3.18). In rapidly dividing cells this lasts for between 16 and 24 h. Interphase commences with the $G_1$ (G = gap) phase during which the chromosomes become thin and extended. This phase of the cycle is very variable in length and is responsible for the variation in generation time between different cell populations. Cells which have stopped dividing, such as neurons, usually arrest in this phase and are said to have entered a non-cyclic stage known as $G_0$.

The $G_1$ phase is followed by the S phase (S = synthesis), when DNA replication occurs and the chromatin of each chromosome is replicated. This results in the formation of two chromatids which give each chromosome its characteristic X-shaped configuration. The process of DNA replication commences at multiple points on a chromosome (p. 15).

Usually homologous pairs of chromosomes replicate in synchrony. However, one of the X chromosomes is

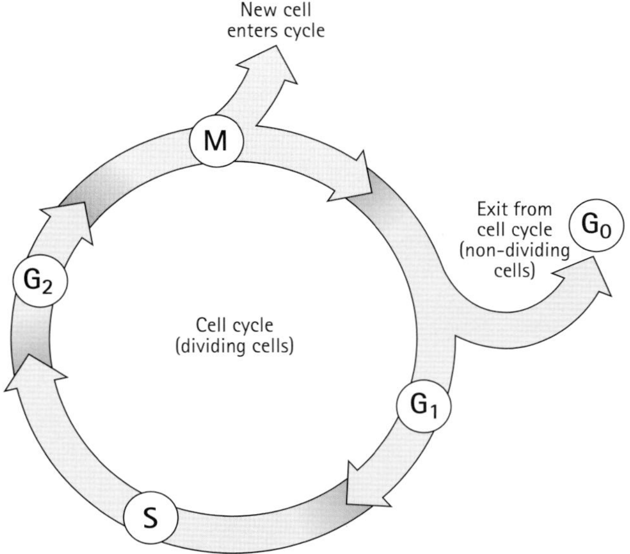


Fig. 3.18
Stages of the cell cycle. $G_1$ and $G_2$ are the first and second 'resting' stages of interphase. S is the stage of DNA replication. M = mitosis.

always late replicating. This is the inactive X chromosome (p. 99) which forms the *sex chromatin*, or the so-called *Barr body*, which can be visualized in interphase in female somatic cells. This used to be the basis of a rather unsatisfactory means of sex determination based on analysis of cells obtained by scraping the buccal mucosa – a 'buccal smear'.

Interphase is completed by a relatively short $G_2$ phase during which the chromosomes begin to condense in preparation for the next mitotic division.

## MEIOSIS

*Meiosis* is the process of nuclear division that occurs during the final stage of gamete formation. Meiosis differs from mitosis in three fundamental ways:

1. Mitosis results in each daughter cell having a diploid chromosome complement (46). During meiosis the diploid count is halved so that each mature gamete receives a haploid complement of 23 chromosomes.
2. Mitosis takes place in somatic cells and during the early cell divisions in gamete formation. Meiosis occurs only at the final division of gamete maturation.
3. Mitosis occurs as a single one-step process. Meiosis can be considered as two cell divisions known as meiosis I and meiosis II, each of which can be considered as having prophase, metaphase, anaphase and telophase stages, as in mitosis (Fig. 3.19).

### Meiosis I

This is sometimes referred to as the reduction division because it is during the first meiotic division that the chromosome number is halved.

### Prophase I

Chromosomes enter this stage already split longitudinally into two chromatids joined at the centromere. Homologous chromosomes pair, and with the exception of the X and Y chromosomes in male meiosis, exchange of homologous segments occurs between non-sister chromatids, that is, chromatids from each of the pair of homologous chromosomes. This exchange of homologous segments between chromatids occurs as a result of a process known as *crossing over* or *recombination*. The importance of crossing over in linkage analysis and risk calculation is considered later (pp. 131, 347).

During prophase I in the male pairing occurs between homologous segments of the X and Y chromosomes at the tip of their short arms, with this portion of each chromosome being known as the *pseudoautosomal* region (p. 105).

The prophase stage of meiosis I is relatively lengthy and can be subdivided into five stages.

#### Leptotene

The chromosomes become visible as they start to condense.

#### Zygotene

Homologous chromosomes align directly opposite each other, a process known as synapsis, and are held together at several points along their length by filamentous structures known as *synaptonemal* complexes.

#### Pachytene

Each pair of homologous chromosomes, known as a *bivalent*, becomes tightly coiled. Crossing over occurs, during which homologous regions of DNA are exchanged between chromatids.

#### Diplotene

The homologous recombinant chromosomes now begin to separate but remain attached at the points where crossing over has occurred. These are known as *chiasmata*. On average small, medium and large chromosomes have one, two and three chiasmata, respectively, giving an overall total of approximately 40 recombination events per meiosis per gamete.

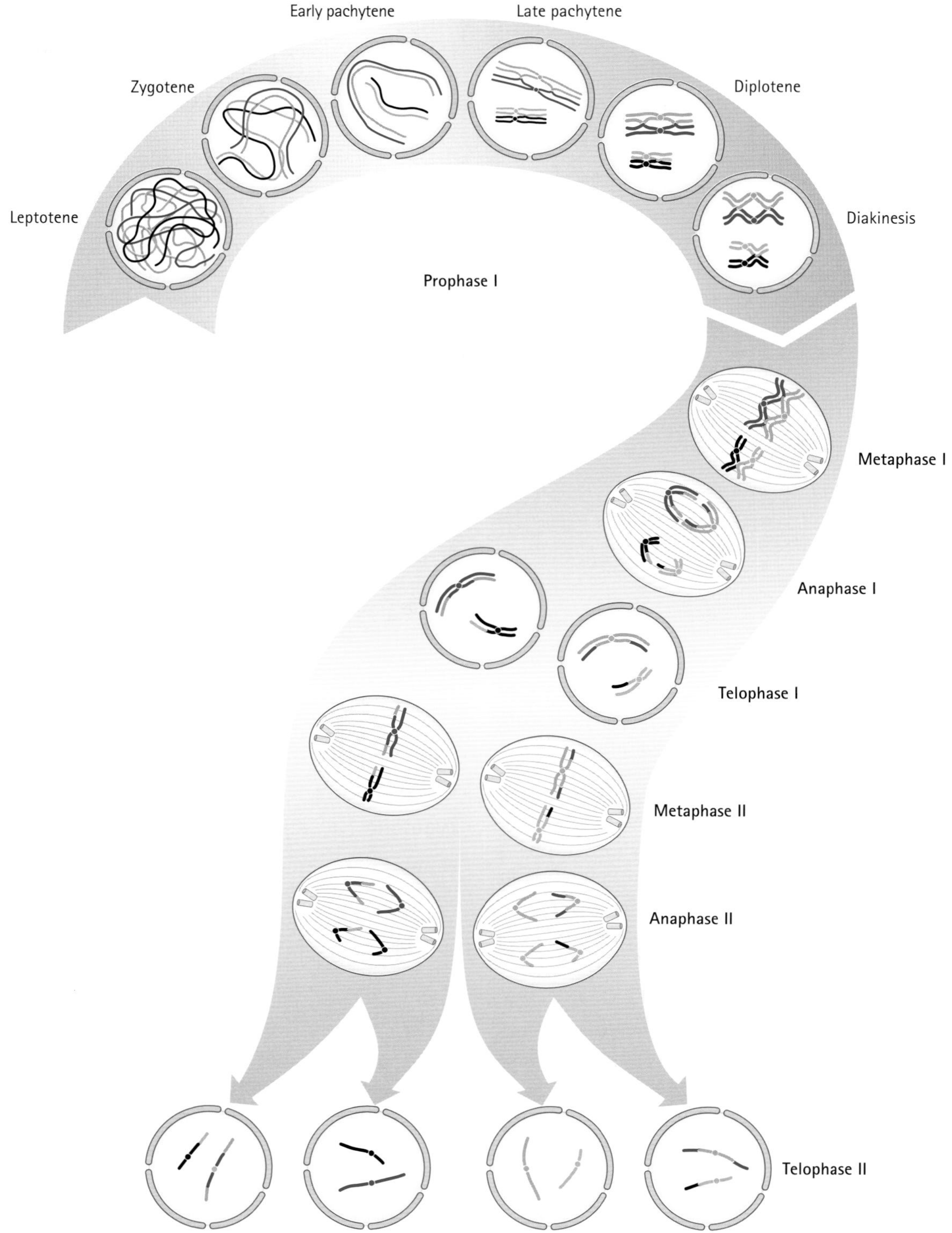


**Fig. 3.19**
Stages of meiosis.

### Diakinesis

Separation of the homologous chromosome pairs proceeds as the chromosomes become maximally condensed.

#### *Metaphase I*

The nuclear membrane disappears and the chromosomes become aligned on the equatorial plane of the cell where they have become attached to the spindle, as in metaphase of mitosis.

#### *Anaphase I*

The chromosomes now separate to opposite poles of the cell as the spindle contracts.

#### *Telophase I*

Each set of haploid chromosomes has now separated completely to opposite ends of the cell, which cleaves into two new daughter gametes, so-called *secondary spermatocytes* or *oocytes*.

### Meiosis II

This is essentially similar to an ordinary mitotic division. Each chromosome, which exists as a pair of chromatids, becomes aligned along the equatorial plane and then splits longitudinally, leading to the formation of two new daughter gametes, known as spermatids or ova.

### The consequences of meiosis

When considered in terms of reproduction and the maintenance of the species, meiosis achieves two major objectives. Firstly it facilitates halving of the diploid number of chromosomes so that each child receives half of its chromosome complement from each parent. Secondly it provides an extraordinary potential for generating genetic diversity. This is achieved in two ways:

1. When the bivalents separate during prophase of meiosis I, they do so independently of one another. This is consistent with Mendel's third law (p. 5). Consequently each gamete receives a selection of parental chromosomes. The likelihood that any two gametes from an individual will contain exactly the same chromosomes equals 1 in $2^{23}$, i.e. approximately 1 in 8 million.
2. As a result of crossing over, each chromatid will usually contain portions of DNA derived from both parental homologous chromosomes. A large chromosome will typically consist of three or more segments of alternating parental origin. The ensuing probability that any two gametes will have an identical genome is therefore infinitesimally small. This dispersion of DNA into different gametes is sometimes referred to as 'gene shuffling'.

## GAMETOGENESIS

The process of gametogenesis shows fundamental differences in males and females (Table 3.2). These have quite distinct clinical consequences if errors occur.

### OOGENESIS

Mature ova develop from oogonia by a complex series of intermediate steps. Oogonia themselves originate from primordial germ cells by a process involving 20–30 mitotic divisions that occur during the first few months of embryonic life. By the completion of embryogenesis at 3 months of intrauterine life, the oogonia have begun to mature into primary oocytes that start to undergo meiosis. At birth all of the primary oocytes have entered a phase of maturation arrest, known as *dictyotene*, in which they remain suspended until meiosis I is completed at the time of ovulation, when a single secondary oocyte is formed. This receives most of the cytoplasm. The other daughter cell from the first meiotic division consists largely of a nucleus and is known as a polar body. Meiosis II then commences, during which fertilization can occur. This second meiotic division results in the formation of a further polar body (Fig. 3.20).

It is probable that the very lengthy interval between the onset of meiosis and its eventual completion, up to 50 years later, accounts for the well-documented increased incidence of chromosome abnormalities in the offspring of older mothers (p. 46). The accumulating effects of wear and tear on the primary oocyte during the dictyotene phase probably damage the cell's spindle formation and repair mechanisms, thereby predisposing to non-disjunction (p. 46).

**Table 3.2 Differences in gametogenesis in male and female**

| | Male | Female |
|---|---|---|
| Commences | Puberty | Early embryonic life |
| Duration | 60–65 days | 10–50 years |
| Numbers of mitoses in gamete formation | 30–500 | 20–30 |
| Gamete production per meiosis | 4 spermatids | 1 ovum + 3 polar bodies |
| Gamete production per ejaculate | 100–200 million cycle | 1 ovum per menstrual |

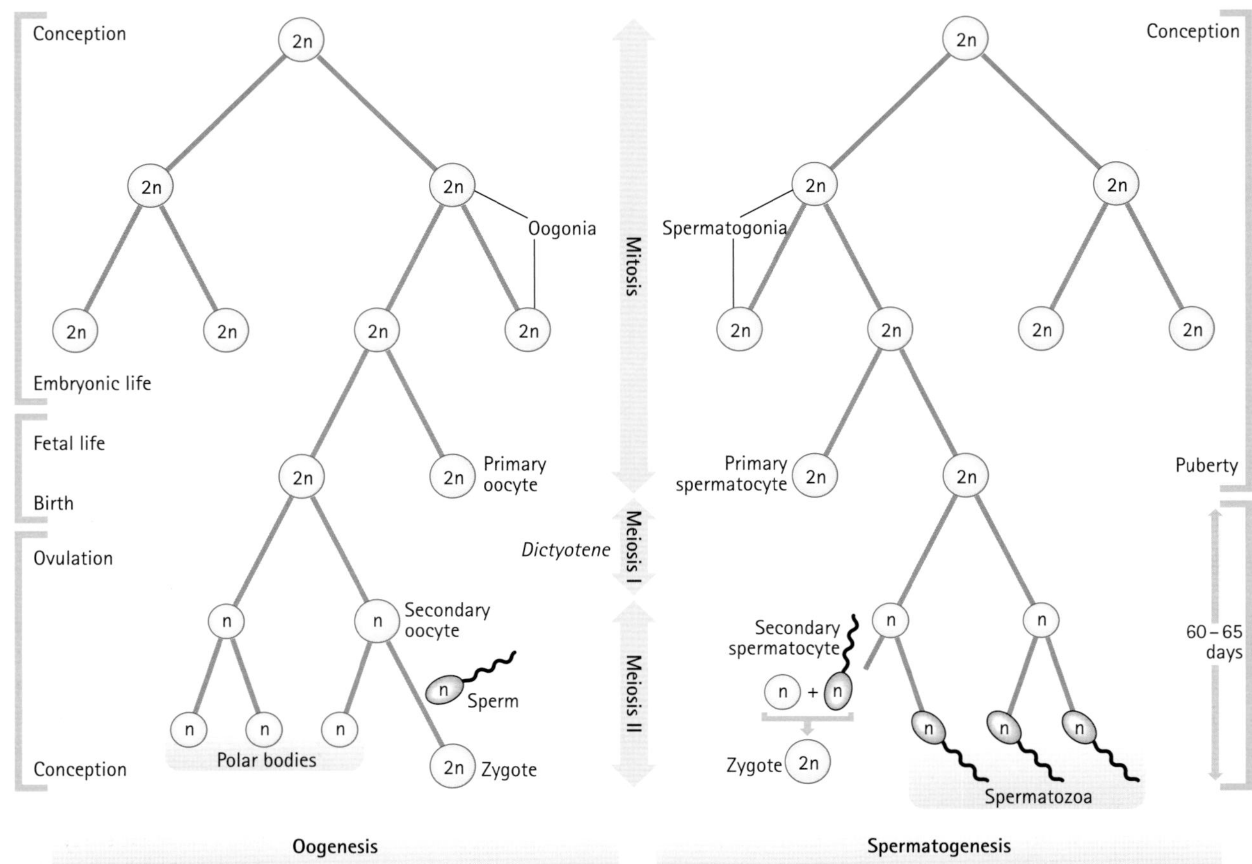


**Fig. 3.20**
Stages of oogenesis and spermatogenesis. n = haploid number.

## SPERMATOGENESIS

In contrast, spermatogenesis is a relatively rapid process with an average duration of 60–65 days. At puberty spermatogonia, which will already have undergone approximately 30 mitotic divisions, begin to mature into primary spermatocytes which enter meiosis I and emerge as haploid secondary spermatocytes. These then undergo the second meiotic division to form spermatids, which in turn develop without any subsequent cell division into mature spermatozoa, of which 100–200 million are present in each ejaculate.

Spermatogenesis is a continuous process involving many mitotic divisions, possibly as many as 20–25 per annum, so that mature spermatozoa produced by a man of 50 years or older could well have undergone several hundred mitotic divisions. The observed paternal age effect for new dominant mutations (p. 108) is consistent with the concept that many mutations arise as a consequence of DNA copy errors occurring during mitosis.

## CHROMOSOME ABNORMALITIES

Specific disorders caused by chromosome abnormalities are considered in Chapter 18. In this section discussion will be restricted to a review of the different types of abnormality that can occur. These can be divided into numerical and structural, with a third category consisting of different chromosome constitutions in two or more cell lines (Table 3.3).

### NUMERICAL ABNORMALITIES

Numerical abnormalities involve the loss or gain of one or more chromosomes, which is referred to as *aneuploidy*, or the addition of one or more complete haploid complements, which is known as *polyploidy*. Loss of a single chromosome results in *monosomy*. Gain of one or two homologous chromosomes is referred to as *trisomy* and *tetrasomy*, respectively.

| Table 3.3 Types of chromosome abnormality | |
|---|---|
| **Numerical** | |
| Aneuploidy | — Monosomy |
| | — Trisomy |
| | — Tetrasomy |
| Polyploidy | — Triploidy |
| | — Tetraploidy |
| **Structural** | |
| Translocations | — Reciprocal |
| | — Robertsonian |
| Deletions | |
| Insertions | |
| Inversions | — Paracentric |
| | — Pericentric |
| Rings | |
| Isochromosomes | |
| **Different cell lines (mixoploidy)** | |
| Mosaicism | |
| Chimerism | |

## Trisomy

The presence of an extra chromosome is referred to as trisomy. Most cases of Down syndrome are due to the presence of an additional number 21 chromosome, hence Down syndrome is often known as trisomy 21. Other autosomal trisomies that are compatible with survival to term are Patau syndrome (trisomy 13) (p. 274) and Edwards syndrome (trisomy 18) (p. 274). Most other autosomal trisomies result in early pregnancy loss, with trisomy 16 being a particularly common finding in first-trimester spontaneous miscarriages. The presence of an additional sex chromosome (X or Y) has only mild phenotypic effects (pp. 281, 283).

Trisomy 21 is usually caused by failure of separation of one of the pairs of homologous chromosomes during anaphase of maternal meiosis I. This failure of the bivalent to separate is called *non-disjunction*. Less often, trisomy can be caused by non-disjunction occurring during meiosis II when a pair of sister chromatids fail to separate. Either way the gamete receives two homologous chromosomes (*disomy*), and if subsequent fertilization occurs a trisomic conceptus results (Fig. 3.21).

### The origin of non-disjunction

The consequences of non-disjunction in meiosis I and meiosis II differ in the chromosomes found in the gamete. An error in meiosis I leads to the gamete containing both homologs of one chromosome pair. In contrast, non-disjunction in meiosis II results in the gamete receiving two copies of one of the homologs of the chromosome pair. Studies using DNA markers have shown that most children with an autosomal trisomy have inherited their additional chromosome as a result of non-disjunction occurring during one of the maternal meiotic divisions (Table 3.4).

Non-disjunction can also occur during an early mitotic division in the developing zygote. This results in the presence of two or more different cell lines, a phenomenon known as *mosaicism* (p. 54).

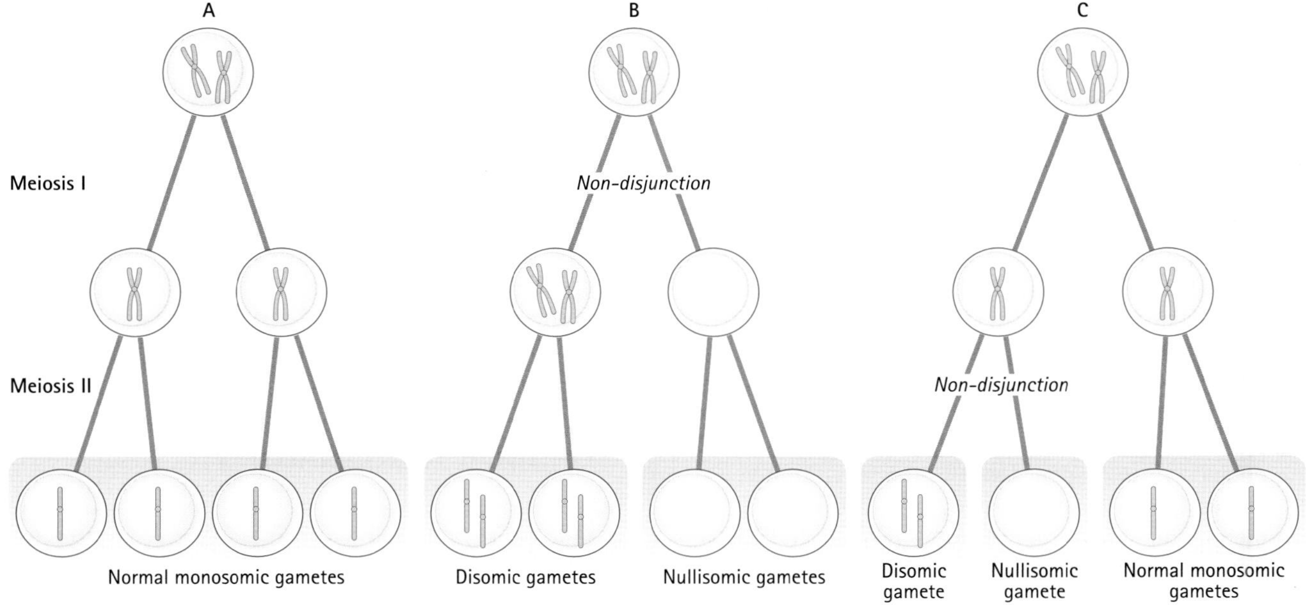


Fig. 3.21
Segregation at meiosis of a single pair of chromosomes in (A) normal meiosis, (B) non-disjunction in meiosis I and (C) non-disjunction in meiosis II.

**Table 3.4 Parental origin of meiotic error leading to aneuploidy**

| Chromosome abnormality | Paternal (%) | Maternal (%) |
|---|---|---|
| Trisomy 13 | 15 | 85 |
| Trisomy 18 | 10 | 90 |
| Trisomy 21 | 5 | 95 |
| 45,X | 80 | 20 |
| 47,XXX | 5 | 95 |
| 47,XXY | 45 | 55 |
| 47,XYY | 100 | 0 |

### *The cause of non-disjunction*

The cause of non-disjunction is uncertain. The most favored explanation is that of an aging effect on the primary oocyte, which can remain in a state of suspended inactivity for up to 50 years (p. 45). This is based on the well-documented association between advancing maternal age and increased incidence of Down syndrome in offspring (Table 18.4, p. 272). A maternal age effect has also been noted for trisomies 13 and 18.

It is not known how or why advancing maternal age predisposes to non-disjunction, although research has shown that absence of recombination in prophase of meiosis I predisposes to subsequent non-disjunction. This is not surprising, as the chiasmata that are formed after recombination are responsible for holding each pair of homologous chromosomes together until subsequent separation occurs in diakinesis. Thus failure of chiasmata formation could allow each pair of homologs to separate prematurely and then segregate randomly to daughter cells. In the female, however, recombination occurs before birth whereas the non-disjunctional event occurs any time between 15 and 50 years later. This suggests that at least two factors can be involved in causing non-disjunction, the first being an absence of recombination between homologous chromosomes in the fetal ovary, and the second an abnormality in spindle formation many years later.

An alternative explanation for the association of advancing maternal age with increased risk of autosomal trisomy is that survival of trisomic embryos could be the result of an age-related reduction in 'immunological' competence. Firm evidence for this theory is limited.

Other factors that have been implicated in causing non-disjunction include radiation and delayed fertilization after ovulation. In animals it has been shown that an increased incidence of aneuploid embryos can result from lengthening of the interval between ovulation and fertilization. It has been suggested that this could account for the relationship between maternal age and the incidence of Down syndrome, as with increasing age intercourse is likely to occur less frequently, with delayed fertilization therefore being more likely. The story is further complicated by the fact that in some species, such as *Drosophila*, non-disjunction is under genetic control. This could account for those occasional families that seem to be prone to recurrent non-disjunction.

### Monosomy

The absence of a single chromosome is referred to as monosomy. Monosomy for an autosome is almost always incompatible with survival to term. Lack of contribution of an X or a Y chromosome results in a 45,X karyotype which causes the condition known as Turner syndrome (p. 282).

As with trisomy, monosomy can result from non-disjunction in meiosis. If one gamete receives two copies of a homologous chromosome (*disomy*), the other corresponding daughter gamete will have no copy of the same chromosome (*nullisomy*). Monosomy can also be caused by loss of a chromosome as it moves to the pole of the cell during anaphase, an event known as 'anaphase lag'.

### Polyploidy

Polyploid cells contain multiples of the haploid number of chromosomes such as 69, *triploidy*, or 92, *tetraploidy*. In humans triploidy is found relatively often in material grown from spontaneous miscarriages, but survival beyond mid-pregnancy is rare. Only a few triploid live births have been described and all have died soon after birth.

Triploidy can be caused by failure of a maturation meiotic division in an ovum or sperm, leading, for example, to retention of a polar body or to the formation of a diploid sperm. Alternatively it can be caused by fertilization of an ovum by two sperm: this is known as *dispermy*. When triploidy results from the presence of an additional set of paternal chromosomes, the placenta is usually swollen with what are known as hydatidiform changes (p. 96). In contrast, when triploidy results from an additional set of maternal chromosomes, the placenta is usually small. Triploidy usually results in early spontaneous miscarriage (Fig. 3.22).

## STRUCTURAL ABNORMALITIES

Structural chromosome rearrangements result from chromosome breakage with subsequent reunion in a different configuration. They can be balanced or unbalanced. In balanced rearrangements the chromosome complement is complete, with no loss or gain of genetic material. Consequently, balanced rearrangements are generally harmless with the exception of rare cases in

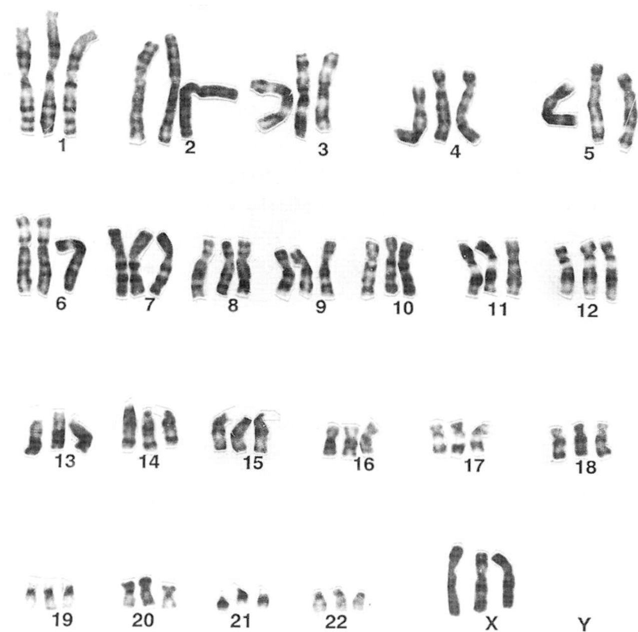


**Fig. 3.22**
Karyotype from products of conception of a spontaneous miscarriage showing triploidy.

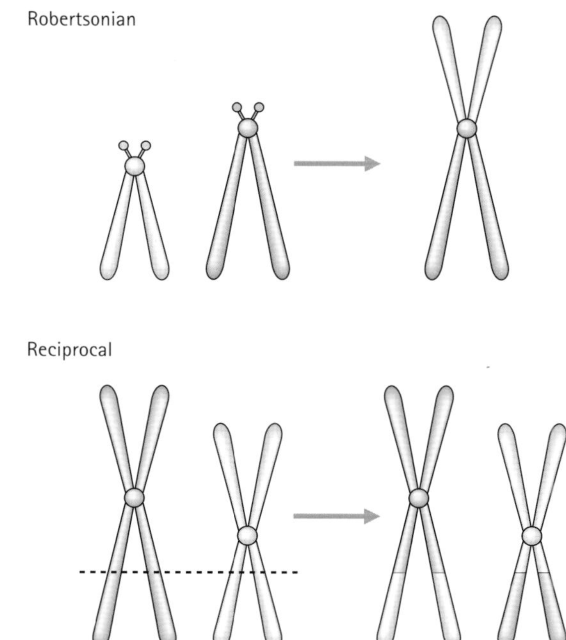


**Fig. 3.23**
Types of translocation.

which one of the break-points damages an important functional gene. However, carriers of balanced rearrangements are often at risk of producing children with an unbalanced chromosomal complement.

When a chromosome rearrangement is unbalanced the chromosomal complement contains an incorrect amount of chromosome material and the clinical effects are usually very serious.

## Translocations

A *translocation* refers to the transfer of genetic material from one chromosome to another. A reciprocal translocation is formed when a break occurs in each of two chromosomes with the segments being exchanged to form two new derivative chromosomes. A Robertsonian translocation is a particular type of reciprocal translocation in which the break-points are located at or close to the centromeres of two acrocentric chromosomes (Fig. 3.23).

### *Reciprocal translocations*

A reciprocal translocation involves breakage of at least two chromosomes with exchange of the fragments. Usually the chromosome number remains at 46, and if the exchanged fragments are of roughly equal size, a reciprocal translocation can only be identified with detailed chromosomal banding studies or FISH (see Fig. 3.11). In general, reciprocal translocations are unique to a particular family, although, for reasons that are unknown, a particular balanced reciprocal translocation involving the long arms of chromosomes 11 and 22 is relatively common. The overall incidence of reciprocal translocations in the general population is approximately 1 in 500.

### Segregation at meiosis

The importance of balanced reciprocal translocations lies in their behavior at meiosis, when they can segregate to generate significant chromosome imbalance. This can lead to early pregnancy loss or to the birth of an infant with multiple abnormalities. Problems arise at meiosis because the chromosomes involved in the translocation cannot pair normally to form bivalents. Instead they form a cluster known as a *pachytene quadrivalent* (Fig. 3.24). The key point to note is that each chromosome aligns with homologous material in the quadrivalent.

*2:2 segregation* When the constituent chromosomes in the quadrivalent separate during the later stages of meiosis I they can do so in several different ways (Table 3.5). If alternate chromosomes segregate to each gamete, then the gamete will carry a normal or balanced haploid complement (Fig. 3.25) and with fertilization the embryo will either have normal chromosomes or carry the balanced rearrangement. If, however, adjacent

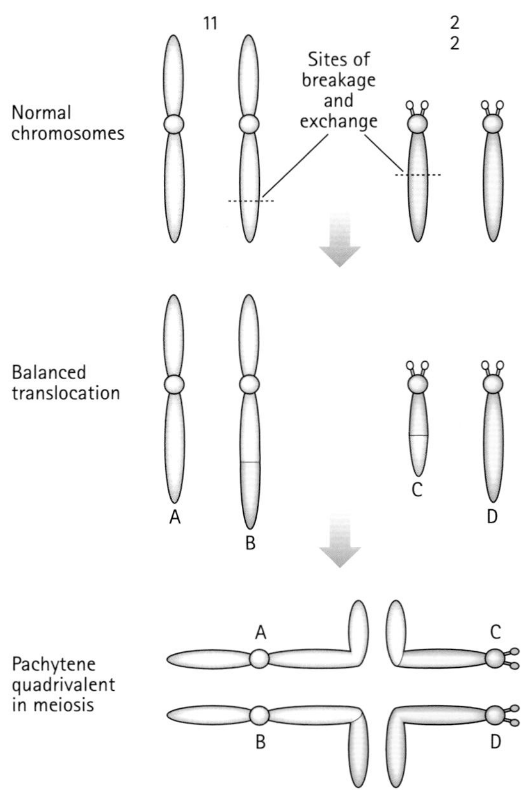


**Fig. 3.24**
Shows how a balanced reciprocal translocation involving chromosomes 11 and 22 leads to the formation of a quadrivalent at pachytene in meiosis I. The quadrivalent is formed to maintain homologous pairing.

chromosomes segregate together, this will invariably result in the gamete acquiring an unbalanced chromosome complement. For example, in Figure 3.24, if the gamete inherits the normal number 11 chromosome (A) and the derivative number 22 chromosome (C), then fertilization will result in an embryo with monosomy for the distal long arm of chromosome 22 and trisomy for the distal long arm of chromosome 11.

*3:1 segregation* Another possibility is that three chromosomes segregate to one gamete with only one chromosome in the other gamete. If, for example, in Figure 3.24 chromosomes 11 (A), 22 (D) and the derivative 22 (C) segregate together to a gamete which is subsequently fertilized, this will result in the embryo being trisomic for the material present in the derivative 22 chromosome. This is sometimes referred to as *tertiary trisomy*. Experience has shown that with this particular reciprocal translocation, tertiary trisomy for the derivative 22 chromosome is the only viable unbalanced product. All other patterns of malsegregation lead to early pregnancy loss. Unfortunately, tertiary trisomy for the derivative 22 chromosome is a serious condition in which affected children have multiple congenital abnormalities and severe learning difficulties.

## Risks in reciprocal translocations

When counseling a carrier of a balanced translocation it is necessary to consider the particular rearrangement to determine whether it could result in the birth of an abnormal baby. This risk will usually lie somewhere

**Table 3.5 Patterns of segregation of a reciprocal translocation (see Figs 3.24 and 3.25)**

| Pattern of segregation | Segregating chromosomes | Chromosome constitution in gamete |
|---|---|---|
| 2:2<br>Alternate | A + D<br>B + C | Normal<br>Balanced translocation |
| Adjacent—1 (non-homologous centromeres segregate together) | A + C<br>or<br>B + D | Unbalanced, leading to a combination of partial monosomy and partial trisomy in the zygote |
| Adjacent—2<br>(homologous centromeres segregate together) | A + B<br>or<br>C + D | |
| 3:1<br>Three chromosomes | A + B + C<br>A + B + D<br>A + C + D<br>B + C + D | Unbalanced, leading to trisomy in the zygote |
| One chromosome | A<br>B<br>C<br>D | Unbalanced, leading to monosomy in the zygote |

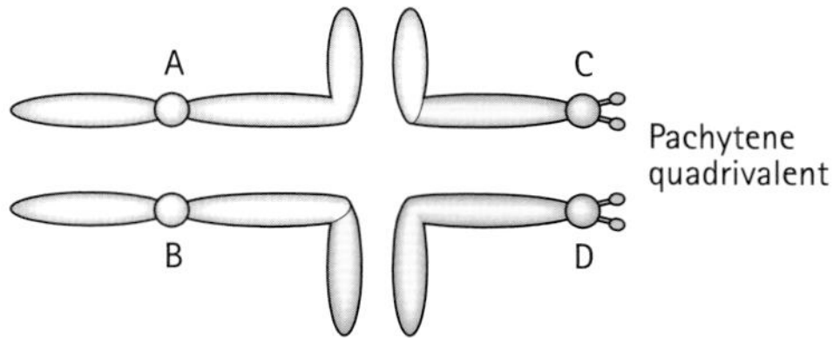


1 Alternate segregation yields normal or balanced haploid complement

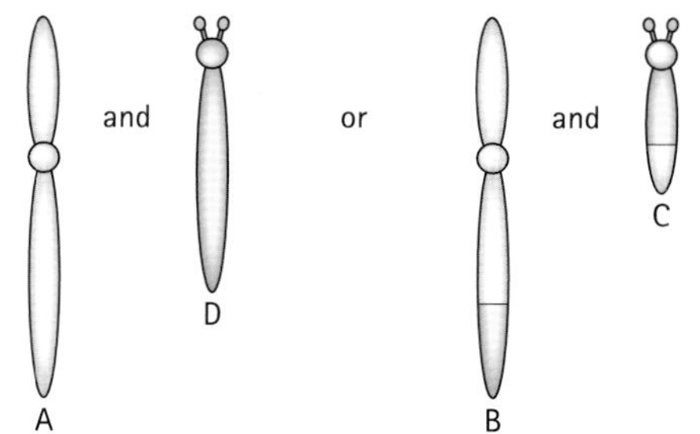


2 Adjacent-1 segregation yields unbalanced haploid complement

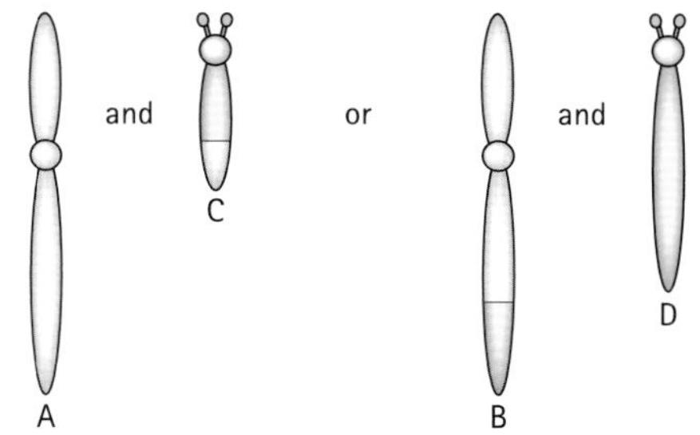


3 Adjacent-2 segregation yields unbalanced haploid complement

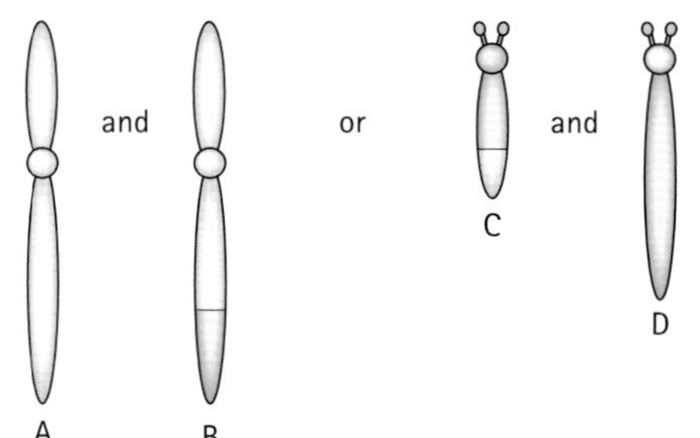


**Fig. 3.25**
Shows the different patterns of 2:2 segregation which can occur from the quadrivalent shown in Figure 3.24. See Table 3.5.

between 1% and 10%. For carriers of the 11;22 translocation discussed, the risk has been shown to be 5%.

### *Robertsonian translocations*

A Robertsonian translocation results from breakage of two acrocentric chromosomes (numbers 13, 14, 15, 21 and 22) at or close to their centromeres, with subsequent fusion of their long arms (see Fig. 3.23). This is also referred to as *centric fusion*. The short arms of each chromosome are lost, this being of no clinical importance as they contain only genes for ribosomal RNA, for which there are multiple copies on the various other acrocentric chromosomes. The total chromosome number is reduced to 45. Since there is no loss or gain of important genetic material this is a functionally balanced rearrangement. The overall incidence of Robertsonian translocations in the general population is approximately 1 in 1000, with by far the most common being fusion of the long arms of chromosomes 13 and 14 (i.e. 13q14q).

### Segregation at meiosis

As with reciprocal translocations, the importance of Robertsonian translocations lies in their behavior at meiosis. For example, a carrier of a 14q21q translocation can produce gametes with (Fig. 3.26):

1. A normal chromosome complement, i.e. a normal 14 and a normal 21.
2. A balanced chromosome complement, i.e. a 14q21q translocation chromosome.
3. An unbalanced chromosome complement possessing both the translocation chromosome and a normal 21. This will result in the fertilized embryo having Down syndrome.
4. An unbalanced chromosome complement with a normal 14 and a missing 21.
5. An unbalanced chromosome complement with a normal 21 and a missing 14.
6. An unbalanced chromosome complement with the translocation chromosome and a normal 14 chromosome.

The last three combinations will result in zygotes with monosomy 21, monosomy 14 and trisomy 14, respectively. All of these combinations are incompatible with survival beyond early pregnancy.

### Translocation down syndrome

The major practical importance of Robertsonian translocations is that they can predispose to the birth of babies with Down syndrome as a result of the embryo inheriting two normal number 21 chromosomes (one from each parent) plus a translocation chromosome involving a number 21 chromosome (Fig. 3.27). The clinical consequences are exactly the same as those seen in pure trisomy 21. However, unlike trisomy 21, the parents of a child with translocation Down syndrome have a relatively high risk of having further affected children if one of them carries the rearrangement in a balanced form.

Consequently the importance of performing a chromosome analysis in a child with Down syndrome lies not only in confirmation of the diagnosis, but also in identification of those children with a translocation. In roughly two-thirds of these latter children with Down syndrome, the translocation will have occurred as a new (de novo)

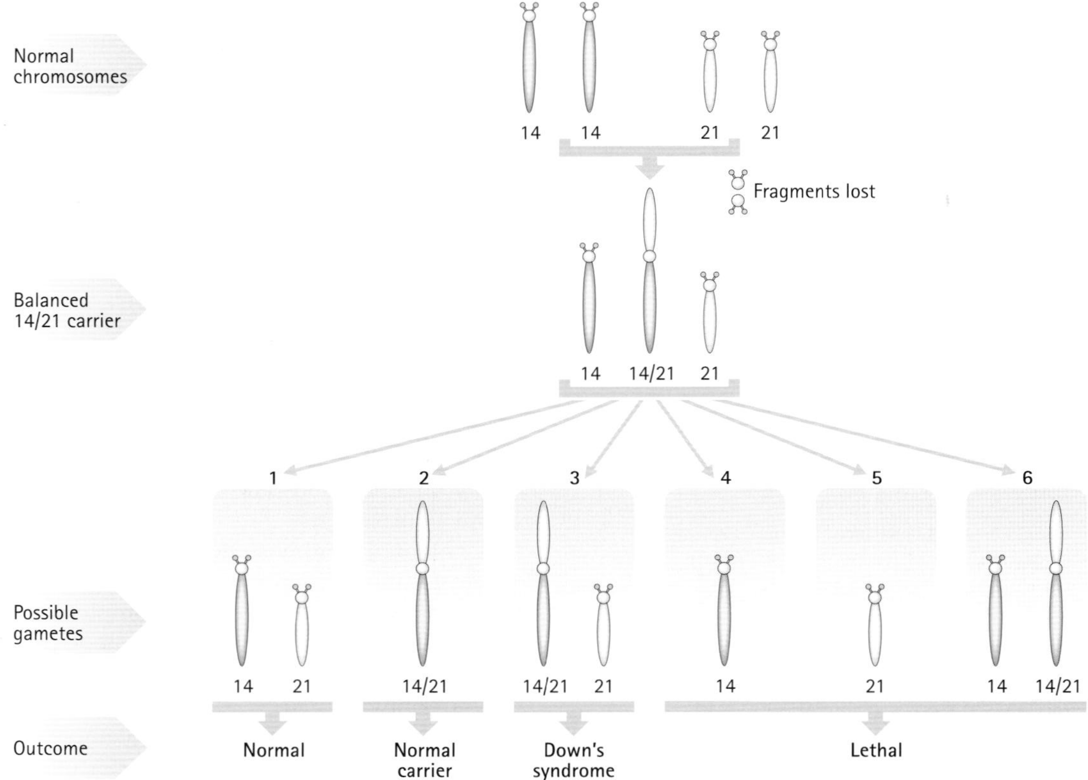


Fig. 3.26
Formation of a 14q21q Robertsonian translocation and the possible gamete chromosome patterns which can be produced at meiosis.

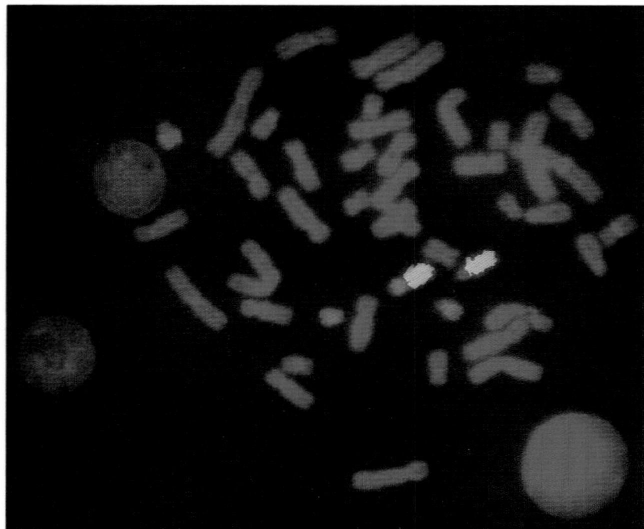

Fig. 3.27
Chromosome painting showing a 14q21q Robertsonian translocation in a child with Down syndrome. Chromosome 21 is shown in blue and chromosome 14 in yellow. (Courtesy of Meg Heath, City Hospital, Nottingham.)

event in the child, but in the remaining one-third one parent will be a carrier. Other relatives can also be carriers. Therefore it is regarded as essential that efforts are made to identify all adult translocation carriers in a family so that they can be alerted to possible risks to future offspring. This is sometimes referred to as translocation tracing or 'chasing'.

## Risks in Robertsonian translocations

Studies have shown that the female carrier of either a 13q21q or a 14q21q Robertsonian translocation runs a risk of approximately 10% for having a baby with Down syndrome, whereas for male carriers the risk is 1–3%. It is worth sparing a thought for the unfortunate carrier of a 21q21q Robertsonian translocation. All gametes will be either nullisomic or disomic for chromosome 21. Consequently all pregnancies will end either in spontaneous miscarriage or in the birth of a child with Down syndrome. This is one of the very rare situations in which offspring are at a risk of greater than 50% for having an abnormality. Other examples are the children of a mother with untreated phenylketonuria (p. 260) and of parents who are both heterozygous for the same autosomal dominant disorder (p. 108).

## Deletions

A *deletion* involves loss of part of a chromosome and results in monosomy for that segment of the chromosome. Usually a very large deletion will be incompatible with survival to term, and as a general rule any deletion resulting in loss of more than 2% of the total haploid genome will have a lethal outcome.

Deletions are now recognized as existing at two levels. A 'large' chromosomal deletion can be visualized under the microscope. Several deletion syndromes have been described, such as the Wolf–Hirschhorn and *Cri du chat* syndromes, which involve loss of material from the short arms of chromosomes 4 and 5, respectively (p. 274). More recently submicroscopic microdeletions have been identified with the help of high-resolution prometaphase cytogenetics augmented by fluorescent in situ hybridization studies (p. 35). For example, it has been shown that several previously unexplained conditions, such as the Prader–Willi and Angelman syndromes, can be caused by microdeletions (p. 276).

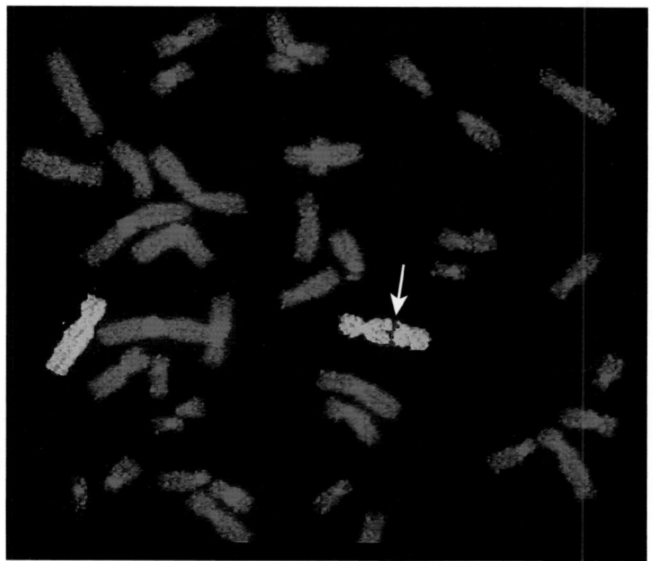

**Fig. 3.28**
Chromosome painting using chromosome 5 paint (CAMBIO) showing a small portion of chromosome 5 (arrowed) which marks the site of an insertion from chromosome 13. See Figure 3.29. (Courtesy of Meg Heath, City Hospital, Nottingham.)

## Insertions

An *insertion* occurs when a segment of one chromosome becomes inserted into another chromosome (Figs 3.28 and 3.29). If the inserted material has moved from elsewhere in another chromosome then the karyotype is balanced. Otherwise an insertion causes an unbalanced chromosome complement. Carriers of a balanced deletion–insertion rearrangement are at a 50% risk of producing unbalanced gametes, as random chromosome segregation at meiosis will result in 50% of the gametes inheriting either the deletion or the insertion but not both.

## Inversions

An *inversion* is a two-break rearrangement involving a single chromosome in which a segment is reversed in position, i.e. inverted. If the inversion segment involves the centromere it is termed a *pericentric inversion* (Fig. 3.30A). If it involves only one arm of the chromosome it is known as a *paracentric inversion* (Fig. 3.30B).

Inversions are balanced rearrangements that rarely cause problems in carriers unless one of the break-points has disrupted an important gene. A pericentric inversion involving chromosome number 9 occurs as a common structural variant or polymorphism (p. 130), also known as a *heteromorphism*, and is not thought to be of any functional importance. However, other inversions, while not causing any clinical problems in balanced carriers, can lead to significant chromosome imbalance in offspring, with important clinical consequences.

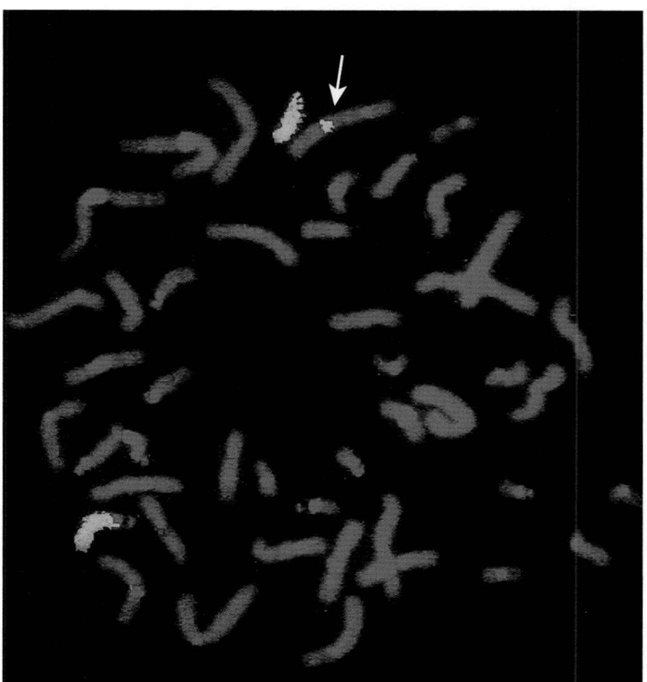

**Fig. 3.29**
Chromosome painting using chromosome 13 paint (CAMBIO) showing material of chromosome 13 origin inserted into chromosome 5 (arrowed). (Courtesy of Meg Heath, City Hospital, Nottingham.)

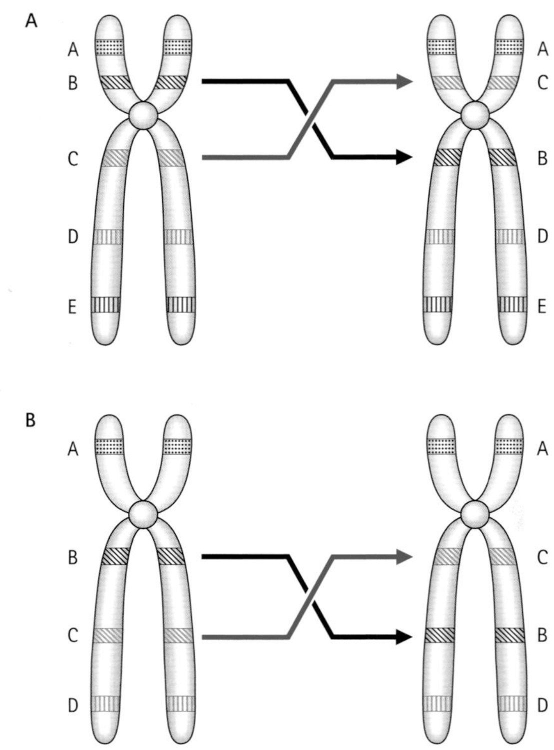


Fig. 3.30
A pericentric (A) and a paracentric (B) inversion. (Courtesy of Dr J Delhanty, Galton Laboratory, London.)

### *Segregation at meiosis*

**Pericentric inversions**

An individual who carries a pericentric inversion can produce unbalanced gametes if a crossover occurs within the inversion segment during meiosis I, when an inversion loop forms as the chromosomes attempt to maintain homologous pairing at synapsis. For a pericentric inversion a crossover within the loop will result in two complementary recombinant chromosomes, one with duplication of the distal non-inverted segment and deletion of the other end of the chromosome, and the other having the opposite arrangement (Fig. 3.31A).

If a pericentric inversion involves only a small proportion of the total length of a chromosome then, in the event of crossing over within the loop, the duplicated and deleted segments will be relatively large. The larger these are then the more likely it is that their effects on the embryo will be so severe that miscarriage ensues. For a large pericentric inversion the duplicated and deleted segments will be relatively small so that survival to term and beyond becomes more likely. Thus in general, the larger the size of a pericentric inversion then the more likely it becomes that it will result in the birth of an abnormal infant.

The pooled results of several studies have shown that a carrier of a balanced pericentric inversion runs a risk of approximately 5–10% for having a child with viable imbalance if that inversion has already resulted in the birth of an abnormal baby. The risk is nearer 1% if the inversion has been ascertained because of a history of recurrent miscarriage.

**Paracentric inversions**

If a crossover occurs in the inverted segment of a paracentric inversion this will result in recombinant chromosomes that are either acentric or dicentric (Fig. 3.31B). Acentric chromosomes, which strictly speaking should be known as chromosomal fragments, cannot undergo mitotic division, so that survival of an embryo with such a rearrangement is extremely uncommon. Dicentric chromosomes are inherently unstable during cell division and are, therefore, also unlikely to be compatible with survival of the embryo. Thus overall the likelihood that a balanced parental paracentric inversion will result in the birth of an abnormal baby is extremely low.

### Ring chromosomes

A *ring chromosome* is formed when a break occurs on each arm of a chromosome leaving two 'sticky' ends on the central portion that reunite as a ring (Fig. 3.32). The two distal chromosomal fragments are lost so that, if the involved chromosome is an autosome, the effects are usually very serious.

Ring chromosomes are often unstable in mitosis so that it is common to find a ring chromosome in only a proportion of cells. The other cells in the individual are usually monosomic because of the absence of the ring chromosome.

### Isochromosomes

An isochromosome shows loss of one arm with duplication of the other. The most probable explanation for the formation of an isochromosome is that the centromere has divided transversely rather than longitudinally. The most commonly encountered isochromosome is that which consists of two long arms of the X chromosome. This accounts for approximately 15% of all cases of Turner syndrome (p. 282).

## MOSAICISM AND CHIMERISM (MIXOPLOIDY)

### Mosaicism

*Mosaicism* can be defined as the presence in an individual or in a tissue of two or more cell lines that differ in their genetic constitution but are derived from a single zygote, i.e. they have the same genetic origin. Chromosome mosaicism usually results from non-disjunction occurring

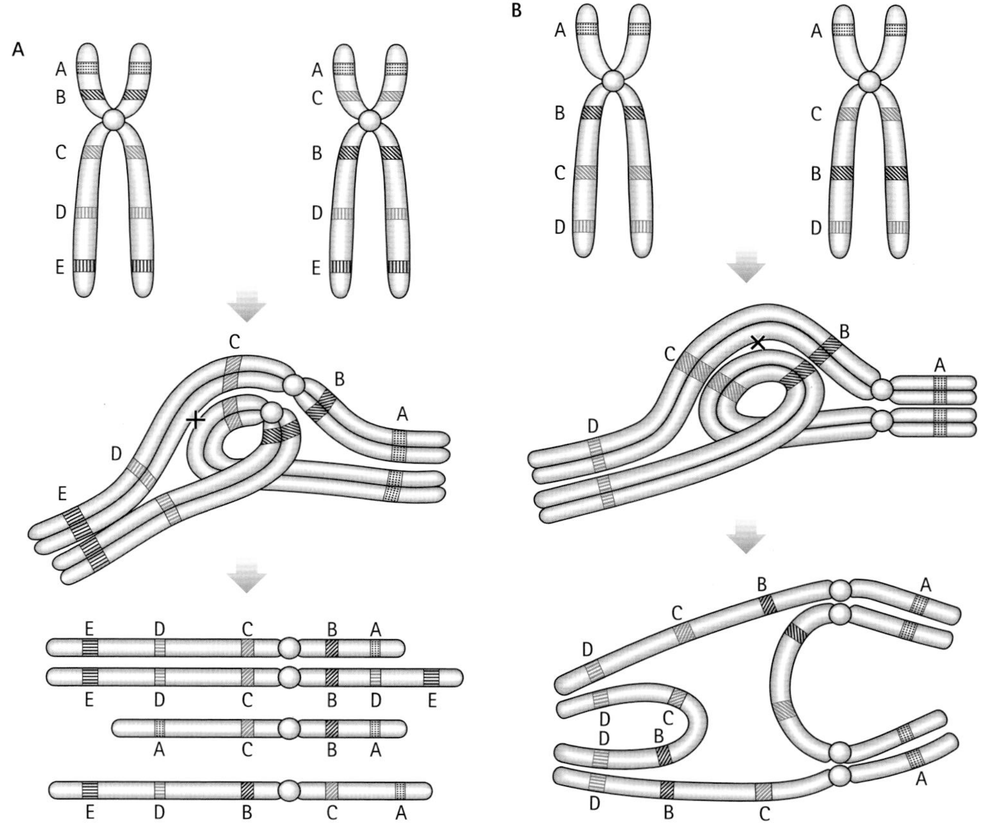


**Fig. 3.31**
Mechanism of production of recombinant unbalanced chromosomes from a pericentric (A) and a paracentric (B) inversion by crossing over in an inversion loop. (Courtesy of Dr J Delhanty, Galton Laboratory, London.)

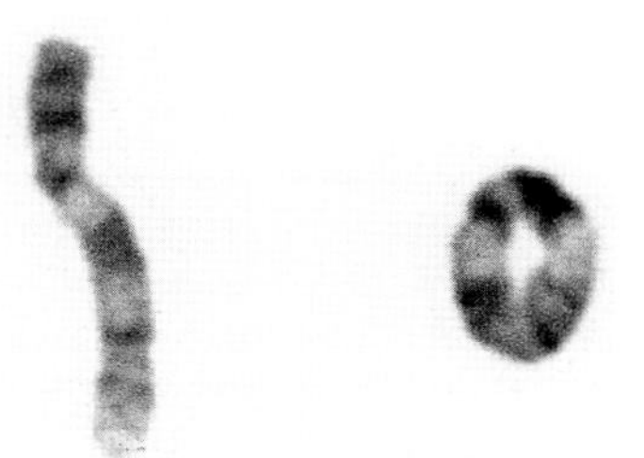

**Fig. 3.32**
Partial karyotype showing a ring chromosome 9. (Courtesy of Meg Heath, City Hospital, Nottingham.)

in an early embryonic mitotic division with the persistence of more than one cell line. If, for example, the two chromatids of a number 21 chromosome failed to separate at the second mitotic division in a human zygote (Fig. 3.33) this would result in the four-cell zygote having two cells with 46 chromosomes, one cell with 47 chromosomes (trisomy 21) and one cell with 45 chromosomes (monosomy

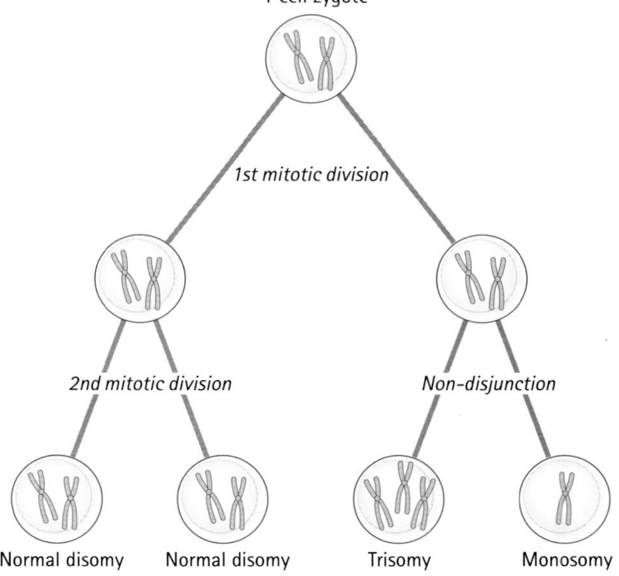


**Fig. 3.33**
Generation of somatic mosaicism caused by mitotic non-disjunction.

21). The ensuing cell line with 45 chromosomes would probably not survive, so that the resulting embryo would be expected to show approximately 33% mosaicism for trisomy 21. Mosaicism accounts for 1–2% of all clinically recognized cases of Down syndrome.

Mosaicism can also exist at a molecular level if a new mutation arises in a somatic or early germ line cell division. The possibility of germ line or gonadal mosaicism is a particular concern when counseling the parents of a child who is an isolated case of a condition such as Duchenne muscular dystrophy (p. 308).

## Chimerism

*Chimerism* can be defined as the presence in an individual of two or more genetically distinct cell lines derived from more than one zygote, i.e. they have a different genetic origin. The word chimera is derived from the mythological Greek monster which had the head of a lion, the body of a goat and the tail of a dragon. In humans chimeras are of two kinds: dispermic chimeras and blood chimeras.

### *Dispermic chimeras*

These are the result of double fertilization whereby two genetically different sperm fertilize two ova and the resulting two zygotes fuse to form one embryo. If the two zygotes are of different sex, the chimeric embryo can develop into an individual with true hermaphroditism (p. 286) and an XX/XY karyotype. Mouse chimeras of this type can now be produced experimentally in the laboratory to facilitate the study of gene transfer.

### *Blood chimeras*

Blood chimeras result from an exchange of cells, via the placenta, between non-identical twins in utero. For example, 90% of one twin's cells can have an XY karyotype with red blood cells showing predominantly blood group B, whereas the other twin can have 90% of cells showing an XX karyotype with red blood cells showing predominantly blood group A. It has long been recognized that when twin calves of opposite sex are born, the female can have ambiguous genitalia. It is now believed that this is because of gonadal chimerism in the female calves that are known as *freemartins*.

## FURTHER READING

Barch M J, Knutsen T, Spurbeck J L (eds) 1997 The AGT cytogenetics laboratory manual, 3rd edn. Lippincott-Raven, Philadelphia
*A large multiauthor laboratory handbook produced by the Association of Genetic Technologists.*

Gersen S L, Keagle M B (eds) 1999 The principles of clinical cytogenetics. Humana Press, Totowa, New Jersey
*A detailed multiauthor guide to all aspects of laboratory and clinical cytogenetics.*

ISCN 1995 Mitelman F (ed) An international system for human cytogenetic nomenclature. Karger, Basel
*An updated report giving details of how chromosome abnormalities including the results of FISH studies should be described.*

Jalal S M, Law M E 1999 Utility of multicolor fluorescent in situ hybridization in clinical cytogenetics. Genet Med 1: 181–186
*A contemporary account of how this new technique can be used to identify subtle and complex chromosome abnormalities.*

Rooney D E, Czepulkowski B H 1997 Human chromosome preparation. Essential techniques. John Wiley, Chichester
*A laboratory handbook describing the different methods available for chromosome analysis.*

Therman E, Susman M 1993 Human chromosomes. Structure, behaviour and effects, 3rd edn. Springer-Verlag, New York
*A useful and comprehensive introduction to human cytogenetics.*

Tjio J H, Levan A 1956 The chromosome number of man. Hereditas 42: 1–6
*A landmark paper that described a reliable method for studying human chromosomes and gave birth to the subject of clinical cytogenetics.*

Vogel F, Motulsky A G 1997 Human genetics, problems and approaches, 3rd edn. Springer-Verlag, Berlin
*An extremely comprehensive textbook of human genetics with a large section devoted to cytogenetics and cell division.*

## WEB-SITES

www.ncbi.nlm.nih.gov/About/primer/microarrays.html
*Microarrays: chipping away at the mysteries of science and medicine.*

## ELEMENTS

1. The normal human karyotype is made up of 46 chromosomes consisting of 22 pairs of autosomes and a pair of sex chromosomes, XX in the female and XY in the male.
2. Each chromosome consists of a short (p) and long (q) arm joined at the centromere. Chromosomes are analyzed using cultured cells and specific banding patterns can be identified using special staining techniques. Molecular cytogenetic techniques, such as fluorescence in situ hybridization (FISH) and comparative genomic hybridization (CGH), can be used to detect and characterize subtle chromosome abnormalities.
3. During mitosis in somatic cell division the two sister chromatids of each chromosome separate, with one chromatid passing to each daughter cell. During meiosis, which occurs during the final stage of gametogenesis, homologous chromosomes pair, exchange segments, and then segregate independently to the mature daughter gametes.
4. Chromosome abnormalities can be structural or numerical. Numerical abnormalities include trisomy and polyploidy. In trisomy a single extra chromosome is present, usually as a result of non-disjunction in the first or second meiotic division. In polyploidy, three or more complete haploid sets are present instead of the usual diploid complement.
5. Structural abnormalities include translocations, inversions, insertions, rings and deletions. Translocations can be balanced or unbalanced. Carriers of balanced translocations are at risk of having children with unbalanced rearrangements who will usually be physically and mentally handicapped.

# CHAPTER 4 DNA technology and applications

In the history of medical genetics, the 'chromosome breakthrough' in the mid-1950s was revolutionary. In the last three decades, DNA technology has had a profound effect, not only in medical genetics (Fig. 4.1), but also in many areas of biological science (Table 4.1).

The identification of restriction endonucleases, the development of the DNA cloning vectors, introduction of the Southern blot technique and Sanger sequencing in the 1970s, and the more recent development of the polymerase chain reaction rank as seminal developments in the field.

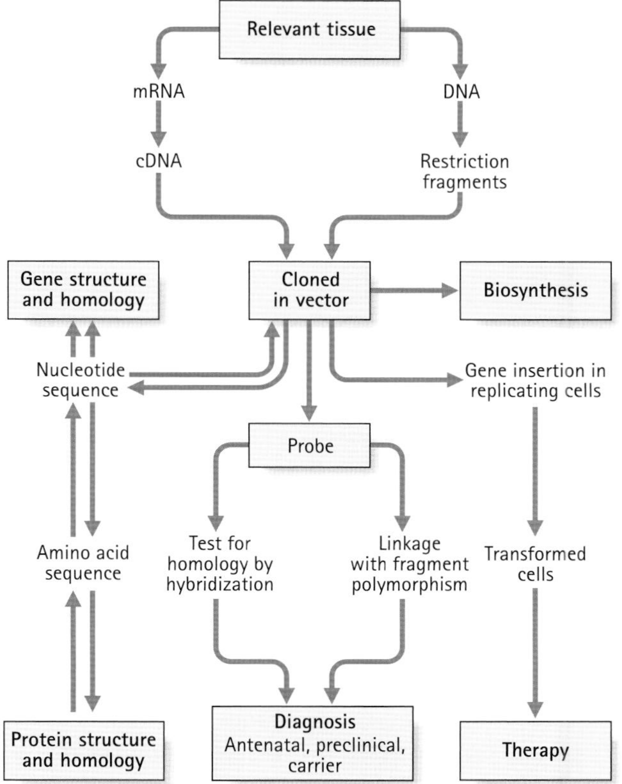


**Fig. 4.1**
Some of the applications of DNA technology in medical genetics.

## PRINCIPLES OF DNA TECHNOLOGY

DNA technology can be split into two main areas: DNA cloning and methods of DNA analysis.

### DNA CLONING

DNA cloning is the selective amplification of a specific DNA fragment or sequence to produce relatively large amounts of a homogeneous DNA fragment that allows its structure and function to be analyzed in detail.

DNA cloning falls into two main types: techniques that use natural in vivo cell-based mechanisms of DNA replication and the more recently developed cell-free or in vitro polymerase chain reaction.

#### In vivo cell-based DNA cloning

There are six basic steps in in vivo cell-based DNA cloning.

##### *Generation of DNA fragments*

Although fragments of DNA can be produced by mechanical shearing techniques, this is a very haphazard process producing fragments which vary in size. In the early 1970s it was recognized that certain microbes contained enzymes that cleave double-stranded DNA in or near a particular sequence of nucleotides. These enzymes restrict the entry of foreign DNA into bacterial cells and were therefore called *restriction enzymes*. They recognize a palindromic nucleotide sequence of DNA between four and eight nucleotides in length, i.e. the same sequence of nucleotides occurring on the two complementary DNA strands when read in one direction of polarity, e.g. 5′ to 3′ (Table 4.2). The longer the nucleotide recognition sequence of the restriction enzyme, the less frequently that particular nucleotide sequence will occur by chance and therefore the larger the average size of the DNA fragments generated.

Well over 300 different restriction enzymes have been isolated from various bacterial organisms. Restriction endonucleases are named according to the organism from which they are derived, e.g. *Eco*ri is from *E. coli* and was the first restriction enzyme isolated from that organism.

**Table 4.1 Applications of DNA technology**

Gene structure/mapping/function
Population genetics
Clinical genetics
  Preimplantation genetic diagnosis
  Prenatal diagnosis
  Presymptomatic diagnosis
  Carrier detection
Diagnosis and pathogenesis of disease
  Genetic
  Acquired — infective, malignant
Biosynthesis
  e.g. insulin, growth hormone, interferon, immunization
Treatment of genetic disease
Gene therapy
Agriculture
  e.g. nitrogen fixation

**Table 4.2 Some examples of restriction endonucleases with their nucleotide recognition sequence and cleavage sites**

| Enzyme | Organism | Cleavage site 5′ 3′ |
|---|---|---|
| *Bam*HI | *Bacillus amyloliquefaciens H* | G • G A T C C |
| *Eco*RI | *Escherichia coli RY 13* | G • A A T T C |
| *Hae*III | *Haemophilus aegyptius* | G G • C C |
| *Hind*III | *Haemophilus influenzae Rd* | A • A G C T T |
| *Hpa*I | *Haemophilus parainfluenzae* | G T T • A A C |
| *Pst*I | *Providencia stuartii* | C T G C A • G |
| *Sma*I | *Serratia marcescens* | C C C • G G G |
| *Sal*I | *Streptomyces albus G* | G • T C G A C |

The complementary pairing of bases in the DNA molecule means that cleavage of double-stranded DNA by a restriction endonuclease always creates double-stranded breaks, which, depending on the cleavage points of the particular restriction enzyme used, results in either a staggered or a blunt end (Fig. 4.2).

Digesting DNA from a specific source with a particular restriction enzyme will produce the same reproducible collection of DNA fragments each time the process is carried out.

## Recombination of DNA fragments

DNA from any source, when digested with the same restriction enzyme, will produce DNA fragments with identical complementary ends or termini. When DNA has been cleaved by a restriction enzyme which produces staggered termini, these are referred to as being 'sticky' or 'cohesive' since they will unite under appropriate conditions with complementary sequences produced by

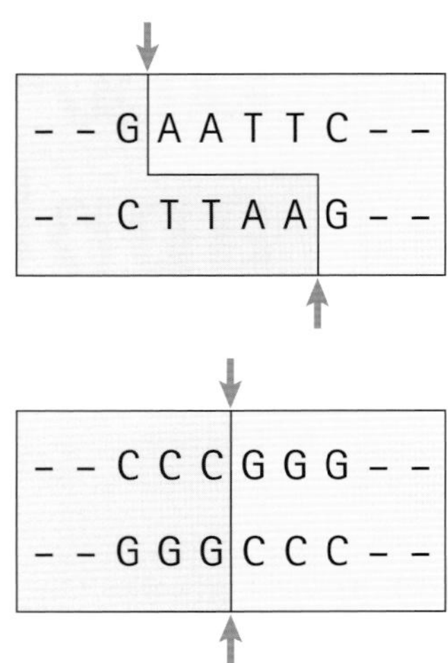


**Fig. 4.2**
The staggered and blunt ends generated by restriction digest of double-stranded DNA by *Eco*RI and *Sma*I. Sites of cleavage of the DNA strands are indicated by arrows.

the same restriction enzyme on DNA from any source. Initially the cohesive termini are held together by hydrogen bonding but are covalently attached with the enzyme called *DNA ligase*. The union of two DNA fragments from different sources produces what is referred to as a *recombinant DNA molecule*.

## Vectors

A *vector*, or *replicon*, is the term for the carrier DNA molecule used in the cloning process which, through its own independent replication within a host organism, will allow the production of multiple copies of itself. The incorporation of the *foreign* or *target* DNA into a vector allows the production of large amounts of that DNA fragment.

In order for naturally occurring vectors to be used for DNA cloning, they need to be modified to ensure that the foreign DNA is inserted at a specific location and that recombinant vectors containing foreign inserted DNA can be detected. Many of the early vectors were constructed so that insertion of the foreign DNA in a gene for antibiotic resistance resulted in loss of that function (Fig. 4.3).

There are five main types of vectors commonly used, which include *plasmids*, *bacteriophages*, *cosmids*, *bacterial* and *yeast artificial chromosomes*. The choice of vector used in cloning depends on a number of factors, such as the particular restriction enzyme being used and the size of the foreign DNA to be inserted. Some of the early vectors, such as plasmids and bacteriophages, were severely limited in the size of the foreign DNA fragment that could be inserted. Later generations of vectors, such as cosmids, can take inserts up to approximately 50 kb in size. A cosmid is essentially a plasmid which has had all

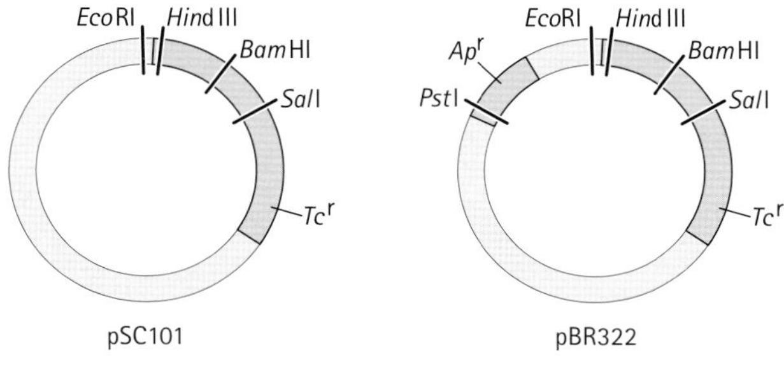


Fig. 4.3
Two plasmids originally used in recombinant DNA technology showing drug resistance genes (Ap$^r$ = ampicillin resistance; Tc$^r$ = tetracycline resistance) and cleavage sites of restriction endonucleases which are present in the DNA only once for use as a cloning site.

but the minimum vector DNA necessary for propagation removed, i.e. the cos sequence, to enable insertion of the largest possible foreign DNA fragment and still allow replication.

More recently, the development of *bacterial* and *yeast artificial chromosomes* (BACs and YACs) allows the possibility of cloning DNA fragments between 300 kb and up to 1000 kb in size. A yeast artificial chromosome consists of a plasmid which contains within it the minimum DNA sequences necessary for centromere and telomere formation plus DNA sequences known as *autonomous replication sequences*, all of which are necessary for accurate replication within yeast. YACs have the advantage that they can incorporate DNA fragments up to 1000 kb in size as well as allow replication of eukaryotic DNA with repetitive DNA sequences, which often cannot take place in bacterial cells. Many eukaryotic genes are very large, being up to 2000 000–3000 000 bp in length (p. 308). YACs allow detailed mapping of genes of this size and their flanking regions, whereas using conventional vectors would require an inordinate number of overlapping clones.

### *Transformation of the host organism*

After introduction of the foreign DNA fragment into the vector, the recombinant vector is introduced into specially modified bacterial or yeast host cells. The bacterial cell membrane is not normally permeable to large molecules such as DNA fragments but can be made permeable by a variety of different methods, including exposure to certain salts or high voltage – what is known as becoming *competent*. Usually only a single DNA molecule will be taken up by a host cell undergoing the process known as *transformation*. If the transformed cells are allowed to multiply, large quantities of identical copies of the original single target DNA or *clones* will be produced (Fig. 4.4).

### *Screening for recombinant vectors*

After the transformed cells have multiplied in culture medium, they are plated out on a master plate of nutrient agar in a Petri dish. Recombinant vectors can be screened for by a detection system, e.g. loss of antibiotic resistance that can be screened for by replica plating on agar which contains the appropriate antibiotic (see Fig. 4.3). Thus, if the enzyme *Pst*I were used to generate DNA fragments and to cut the plasmid pBR322, any recombinant plasmids produced would make the bacterial host cells they transform sensitive to ampicillin, since this gene would no longer be functional, but they would remain resistant to tetracycline. Replica plating of the master plates from the cultures allows identification of individual specific recombinant clones.

### *Selection of specific clones*

A number of techniques have been developed to detect the presence of clones with specific DNA sequence inserts. The most widely used method is nucleic acid hybridization (p. 64). Colonies of transformed host bacteria with recombinant clones are used to make replica plates that are lyzed and then blotted on to a nitrocellulose filter to which nucleic acid binds. The DNA of the replica blot is then denatured to make the DNA single stranded, which will allow it to hybridize with single-stranded, radioactively labeled DNA or RNA probes (p. 64) that can then be detected by exposure to an X-ray film, or what is known as *autoradiography*. In this way a transformed host bacterial colony containing a sequence complementary to the probe can be detected and, from its position on the replica plate, the colony containing that clone can be identified on the master plate, 'picked' and cultured separately (Fig. 4.5).

Alternatively, if an antibody is available to a protein and an expression vector is used for the DNA cloning, then the replica filter clones can be screened for by the presence or absence of binding of the antibody to detect clones containing recombinant vectors with the DNA fragment containing the gene (or part of) of interest.

## DNA libraries

Different sources of DNA can be used to make recombinant DNA molecules. DNA from nucleated cells is termed *total* or *genomic* DNA. DNA made by the action of the enzyme reverse transcriptase on mRNA is called *complementary DNA* or *cDNA*. It is possible to enrich for DNA sequences of particular interest by using a specific tissue or cell type as a source of mRNA, e.g. immature red blood cells (reticulocytes) containing predominantly globin mRNA resulted in cloning of the genes for the globin chains of hemoglobin (p. 149).

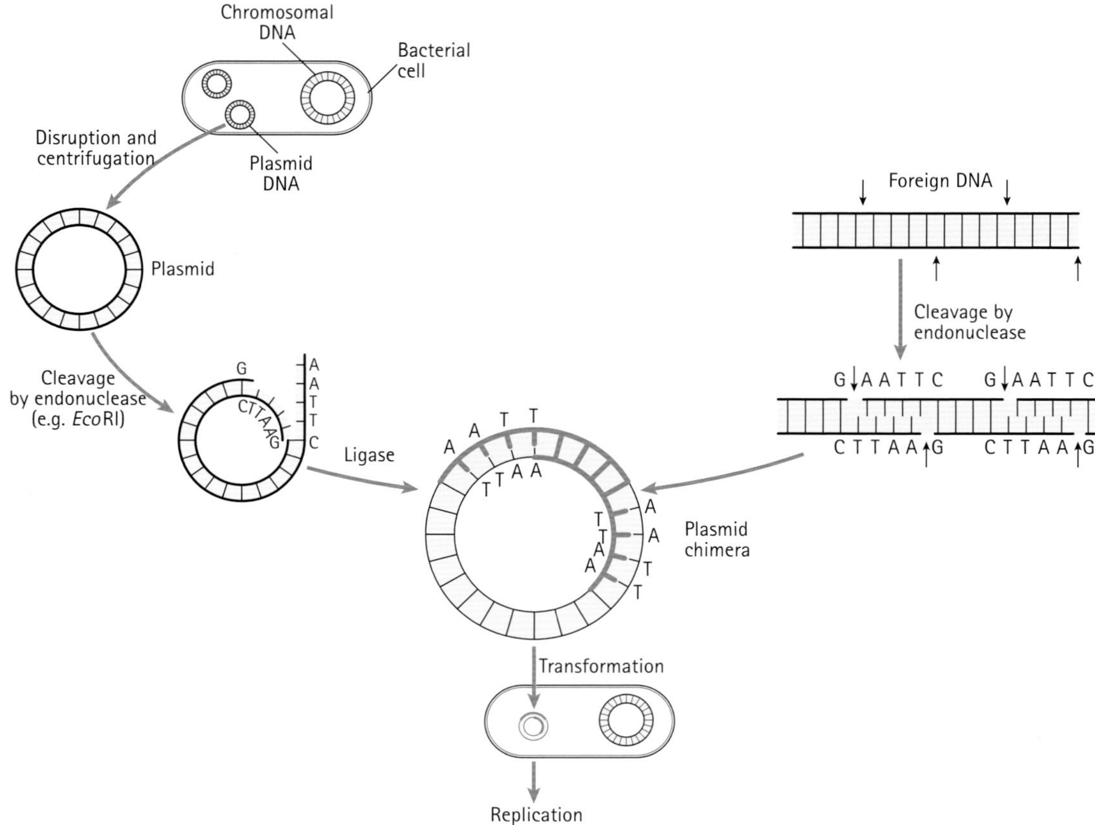


Fig. 4.4
Generation of a recombinant plasmid using *Eco*RI and transformation of the host bacterial organism. (From Emery A E H 1981 Lancet ii: 1406, with permission.)

The collection of recombinant DNA molecules generated from a specific source is referred to as a *DNA library*, e.g. a genomic or cDNA library. A DNA library of the human genome using plasmids as a vector would need to consist of several hundred thousand clones to be likely to contain the whole of the human genome. The use of YACs as cloning vectors with DNA digested by infrequently cutting restriction enzymes means that the whole of the human genome can be contained in a library of 13 000–14 000 clones.

## Cell-free DNA cloning

One of the most revolutionary developments in DNA technology is the technique first developed in the mid-1980s known as the *polymerase chain reaction* or *PCR*. PCR can be used to produce vast quantities of a target DNA fragment provided that the DNA sequence of that region is known.

### *The polymerase chain reaction*

DNA sequence information is used to design two oligonucleotide primers (*amplimers*) of approximately 20 bp in length complementary to the DNA sequences flanking the target DNA fragment. The primers, when added to denatured DNA, will bind to the complementary DNA sequences that, with the action of DNA polymerase, will result in extension of the primer DNA on the single-stranded DNA template in the presence of the deoxynucleotide triphosphates (dATP, dCTP, dGTP and dTTP) to synthesize the complementary DNA sequence. Subsequent heat denaturation of the double-stranded DNA, followed by annealing of the same primer sequences to the resulting single-stranded DNA, will result in synthesis of further copies of the target DNA. Thirty to 35 successive repeated cycles results in over 1 million copies (*amplicons*) of the DNA target, sufficient for direct visualization by ultraviolet fluorescence after ethidium bromide staining, without the need to use indirect detection techniques (Fig. 4.6).

The polymerase chain reaction (PCR) allows analysis of DNA from any cellular source containing nuclei and, in addition to blood, can include less invasive samples such as buccal scrapings or pathological archival material. It is also possible to start with quantities of DNA as small as that from a single cell, as is the case in preimplantation genetic diagnosis (p. 336). Great care has to be taken with PCR, however, since DNA from a contaminating

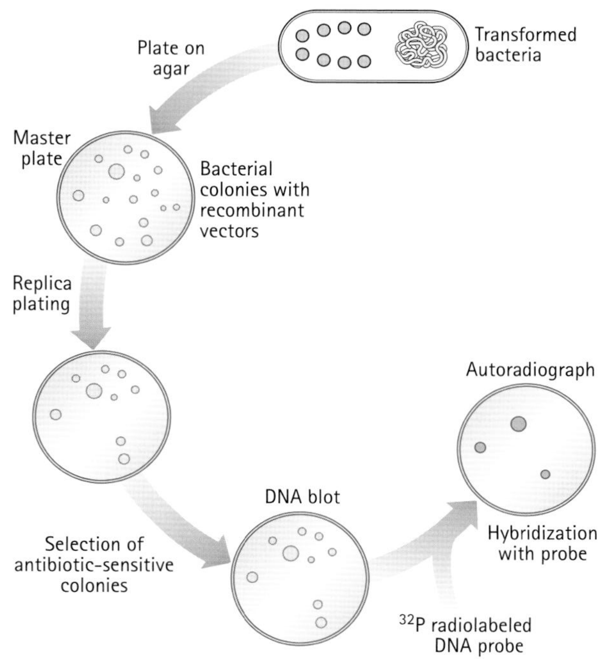


Fig. 4.5
Identification of recombinant DNA clones with specific DNA inserts by loss of antibiotic resistance, nucleic acid hybridization and autoradiography.

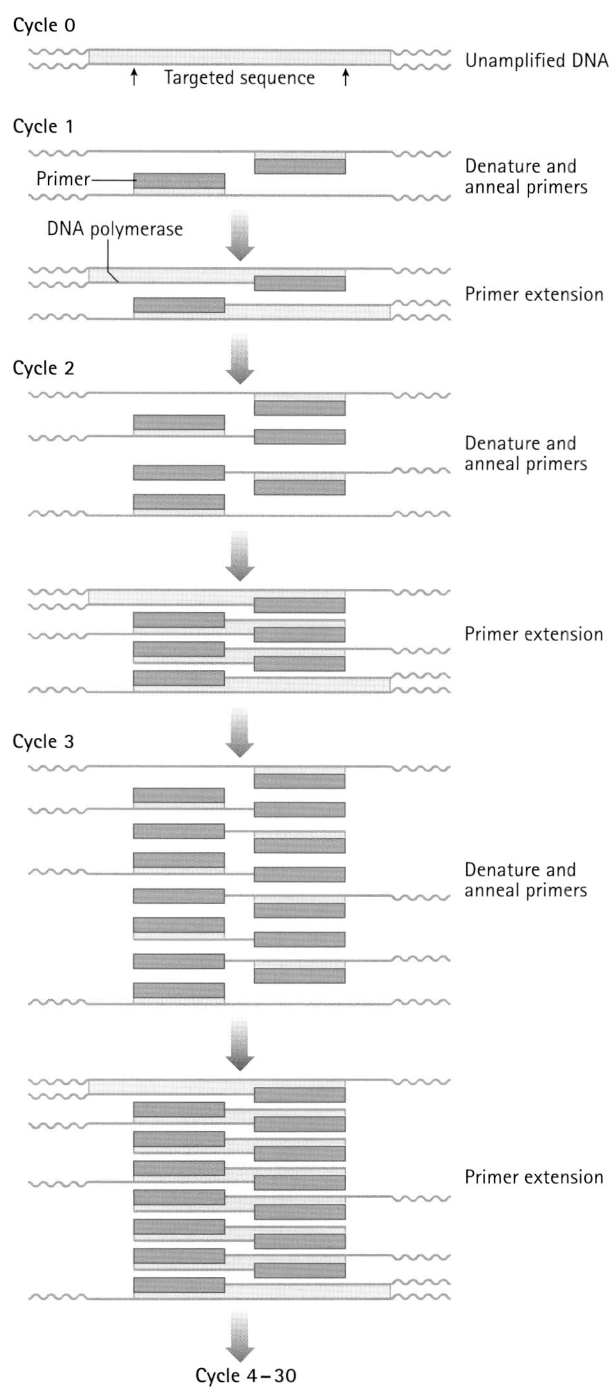


Fig. 4.6
Diagram of the polymerase chain reaction showing serial denaturation of DNA, primer annealing, and extension with doubling of the target DNA fragment numbers in each cycle.

extraneous source, such as desquamated skin from a laboratory worker, will also be amplified. This can lead to false-positive results unless the appropriate control studies are used to detect this possible source of error.

Another advantage of PCR is the rapid turn-round time of samples for analysis. Use of the heat stable *Taq* DNA polymerase isolated from the bacterium *Thermophilus aquaticus*, which grows naturally in hot springs, generates PCR products in a matter of hours rather than the days or weeks required for cell-based in-vivo DNA cloning techniques.

Real-time PCR machines have reduced this time to less than 1 h, and fluorescent technology is used to monitor the generation of PCR products during each cycle, thus eliminating the need for gel electrophoresis.

DNA cloning by PCR, in contrast to in-vivo cell-based techniques, has the disadvantage that it requires knowledge of the nucleotide sequence of the target DNA fragment and is best used to amplify DNA fragments up to 1 kb, although long-range PCR allows the amplification of larger DNA fragments up to 20–30 kb.

## TECHNIQUES OF DNA ANALYSIS

Many methods of DNA analysis involve the use of nucleic acid probes and the process of nucleic acid hybridization.

## NUCLEIC ACID PROBES

Nucleic acid probes are usually single-stranded DNA sequences that have been radioactively or non-radioactively labeled and can be used to detect DNA or RNA fragments with sequence homology. DNA probes can come from a variety of sources, including random genomic DNA sequences, specific genes, cDNA sequences or oligonucleotide DNA sequences produced synthetically based on knowledge of the protein amino acid sequence. A DNA probe can be labeled by a variety of processes, including isotopic labeling with $^{32}$P and non-isotopic methods using modified nucleotides containing fluorophores, e.g. fluorescein or rhodamine. Hybridization of a radioactively labeled DNA probe with complementary DNA sequences on a nitrocellulose filter can be detected by autoradiography, whereas DNA fragments that are fluorescently labeled can be detected by exposure to the appropriate wavelength of light, e.g. fluorescent in situ hybridization (p. 35).

## NUCLEIC ACID HYBRIDIZATION

Nucleic acid hybridization involves mixing DNA from two sources that have been denatured by heat or alkali to make them single stranded and then, under the appropriate conditions, allowing complementary base pairing of homologous sequences. If one of the DNA sources has been labeled in some way, i.e. is a DNA probe, this allows identification of specific DNA sequences in the other source. The two main methods of nucleic acid hybridization most commonly used are Southern and Northern blotting.

### Southern blotting

Southern blotting, named after Edwin Southern who developed the technique, involves digesting DNA by a restriction enzyme which is then subjected to electrophoresis on an agarose gel. This separates the DNA or restriction fragments by size, the smaller fragments migrating faster than the larger ones. The DNA fragments in the gel are then denaturated with alkali, making them single stranded. A 'permanent' copy of these single-stranded fragments is made by transferring them on to a nitrocellulose filter which binds the single-stranded DNA, the so-called *Southern blot*. A particular target DNA fragment of interest from the collection on the filter can be visualized by adding a single-stranded $^{32}$P radioactively labeled DNA probe that will hybridize with homologous DNA fragments in the Southern blot, which can then be detected by autoradiography (Fig. 4.7). An example of the use of Southern blotting for diagnostic testing in patients with Fragile X is shown in Figure 4.8.

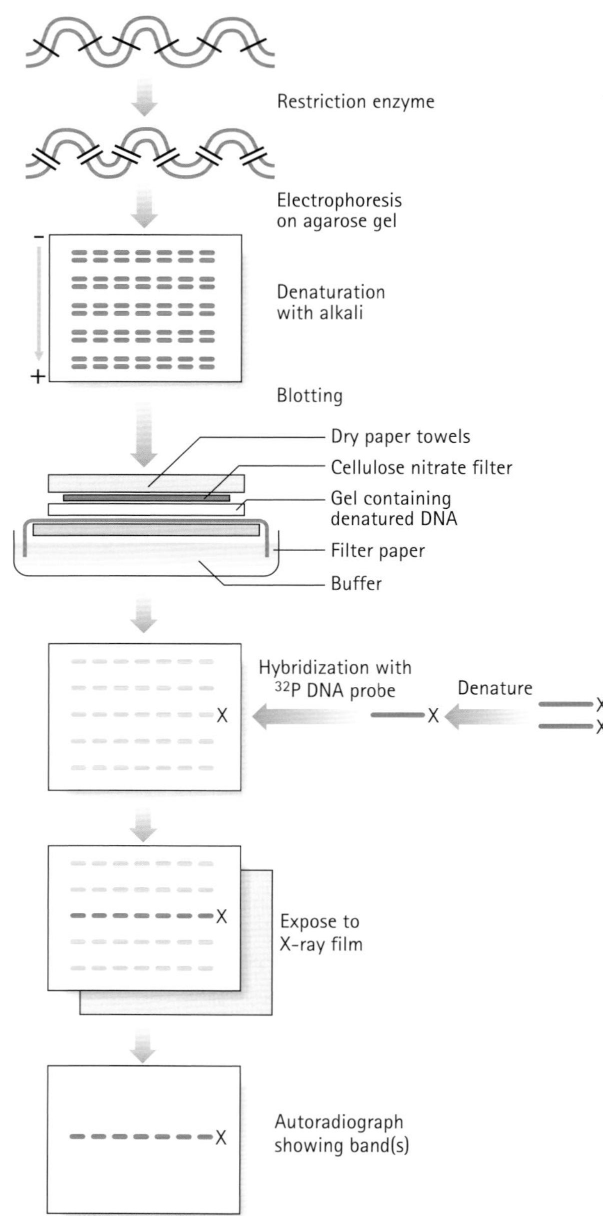


**Fig. 4.7**
Diagram of the Southern blot technique showing size fractionation of the DNA fragments by gel electrophoresis, denaturation of the double-stranded DNA to become single stranded, and transfer to a nitrocellulose filter that is hybridized with a $^{32}$P radioactively labeled DNA probe.

### Northern blotting

Northern blotting differs from Southern blotting by the use of mRNA as the target nucleic acid in the same procedure; mRNA is very unstable because of intrinsic cellular ribonucleases. Use of ribonuclease inhibitors allows isolation of mRNA that, if run on an electrophoretic gel, can be transferred to a filter. Hybridizing the blot with a radiolabeled DNA probe allows determination of the size

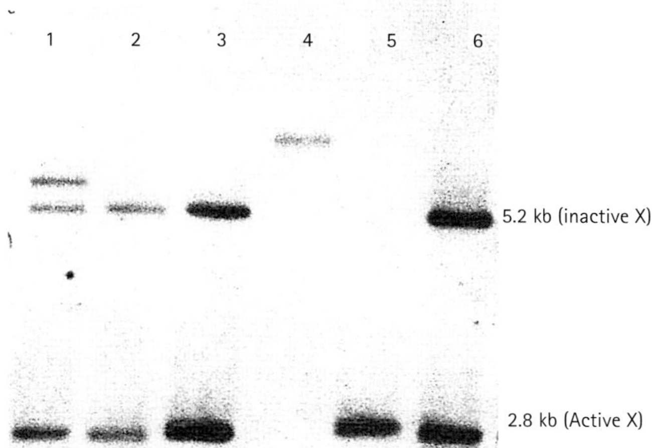


**Fig. 4.8**
Southern blot to detect methylation of the FMR-1 promoter in patients with fragile X. DNA digested with *Eco*R1 and the methylation sensitive enzyme *Bst* Z1 was probed with Ox1.9 which hybridizes to a CpG island within the FMR-1 promoter. Patient 1 is a female with a methylated expansion, patients 2, 3 and 6 are normal females, patient 4 is an affected male and patient 5 is a normal male. (Courtesy of A. Gardner, Department of Molecular Genetics, Southmead Hospital, Bristol.)

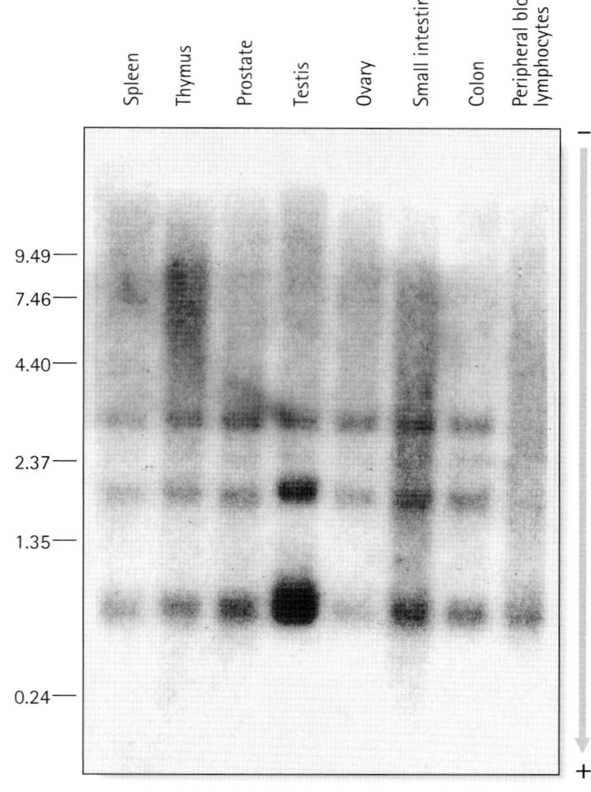


**Fig. 4.9**
Representation of a Northern blot analysis of the ubiquitin conjugating enzyme gene *UBE2L3* probed with cDNA to the human gene showing expression of three transcripts of approximately 2.7, 1.5 and 0.5 kb in multiple tissues, with the 0.5 kb transcript being more abundantly expressed in testis (courtesy of Dr T. Moynihan, Dept of Molecular Medicine, St James's Hospital, Leeds).

and quantity of the mRNA transcript, a so-called *Northern blot* (Fig. 4.9). In a gene disorder in which a mutation has not been identified in the coding sequences, an alteration in the size of the mRNA transcript suggests the possibility of a mutation in a non-coding region of the gene, such as the splice junction of the intron–exon border. Northern blotting can also be used to demonstrate the differential pattern of expression of a gene in different tissues or at different times of development.

### DNA microarrays

DNA microarrays are based on the same principle of hybridization but on a miniaturized scale, which allows simultaneous analysis of tens or hundreds of thousands of targets. Short, fluorescently labeled oligonucleotides attached to a glass microscope slide can be used to detect hybridization of target DNA under appropriate conditions. The color pattern of the microarray is then analyzed automatically by computer. Two classes of application have been described: expression studies to look at the differential expression of thousands of genes at the mRNA level, and analysis of DNA variation for mutation detection and SNP typing (p. 70).

## MUTATION DETECTION

The choice of method will depend primarily upon whether the test is for a known sequence change or to identify the presence of any mutation within a particular gene. There are a number of techniques that can be used to screen for mutations which differ in their ease of use and reliability. The choice of assay will depend on many factors, including sensitivity required, cost, equipment, and the size and structure (including number of polymorphisms) of the gene (see Table 4.3). Identification of a possible sequence variant by one of the mutation screening methods requires confirmation by DNA sequencing. Some of the most common techniques in current use are described below.

### Size analysis of polymerase chain reaction (PCR) products

Deletion or insertion mutations can sometimes be detected by simply determining the size of a PCR product. For example, the most common mutation that causes cystic fibrosis, ΔF508, is a 3 bp deletion that can be detected on a polyacrylamide gel (p. 304). Some trinucleotide repeat expansion mutations can be amplified by PCR (see Fig. 4.10).

**Table 4.3 Methods for detecting mutations**

| Method | Known/unknown mutations | Example | Advantages/disadvantages |
|---|---|---|---|
| Southern blot | Known (or unknown rearrangement) | Trinucleotide expansions in Fragile X and myotonic dystrophy | Laborious |
| Sizing of PCR products | Known | ΔF508, Trinucleotide expansions in HD and SCA genes | Simple, cheap |
| ARMS PCR | Known | *CFTR* mutations | Multiplex possible |
| Oligonucleotide ligation | Known | *CFTR* mutations | Multiplex possible |
| Real-time PCR | Known | Factor V Leiden | Expensive equipment |
| Single-strand conformation polymorphism (SSCP) | Unknown | Any gene | Cheap, limited sensitivity |
| Denaturing HPLC | Unknown | Any gene | High throughput, more sensitive than SSCP |
| Sequencing | Known or unknown | Any gene | Gold standard but expensive |
| DNA microarray | Known or unknown | Any gene | High throughput, expensive equipment. Sensitivity for unknown mutations may be limited |
| Mass spectroscopy | Known or unknown | Any gene | High throughput, expensive equipment |

## Restriction fragment length polymorphism

If a base substitution creates or abolishes the recognition site of a restriction enzyme, it is possible to test for the mutation by digesting a PCR product with the appropriate enzyme and separating the products by electrophoresis (see Fig. 4.11).

## Amplification-refractory mutation system (ARMS) PCR

Allele-specific PCR utilizes primers specific for the normal and mutant sequences. The most common design is a two-tube assay with normal and mutant primers in separate reactions together with control primers to ensure that the PCR reaction has worked. An example of a multiplex ARMS assay to detect 12 different cystic fibrosis mutations is shown in Figure 4.12.

## Oligonucleotide ligation assay (OLA)

A pair of oligonucleotides are designed to anneal to adjacent sequences within a PCR product. If they are perfectly hybridized they can be joined by DNA ligase. Oligonucleotides complementary to the normal and mutant sequences are differentially labeled and the products identified by computer software (see Fig. 4.13).

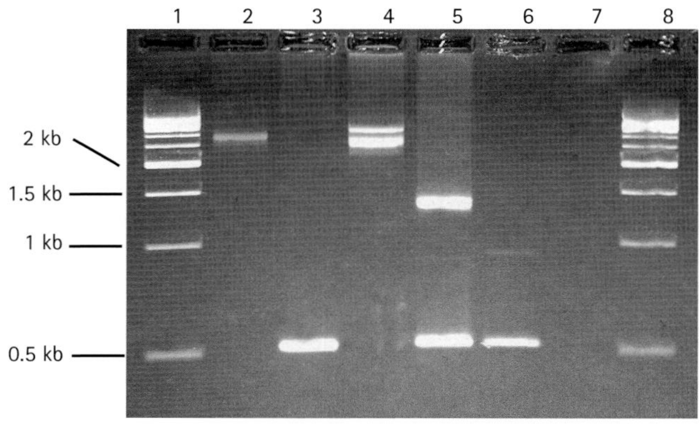


**Fig. 4.10**
Amplification of the GAA repeat expansion mutation by PCR to test for Friedreich ataxia. Products are stained with ethidium bromide and electrophoresed on a 1.5% agarose gel. Lanes 1 and 8 show 500 bp ladder size standards, lanes 2 and 4 show patients with homozygous expansions, lanes 3 and 6 show unaffected controls, lane 5 shows a heterozygous expansion carrier and lane 7 is the negative control. (Courtesy of K. Thomson, Department of Molecular Genetics, Royal Devon & Exeter Hospital.)

## Real-time (PCR)

The TaqMan™ and LightCycler™ use fluorescent technology to detect mutations by allelic discrimination of PCR products. See Figure 4.14 for an example of the FRET probe detection of the Factor V Leiden mutation.

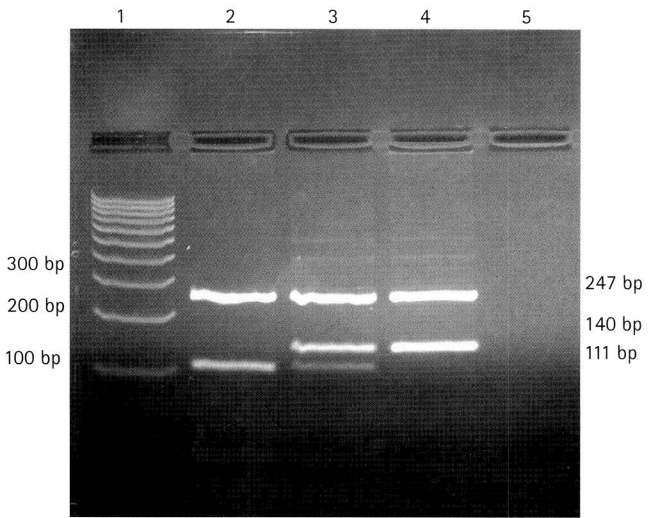


Fig. 4.11
Detection of the *HFE* gene mutation C282Y by RFLP. The normal 387 bp PCR product is digested with *Rsa*I to give products of 247 and 140 bp. The C282Y mutation creates an additional recognition site for *Rsa*I, giving products of 247, 111 and 29 bp. Lane 1 shows a 100 bp ladder size standard, lanes 24-4 show patients homozygous, heterozygous and normal for the C282Y mutation, respectively. Lane 5 is the negative control. (Courtesy of N. Goodman, Department of Molecular Genetics, Royal Devon & Exeter Hospital.)

## DNA microarrays (DNA 'CHIPS')

DNA microarrays hold the promise of rapid mutation testing. They involve synthesizing custom-designed 20–25 base pair oligonucleotide sequences for both the normal DNA sequence and known and/or possible single nucleotide substitutions of a gene. These are attached to a 'chip' in a structured arrangement in what is known as a *microarray*. The sample DNA being screened for a mutation is amplified by PCR, fluorescently labeled and hybridized with the oligonucleotides in the microarray (Fig. 4.15). Analysis of the color pattern of the microarray generated after hybridization by a computer allows rapid automated mutation testing. The prospect of gene-specific DNA chip microarrays may lead to a revolution in the speed and reliability of mutation screening, provided the technology is affordable and the technique can be demonstrated to be robust. The detection of known base substitutions or SNPs (single nucleotide polymorphisms) has been very successful, but screening for unknown mutations has proved more difficult.

## Single-stranded conformational polymorphism (SSCP)

PCR products of double-stranded DNA, if made single stranded, fold up, making a three-dimensional structure. An alteration in the DNA sequence can result in a different conformation which, under appropriate gel conditions, results in a different electrophoretic mobility, a so-called single-stranded conformational polymorphism (SSCP).

## Denaturing high-performance liquid chromatography (DHPLC)

This technique detects the presence of heteroduplexes owing to their abnormal denaturing profiles. PCR products from patients with heterozygous mutations will form heteroduplexes if denatured by heating (to separate the double-stranded DNA) and then cooled slowly. Homozygous mutations can be detected by mixing the PCR products with normal sequence products to generate heteroduplexes. DHPLC provides a sensitive detection platform with relatively high throughput capacity.

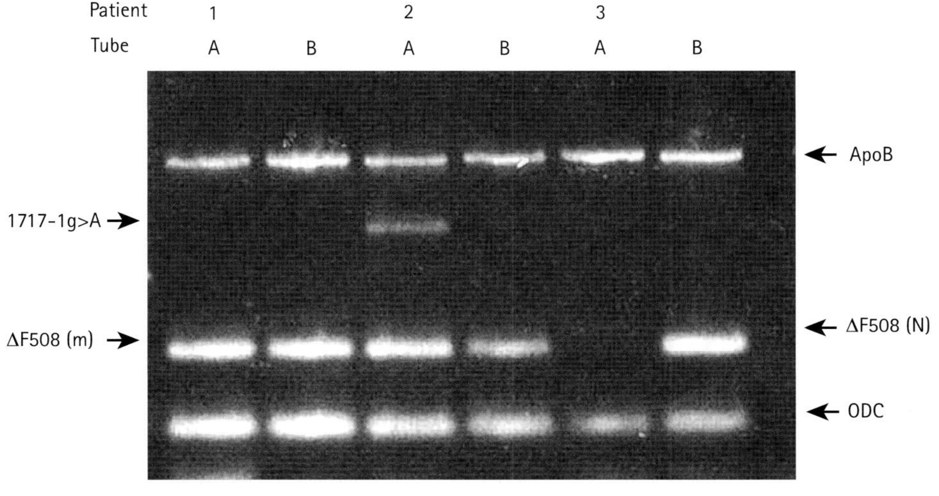


Fig. 4.12
Detection of *CFTR* mutations by two-tube ARMS-PCR. Patient 1 is heterozygous for ΔF508, patient 2 is a compound heterozygote for ΔF508 and 1717-1G>A, patient 3 is homozygous normal for the 12 mutations tested. Primers for two internal controls (ApoB and ODC) are included in each tube.

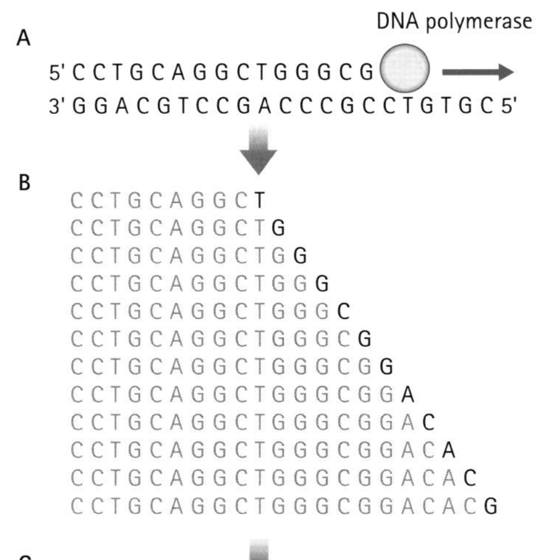


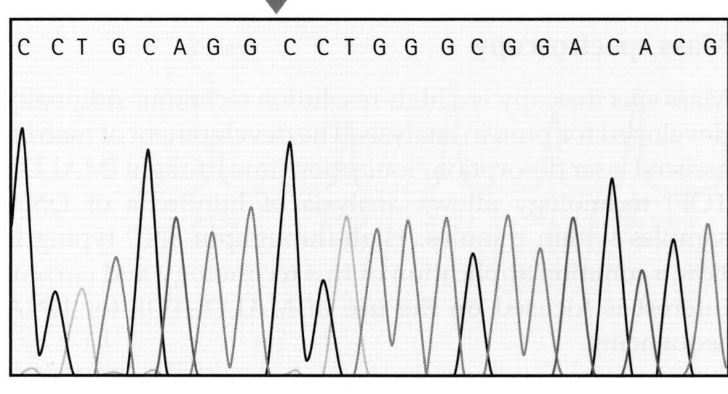


D

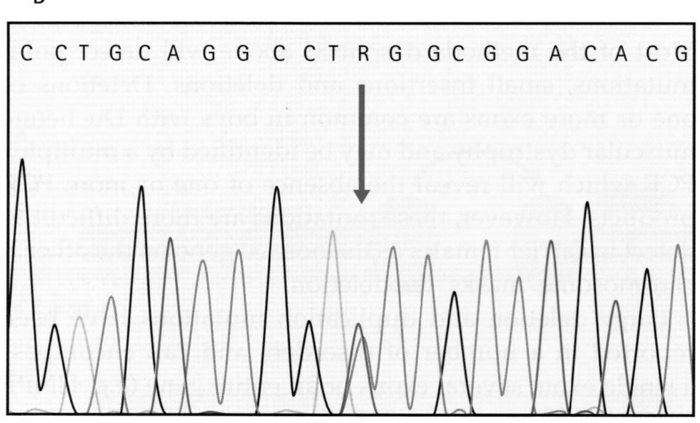


**Fig. 4.16**
Fluorescent dideoxy DNA sequencing. The sequencing primer (shown in italics) binds to the template and primes synthesis of a complementary DNA strand in the direction indicated (A). The sequencing reaction includes four dNTPs and four ddNTPs, each labeled with a different fluorescent dye. Competition between the dNTPs and ddNTPs results in the production of a collection of fragments (B) which are then separated by electrophoresis to generate an electropherogram (C). A heterozygous mutation (TGG>TAG; tryptophan>stop) is shown in (D).

## APPLICATION OF DNA SEQUENCE POLYMORPHISMS

There is an enormous amount of DNA sequence variation in the human genome (p. 18). Two main types, single nucleotide polymorphisms (SNPs) and hypervariable tandem repeat DNA length (VNTR) polymorphisms are predominately used in genetic analysis.

### Single nucleotide polymorphisms

Around 1 in 1000 bases within the human genome shows variation. Single nucleotide polymorphisms (SNPs) are most frequently biallelic and occur in coding and non-coding regions. If an SNP lies within the recognition sequence of a restriction enzyme, the DNA fragments produced by that restriction enzyme will be of different lengths in different people. This can be recognized by the altered mobility of the restriction fragments on gel electrophoresis, so-called *restriction fragment length polymorphisms*, RFLPs. Early genetic mapping studies used Southern blotting to detect RFLPs but current technology enables the detection of any SNP. New high-throughput methods (e.g. DNA microarrays) have led to the creation of a dense SNP map of the human genome and will assist genome searches for linkage studies in mapping single-gene disorders (p. 131) and association studies in common diseases.

### Variable number tandem repeats

Variable number tandem repeats (VNTRs) are highly polymorphic and are due to the presence of variable numbers of tandem repeats of a short DNA sequence that have been shown to be inherited in a Mendelian codominant fashion (p. 18). The advantage of using VNTRs over SNPs is the large number of alleles for each VNTR compared to SNPs, which are mostly biallelic.

### Minisatellites

Jeffreys identified a short 10–15 bp 'core' sequence with homology to many highly variable loci spread throughout the human genome (p. 18). Using a probe containing tandem repeats of this core sequence, a pattern of hypervariable DNA fragments is identified. The multiple variable-size repeat sequences identified by the core sequence are known as *minisatellites*. These minisatellites are highly polymorphic and a profile unique to an individual (unless they have an identical twin!) is described as a *DNA fingerprint*. The technique of DNA fingerprinting has been widely used in paternity testing (see Fig 4.19) and for forensic purposes.

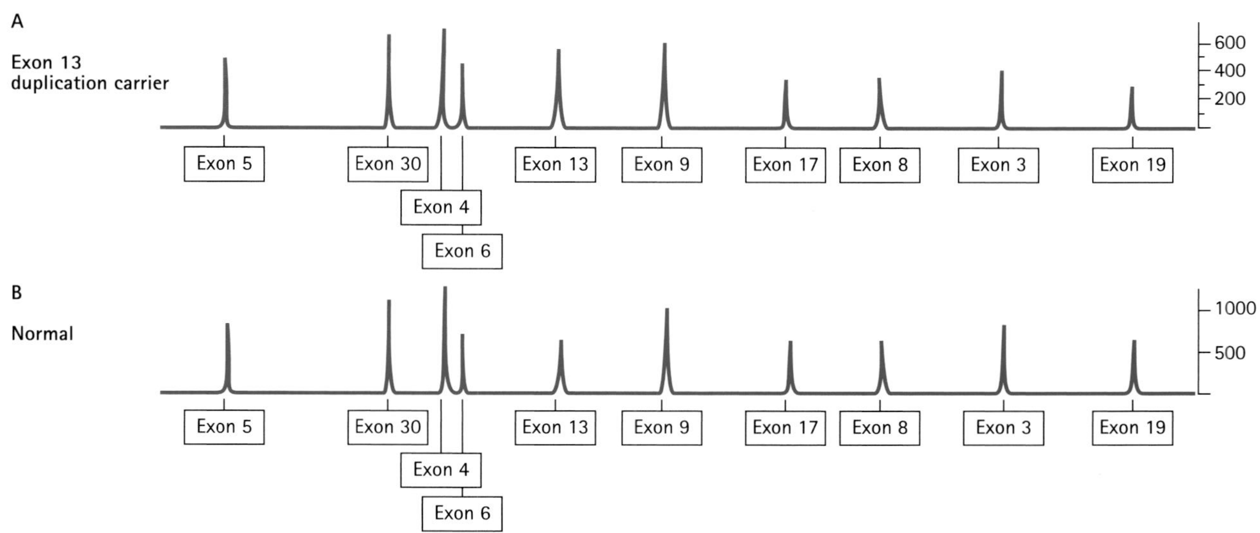


Fig. 4.17
Detection of a dystrophin duplication carrier by quantitative fluorescent PCR (QF-PCR). Ten exons of the dystrophin gene were amplified by multiplex fluorescent PCR. Comparison of the peak heights reveals a raised peak for exon 13 in the female carrier (A) compared to the normal control (B). (Courtesy of R. Butler, Institute of Medical Genetics, University Hospital of Wales.)

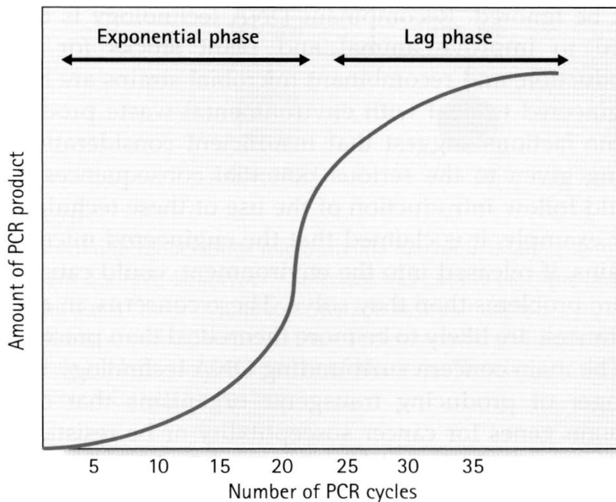


Fig. 4.18
Accumulation of PCR product during exponential and lag phases.

## Microsatellites

The human genome contains some 50 000–100 000 blocks of a variable number of tandem repeats of the dinucleotide CA:GT, so-called CA repeats or *microsatellites* (p. 18). The difference in the number of CA repeats at any one site between individuals is very highly polymorphic and these have been shown to be inherited in a Mendelian codominant manner. In addition, highly polymorphic tri- and tetranucleotide repeats have also been identified, which can be used in a similar way (Fig. 4.20). These microsatellites can be analyzed by PCR and the use of fluorescent detection systems allows relatively high-throughput analysis. Consequently, microsatellite analysis has largely replaced DNA fingerprinting in the applications of paternity testing and establishing zygosity.

## Clinical applications of gene tracking

If a gene has been mapped by linkage studies but not identified it is possible to use the linked markers to 'track' the mutant haplotype within a family. This approach may also be used for known genes where a mutation has not been found within a family. Closely flanking or intragenic microsatellites are most commonly used because of the lower likelihood of finding informative SNPs within families. Figure 4.21 illustrates a family where gene tracking has been used to determine carrier risk in the absence of a known mutation. There are some pitfalls associated with this method: recombination between the microsatellite and the gene may give an incorrect risk estimate, and the possibility of genetic heterogeneity (where mutations in more than one gene cause a disease) should be borne in mind.

# DIAGNOSIS IN NON-GENETIC DISEASE

DNA technology, especially PCR, has found application in the diagnosis and management of both infectious and malignant disease.

## FURTHER READING

Elles R, Mountford R 2003 Molecular diagnosis of genetic disease, 2nd edn. Humana Press, New Jersey
*Key techniques used for genetic testing of common disorders in diagnostic laboratories.*
Emery A E H, Malcolm S 1995 An introduction to recombinant DNA medicine, 2nd edn. John Wiley, Chichester
*The second edition of this text which covers the techniques and applications of DNA technology in clinical medicine.*
McKusick V A 1998 Mendelian inheritance in man, 12th edn. Johns Hopkins University Press, Baltimore
*A computerized catalog of the dominant, recessive and X-linked Mendelian traits and disorders in humans with a brief clinical commentary and details of the mutational basis if known. Also available online, updated regularly.*
Strachan T, Read A P 2004 Human molecular genetics, 3rd edn. Garland Science, London and New York
*A comprehensive textbook of all aspects of molecular and cellular biology as it relates to inherited disease in humans.*
Weatherall D J 1991 The new genetics and clinical practice, 3rd edn. Oxford Medical, Oxford
*One of the original texts that provided a lucid overview of the application of DNA techniques in clinical medicine.*

## ELEMENTS

1. Restriction enzymes allow DNA from any source to be cleaved into reproducible fragments based on the presence of specific nucleotide recognition sequences. These fragments can be made to recombine, enabling their incorporation into a suitable vector, with subsequent transformation of a host organism by the vector leading to the production of clones containing a particular DNA sequence.

2. The polymerase chain reaction (PCR) has revolutionized medical genetics. More than a million copies of a gene can be amplified from a patient's DNA sample within hours. The PCR product may be analyzed for the presence of a pathogenic mutation, gene rearrangement or infectious agent.

3. Techniques including Southern and Northern blotting, DNA sequencing and mutation screening can be used to identify or analyze specific DNA sequences of interest. These techniques can be used for analyzing normal gene structure and function as well as revealing the molecular pathology of inherited disease. This provides a means for presymptomatic diagnosis, carrier detection and prenatal diagnosis, either by direct mutational analysis or indirectly using polymorphic markers in family studies.

4. Recombinant DNA technology is potentially biologically hazardous but these risks can be minimized by physical and biological containment methods.

CHAPTER 5

# Mapping and identifying genes

The identification of the gene responsible for an inherited single-gene disorder, as well as having immediate clinical diagnostic application, will enable an understanding of the developmental basis of the pathology (p. 83) with the prospect of possible therapeutic interventions (p. 355).

The first human disease genes identified were those with a biochemical basis where it was possible to purify and sequence the gene product. The development of recombinant DNA techniques in the 1980s enabled physical mapping strategies and led to a new approach, positional cloning. This describes the identification of a gene based purely on the basis of its location, without any prior knowledge of its function. Notable early successes were the identification of the dystrophin gene (mutated in Duchenne muscular dystrophy), the cystic fibrosis transmembrane regulatory gene and the retinoblastoma gene.

In the 1990s a genome-wide set of microsatellites was constructed with approximately 1 marker per 10 cM. These 350 markers could be amplified by PCR and facilitated genetic mapping studies that led to the identification of thousands of genes. This approach is likely to be superseded by DNA microarrays or 'SNP chips'. Although SNPs (p. 70) are less informative than microsatellites, they can be scored automatically and microarrays are commercially available with approximately 10 000 SNPs distributed evenly throughout the genome.

Developments in mutation screening techniques assisted in the identification of pathogenic mutations in candidate genes. With the sequencing of the human genome now complete, it is possible to find new disease genes by searching through genetic databases, i.e. 'in silico'.

## GENE MAPPING

There are two different approaches for assembling gene maps of human chromosomes: *physical mapping* and *genetic mapping*. These maps are interdependent and complementary. Physical mapping permits assignment of genes to a chromosomal location on a map, which is determined by physical distances (measured in base pairs) between genes. It is commonly divided into low-resolution mapping (1–several megabases) or high-resolution mapping (from hundreds of kilobases down to a single nucleotide). Genetic mapping, or linkage analysis (p. 131), is based on genetic distances which are measured in centimorgans (cM). A genetic distance of 1 cM is the distance between two genes that show 1% recombination, i.e. in 1% of meioses the genes will not be co-inherited.

### LOW-RESOLUTION PHYSICAL MAPPING

Low-resolution physical mapping techniques include somatic cell hybridization, chromosome-specific libraries and fluorescence in situ hybridization. Location of genes to specific chromosomes or chromosome regions is possible using these methods.

#### Somatic cell hybridization

*Somatic cell hybridization* involves taking cells from two different species and fusing them, a process facilitated by the presence of the Sendai virus or by the use of the chemical polyethylene glycol. The chromosome constitution of the resulting somatic cell hybrid shows a preferential loss of the human chromosomes from the cells (Fig. 5.1). It is possible to determine which human chromosomes have been retained and to select interspecific hybrids that contain different human chromosome(s). A panel of somatic cell hybrid clones that retain different human chromosomes can be selected that will enable assignment of any DNA sequence or expressed enzyme or protein to a particular human chromosome. Cells from individuals with chromosome rearrangments, e.g. deletions or translocations, can be used to more precisely map a gene to a particular region of a chromosome. As a further refinement of this approach, cells exposed to radiation that fragments their chromosomes allow the establishment of so-called *radiation hybrids*. These contain subchromosomal fragments enabling assignment of a particular gene or DNA sequence to a specific region of a chromosome.

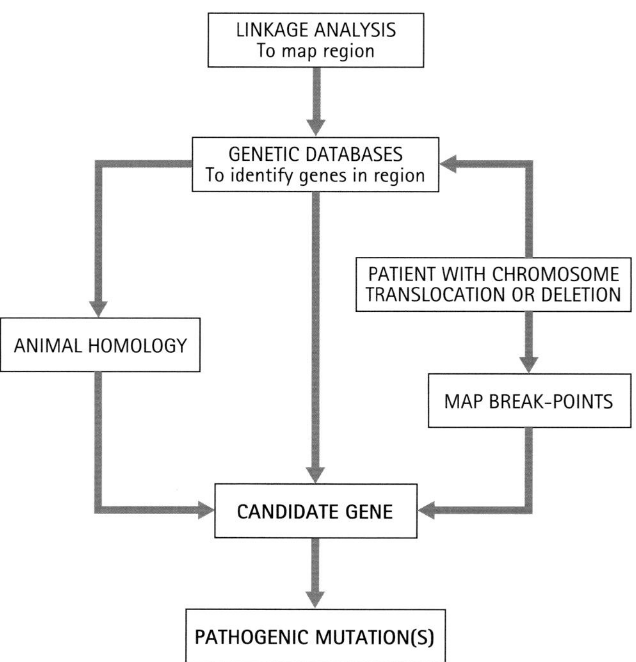


**Fig. 5.3**
Pathways towards human disease gene identification.

sequences specific to all genes, such as the conserved intron–exon splice junctions, promoter sequences, polyadenylation sites and stretches of open reading frames (ORFs).

## IDENTIFICATION OF HUMAN DISEASE GENES

Nearly 1500 human disease genes have been identified using a variety of approaches. The common step is arriving at a potential candidate gene (Fig. 5.3). The term 'positional cloning' is used to describe the approach of identifying a gene purely on the basis of its chromosomal location. This may be achieved through a genome-wide scan where a set of genetic markers that cover all the chromosomes is used for linkage mapping (p. 131). Short cuts are sometimes possible: for example, patients with cytogenetic abnormalities have assisted studies by highlighting the likely chromosome region. Candidate genes may be suggested from animal models of disease or by *homology*, either to a *paralogous* human gene (e.g. where multigene families exist), or to an *orthologous* gene in another species.

The timescale for identifying human disase genes has decreased dramatically from a period of years (e.g. the search for the cystic fibrosis gene in the 1980s) to weeks or maybe even days, now that the human genome sequence is available in public databases.

### POSITIONAL CLONING BY LINKAGE ANALYSIS

Linkage of cystic fibrosis (CF) to chromosome 7 was found by testing nearly 50 Caucasian families with hundreds of DNA markers. The gene was mapped to a region of 500 kb between markers *MET* and *D7S8* at chromosome band 7q31-32 when it became evident that the majority of CF chromosomes had a particular set of alleles for these markers (shared haplotype), which was only found in 25% of non-CF chromosomes. This finding is described as *linkage disequilibrium* and suggests a common mutation due to a founder effect (p. 303). Extensive physical mapping studies eventually led to the identification of four genes within the genetic interval identified by linkage analysis, and in 1989 a 3 bp deletion was found within the cystic fibrosis transmembrane receptor (*CFTR*) gene. This mutation (ΔF508) was present in approximately 70% of CF chromosomes and 2–3% of non-CF chromosomes, consistent with the carrier frequency of 1 in 25 in Caucasians.

### POSITIONAL CLONING ASSISTED BY CHROMOSOME ABNORMALITIES

Occasionally, individuals are recognized with single-gene disorders who are also found to have structural chromosomal abnormalities. The first clue that the gene responsible for Duchenne muscular dystrophy (DMD) (p. 308), was located on the short arm of the X chromosome was the identification of a number of females with DMD who were also found to have a chromosomal rearrangement between an autosome and a specific region of the short arm of one of their X chromosomes. Isolation of DNA clones spanning the region of the X chromosome involved in the rearrangement led in one such female to more detailed gene mapping information as well as to the eventual cloning of the DMD or dystrophin gene (p. 309).

At the same time as these observations, a male was reported with three X-linked disorders: Duchenne muscular dystrophy, chronic granulomatous disease and retinitis pigmentosa. He also had an unusual X-linked red cell group known as the McLeod phenotype. It was suggested that he could have a deletion of a number of genes of the short arm of his X chromosome, including the Duchenne muscular dystrophy gene, or what is now termed a *contiguous gene syndrome*. Detailed prometaphase chromosome analysis revealed this to be the case. DNA from this individual was used in vast excess to hybridize in competitive reassociation, under special conditions, with DNA from persons with multiple X chromosomes to enrich for DNA sequences that he lacked, the so-called phenol enhanced reassociation technique, or pERT, which allowed isolation of DNA clones containing portions of the DMD gene.

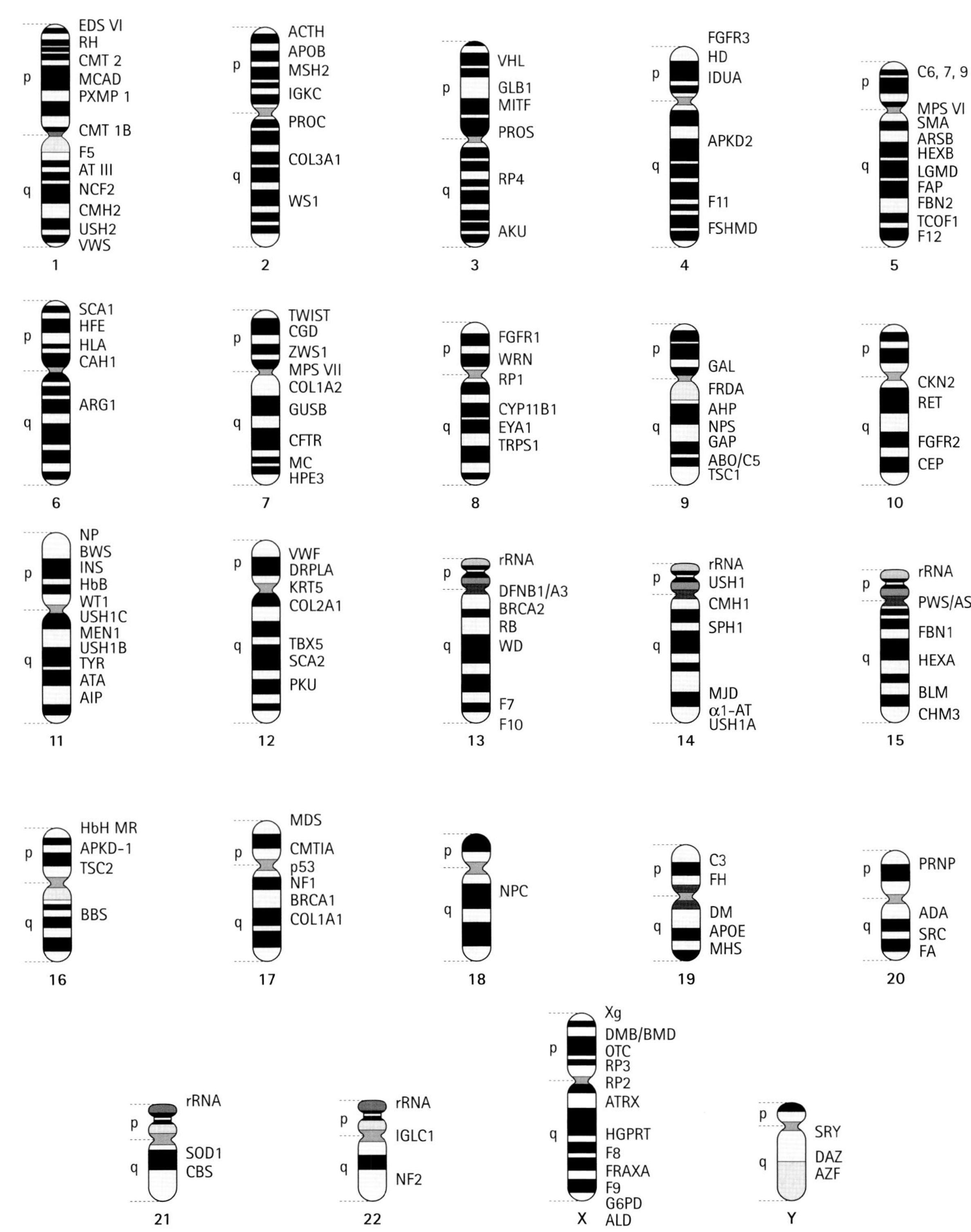


**Fig. 5.4**
A gene map of the human genome with examples of some of the more common or important single genes and disorders.

α1-AT – 14q32 – $\alpha_1$-antitrypsin deficiency
ABO – 9q34 – ABO blood group
ACTH – 2p25 – Adrenocorticotrophic hormone deficiency
ADA – 20q13.11 – Severe combined immunodeficiency, ADA deficiency
AHP – 9q34 – Acute hepatic porphyria
AIP – 11q23.3 – Acute intermittent porphyria
AKU – 3q2 – Alkaptonuria
ALD – Xq28 – Adrenoleukodystrophy
APKD1 – 16p13 – Adult polycystic kidney disease, locus 1

in another species which is shown to exhibit similar phenotypic features to those seen in persons affected with the disorder or restoration of the normal phenotype by transfection of the normal gene into a cell line, provides final proof that the candidate gene and the disease gene are one and the same.

## THE HUMAN GENE MAP

The rate at which single-gene disorders and their genes are being mapped in humans is increasing exponentially (see Fig. 1.6, p. 8). Many of the more common and clinically important single-gene disorders have been mapped to produce the 'morbid anatomy of the human genome' (Fig. 5.4).

## FURTHER READING

Botstein D, White R L, Skolnick M, Davis R W 1980 Construction of a genetic linkage map in man using restriction fragment length polymorphisms. Am J Hum Genet 32: 314-331
*One of the original papers describing the concept of linked RFLPs.*

Kerem B, Rommens JM, Buchanan JA, Markiewicz D et al 1989 Identification of the cystic fibrosis gene. Genetic analysis. Science 245:1073–1080
*Original paper describing cloning of the cystic fibrosis gene.*

McKusick V A 1998 Mendelian inheritance in man, 12th edn. Johns Hopkins University Press, London
*A computerized catalogue of the dominant, recessive and X-linked Mendelian traits and disorders in humans with a brief clinical commentary and details of the mutational basis if known. Also available online, updated regularly.*

Strachan T, Read A P 2004 Human molecular genetics, 3rd edn. Garland Science, London and New York
*A comprehensive textbook of all aspects of molecular and cellular biology as it relates to inherited disease in humans.*

## ELEMENTS

1. Low-resolution mapping techniques, which include somatic cell hybridization, chromosome-specific libraries and in-situ hybridization, enable assignment of a gene to a chromosome or a region of a chromosome. Pulsed field gel electrophoresis, chromatin fiber FISH and analysis of yeast artificial chromosome contigs allow high-resolution mapping.

2. Identification of DNA fragments containing genes is facilitated by identification of HTF/CpG islands, demonstration of their presence in zoo blots, exon trapping, expressed sequence tags, homology to genes in model organisms and analysis of Human Genome Project databases.

3. Positional cloning describes the identification of a gene on the basis of its chromosomal location. Chromosome abnormalities or animal models may assist this approach by highlighting particular chromosome regions of interest. Genetic databases with human genome sequence data now make the possibility of identifying genes 'in silico' a reality.

4. Confirmation that a specific gene is responsible for a particular inherited disorder can be obtained by tissue and developmental expression studies, in-vitro cell-culture studies, or the introduction and analysis of mutations in a homologous gene in another species. As a consequence the 'anatomy of the human genome' is continually being unraveled.

CHAPTER 6

# Developmental genetics

*"The history of man for the nine months preceding his birth would, probably, be far more interesting and contain events of greater moment than all the three score and ten years that follow it."*

Samual Taylor Coleridge

The formation and subsequent development of a human being are extremely complex processes that are still only poorly understood. Both genetic and environmental factors play important roles. Given a suitable environment, genes inherited from both parents determine how a small cluster of undifferentiated cells derived from the fertilized egg or zygote develops over a period of approximately 12 weeks into a recognizably human fetus. The developmental processes that take place within these first 12 weeks following conception fall within the realm of embryology. In this chapter we are not concerned so much with the mechanics of these structural changes as with the way these processes are under genetic control. It is this aspect of biology that constitutes the field of developmental genetics.

Prenatal life can be divided into three main stages – *pre-embryonic*, *embryonic* and *fetal* (Table 6.1). During the pre-embryonic stage a small collection of cells becomes distinguishable, firstly as a double-layered or *bilaminar disc*, and then as a triple-layered or *trilaminar disc* (Fig. 6.1) that is destined to develop into the human

**Table 6.1 Main events in the development of a human infant**

| Stage | Time from conception | Length of embryo/fetus |
|---|---|---|
| **Pre-embryonic** | | |
| First cell division | 30 hours | |
| Zygote reaches uterine cavity | 4 days | |
| Implantation | 5–6 days | |
| Formation of bilaminar disc | 12 days | 0.2 mm |
| Lyonization in female | 16 days | |
| Formation of trilaminar disc and primitive streak | 19 days | 1 mm |
| **Embryonic stage** | | |
| Organogenesis | 4–8 weeks | |
| Brain and spinal cord are forming | 4 weeks | 4 mm |
| First signs of heart and limb buds | | |
| Brain, eyes, heart and limbs developing rapidly | 6 weeks | 17 mm |
| Bowel and lungs beginning to develop | | |
| Digits have appeared. Ears, kidneys, liver and muscle are developing | 8 weeks | 4 cm |
| Palate closes and joints form | 10 weeks | 6 cm |
| Sexual differentiation almost complete | 12 weeks | 9 cm |
| **Fetal stage** | | |
| Fetal movements felt | 16–18 weeks | 20 cm |
| Eyelids open. Fetus is now viable with specialized care | 24–26 weeks | 35 cm |
| Rapid weight gain due to growth and accumulation of fat as lungs mature | 28–38 weeks | 40–50 cm |

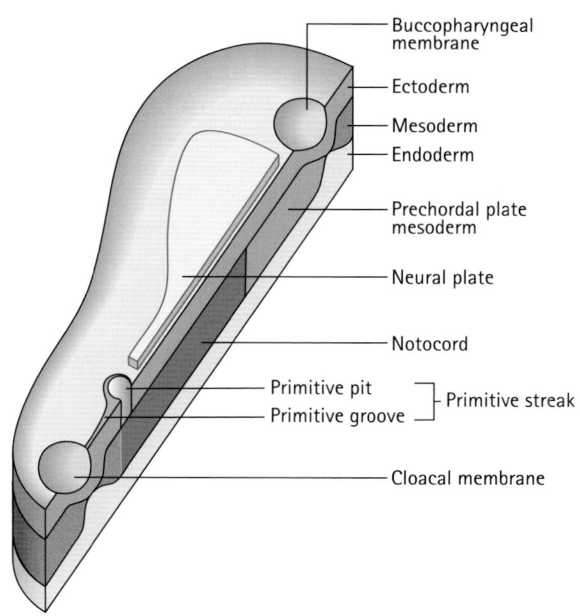


**Fig. 6.1**
A schematic trilaminar disc, sectioned along the rostro-caudal axis. Cells from the future ectoderm (mid blue) migrate through the primitive streak to form the endoderm (light blue) and mesoderm (gray). Formation of the neutral plate in the overlying ectoderm, destined to be the CNS, involves sonic hedgehog signaling (see p. 86) from the notochord and prechordial plate mesoderm. (Redrawn with permission from *Essentials of human embryology*, Larsen W. J., 1998 Churchill Livingstone, New York)

infant. During the embryonic stage, cranio-caudal, dorsoventral, and proximo-distal axes are established, as cellular aggregation and differentiation lead to tissue and organ formation. The final fetal stage is characterized by rapid growth and development as the embryo, now known as a fetus, matures into a viable human infant.

On average, this extraordinary process takes approximately 38 weeks. By convention pregnancy is usually dated from the first day of the last menstrual period (LMP), which usually precedes conception by around 2 weeks so that the normal period of gestation is often stated incorrectly as lasting for 40 weeks.

**Table 6.2 Organ and tissue origins**

| |
|---|
| **Ectodermal** |
| Central nervous system |
| Peripheral nervous system |
| Epidermis, including hair and nails |
| Subcutaneous glands |
| Dental enamel |
| **Mesodermal** |
| Connective tissue |
| Cartilage and bone |
| Smooth and striated muscle |
| Cardiovascular system |
| Urogenital system |
| **Endodermal** |
| Thymus and thyroid |
| Gastrointestinal system |
| Liver and pancreas |

## FERTILIZATION AND GASTRULATION

Fertilization, the process by which the male and female gametes fuse, occurs in the fallopian tube. Of the 100–200 million spermatozoa deposited in the female genital tract only a few hundred reach the site of fertilization. Of these, usually only a single spermatozoon succeeds in penetrating first the corona radiata, then the zona pellucida and finally the oocyte cell membrane, whereupon the oocyte completes its second meiotic division (Fig. 3.19, p. 44).

After the sperm has penetrated the oocyte and the meiotic process has been completed, the two nuclei, now known as pronuclei, fuse, thereby restoring the diploid number of 46 chromosomes. The fertilized ovum or zygote then undergoes a series of mitotic divisions to consist of two cells by 30 h, four cells by 40 h and 12–16 cells by 3 days, when it is known as a morula. A key concept in development at all stages is the emergence of *polarity* within groups of cells, part of the process of differentiation that generates multiple cell types with unique identities. Whilst precise mechanisms remain elusive, observations suggest this begins at the very outset – in the fertilized egg of the mouse the point of entry of the sperm determines the plane through which the first cell cleavage division occurs. This seminal event is the first step in the development of the so-called dorsoventral, or primary body, axis in the embryo.

Further cell division leads to formation of a *blastocyst*, which consists of an inner cell mass or *embryoblast*, destined to form the embryo, and an outer cell mass or *trophoblast*, which gives rise to the placenta. The process of converting the inner cell mass into firstly a bilaminar and then a trilaminar disc (Fig. 6.1) is known as *gastrulation*, and takes place between the beginning of the second and the end of the third weeks.

Between 4 and 8 weeks the body form is established, beginning with the formation of the primitive streak at the caudal end of the embryo. The germinal layers of the trilaminar disc give rise to *ectodermal*, *mesodermal* and *endodermal* structures (Table 6.2). The neural tube is formed and neural crest cells migrate to form sensory ganglia, the sympathetic nervous system, pigment cells, and both bone and cartilage in parts of the face and branchial arches.

Disorders involving cells of neural crest origin, such as neurofibromatosis (p. 298), are sometimes referred to as *neurocristopathies*. This period between 4 and 8 weeks is referred to as the period of organogenesis as it is during this interval that all of the major organs are formed as regional specialization proceeds in a cranio-caudal direction down the axis of the embryo.

## DEVELOPMENTAL GENE FAMILIES

Information about the genetic factors that initiate, maintain and direct embryogenesis is limited. However, extensive genetic studies of the fruit fly, *Drosophila melanogaster*, and vertebrates such as mouse, chick and zebrafish, have identified several genes and gene families that play important roles in the early developmental processes. It has also been possible through painstaking gene expression studies to identify several key developmental pathways, or cascades, to which more detail and complexity is continually being added. The gene families identified in vertebrates usually show strong sequence homology with developmental regulatory genes in *Drosophila*. Recent studies in humans have revealed that mutations in various members of these gene families can result in either isolated malformations or multiple congenital anomaly syndromes (Table 16.5, p. 253). Many developmental genes produce proteins called transcription factors (p. 22), which control RNA transcription from the DNA template by binding to specific regulatory DNA sequences to form complexes that initiate transcription by RNA polymerase.

Transcription factors can switch genes on and off by activating or repressing gene expression. It is likely that important transcription factors control many other genes in coordinated sequential cascades and feedback loops involving the regulation of fundamental embryological processes such as *segmentation, induction, migration, differentiation* and *programmed cell death* (known as *apoptosis*). It is believed that these processes are mediated by growth factors, cell receptors and chemicals known as *morphogens*. Across species the signaling molecules involved are very similar. The protein signals identified over and over again tend to be members of the *transforming growth factor-beta* (*TGF-β*) family, the *wingless* (*Wnt*) family, and the *hedgehog* (*HH*) family. Also, it is clear within any given organism that the same molecular pathways are reused in different developmental domains.

## EARLY PATTERNING AND SEGMENTATION GENES

Insect bodies consist of series of repeated body segments that differentiate into particular structures according to their position. Three main groups of segmentation-determining genes have been classified on the basis of their mutant phenotypes. These are gap mutants, which delete groups of adjacent segments, pair-rule mutants, which delete alternate segments, and segment polarity mutants, which cause portions of each segment to be deleted and duplicated on the wrong side. In vertebrates, dorsoventral axis specification is dependent on normal activity of the *Wnt signaling pathway*. It is not clear how this pathway is activated, but when this occurs down-regulation of glycogen synthase kinase-3β (*GSK3β*) follows, which in turn stabilizes β-catenin. As a result, β-catenin accumulates in dorsal, rather than ventral, nuclei, where it activates the transcription of dorsal-specific regulatory genes. Another group of proteins key to dorsoventral patterning at this stage are those of the *bone morphogenetic pathway* (BMP), as well as their inhibitors, which play an important role in the induction of neural tissue. There is no known human disease phenotype due to mutated *WNT* genes but overexpression of *BMP4* has been found in the rare bony condition fibrodyplasia ossificans progressiva (FOP). BMPs are part of the *TGF-β* superfamily.

## SOMITOGENESIS AND THE AXIAL SKELETON

The vertebrate axis is closely linked to the development of the primary body axis during gastrulation, and during this process the paraxial mesoderm (PSM), where somites arise, is laid down in higher vertebrates. Wnt and fibroblast growth factor signals (FGF) signals play vital roles in the specification of the PSM. The somites form as blocks of tissue from the PSM in a rostro-caudal direction (Fig. 6.2), each being laid down with a precise periodicity that in the 1970s gave rise to the concept of the 'clock and wavefront' model. Since then molecular techniques have given substance to this concept, and the key pathway here is *notch-delta signaling* and the 'oscillation clock' – a precise temporally defined wave of gene expression (*lunatic fringe* (!) in the mouse) that sweeps from the tail-bud region in a rostral direction and has a key role in the process leading to the defining of somite boundaries. Once again, not all the components are fully understood, but the *notch receptor* and its ligands, *delta-like-1* and *delta-like-3*, together with *presenilin-1* and *mesoderm posterior-2*, work in concert to establish rostro-caudal polarity within the PSM such that somite blocks are formed. Human phenotypes due to mutated genes in this pathway are now well known and include presenile dementia (*presenilin-1*), which is dominantly inherited, and spondylocostal dysostosis (*delta-like-3*) – recessively inherited (Fig. 6.3). Another component of the pathway is *JAGGED1*, and when mutated the dominantly inherited and very variable condition Alagille syndrome (arterio-hepatic dysplasia) results (Fig. 6.4).

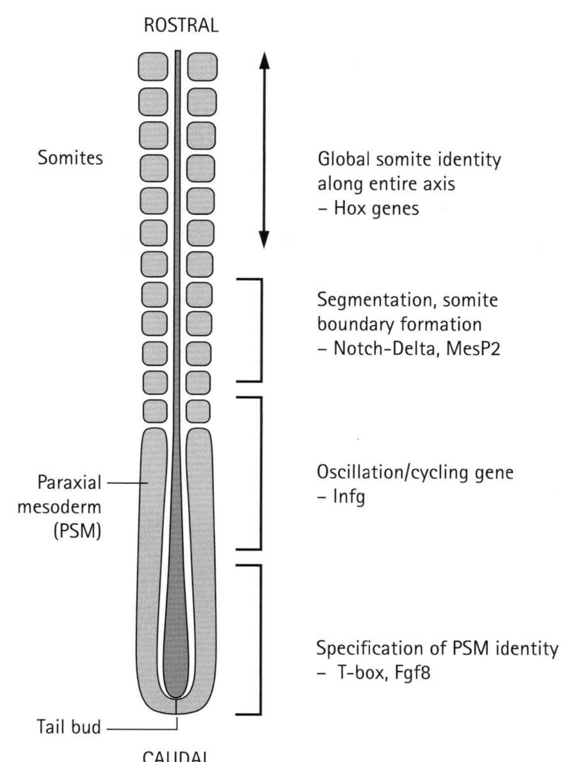


**Fig. 6.2**
Somitogenesis and Notch–Delta pathway. T-box have a role in PSM specification whilst the segmentation clock depends on oscillation, or cycling, genes that are important in somite boundary formation where genes of the Notch–Delta pathway establish rostro-caudal polarity. *HOX* genes have a global function in establishing somite identity along the entire rostro-caudal axis. (Adapted from *Patterning in Vertebrate Development*, ed. Trickle C, 2003, Oxford University Press)

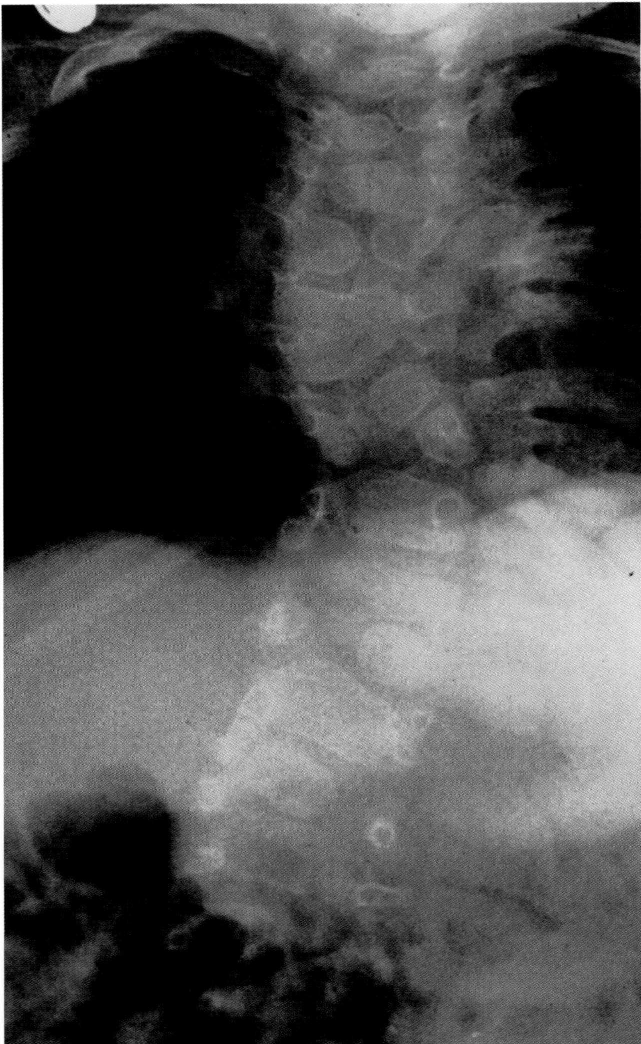

Fig. 6.3
Disrupted development of the vertebrae in patient with spondylocostal dysostosis type 1, due to mutations in the *delta-like3* gene, part of the notch signaling pathway. (Courtesy of Dr Meriel McEntagart, Kennedy-Galton Centre, London)

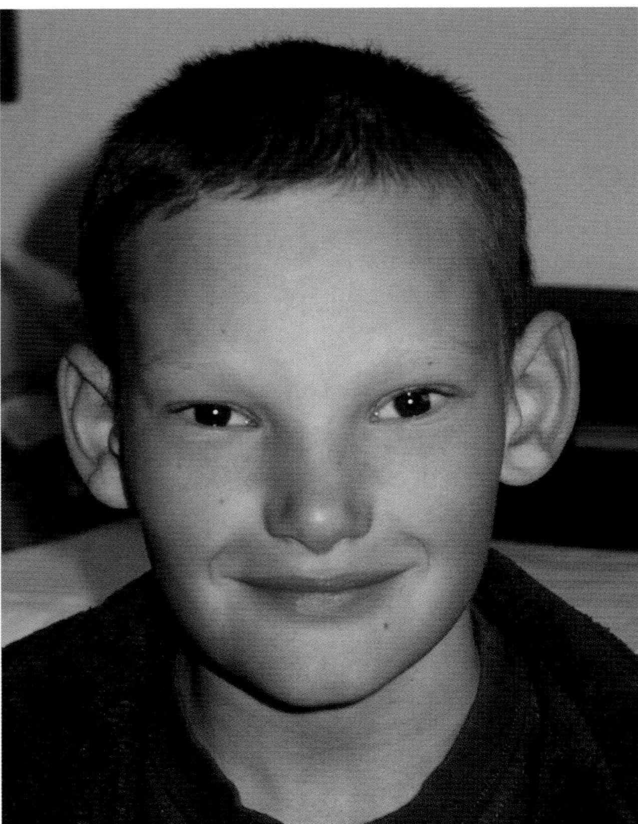

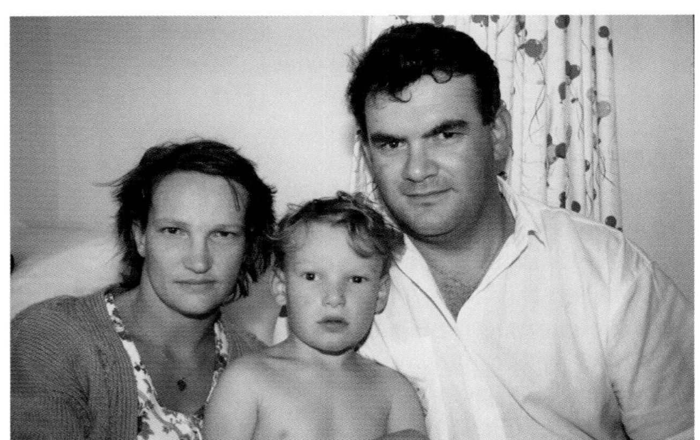

Fig. 6.4
(A) A boy with Alagille syndrome and confirmed mutation in *JAGGED1* who presented with congenital heart disease. (B) The same boy a few years earlier with his parents. His mother has a pigmentary retinopathy and was positive for the same gene mutation

## THE SONIC HEDGEHOG-PATCHED-GLI PATHWAY

The Sonic hedgehog gene (*SHH*) is as well known for its quirky name as for its function. *SHH* induces cell proliferation in a tissue-specific distribution and is expressed in the notochord, the brain, and the zone of polarizing activity of developing limbs. Following cleavage and modification by the addition of a cholesterol moiety, the SHH protein binds with its receptor, Patched (Ptch), a transmembrane protein. The normal action of Ptch is to inhibit another transmembrane protein called Smoothened (Smo), but when bound by Shh this inhibition is released and a signaling cascade within the cell activated. The key intracellular targets are the *GLI* family of transcription factors (Fig. 6.5).

Molecular defects in any part of this pathway lead to a number of apparently diverse malformation syndromes (Fig. 6.5). Mutations in, or deletions of, *SHH* (chromosome 7q36) cause holoprosencephaly (Fig. 6.6), in which

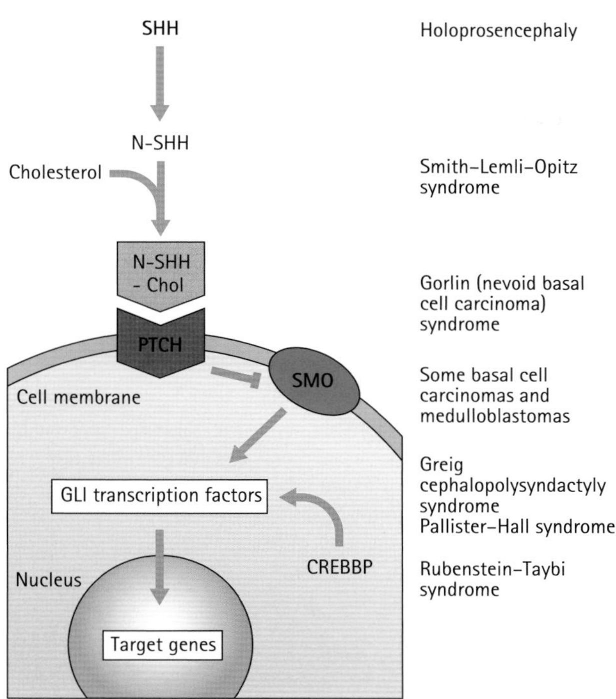


**Fig. 6.5**
The Sonic hedgehog (*SHH*)-patched (*PTCH*)-Gli pathway and connection with disease. Different elements in the pathway act as activators (arrows) or inhibitors (bars). The normal action of *PTCH* is to inhibit *SMO*, but when *PTCH* is bound by *SHH*, this inhibition is removed and the downstream signaling proceeds.

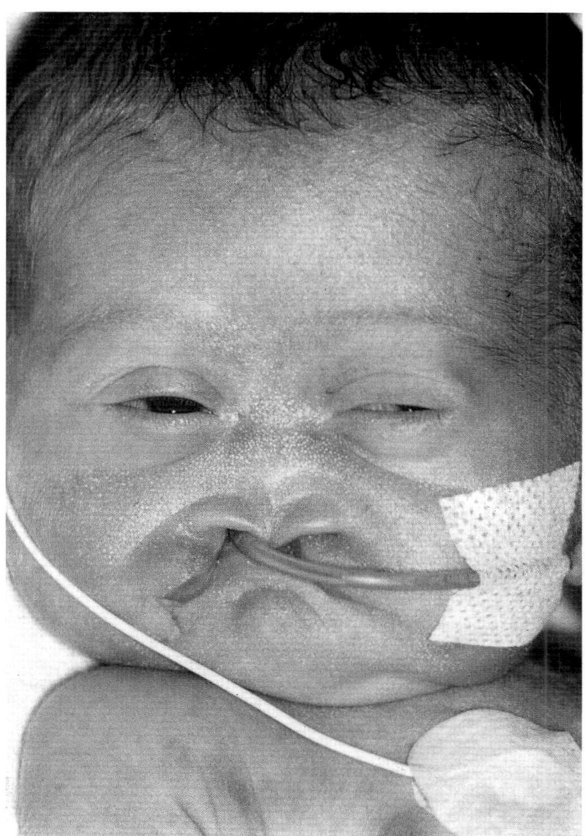

**Fig. 6.6**
The facial features in holoprosencephaly. The eyes are close together and there is a midline cleft lip due to failure of normal prolabia development.

the primary defect is incomplete cleavage of the developing brain into separate hemispheres and ventricles. The most severe form of this malformation is cyclopia, i.e. the presence of a single central eye. (The complexity of early development can be appreciated by the fact that a dozen or so chromosomal regions have so far been implicated in the pathogenesis of holoprosencephaly (p. 256).) Mutations in *PTCH* (9q22) cause Gorlin syndrome (Fig. 6.7) – nevoid basal cell carcinoma syndrome – comprising multiple basal cell carcinomas, odontogenic keratocysts, bifid ribs, calcification of the falx cerebri and ovarian fibromata. Mutations in *SMO* (7q31) are found in some basal cell carcinomas and medulloblastomas. Mutations in *GLI3* (7p13) cause Pallister–Hall syndrome and Grieg syndrome – distinct entities with more or less the same body systems affected. But there are also links to other conditions, in particular the very variable Smith–Lemli–Opitz syndrome (SLOS), which may include holoprosencephaly as well as some characteristic facial features, genital anomalies and syndactyly. It is due to a defect in the final step of cholesterol biosynthesis, which in turn may disrupt the binding of Shh with its receptor Ptch. Some, or all, of the features of SLOS may therefore be due to loss of integrity in this pathway (p. 256). Furthermore, a co-factor for the Gli proteins, *CREBBP* (16p13) is mutated in Rubenstein–Taybi syndrome.

## HOMEOBOX (*HOX*) GENES

In *Drosophila* a class of genes known as the homeotic genes have been shown to determine segment identity. Incorrect expression of these genes results in major structural abnormalities; the *Antp* gene, for example, which is normally expressed in the second thoracic segment, will transform the adult fly's antennae into legs if incorrectly expressed in the head. Homeotic genes contain a conserved 180 bp sequence known as the homeobox, which is believed to be characteristic of genes involved in spatial pattern control and development. This encodes a 60 amino acid domain which binds to DNA. Proteins from homeobox (or *HOX*)-containing genes are therefore important transcription factors that specify cell fate and help to establish the embryonic pattern along the primary

A

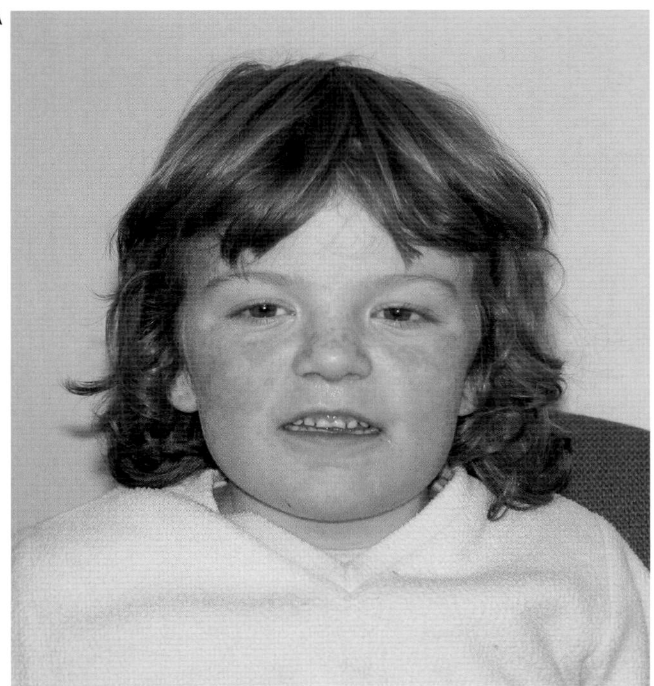

B

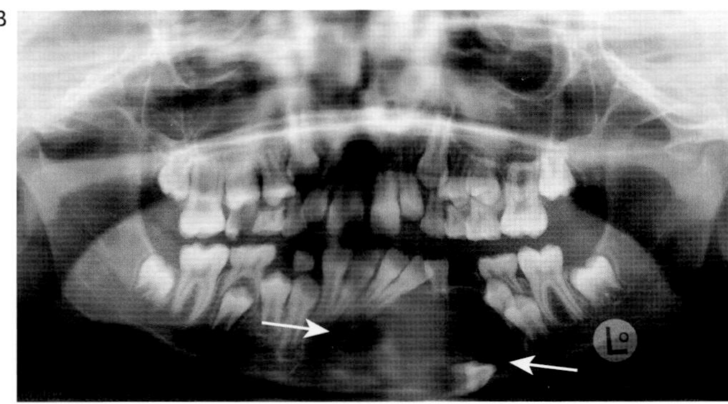


**Fig. 6.7**
Gorlin (nevoid basal cell carcinoma) syndrome. (A) This 6-year-old girl from a large family with Gorlin syndrome has macrocephaly and a cherubic appearance. Her affected sister (B) developed a rapidly enlarging odontogenic keratocyst (arrowed) in her mandible at the age of 9 years, displacing the roots of her teeth.

(rostro-caudal) axis as well as the secondary (genital and limb bud) axis. They therefore play a major part in development of the CNS, axial skeleton and limbs, the gastrointestinal and urogenital tracts, and external genitalia.

*Drosophila* has eight *Hox* genes arranged in a single cluster but in man, as in most vertebrates, there are four homeobox gene clusters containing a total of 39 *HOX* genes (Fig. 6.8). Each cluster contains a series of closely linked genes. In vertebrates such as mice it has been shown that these genes are expressed in segmental units in the hindbrain and in global patterning of the somites formed from axial presomitic mesoderm. In each *HOX* cluster there is a direct linear correlation between the position of the gene and its temporal and spatial expression. These observations indicate that these genes play a crucial role in early morphogenesis. Thus in the developing limb bud (p. 94) *HOXA9* is expressed both anteriorly to, and before, *HOX10*, and so on.

Mutations in *HOXA13* cause a rare condition known as the hand–foot–genital syndrome. This shows autosomal dominant inheritance and is characterized by shortening of the first and fifth digits, with hypospadias in males and bicornuate uterus in females. Mutations in *HOXD13* result in an equally rare limb developmental abnormality known as synpolydactyly. This also shows autosomal dominant inheritance and is characterized by insertion of an additional digit between the third and fourth fingers and the fourth and fifth toes, which are webbed (Fig. 6.9). The phenotype in homozygotes is more severe, with the metacarpals and metatarsals being converted into short carpal and tarsal-like bones, respectively. Reported mutations take the form of an increase in the number of residues in a polyalanine tract. This triplet repeat expansion probably alters the structure and function of the protein, thereby constituting a gain-of-function mutation (p. 26). To date, these are the only two *HOX* genes proved to be mutated in human malformations. They are each located at the 5′ end of their respective clusters and co-operate in the development of caudal structures along the primary body axis, the most distal part of the limb, and the genital tubercle.

Given that there are 39 *HOX* genes in mammals it is surprising that no other recognized syndromes or malformations have been attributed to *HOX* gene mutations. One possible explanation is that most *HOX* mutations are so devastating that the embryo cannot survive. Alternatively, the high degree of homology between *HOX* genes in the different clusters could lead to functional redundancy so that one *HOX* gene could compensate for a loss-of-function mutation in another. In this context *HOX* genes are said to be paralogous because family members from different clusters, such as *HOXA13* and *HOXD13*, are more similar than adjacent genes in the same cluster.

Several other developmental genes also contain a homeobox-like domain. These include *MSX2* and *EMX2*. Mutations in *MSX2* can cause craniosynostosis, i.e. premature fusion of the cranial sutures. Mutations in *EMX2* cause a severe cerebral malformation known as

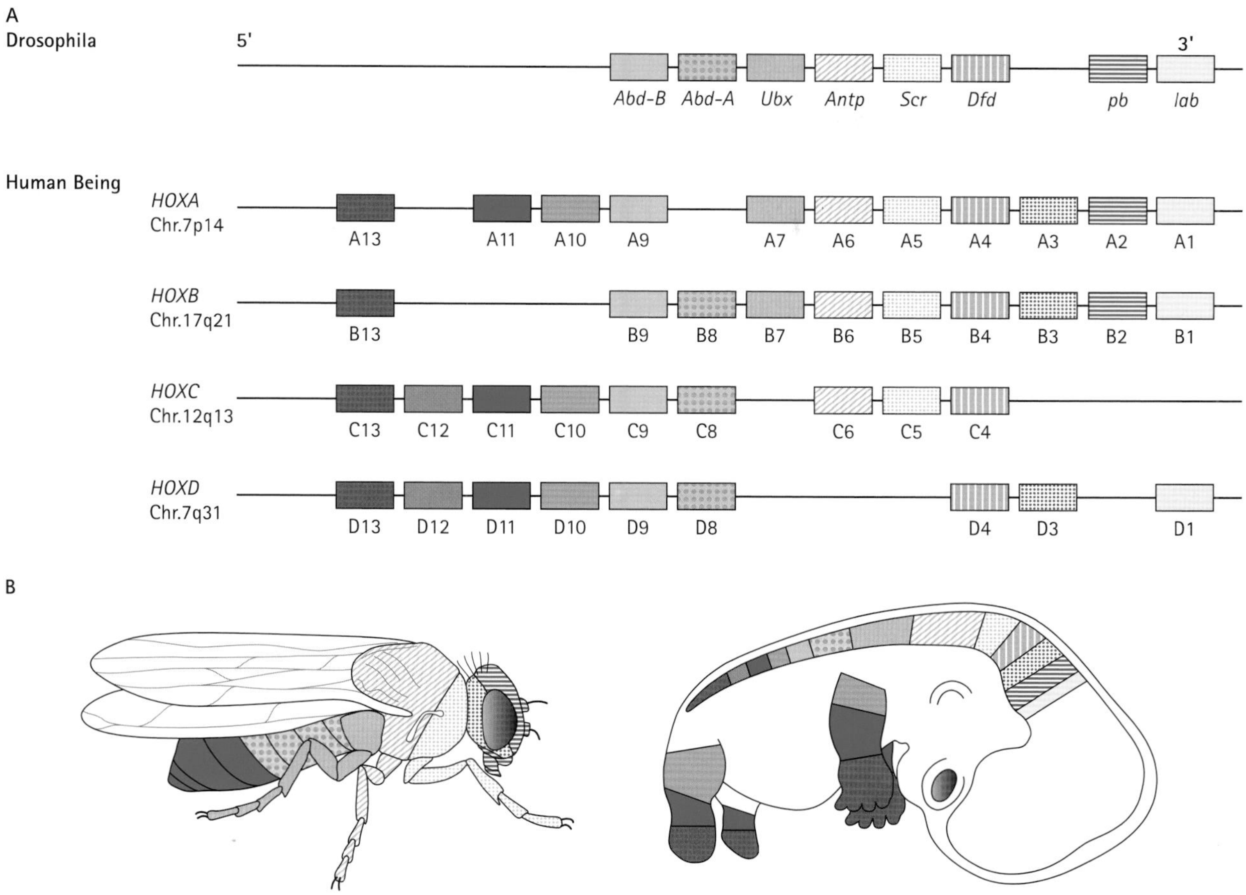

A

Drosophila 5' 3'

*Abd-B* *Abd-A* *Ubx* *Antp* *Scr* *Dfd* *pb* *lab*

Human Being

*HOXA* Chr.7p14

A13 A11 A10 A9 A7 A6 A5 A4 A3 A2 A1

*HOXB* Chr.17q21

B13 B9 B8 B7 B6 B5 B4 B3 B2 B1

*HOXC* Chr.12q13

C13 C12 C11 C10 C9 C8 C6 C5 C4

*HOXD* Chr.7q31

D13 D12 D11 D10 D9 D8 D4 D3 D1

B

**Fig. 6.8**
(A) *Drosophilia* has eight *Hox* genes in a single cluster whereas there are 39 *HOX* genes in man, arranged in four clusters located on chromosomes 7p, 17q, 12q and 2q for the A, B, C and D clusters, respectively. (B) The expression patterns of the *Hox/HOX* genes are along the rostro-caudal axis in both invertebrates and vertebrates, respectively. In vertebrates the clusters are *paralogous* and appear to compensate for each other.
(Redrawn with permission from, Verasaka, A. *et al.* (2000) Developmental patterning genes and their conserved functions: from model organisms to humans. *Molecular Genetics and Metabolism* **69**: 85–100)

A

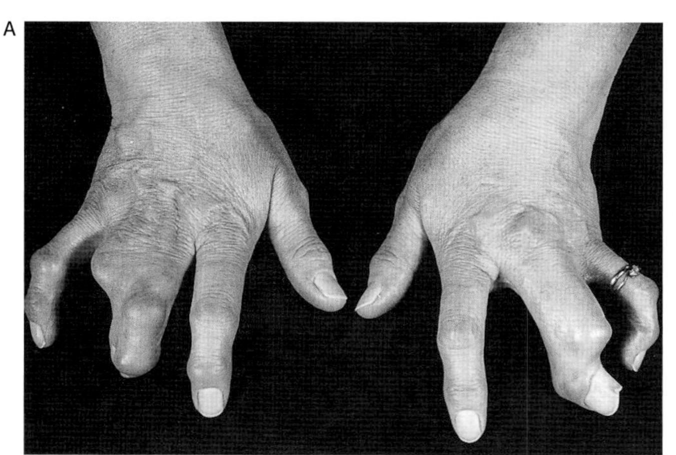

B

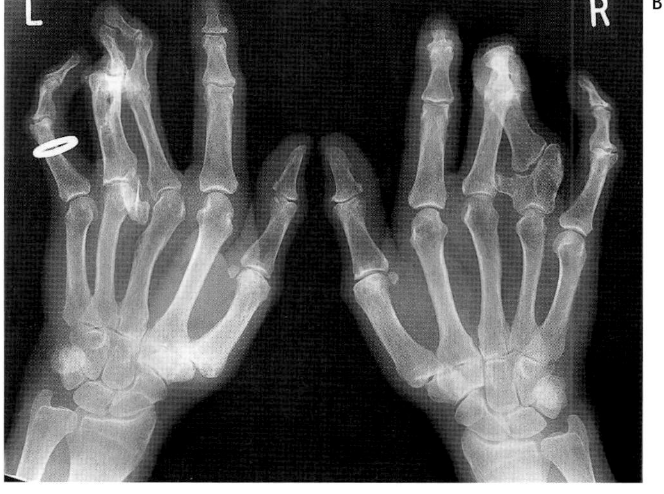


**Fig. 6.9**
(A) Clinical and (B) X-ray views of the hands in synpolydactyly.

**Table 6.3 Developmental abnormalities associated with *PAX* gene mutations**

| Gene | Chromosome location | Developmental abnormality |
|---|---|---|
| *PAX2* | 10q24 | Renal-coloboma syndrome |
| *PAX3* | 2q35 | Waardenburg syndrome type 1 |
| *PAX6* | 11p13 | Aniridia |
| *PAX8* | 2q12 | Absent or ectopic thyroid gland |
| *PAX9* | 14q12 | Oligodontia |

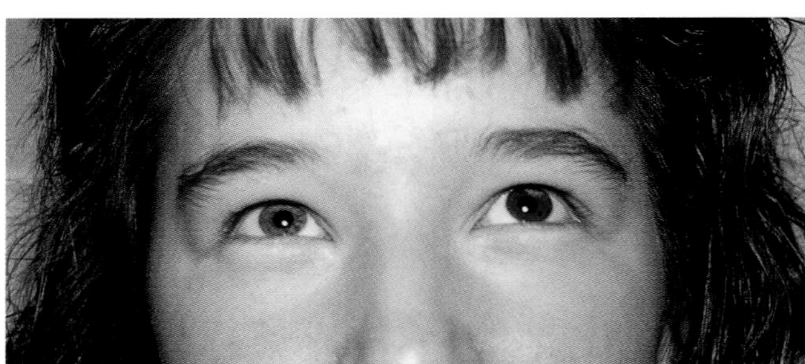

Fig. 6.10
Iris heterochromia in a person with Waardenburg syndrome. (Courtesy of Dr C. P. Bennett, St James's Hospital, Leeds.)

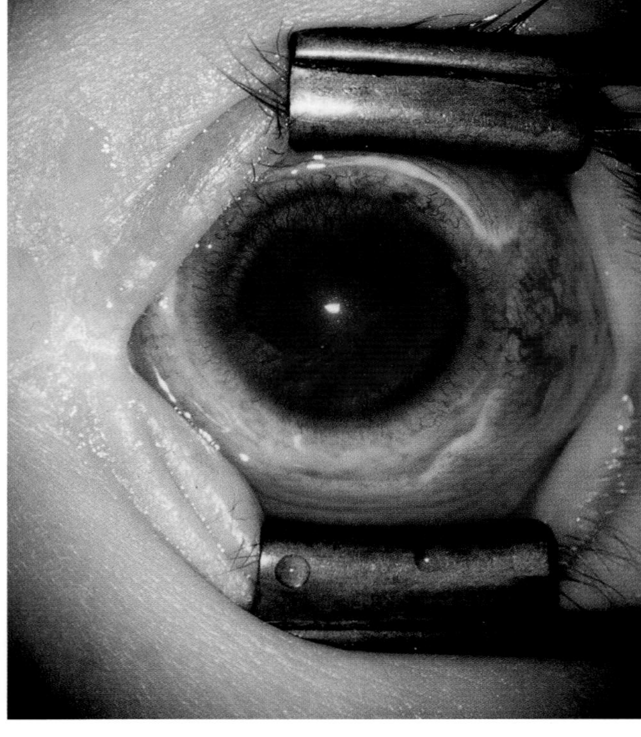

Fig. 6.11
An eye showing absence of the iris (aniridia). The cornea shows abnormal vascularization. (Courtesy of Mr R. Gregson, Queen's Medical Centre, Nottingham.)

schizencephaly, in which there is a large full-thickness cleft in one or both cerebral hemispheres.

## PAIRED-BOX (*PAX*) GENES

The paired-box is a highly conserved DNA sequence that encodes a 130 amino acid DNA-binding transcription regulator domain. Nine *PAX* genes have been identified in mice and humans. In mice these have been shown to play important roles in the developing nervous system and vertebral column. In humans loss-of-function mutations in five *PAX* genes have been identified in association with developmental abnormalities (Table 6.3). Waardenburg syndrome type 1 is caused by mutations in *PAX3*. It shows autosomal dominant inheritance and is characterized by sensorineural hearing loss, areas of depigmentation in hair and skin, abnormal patterns of pigmentation in the iris, and widely spaced inner canthi (Fig. 6.10). Waardenburg syndrome shows genetic heterogeneity with the more common type 2 form, in which the inner canthi are not widely separated, some cases being caused by mutations in the human microphthalmia (*MITF*) gene on chromosome 3, and still others by additional genes.

The importance of expression of the *PAX* gene family in eye development is illustrated by the effects of mutations in *PAX2* and *PAX6*. Mutations in *PAX2* cause the renal-coloboma syndrome, in which renal malformations occur in association with structural defects in various parts of the eye, including the retina and optic nerve. Mutations in *PAX6* lead to absence of the iris, which is known as aniridia (Fig. 6.11). This is a key feature of the WAGR syndrome (p. 276), which results from a contiguous gene deletion involving the *PAX6* locus on chromosome 11.

## SRY-TYPE HMG BOX (*SOX*) GENES

*SRY* is the Y-linked gene that plays a major role in male sex determination (p. 97). A series of genes known as the *SOX* genes show homology with *SRY* by sharing a 79 amino acid domain known as the HMG (high-mobility group) box. This HMG domain activates transcription by bending DNA in such a way that other regulatory factors can bind with the promoter regions of genes which encode for important structural proteins. These *SOX* genes are thus transcription regulators and are expressed in specific tissues during embryogenesis. For example,

*SOX1*, *SOX2* and *SOX3* are expressed in the developing mouse nervous system.

In humans it has been shown that loss-of-function mutations in *SOX9* on chromosome 17 cause campomelic dysplasia. This very rare disorder is characterized by bowing of the long bones, sex reversal in chromosomal males and very poor long-term survival. In-situ hybridization studies in mice have shown that *SOX9* is expressed in the developing embryo in skeletal primordial tissue, where it regulates type II collagen expression, as well as in the genital ridges and early gonads. *SOX9* is now thought to be one of several genes that are expressed downstream of *SRY* in the process of male sex determination (p. 97). Mutations in *SOX10* on chromosome 22 cause a rare form of Waardenburg syndrome in which affected individuals have a high incidence of Hirschsprung disease.

## T-BOX (*TBX*) GENES

The T gene in mice plays an important role in specification of the paraxial mesoderm and notochord differentiation. Heterozygotes for loss-of-function mutations have a short tail and malformed sacral vertebrae. This gene, which is also known as *Brachyury*, encodes a transcription factor that contains both activator and repressor domains. It shows homology with a series of genes through the shared possession of the T domain, which is also referred to as the T-box. These T-box or *TBX* genes are dispersed throughout the human genome, with some family members existing in small clusters. One of these clusters on chromosome 12 contains *TBX3* and *TBX5*. Loss-of-function mutations in *TBX3* cause the ulnar-mammary syndrome in which ulnar ray developmental abnormalities in the upper limbs are associated with hypoplasia of the mammary glands. Loss-of-function mutations in *TBX5* cause the Holt–Oram syndrome. This autosomal dominant disorder is characterized by congenital heart abnormalities, most notably atrial septal defects, and upper limb radial ray reduction defects that can vary from mild hypoplasia (sometimes duplication) of the thumbs to almost complete absence of the forearms.

## ZINC FINGER GENES

The term *zinc finger* refers to a finger-like loop projection that is formed by a series of four amino acids that form a complex with a zinc ion. Genes that contain a zinc finger motif act as transcription factors through binding of the zinc finger to DNA. Consequently they are good candidates for single-gene developmental disorders (Table 6.4).

For example a zinc finger motif containing a gene known as *GLI3* on chromosome 7 has been implicated as the cause of two developmental disorders. Large deletions or translocations involving *GLI3* cause Greig cephalopolysyndactyly, which is characterized by head, hand and foot abnormalities such as polydactyly and syndactyly (Fig. 6.12). In contrast, frameshift mutations in *GLI3* have been reported in the Pallister–Hall syndrome, in which the key features are polydactyly, hypothalamic hamartomata and imperforate anus.

**Table 6.4 Developmental abnormalities associated with genes containing a zinc finger motif**

| Gene | Chromosome location | Developmental abnormality |
|---|---|---|
| *GLI3* | 7p13 | Greig syndrome and Pallister–Hall syndrome |
| *WT1* | 11p13 | Denys–Drash syndrome |
| *ZIC2* | 13q32 | Holoprosencephaly |
| *ZIC3* | Xq26 | Laterality defects |

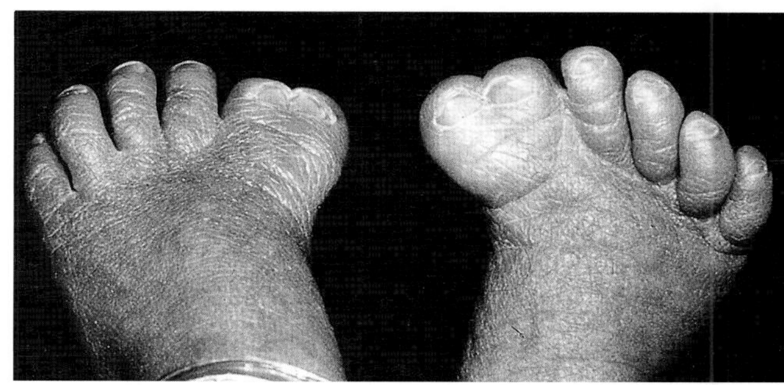

Fig. 6.12
The feet of a child with Greig cephalopolysyndactyly. Note that they show both polydactyly (extra digits) and syndactyly (fused digits).

Mutations in another zinc finger motif containing a gene known as *WT1* on chromosome 11 can cause both Wilms' tumour and a rare developmental disorder, the Denys–Drash syndrome, in which the external genitalia are ambiguous and there is progressive renal failure as a result of nephritis. Mutations in two other zinc finger motif containing genes, *ZIC2* and *ZIC3*, have recently been shown to cause holoprosencephaly and laterality defects, respectively. Just as *polarity* is a key concept in development, so too is *laterality*, with implications for the establishment of a normal left–right body axis. *Situs solitus* is the term given to normal left–right asymmetry and *situs inversus* to reversal of the normal arrangement. Up to 25% of individuals with situs inversus have an autosomal recessive condition – Kartagener syndrome, or ciliary dyskinesia. Other terms used are *isomerism sequence*, *heterotaxy*, *asplenia/polyasplenia*, and *Ivemark syndrome*. Laterality defects are characterized by abnormal positioning of unpaired organs such as the heart, liver and spleen, and more than 20 genes are now implicated from studies in vertebrates, with a number identified in humans through studying affected families, with all the main patterns of inheritance represented.

## SIGNAL TRANSDUCTION ('SIGNALING') GENES

Signal transduction is the process whereby extracellular growth factors regulate cell division and differentiation by a complex pathway of genetically determined intermediate steps. Mutations in many of the genes involved in signal transduction play a role in causing cancer (p. 207). In some cases they can also cause developmental abnormalities.

### The *RET* proto-oncogene

The proto-oncogene *RET* on chromosome 10q11.2 encodes a cell surface tyrosine kinase. Gain-of-function mutations, whether inherited or acquired, are found in a high proportion of thyroid cancers. Loss-of-function mutations in *RET* have been identified in approximately 50% of familial cases of Hirschsprung disease, in which there is failure of migration of ganglionic cells to the submucosal and myenteric plexuses of the large bowel. The clinical consequences are usually apparent shortly after birth when the child presents with abdominal distension and intestinal obstruction.

### Fibroblast growth factor receptors

Fibroblast growth factors (FGFs) play key roles in embryogenesis, including cell division, migration and differentiation. The transduction of extracellular FGF signals is mediated by a family of four transmembrane tyrosine kinase receptors. These are the fibroblast growth factor receptors (FGFRs), each of which contains three main components – an extracellular region with three immunoglobulin-like domains, a transmembrane segment and two intracellular tyrosine kinase domains (Fig. 6.13).

Mutations in the genes that code for FGFRs have been identified in two groups of developmental disorders (Table 6.5). These are the craniosynostosis syndromes and the achondroplasia family of skeletal dysplasias. The craniosynostosis syndromes, of which Apert syndrome (Fig. 6.14) is the best known, are characterized by premature fusion of the cranial sutures, often in association with hand and foot abnormalities such as syndactyly (fusion of the digits). Apert syndrome is caused by a mutation in one of the adjacent *FGFR2* residues in the peptides that link the second and third immunoglobulin loops (Fig. 6.13). In contrast mutations in the third immunoglobulin loop can cause either Crouzon syndrome, in which the limbs are normal, or Pfeiffer syndrome in which usually only the thumbs and big toes are abnormal.

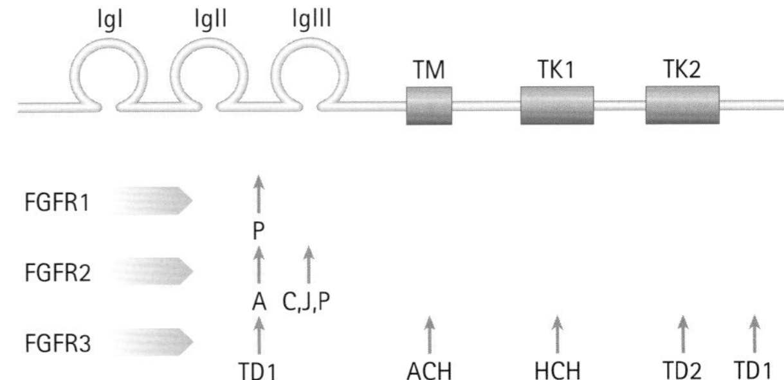


**Fig. 6.13**
Fibroblast growth factor receptor (*FGFR*) structure. Arrows indicate the location of mutations in the craniosynostosis syndromes and achondroplasia group of skeletal dysplasias. Ig = immunoglobulin-like domain; TM = transmembrane domain; TK = tyrosine kinase domain; P = Pfeiffer syndrome; A = Apert syndrome; C = Crouzon syndrome; J = Jackson–Weiss syndrome; TD = thanatophoric dysplasia; ACH = achondroplasia, HCH = hypochondroplasia.

**Table 6.5 Developmental disorders caused by mutations in fibroblast growth factor receptors**

| Gene | Chromosome | Syndrome |
|---|---|---|
| **Craniosynostosis syndromes** | | |
| *FGFR1* | 8p11 | Pfeiffer |
| *FGFR2* | 10q25 | Apert |
| | | Crouzon |
| | | Jackson–Weiss |
| | | Pfeiffer |
| *FGFR3* | 4p16 | Crouzon (with acanthosis nigricans) |
| **Skeletal dysplasias** | | |
| *FGFR3* | 4p16 | Achondroplasia |
| | | Hypochondroplasia |
| | | Thanatophoric dysplasia |

At present the relationship between genotype and phenotype in this group of disorders is not well understood.

Achondroplasia is the most commonly encountered form of genetic short stature (Fig. 6.15). The limbs show proximal ('rhizomelic') shortening and the head is enlarged with frontal bossing. Intelligence and life expectancy are entirely normal. Achondroplasia is almost always caused by a mutation in or close to the transmembrane (TM) domain of *FGFR3*. The common TM domain mutation leads to the replacement of a glycine amino acid residue by an arginine – an amino acid that is never normally found in cell membranes. This in turn appears to enhance dimerization of the protein that catalyses downstream signaling. Hypochondroplasia, a milder form of skeletal dysplasia with similar trunk and limb changes but normal head shape and size, is caused by mutations in the proximal tyrosine kinase domain (intracellular) of *FGFR3*. Finally, thanatophoric dysplasia, a much more severe and invariably lethal form of skeletal

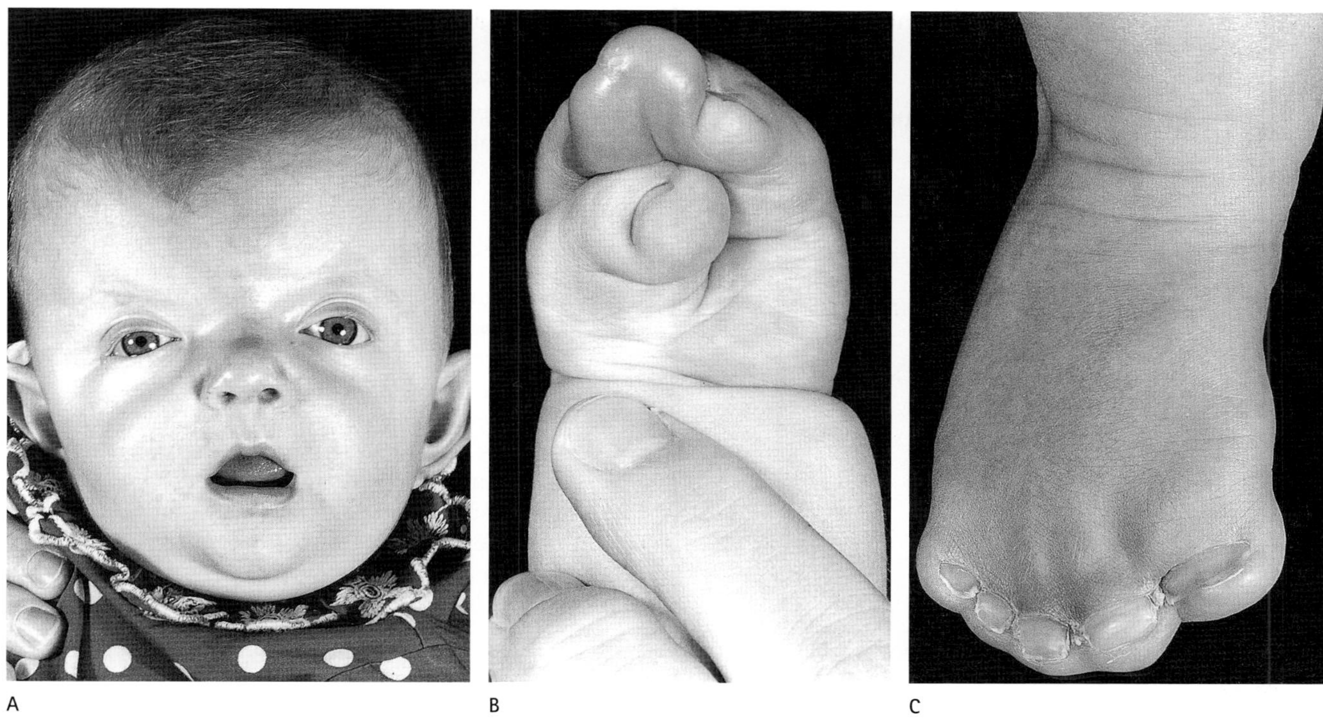


Fig. 6.14
Views of (A) the face, (B) the hand and (C) the foot of a child with Apert syndrome.

dysplasia, is caused by mutations in either the peptides linking the second and third immunoglobulin domains (extracellular) of *FGFR3*, or the distal *FGFR3* tyrosine kinase domain.

The mechanism by which these mutations cause skeletal shortening is not understood at present. The mutations cannot have loss-of-function effects as children with the Wolf–Hirschhorn syndrome (p. 274), due to chromosome microdeletions which include *FGFR3*, do not show similar skeletal abnormalities. Instead, the mutations probably involve a gain-of-function mediated by increased ligand binding or receptor activation.

## THE PHARYNGEAL ARCHES

The pharyngeal (or branchial) arches correspond to the gill system of lower vertebrates. Five (segmented) pharyngeal arches in man arise lateral to the structures of the head (Fig. 6.16) and each comprises cells from the three germ layers and the neural crest. From the *endoderm* will arise the lining of the pharynx, the thyroid and parathyroids, and the outer epidermal layer arises from the *ectoderm*. The musculature arises from the *mesoderm*, and bony structures from *neural crest* cells. Separating the arches are the pharyngeal clefts externally and the pharyngeal pouches internally, which have important destinies. Numbered from the rostral end, the first arch forms the jaw, the first cleft is destined to be the external auditory meatus, and the first pouch the middle ear apparatus. The second arch forms the hyoid apparatus, whilst the third pouch develops into the thymus, and the third and fourth pouches become the parathyroids. The arteries within the arches have important destinies too and, after remodelling, give rise to the aortic and pulmonary arterial systems.

The most well known, and probably most common, condition due to disturbed development of pharyngeal structures is DiGeorge syndrome (DGS), also known as velocardiofacial syndrome (VCFS), and well described even earlier by Sedlácková of Prague in 1955. This is described in more detail in Chapter 18 (p. 277) but it results from a submicroscopic chromosome deletion of band 22q11 with the loss of some 30 genes. Studies in mice (the equivalent, or *syntenic* region is on mouse chromosome 16) suggest that the most significant gene loss is that of *Tbx1*, strongly expressed throughout the pharyngeal apparatus. Heterozygous *Tbx1* knock-out mice show hypoplastic or absent fourth pharyngeal arch arteries, suggesting that *TBX1* in humans is the key. Indeed, mutations in this gene have now been found in some congenital heart abnormalities and it is possible that *TBX1* is the key gene for other elements of the phenotype. However, there are still unanswered questions in the whole DGS/VCFS/Sedlácková story.

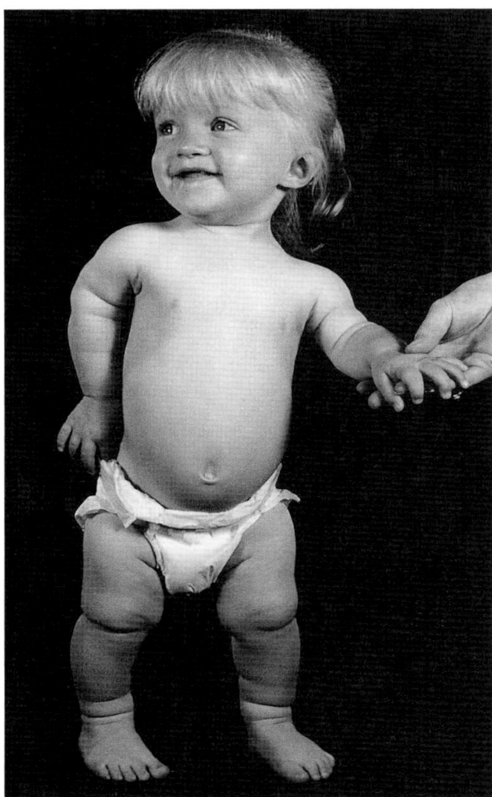

Fig. 6.15
A young child with achondroplasia.

Nevertheless, there are many examples of developmental genes in lower organisms whose homologs in man are linked to malformation syndromes, and in the first branchial arch one such is *EYA1*. In *Drosophila* this is the *eyes absent* gene, but in humans when mutated it causes branchio-oto-renal syndrome, consisting of branchial sinuses, external ear malformations and abnormal renal development.

## THE LIMB AS A DEVELOPMENTAL MODEL

Four main phases are recognized in limb development. These are (1) initiation, (2) specification, (3) tissue differentiation and (4) growth. Although none of these stages is fully understood, insight into the probable underlying mechanisms has been gleaned from the study of limb development in chicks and mice in particular.

### INITIATION AND SPECIFICATION

Limb bud formation is thought to be initiated at around 28 days by a member of the *FGF* family as illustrated by the development of an extra limb if *FGF1*, *-2* or *-4* is applied to the side of a developing chick embryo. During normal limb initiation *FGF8* transcripts have been identified in mesenchyme near the initiation site. *FGF8* expression is probably controlled by *HOX* genes, which determine limb type (i.e. forelimb or hindlimb) and number.

### TISSUE DIFFERENTIATION AND GROWTH

Once limb formation has been initiated a localized area of thickened ectoderm at the limb tip, known as the *apical ectodermal ridge* (AER), produces growth signals such as *FGF4* and *FGF8*, which maintain further growth and establish the proximo-distal axis (Fig. 6.17). Expression of the gene *p63* is crucial for sustaining the AER and, when this gene is mutated, split hand–foot (ectrodactyly) malformations result, often together with oral clefting and other anomalies. Signals from another localized area on the posterior margin of the developing bud, known as the *zone of polarizing activity* (ZPA), determine the antero-posterior axis. One of these signals is Sonic Hedgehog (*SHH*) (p. 86), which acts in concert with other *FGF* genes, *GLI3* and another gene family, which produces bone morphogenetic proteins (BMPs). Another morphogen, retinoic acid, is believed to play a major role at this stage in determining development at the anterior margin of the limb bud.

Subsequent development involves the activation of genes from the *HOXA* and *HOXD* clusters in the undifferentiated proliferating mesenchymal cells beneath the AER. This area is known as the progress zone. Cells in different regions express different combinations of *HOX* genes that determine local cell proliferation, adhesion and differentiation. Downstream targets of the *HOX* gene clusters remain to be identified. Other genes that clearly have a key role are those of the *T-box* family, already discussed, and *SALL4*, recently shown to be mutated in Okihiro syndrome (radial ray defects with abnormal eye movements due to congenital palsy affecting the sixth cranial nerve).

Fibroblast growth factors continue to be important during the later stages of limb development. In this context it becomes easy to understand why limb abnormalities are a feature of disorders such as Apert syndrome (see Fig. 6.14), in which mutations have been identified in the extracellular domains of *FGFR2*.

## DEVELOPMENTAL GENES AND CANCER

Several genes that play important roles in embryogenesis have also been shown to play a role in causing cancer (Table 6.6). This is not surprising, given that many developmental genes are expressed throughout life in

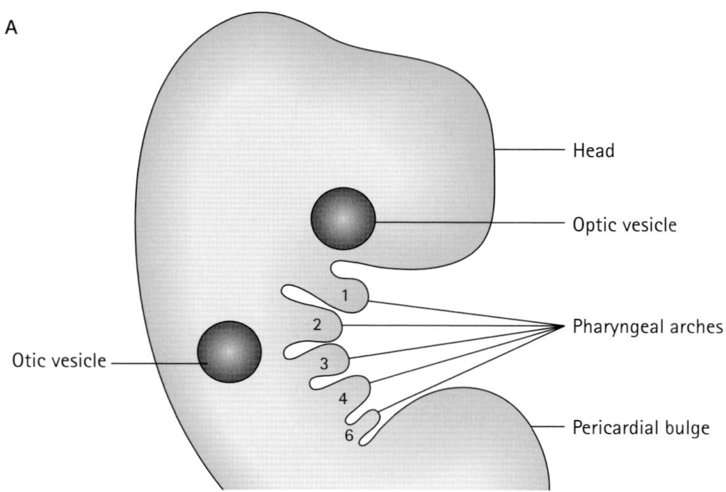


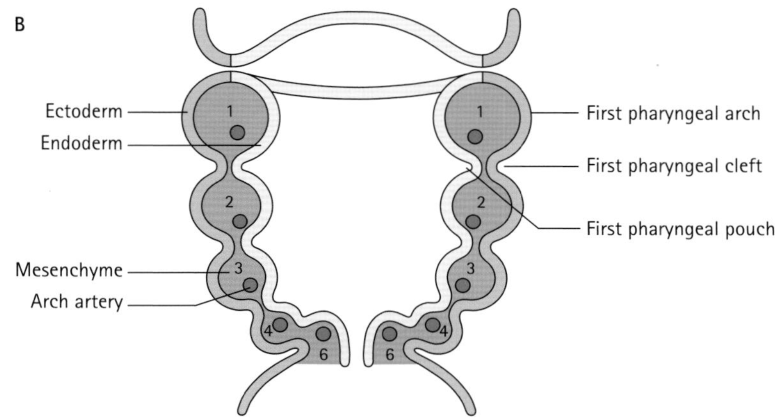


**Fig. 6.16**
The pharyngeal (or branchial) apparatus. The lateral view shows the five pharyngeal arches close to the embryonic head whilst the cross-section show the basic arrangement from which many head and neck structures, as well as the heart, develop. Humans and mice do not have arch no. 5.
(Redrawn from, Graham, A. & Smith, A. (2001) Patterning the pharyngeal arches. *Bioessays* **23**:54–61 with permission of Wiley-Liss Inc. a subsidiary of John Wiley & Sons, Inc.)

processes such as signal transduction and signal transcription (p. 207). It has been shown that several different mechanisms can account for the phenotypic diversity demonstrated by these so-called teratogenes.

## GAIN-OF-FUNCTION VS LOSS-OF-FUNCTION MUTATIONS

Mention has already been made of the causal role of the *RET* proto-oncogene in familial Hirschsprung, disease as well as in both inherited and sporadic thyroid cancer (pp. 92, 219). The protein product encoded by *RET* consists of three main domains: an extracellular domain that binds to a glial cell line-derived neurotrophil factor, a transmembrane domain, and an intracellular tyrosine kinase domain that activates signal transduction (Fig. 6.18). Mutations which cause loss-of-function result in Hirschsprung disease. These include whole gene deletions, small intragenic deletions, nonsense mutations and splicing mutations leading to synthesis of a truncated protein.

In contrast, mutations which cause a gain-of-function effect result in either type 2A or type 2B multiple endocrine neoplasia (MEN) (p. 219). These disorders are characterized by a high incidence of medullary thyroid carcinoma and pheochromocytoma. The activating mutations which cause MEN 2A are clustered in five cysteine residues in the extracellular domain. MEN 2B, which differs from MEN 2A in that affected individuals are tall and thin, is usually caused by a unique mutation in a methionine residue in the tyrosine kinase domain.

## SOMATIC REARRANGEMENTS

Activation of the *RET* proto-oncogene can occur by a different mechanism whereby the genomic region

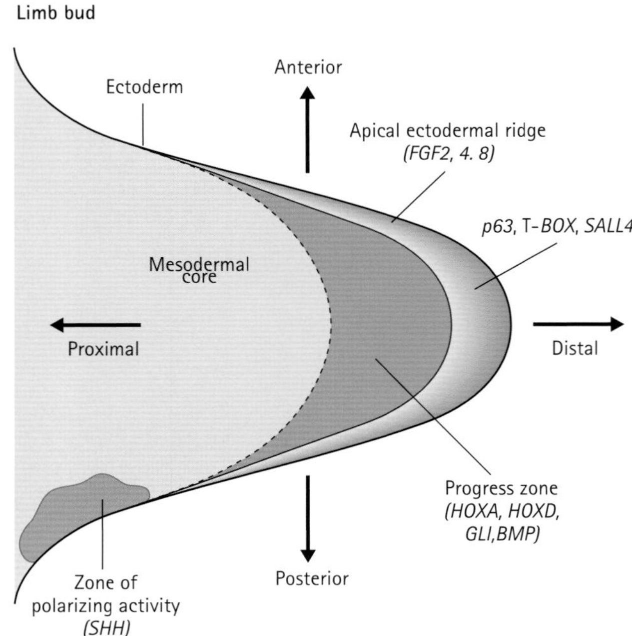


**Fig. 6.17**
Simplified representation of vertebrate limb development.

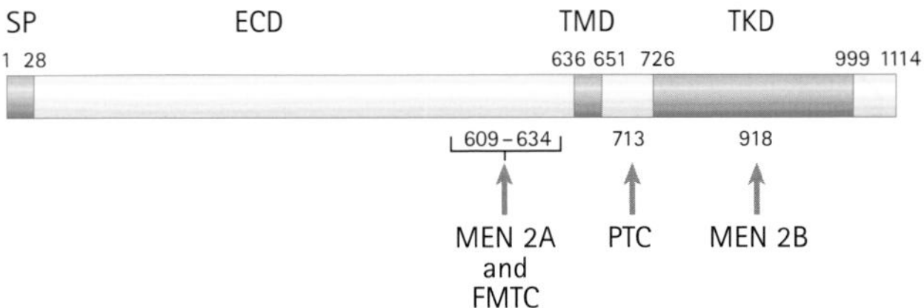


**Fig. 6.18**
The RET proto-oncogene. The most common mutation sites in the different clinical entities associated with *RET* are indicated. Numbers refer to amino acid residues. SP = signal peptide; ECD = extracellular domain; TMD = transmembrane domain; TKD = tyrosine kinase domain; MEN = multiple endocrine adenomatosis; FMTC = familial medullary thyroid carcinoma. The arrow above PTC (= papillary thyroid carcinoma) indicates the somatic rearrangement site for the formation of new hybrid forms of *RET*. (Adapted from Pasini B, Ceccherini I, Romeo G 1996 RET mutations in human disease. Trends in Genetics 12: 138-144.)

**Table 6.6 Genes which can cause both developmental anomalies and cancer**

| Gene | Chromosome | Developmental anomaly | Cancer |
|---|---|---|---|
| *PAX3* | 2q35 | Waardenburg syndrome type 1 | Alveolar rhabdomyosarcoma |
| *KIT* | 4q12 | Piebaldism | Mast cell leukemia |
| *PTCH* (Patched) | 9q22 | Gorlin syndrome | Basal cell carcinoma |
| *RET* | 10q11 | Hirschsprung disease thyroid carcinoma | MEN 2A, MEN 2B, |
| *WT1* | 11p13 | Denys–Drash syndrome | Wilms' tumour |

encoding the intracellular domain is juxtaposed to one of several activating genes that are normally preferentially expressed in the thyroid gland. The newly formed hybrid *RET* gene produces a novel protein whose activity is not ligand dependent. These somatic rearrangements are found in a high proportion of papillary thyroid carcinomas, which show a particularly high incidence in children who were exposed to radiation following the Chernobyl accident in 1986.

*PAX3* provides another example of a developmental gene that can cause cancer if it is fused to new DNA sequences. A specific translocation between chromosomes 2 and 13 that results in a new chimeric transcript leads to the development in children of a rare lung tumor called alveolar rhabdomyosarcoma.

## POSITIONAL EFFECTS AND DEVELOPMENTAL GENES

The discovery of a chromosomal abnormality, such as a translocation or inversion, in a person with a single-gene developmental syndrome provides a strong indication of the probable position of the disease locus as it is likely that one of the break-points involved in the rearrangement will have disrupted the relevant gene. However, in a few instances it has emerged that the chromosome break-point actually lies approximately 10–1000 kb upstream or downstream of the gene that is subsequently shown to be mutated in other affected individuals (Table 6.7). The probable explanation is that the break-point has separated the coding part of the gene from contiguous regulatory elements (p. 22). These observations have created obvious difficulties for those carrying out the original research when the putative disease gene in translocation families has been found not to contain an intragenic mutation.

## HYDATIDIFORM MOLES

Occasionally conception results in an abnormal pregnancy in which the placenta consists of a proliferating disorganized mass known as a hydatidiform mole. These changes can be either partial or complete (Table 6.8).

**Table 6.7 Developmental genes which show a position effect**

| Gene | Chromosome | Developmental anomaly |
|---|---|---|
| *GLI3* | 7p13 | Greig cephalopolysyndactyly |
| *SHH* | 7q36 | Holoprosencephaly |
| *PAX6* | 11p13 | Aniridia |
| *SOX9* | 17q24 | Campomelic dysplasia |

**Table 6.8 Characteristics of partial and complete hydatidiform moles**

| | Partial | Complete |
|---|---|---|
| Number of chromosomes | 69 | 46 |
| Parental origin of chromosomes | 23 — maternal<br>46 — paternal | All 46 paternal |
| Fetus present | Yes — but not viable | No |
| Malignant potential | Very low | High |

## PARTIAL HYDATIDIFORM MOLE

Chromosome analysis of tissue from partial moles reveals the presence of 69 chromosomes, i.e. triploidy (p. 280). Using DNA polymorphisms it has been shown that 46 of these chromosomes are always derived from the father, with the remaining 23 being maternal in origin. This doubling of the normal haploid paternal contribution of 23 chromosomes can be due to either fertilization by two sperm, which is known as *dispermy*, or to duplication of a haploid sperm chromosome set by a process known as *endoreduplication*.

In these pregnancies the fetus rarely if ever survives to term. Triploid conceptions only survive to term if the additional chromosome complement is maternally derived, in which cases partial hydatidiform changes do not occur. Even in these situations it is extremely uncommon for a triploid infant to survive for more than a few hours or days after birth.

## COMPLETE HYDATIDIFORM MOLE

Complete moles have only 46 chromosomes, but these are exclusively paternal in origin. A complete mole is caused by fertilization of an empty ovum either by two sperm or by a single sperm that undergoes endoreduplication. The opposite situation of an egg undergoing development without being fertilized by a sperm, a process known as parthenogenesis, occurs in lower animals such as arthropods but has been reported in a human on only one occasion, this being in the form of chimeric fusion with another cell line that had a normal male-derived complement.

The main importance of complete moles lies in their potential to undergo malignant change into invasive choriocarcinoma. This can usually be treated very successfully by chemotherapy, but if untreated the outcome can be fatal. Malignant change is seen only very rarely with partial moles.

## DIFFERENT PARENTAL EXPRESSION IN TROPHOBLAST AND EMBRYOBLAST

Studies in mice have shown that when all nuclear genes in a zygote are derived from the father, the embryo fails to develop, whereas trophoblast development proceeds relatively unimpaired. In contrast, if all of the nuclear genes are maternal in origin, the embryo develops normally but extra-embryonic development is very poor. The observations outlined above on partial and complete moles indicate that a comparable situation exists in humans, with paternally derived genes being essential for trophoblast development and maternally derived genes being necessary for early embryonic development. These phenomena are relevant to the concept of genomic imprinting (p. 118).

# SEXUAL DIFFERENTIATION AND DETERMINATION

The sex of an individual is determined by the X and Y chromosomes (p. 33). The presence of an intact Y chromosome leads to maleness regardless of the number of X chromosomes present. Absence of a Y chromosome results in female development.

Although the sex chromosomes are present from conception, differentiation into a phenotypic male or female does not commence until approximately 6 weeks. Up to this point both the müllerian and wolffian duct systems are present and the embryonic gonads, although consisting of cortex and medulla, are still undifferentiated. From 6 weeks onwards the embryo develops into a female unless the testis-determining factor initiates a sequence of events that prompt the undifferentiated gonads to develop into testes.

## THE TESTIS-DETERMINING FACTOR – *SRY*

In 1990 it was shown that the testis-determining factor or gene is located on the short arm of the Y chromosome close to the pseudoautosomal region (p. 114). This gene is now referred to as being located in the sex-determining region of the Y chromosome (*SRY*). It consists of a single exon that encodes a protein of 204 amino acids which include a 79 amino acid HMG box (p. 87), indicating that it is likely to be a transcription regulator.

Evidence that the SRY gene is the primary factor that determines maleness comes from several observations:

1. *SRY* sequences are present in XX males. These are infertile phenotypic males who appear to have a normal 46,XX karyotype.
2. Mutations or deletions in the SRY sequences are found in many XY females. These are infertile phenotypic females who are found to have a 46,XY karyotype.
3. In mice the *SRY* gene is expressed only in the male gonadal ridge as the testes are developing in the embryo.
4. Transgenic XX mice that have a tiny portion of the Y chromosome containing the *SRY* region develop into males with testes.

Considered from the evolutionary point of view and for the maintenance of the species, it would clearly be impossible for the *SRY* gene to be involved in crossing over with the X chromosome during meiosis I. Hence *SRY* has to lie outside the pseudoautosomal region.

However, there has to be pairing of the X and Y chromosomes, as otherwise they would segregate together into the same gamete during, on average, 50% of meioses. Nature's compromise has been to ensure that only a small portion of the X and Y chromosomes are homologous and therefore pair during meiosis I. Unfortunately the close proximity of *SRY* to the pseudoautosomal region means that, occasionally, it can get caught up in a recombinational event. This almost certainly accounts for the majority of XX males, in whom molecular and FISH studies show evidence of Y chromosome sequences at the distal end of one X chromosome short arm (Fig. 18.22, p. 286).

Expression of *SRY* triggers off a series of events, which involves other genes such as *SOX9*, leading to the medulla of the undifferentiated gonad developing into a testis, in which the Leydig cells begin to produce testosterone (Fig. 6.19). This leads to stimulation of the wolffian ducts, which form the male internal genitalia, and also to masculinization of the external genitalia. This latter step

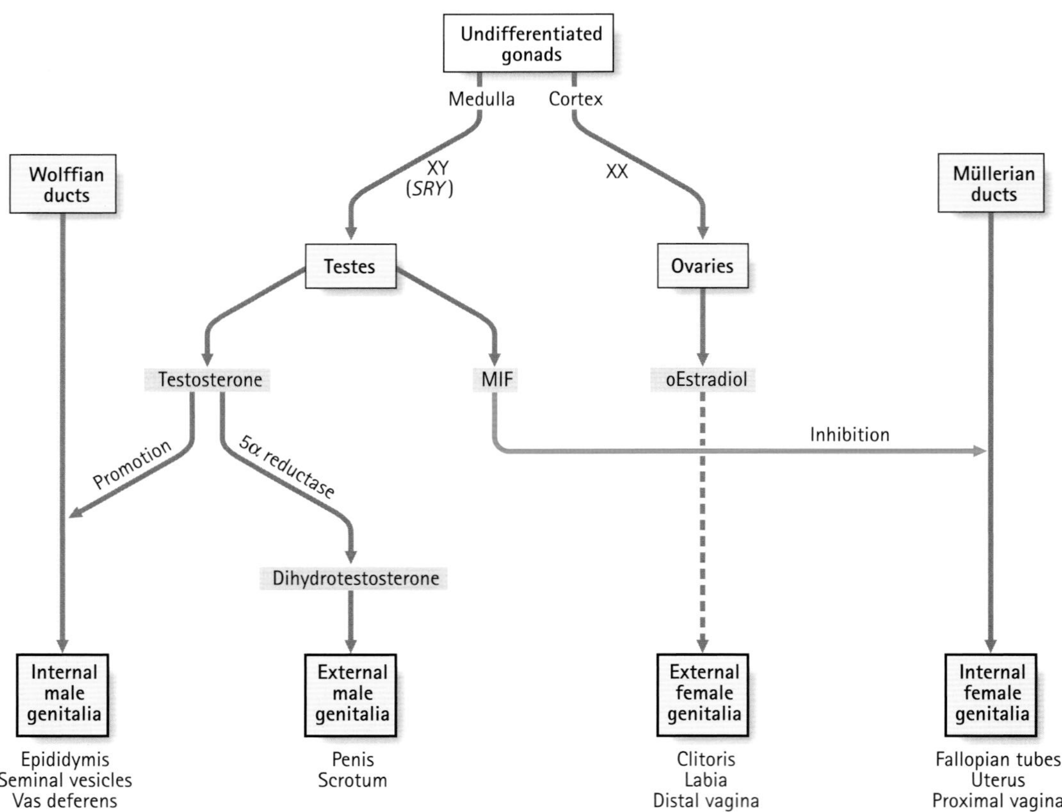


**Fig. 6.19**
Summary of the main events involved in sex determination. *SRY* = sex determining region of the Y chromosome; MIF = müllerian inhibitory factor.

is mediated by dihydrotestosterone, which is produced from testosterone by the action of 5α-reductase (p. 169, 286). The Sertoli cells in the testes produce a hormone known as müllerian inhibitory factor that causes the müllerian duct system to regress.

In the absence of normal *SRY* expression, the cortex of the undifferentiated gonad develops into an ovary. The müllerian duct forms the internal genitalia. The external genitalia fail to fuse and grow as in the male, and instead evolve into normal female external genitalia. This normal process of female development is sometimes referred to rather chauvinistically as the 'default' pathway. Without the stimulating effects of testosterone, the wolffian duct system regresses.

Normally sexual differentiation is complete by 12–14 weeks gestation, although the testes do not migrate into the scrotum until late pregnancy. Abnormalities of sexual differentiation are uncommon but they are important causes of infertility and sexual ambiguity and are considered further in Chapter 18.

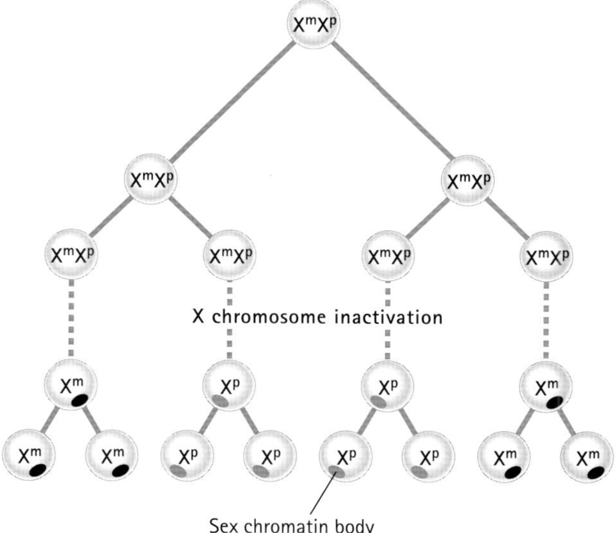


Fig. 6.20
X chromosome inactivation during development. The maternally and paternally derived X chromosomes are represented as Xm and Xp, respectively.

## X CHROMOSOME INACTIVATION

As techniques were developed for studying chromosomes it was noted that in female mice one of the X chromosomes often differed from all other chromosomes in the extent to which it was condensed. In 1961 Dr Mary Lyon proposed that this heteropyknotic X chromosome was inactivated, citing as evidence her observations on the mosaic pattern of skin coloration seen in mice known to be heterozygous for X-linked genes that influence coat color. Subsequent events have confirmed the validity of Dr Lyon's hypothesis, and in recognition of her foresight the process of X-inactivation is often referred to as lyonization.

The process of X-inactivation occurs early in development at around 15–16 days gestation, when the embryo consists of approximately 5000 cells. Normally either of the two X chromosomes can be inactivated in any particular cell. Thereafter the same X chromosome is inactivated in all daughter cells (Fig. 6.20). This differs from marsupials, in which the paternally derived X chromosome is consistently inactivated.

The inactive X chromosome exists in a condensed form during interphase when it appears as a darkly staining mass of chromatin known as the sex chromatin or Barr body. During mitosis the inactive X chromosome is late replicating. Laboratory techniques have been developed for distinguishing which X chromosome is late replicating in each cell. This can be useful for confirming that one of the X chromosomes is structurally abnormal, as usually an abnormal X chromosome will be preferentially inactivated, or more correctly, only those hematopoietic stem cells in which the normal X chromosome is active will have survived. Apparent non-random inactivation also occurs if one of the X chromosomes is involved in a translocation with an autosome (p. 112).

The process of X-inactivation is achieved by differential methylation (a form of imprinting – p. 118) and is initiated by a gene, *XIST* ('X inactivation specific transcript'), which maps within the X-inactivation centre at Xq13.3. *XIST* is expressed only from the inactive X chromosome and produces RNA that spreads an inactivation methylation signal up and down the X chromosome on which it is located. This differential methylation of the X chromosomes has been utilized in carrier detection studies for X-linked immunodeficiency diseases, e.g. Wiskott–Aldrich syndrome, using methylation-sensitive restriction enzymes (p. 198). Not all of the X chromosome is inactivated. Genes in the pseudoautosomal region at the tip of the short arm remain active, as do other loci elsewhere on the short and long arms, such as *XIST*. If all loci on the X chromosome were inactivated then all women would have the clinical features of Turner syndrome and the presence of more than one X chromosome in a male, e.g. 47,XXY or two in a female, e.g. 47,XXX, would have no phenotypic effects. There are, in fact, quite characteristic clinical features in these disorders (p. 281).

X chromosome inactivation provides a satisfactory explanation for several observations:

1. Barr bodies – In men and women with more than one X chromosome, the number of Barr bodies (p. 43) visible at interphase is always one less than the total number of X chromosomes. For example, men with a 47,XXY karyotype have a single Barr body, whereas

women with a 47,XXX karyotype have two Barr bodies.

2. Dosage compensation – Women with two normal X chromosomes have the same blood levels of X chromosome protein products, such as factor VIII, as normal men, who of course have only one X chromosome. An exception to this phenomenon of dosage compensation is the level of steroid sulphatase in blood, which is increased in women compared to men. Not surprisingly it has been shown that the locus for steroid sulphatase, deficiency of which causes a skin disorder known as ichthyosis, is in the pseudo-autosomal region.
3. Mosaicism – Mice which are heterozygous for X-linked genes affecting coat color show mosaicism with alternating patches of different color rather than a homogeneous pattern. This is consistent with patches of skin being clonal in origin in that they are derived from a single stem cell in which one or other of the X chromosomes is expressed but not both. Thus, each patch reflects which of the X chromosomes was active in the original stem cell. Similar effects are seen in tissues of clonal origin in women who are heterozygous for X-linked mutations such as ocular albinism (Fig. 6.21). Other evidence confirming that X-inactivation leads to mosaicism in females comes from studies of the expression of the enzyme glucose-6-phosphate dehydrogenase (p. 183) in clones of cultured fibroblasts from women heterozygous for variants of this gene. Each clone is derived from a single cell and expresses one of the variants but never both. The clonal origin of tumors can be confirmed in women who are heterozygous for such variants by demonstration of expression of only one of the variants in the tumor.
4. Problems of carrier detection – Carrier detection for X-linked recessive disorders based only on examination of clinical features or on indirect assay of gene function is notoriously difficult and unreliable. Cells in which the X chromosome with the normal gene is active can have a selective advantage, or they can correct the defect in closely adjacent cells in which the X chromosome with the mutant gene is active. For example, only a proportion of carriers of Duchenne muscular dystrophy (DMD) show evidence of muscle damage as indicated by measurement of creatine kinase in serum (p. 316). Similarly, distorted very long chain fatty acid (VLCFA) ratios are seen in many, but not all, carriers of X-linked adrenoleukodystrophy (XLALD). Fortunately, the development of molecular methods for carrier detection in X-linked disorders can bypass these problems as techniques such as Southern blotting are not influenced by methylation unless methylation-sensitive restriction enzymes are used. When methylation-sensitive enzymes are used this can in fact provide a means of carrier detection if there has been strong selection against the cell line in which the mutant-bearing X chromosome is active (Fig. 6.22).

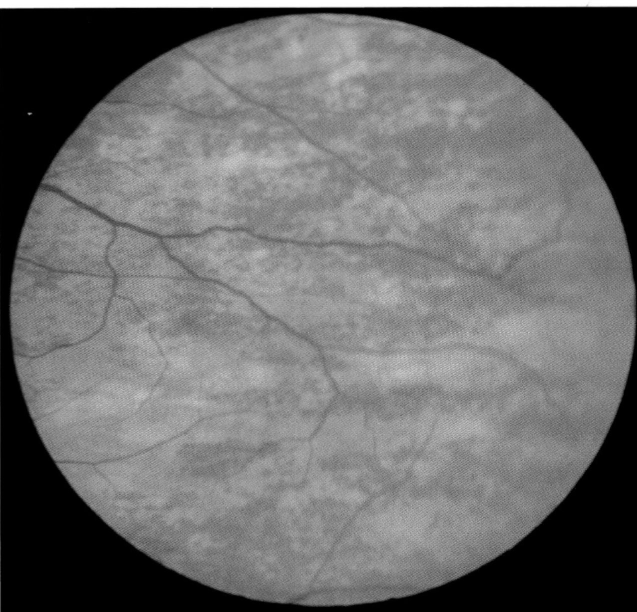

**Fig. 6.21**
The fundus of a carrier of X-linked ocular albinism showing a mosaic pattern of retinal pigmentation. (Courtesy of Mr S. J. Charles, The Royal Eye Hospital, Manchester.)

5. Manifesting heterozygotes – Occasionally a woman is encountered who shows mild or even full expression of an X-linked recessive disorder, e.g. DMD or XLALD. One possible explanation is that she is a manifesting heterozygote in whom, by chance, the X chromosome bearing the normal gene has been inactivated in significantly more than 50% of relevant cells. This is referred to as skewed X-inactivation (p. 112). There is some evidence that X chromosome inactivation can itself be under genetic control, as families with several manifesting carriers of disorders such as Duchenne muscular dystrophy and Fabry disease have been reported. In a few families marked skewing of X-inactivation in several females has been shown to be associated with an underlying mutation in *XIST*.
6. The 46,Xr(X) phenotype – A 46,Xr(X) karyotype is found in some women with typical Turner syndrome features. This is consistent with the ring lacking X sequences, which are normally not inactivated and which are needed for a normal phenotype. Curiously a few 46,Xr(X) women have congenital abnormalities and show mental retardation. In these women it has been shown that *XIST* is not expressed on the ring X, so that it is likely that their relatively severe phenotype is caused by functional disomy for those genes present on their ring X chromosome. Other studies in Turner

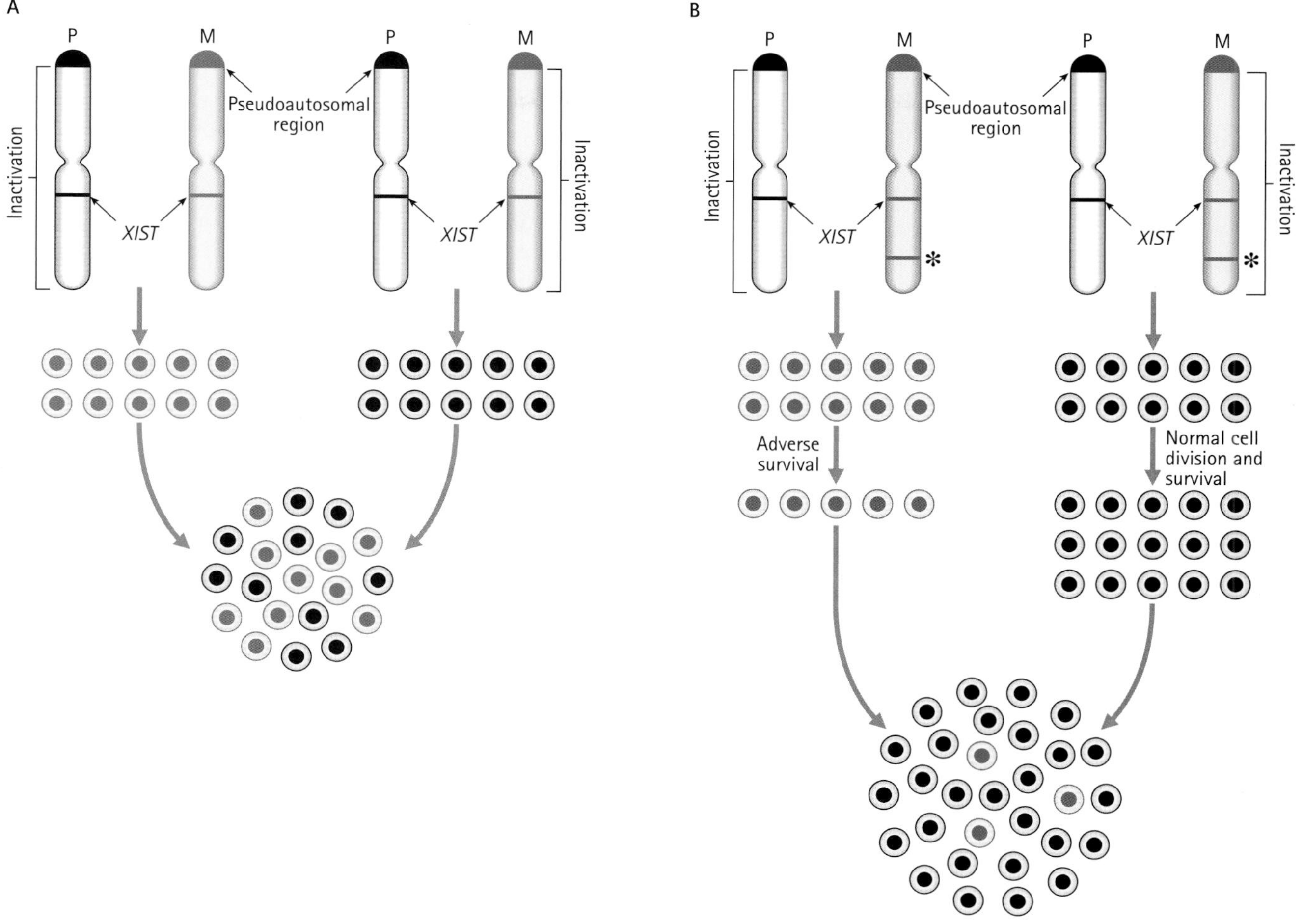


Fig. 6.22
(A) Normal X chromosome inactivation resulting in survival of roughly equal numbers of cells with the paternally (P) and maternally (M) derived X chromosome active. (B) In this situation the maternally derived X chromosome has a mutation* which results in selection against those cells in which it is active. Thus surviving cells show preferential expression of the paternally derived X chromosome.

syndrome, this time pure 45,X cases, have shown some differences in social cognition and higher-order executive function skills according to whether their X chromosome was paternal or maternal in origin. Cases with a *paternal* X scored better, from which the existence of a locus for social cognition on the X chromosome can be postulated. If such a locus is not expressed from the maternal X, this could provide at least part of the explanation for the excess difficulty with language and social skills observed in 46,XY males, since their X is always maternal in origin.

## TWINNING

Twinning occurs frequently in humans, although the incidence in early pregnancy as diagnosed by ultrasonography is greater than at delivery, presumably as a result of death and subsequent resorption of one of the twins in a proportion of twin pregnancies. The overall incidence of twinning in the UK is approximately 1 in 80 of all pregnancies, so that approximately 1 in 40 (i.e. 2 out of 80) of all individuals is a twin. However, the spontaneous twinning rate varies enormously, from approximately 1 in 125 pregnancies in Japan to 1 in 22 in Nigeria.

Twins can be identical or non-identical – *monozygotic* (MZ) (uniovular) or *dizygotic* (DZ) (biovular) – depending on whether they originate from a single conception or from two separate conceptions (Table 6.9). Comparison of the incidence of disease in identical and non-identical twins reared apart and together can provide information about the relative contributions of genetics and environment to the cause of many of the common diseases of adult life, as discussed in Chapter 15.

**Table 6.9 Summary of differences between monozygotic and dizygotic twins**

| | Monozygotic | Dizygotic |
|---|---|---|
| *Origin* | Single egg fertilized | Two eggs, each fertilized by a single sperm |
| *Incidence* | 1 in 300 pregnancies | Varies from 1 in 100 to 1 in 500 pregnancies |
| *Proportion of genes in common* | 100% | 50% (on average) |
| *Fetal membranes* | 70% monochorionic and diamniotic 30% dichorionic and diamniotic, rarely monochorionic and monoamniotic | Always dichorionic and diamniotic |

## MONOZYGOTIC TWINS

MZ twinning occurs in about 1 in 300 births in all populations that have been studied. MZ twins originate from a single egg that has been fertilized by a single sperm. A very early division, occurring in the zygote before separation of the cells that make the chorion, results in dichorionic twins. Division during the blastocyst stage from days 3 to 7 results in monochorionic diamniotic twins. Division after the first week leads to monoamniotic twins. However, the reason(s) why MZ twinning occurs at all in humans is not clear. As an event, the incidence is increased 2–5 times in babies born by in-vitro fertilization. There are rare cases of familial MZ twinning that can be transmitted by the father or mother, suggesting a single-gene defect that predisposes to the phenomenon.

MZ twins are genetically identical, although occasionally they can be discordant for structural birth defects that may be linked to the twinning process itself – especially those anomalies affecting midline structures. There is probably a two- to three-fold increased risk of congenital anomalies in MZ twins, i.e. 5–10% of MZ twins overall. Discordance for single-gene traits or chromosome abnormalities may occur because of a post-zygotic somatic mutation or non-disjunction, respectively. One example of the latter is the rare occurrence of MZ twins of different sex – one 46,XY and the other 45,X. Curiously, MZ female twins can show quite striking discrepancy in X chromosome inactivation. There are several reports of female MZ twin pairs only one of whom is affected with an X-linked recessive condition such as Duchenne muscular dystrophy or hemophilia. In these rare examples both twins have the mutation and both show non-random X-inactivation but in opposite directions.

Very late division occurring more than 14 days after conception can result in conjoined twins. This occurs in about 1 in 100 000 pregnancies, or approximately 1 in 400 MZ twin births. Conjoined twins are sometimes referred to as Siamese, in memory of Chang and Eng, who were born in 1811 in Thailand, then known as Siam, joined at the upper abdomen. Chang and Eng made a successful living out of showing themselves at traveling shows in the USA, where they settled and married. Somehow they both managed to have large numbers of children despite remaining conjoined until they died within a few hours of each other at the age of 61 years. The sex ratio for conjoined twins is markedly distorted, with about 75% being female. The later the twinning event, the more distorted the sex ratio in favor of females, and X-inactivation studies suggest that MZ twinning occurs around the time of X-inactivation, a phenomenon limited to female zygotes of course.

## DIZYGOTIC TWINS

DZ twins result from the fertilization of two ova by two sperm and are no more closely related genetically than brothers and sisters, i.e. they share, on average, 50% of the same genes from each parent. Hence they are sometimes referred to as *fraternal twins*. DZ twins are dichorionic and diamniotic, although they can have a single fused placenta if implantation occurs at closely adjacent sites. The incidence varies from approximately 1 in 100 deliveries in Afro-Caribbean populations to 1 in 500 deliveries in Asia and Japan. In Western European Caucasians the incidence is approximately 1 in 120 deliveries and has been observed to fall with both urbanization and starvation, but increases in relation to the amount of seasonal light – for example, in northern Scandanavia during the summer. Factors that convey an increased risk for DZ twinning are increased maternal age, a positive family history (due to a familial increase in FSH levels) and the use of ovulation-inducing drugs such as clomiphene.

## DETERMINATION OF ZYGOSITY

This used to be established by study of the placenta and membranes and also by analysis of polymorphic systems such as the blood groups, the HLA antigens and other biochemical markers. Now zygosity is most reliably determined using highly polymorphic molecular markers (p. 72).

## FURTHER READING


Dreyer S D, Zhou G, Lee B 1998 The long and the short of it: developmental genetics of the skeletal dysplasias. Clin Genet 54: 464–473

*A short review of developmental genes known to cause abnormal skeletal development.*

Hall J G 2003 Twinning. Lancet 362:735–743

Hammerschmidt M, Brook A, McMahon A P 1997 The world according to hedgehog. Trends Genet 13: 14–20

*A comprehensive account of the role of the hedgehog gene family in early vertebrate development.*

Kleinjan D J, van Heyningen V 1998 Position effect in human genetic disease. Hum Mol Genet 7: 1611–1618

*An outline of the various theories and mechanisms which have been proposed to account for observed positional effects in developmental gene expression.*

Kornak U, Mundlos S 2003 Genetic disorders of the skeleton: a developmental approach. Am J Hum Genet 73: 447–474

*An up-to-date summary of current knowledge.*

Lacombe D 1999 Transcription factors in dysmorphology. Clin Genet 55: 137–143

*As the title indicates a description of the role of transcription regulatory genes in causing multiple congenital abnormality syndromes.*

Lindor N M, Ney J A, Gaffey T A et al 1992 A genetic review of complete and partial hydatidiform moles and nonmolar triploidy. Mayo Clin Proc 67: 791–799

*A detailed review of the mechanisms that can lead to the formation of hydatidiform moles.*

Lyon M F 1961 Gene action in the X chromosome of the mouse (*Mus musculus L*). Nature 190: 372–373

*The original proposal of X-inactivation. Very short and easily understood.*

Manouvrier-Hanu S, Holder-Espinasse M, Lyonnet S 1999 Genetics of limb anomalies in humans. Trends Genet 15: 409–417

*A detailed and well illustrated account of vertebrate limb development.*

Muenke M, Schell U 1995 Fibroblast-growth-factor receptor mutations in human skeletal disorders. Trends Genet 11: 308–313

*A concise review of the functions of the fibroblast growth factors and their receptors.*

Muragaki Y, Mundlos S, Upton J, Olsen B R 1996 Altered growth and branching patterns in synpolydactyly caused by mutations in HOXD13. Science 272: 548–551

*The long-awaited first report of a human malformation caused by a mutation in a* HOX *gene.*

Saga Y, Takeda H 2001 The making of the somite: molecular events in vertebrate segmentation. Nature Rev Genet 2: 835–844

*An excellent review of somite development.*

Tickle C (ed) 2003 Patterning in vertebrate development. Oxford University Press, Oxford

*A detailed, multi-author collection handling very early development, mainly from molecular perspectives.*


## ELEMENTS

1. Several developmental gene families first identified in *Drosophila* and mice also play important roles in human morphogenesis. These include segment polarity genes, homeobox containing genes (*HOX*), and paired-box containing genes (*PAX*). Many of these genes act as transcription factors that regulate sequential developmental processes. Others are important in cell signaling. It has recently been shown that several human malformations and multiple malformation syndromes are caused by mutations in these genes.

2. For normal development a haploid chromosome set must be inherited from each parent. A paternal diploid complement results in a complete hydatidiform mole if there is no maternal contribution, and in triploidy with a partial hydatidiform mole if there is a haploid maternal contribution.

3. A testis-determining factor on the Y chromosome, known as *SRY*, stimulates the undifferentiated gonads to develop into testes. This, in turn, sets off a series of events leading to male development. In the absence of *SRY* expression the human embryo develops into a female.

4. In females one of the X chromosomes is inactivated in each cell in early embryogenesis. This can be either the maternally derived or the paternally derived X chromosome. Thereafter, in all daughter cells the same X chromosome is inactivated. This process, known as lyonization, explains the presence of the Barr body in female nuclei and achieves dosage compensation of X chromosome gene products in males and females.

5. Twins can be monozygotic (identical) or dizygotic (fraternal). Monozygotic twins originate from a single zygote that divides into two during the first 2 weeks after conception. Monozygotic twins are genetically identical. Dizygotic twins originate from two separate zygotes and are no more genetically alike than brothers and sisters.

CHAPTER

# 7 Patterns of inheritance

## FAMILY STUDIES

If we wish to investigate whether a particular trait or disorder in humans is genetic and hereditary, we usually have to rely either on observation of the way in which it is transmitted from one generation to another, or on study of its frequency among relatives.

An important reason for studying the pattern of inheritance of disorders within families is to enable advice to be given to members of a family regarding the likelihood of their developing it or passing it on to their children, i.e. *genetic counseling* (Ch. 17). Taking a family history can, in itself, provide a diagnosis. For example, a child could come to the attention of a doctor having a fracture after a seemingly trivial injury. A family history of relatives with a similar tendency to fracture and blue sclerae would suggest the diagnosis of osteogenesis imperfecta. In the absence of a positive family history other diagnoses would have to be considered.

## PEDIGREE DRAWING AND TERMINOLOGY

A family tree is a shorthand system of recording the pertinent information about a family. It usually begins with the person through whom the family came to the attention of the investigator. This person is referred to as the *index* case, *proband* or *propositus*, or if female, the *proposita*. The position of the proband in the family tree is indicated by an arrow. Information about the health of the rest of the family is obtained by asking direct questions about brothers, sisters, parents and maternal and paternal relatives, with the relevant information about the sex of the individual, affection status and relationship to other individuals being carefully recorded in the pedigree chart (Fig. 7.1). Attention to detail can be crucial because patients do not always appreciate the important difference between siblings and *half*-siblings, or might overlook the fact, for example, that the child of a brother who is at risk of Huntington disease is actually a *step*-child and not a biological relative.

## MENDELIAN INHERITANCE

Over 11 000 traits or disorders in humans exhibit single gene *unifactorial* or *Mendelian inheritance*. However, characteristics such as height, and many common familial disorders, such as diabetes, hypertension, etc., do not usually follow a simple pattern of Mendelian inheritance (Ch. 9).

A trait or disorder that is determined by a gene on an autosome is said to show *autosomal inheritance*, whereas a trait or disorder determined by a gene on one of the sex chromosomes is said to show *sex-linked inheritance*.

## AUTOSOMAL DOMINANT INHERITANCE

An autosomal dominant trait is one which manifests in the heterozygous state, i.e. in a person possessing both an abnormal or mutant allele and the normal allele. It is often possible to trace a dominantly inherited trait or disorder through many generations of a family (Fig. 7.2). In South Africa the vast majority of cases of porphyria variegata can be traced back to one couple in the late seventeenth century. This is a metabolic disorder characterized by skin blistering through increased sensitivity to sunlight and the excretion of urine that becomes 'port wine' colored on standing as a result of the presence of porphyrins (p. 175) (Fig. 7.3). This pattern of inheritance is sometimes referred to as 'vertical' transmission and is confirmed when male–male (i.e. father to son) transmission is observed.

### Genetic risks

Each gamete from an individual with a dominant trait or disorder will contain either the normal allele or the mutant allele. If we represent the dominant mutant allele as 'A' and the recessive normal allele as 'a', then the various possible combinations of the gametes can be represented in a Punnett's square (Fig. 7.4). Any child born to a person affected with a dominant trait or disorder has a 1 in 2 (50%) chance of inheriting it and being similarly affected.

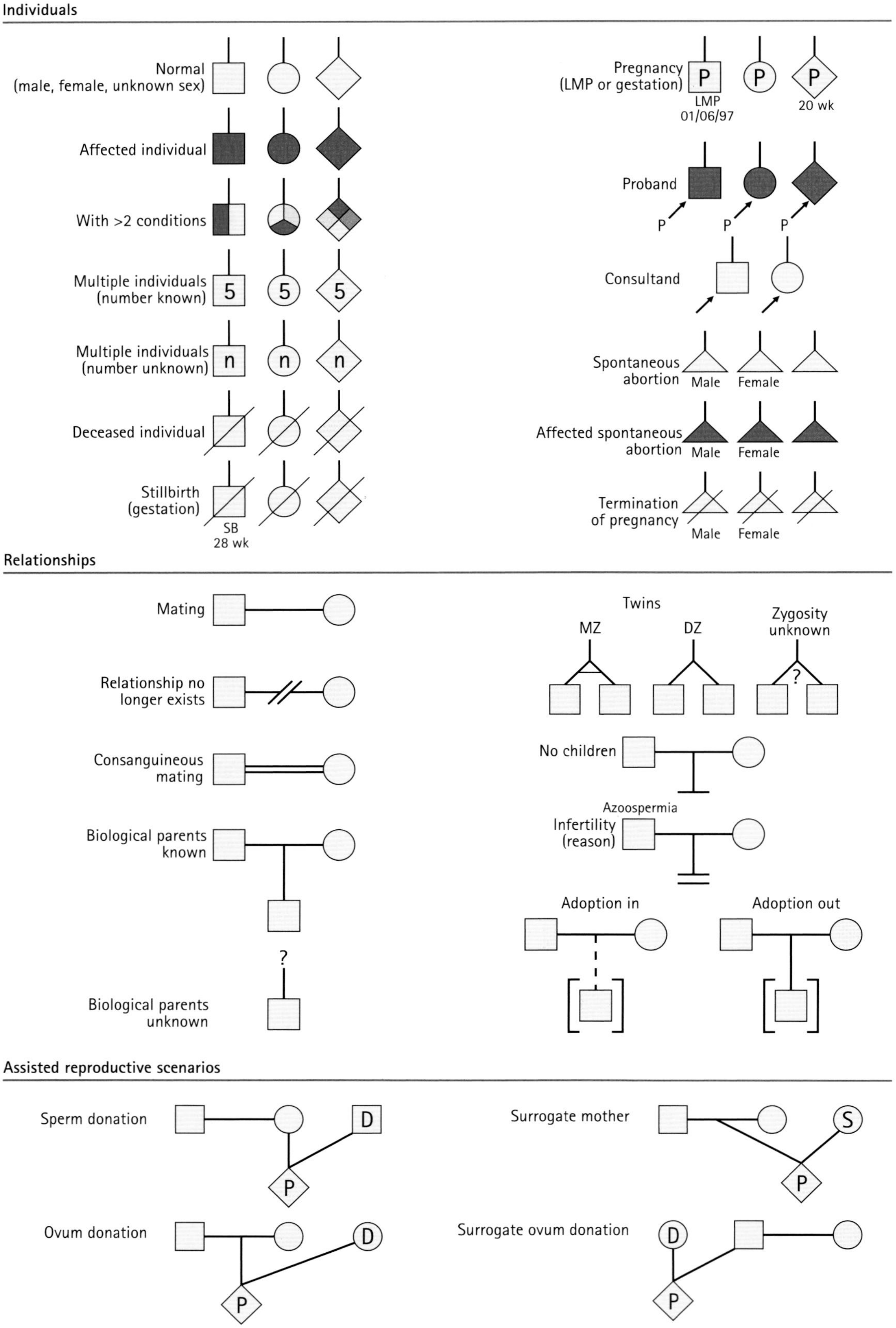

**Individuals**

Normal (male, female, unknown sex)

Affected individual

With >2 conditions

Multiple individuals (number known) 5 5 5

Multiple individuals (number unknown) n n n

Deceased individual

Stillbirth (gestation) SB 28 wk

Pregnancy (LMP or gestation) P P P LMP 01/06/97 20 wk

Proband P P P

Consultand

Spontaneous abortion Male Female

Affected spontaneous abortion Male Female

Termination of pregnancy Male Female

**Relationships**

Mating

Relationship no longer exists

Consanguineous mating

Biological parents known

?

Biological parents unknown

Twins

MZ DZ Zygosity unknown

?

No children

Azoospermia

Infertility (reason)

Adoption in

Adoption out

**Assisted reproductive scenarios**

Sperm donation D P

Ovum donation D P

Surrogate mother S P

Surrogate ovum donation D P

**Fig. 7.1**
Symbols used to represent individuals and relationships in family trees.

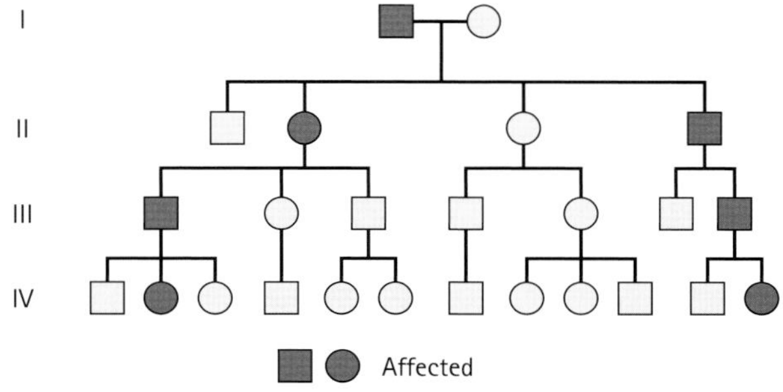


**Fig. 7.2**
Family tree of an autosomal dominant trait. Note the presence of male-to-male transmission.

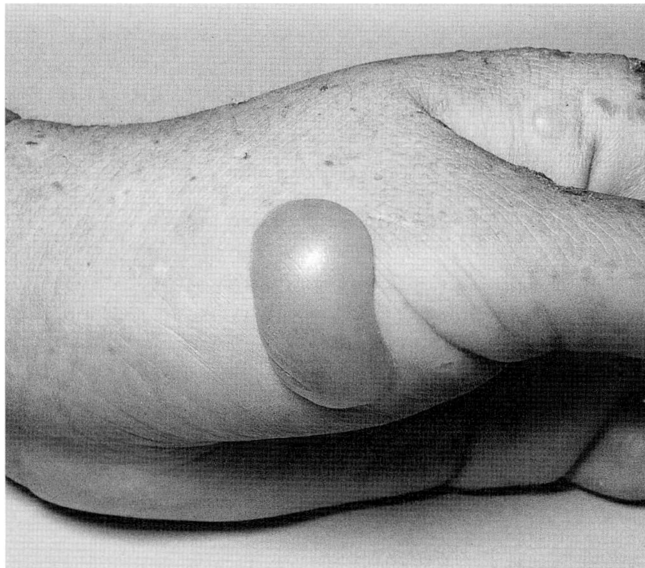

**Fig. 7.3**
Blistering skin lesions on the hand in porphyria variegata.

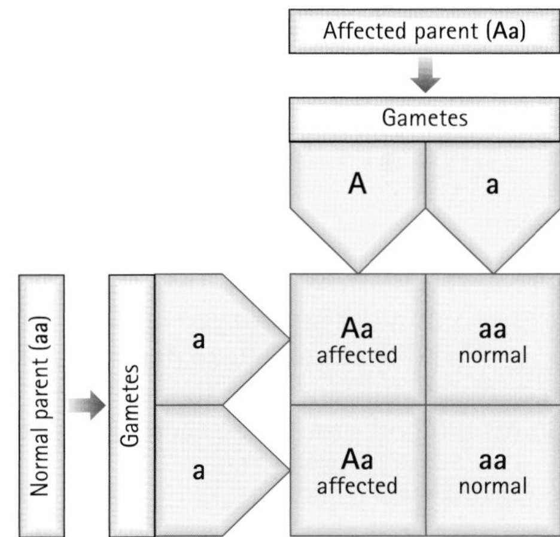


**Fig. 7.4**
Punnett's square showing possible gamete combinations for an autosomal dominant allele.

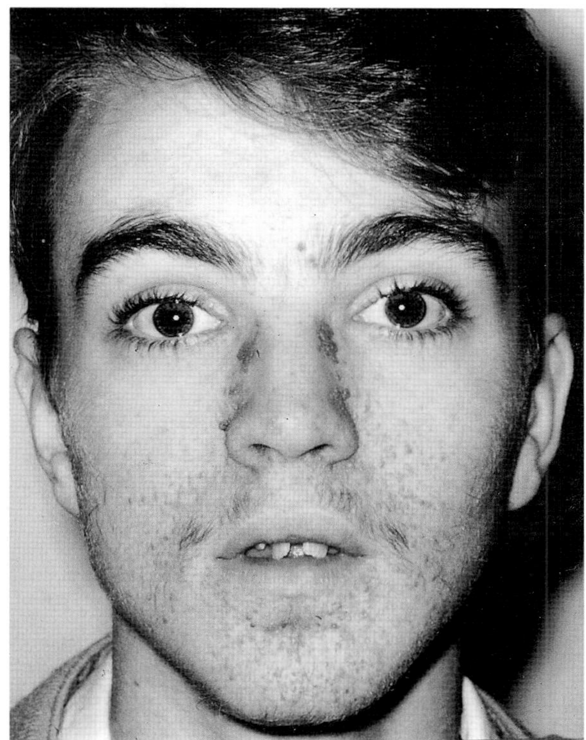

**Fig. 7.5**
Facial rash of angiokeratoma in a male with tuberous sclerosis.

## Pleiotropy

Autosomal dominant traits may involve only one organ or part of the body, for example the eye in congenital cataracts. It is common, however, for autosomal dominant disorders to manifest in different systems of the body in a variety of ways. This is pleiotropy – a single gene that may give rise to two or more apparently unrelated effects. In tuberous sclerosis affected individuals can present with either learning difficulties, epilepsy, or a facial rash known as adenoma sebaceum (Fig. 7.5) (histologically composed of blood vessels and fibrous tissue known as angiokeratoma); some affected individuals have all features (see also p. 318). Recently, our conceptual understanding of the term *pleiotropy* has been challenged by the remarkably diverse syndromes that can result from different mutations in the same gene, for example the *LMNA* gene (which encodes Lamin A/C) and the X-linked Filamin A gene. Mutations in *LMNA* may cause Emery–Dreifuss muscular dystrophy, a form of limb girdle muscular dystrophy, a form of Charcot–Marie–Tooth disease (p. 297), dilated cardiomyopathy (p. 305), Dunnigan-type familial partial lipodystrophy (Fig. 7.6), mandibuloacral dysplasia, and the very rare condition that has always been a great curiosity – Hutchinson–Gilford progeria. These are due to heterozygous mutations, with the exception of the Charcot–Marie–Tooth disease

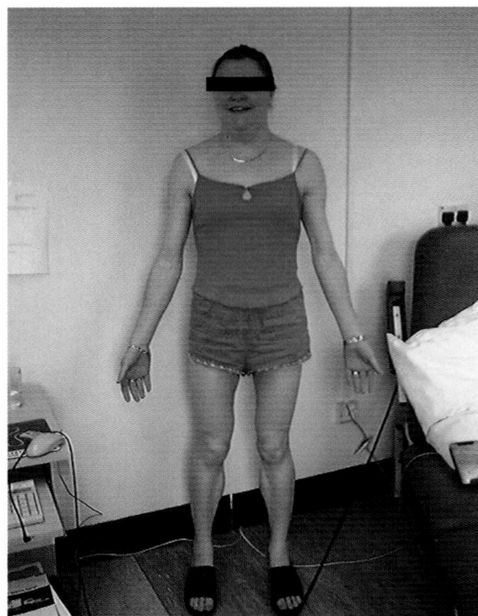

Fig. 7.6
Dunnigan-type familial partial lipodystrophy due to a mutation in the Lamin A/C gene. The patient lacks adipose tissue, especially in the distal limbs. A wide variety of clinical phenotypes are associated with mutations in this one gene.

and mandibuloacral dysplasia, which are recessive, and therefore homozygous for *LMNA* mutations. Sometimes an individual with a mutation is entirely normal. Mutations in the Filamin A gene have recently been implicated in the distinct, though overlapping, X-linked dominant dysmorphic conditions oto-palato-digital syndrome, Melnick–Needles syndrome and frontometaphyseal dysplasia. In addition, however, it would not have been foreseen that a form of X-linked dominant epilepsy in women, called periventricular nodular heterotopia, is also due to mutations in this gene.

## Variable expressivity

The clinical features in autosomal dominant disorders can show striking variation from person to person, even in the same family. This difference between individuals is referred to as *variable expressivity*. In autosomal dominant polycystic kidney disease, for example, some affected individuals develop renal failure in early adulthood whilst others have just a few renal cysts that do not significantly affect renal function.

## Reduced penetrance

In some individuals heterozygous for gene mutations giving rise to certain autosomal dominant disorders there may be no abnormal clinical features, representing so-called *reduced penetrance* or what is commonly referred to in lay terms as 'skipping a generation'. Reduced penetrance is thought to be the result of the modifying effects of other genes, as well as being due to interaction of the gene with environmental factors. An individual who has no features of a disorder despite being heterozygous for a particular gene mutation is said to represent *non-penetrance*.

Reduced penetrance and variable expressivity, together with the pleiotropic effects of a mutant allele, all need to be taken into account when providing genetic counseling to individuals at risk for autosomal dominantly inherited disorders.

## New mutations

In autosomal dominant disorders an affected person will usually have an affected parent. However, this is not always the case and it is not unusual for a trait to appear in an individual when there is no family history of the disorder. A striking example is achondroplasia, a form of short-limbed dwarfism (p. 92), in which the parents usually have normal stature. The sudden unexpected appearance of a condition arising as a result of a mistake occurring in the transmission of a gene is called a *new mutation*. The dominant mode of inheritance of achondroplasia could only be confirmed by the observation that the offspring of persons with achondroplasia had a 50% chance of having achondroplasia or being of normal stature.

In less striking examples other possible explanations for the 'sudden' appearance of a disorder must be considered. One of the parents might be heterozygous for the mutant allele but so mildly affected that it has not previously been detected, i.e. non-penetrance. The possibility of variable expression also needs to be considered, as well as the family relationships not being as stated, i.e. *non-paternity* (p. 269) (and occasionally *non-maternity*).

New dominant mutations, in certain instances, have been associated with an increased age of the father. It is believed that this is because of the large number of mitotic divisions that male gamete stem cells undergo during a man's reproductive lifetime (p. 46).

## Codominance

*Codominance* is the term used for two allelic traits that are both expressed in the heterozygous state. In persons with blood group AB it is possible to demonstrate both A and B blood group substances on the red blood cells, so that the A and B blood groups are therefore codominant (p. 198).

## Homozygosity for autosomal dominant traits

The rarity of most autosomal dominant disorders and diseases means that they usually only occur in the

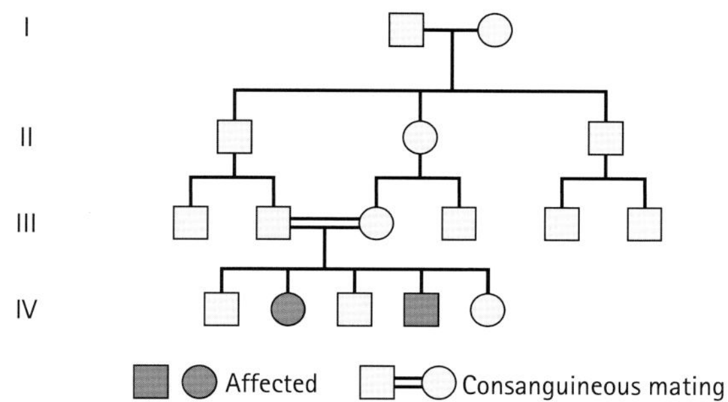


Fig. 7.7
Family tree of an autosomal recessive trait.

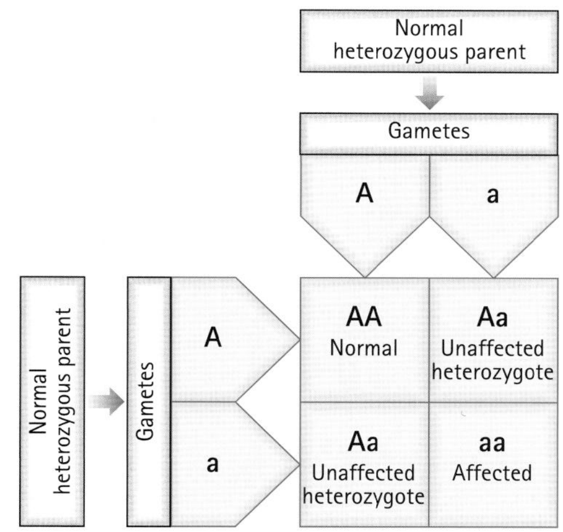


Fig. 7.8
Punnett's square showing possible gametic combinations for heterozygous carrier parents of an autosomal recessive allele.

heterozygous state. There are, however, a few reports of children born to couples where both parents are heterozygous for a dominantly inherited disorder. Offspring of such couples are, therefore, at risk of being homozygous. In some instances affected individuals appear to be either more severely affected, as has been reported with achondroplasia, or have an earlier age of onset, as in familial hypercholesterolemia (p. 170). The heterozygote having a phenotype intermediate between the homozygotes for the normal and mutant alleles is consistent with a haploinsufficiency loss-of-function mutation (p. 26).

Conversely, with other dominantly inherited disorders, homozygous individuals are not more severely affected than heterozygotes, e.g. Huntington disease (p. 293) and myotonic dystrophy (p. 295).

## AUTOSOMAL RECESSIVE INHERITANCE

Recessive traits and disorders are only manifest when the mutant allele is present in a double dose, i.e. homozygosity. Individuals heterozygous for such mutant alleles show no features of the disorder and are perfectly healthy, i.e. they are *carriers*. The family tree for recessive traits differs markedly from that seen in autosomal dominant traits (Fig. 7.7). It is not possible to trace an autosomal recessive trait or disorder through the family, i.e. all the affected individuals in a family are usually in a single *sibship*, i.e. brothers and sisters. This is sometimes referred to as 'horizontal' transmission (an inappropriate and misleading term).

### Consanguinity

Enquiry into the family history of individuals affected with rare recessive traits or disorders might reveal that their parents are related, i.e. *consanguineous*. The rarer a recessive trait or disorder, the greater the frequency of consanguinity among the parents of affected individuals. In cystic fibrosis, the commonest 'serious' autosomal recessive disorder in persons of Western European origin (p. 302), the frequency of parental consanguinity is only slightly greater than that seen in the general population. By contrast, in alkaptonuria, one of the original inborn errors of metabolism (p. 165), which is an exceedingly rare recessive disorder, Bateson and Garrod, in their original description of the disorder, observed that one-quarter or more of the parents were first cousins. They reasoned that rare alleles for disorders such as alkaptonuria are more likely to 'meet up' in the offspring of cousins than in the offspring of parents who are unrelated.

### Genetic risks

If we represent the normal dominant allele as 'A' and the recessive mutant allele as 'a', then each parental gamete carries either the mutant or the normal allele (Fig. 7.8). The various possible combinations of gametes mean that the offspring of two heterozygotes have a 1 in 4 (25%) chance of being homozygous affected, a 1 in 2 (50%) chance of being heterozygous unaffected, and a 1 in 4 (25%) chance of being homozygous unaffected.

### Pseudodominance

If an individual who is homozygous for an autosomal recessive disorder marries a carrier of the same disorder, their children have a 1 in 2 (50%) chance of being affected. Such a pedigree is said to exhibit *pseudodominance* (Fig. 7.9).

### Locus heterogeneity

A disorder inherited in the same manner can be due to mutations in more than one gene, or what is known as *locus heterogeneity*. For example, it is recognized that

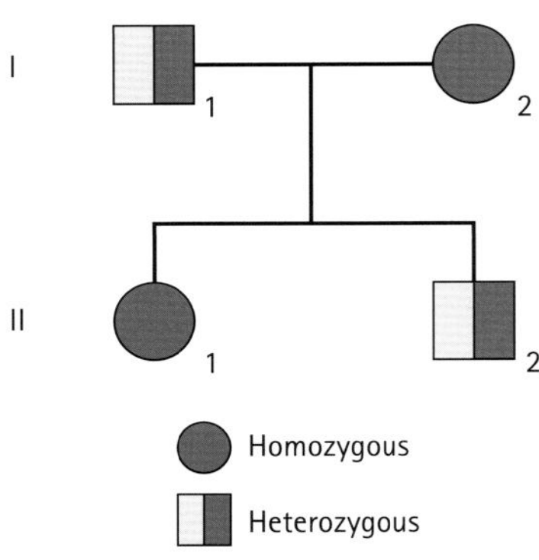


**Fig. 7.9**
A pedigree with a woman ($I_2$) homozygous for an autosomal recessive disorder whose husband is heterozygous for the same disorder. They have a homozygous affected daughter so that the pedigree shows pseudodominant inheritance.

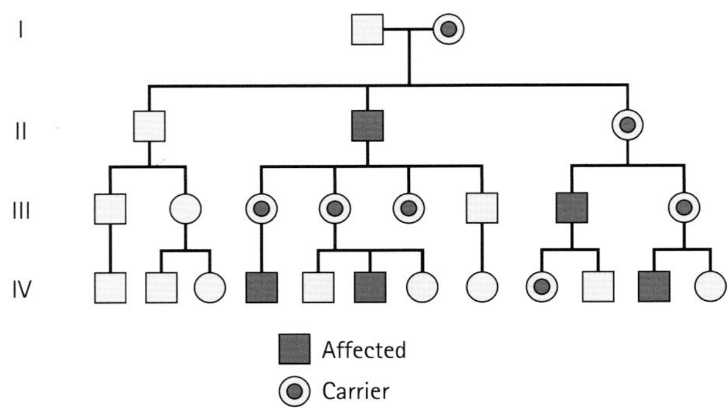


**Fig. 7.10**
Family tree of an X-linked recessive trait in which affected males reproduce.

sensorineural hearing impairment/deafness most commonly shows autosomal recessive inheritance. Deaf persons, by virtue of their schooling and involvement in the deaf community, often choose to have children with another deaf person. It would be expected that if two deaf persons were homozygous for the same recessive gene, all of their children would be similarly affected. Families have been described in which all the children born to parents deaf due to autosomal recessive genes have had perfectly normal hearing and are what is known as *double heterozygotes*. The explanation for this must be that the parents were homozygous for mutant alleles at different loci, i.e. that a number of different genes can cause autosomal recessive sensorineural deafness. In fact, over the past 10–15 years, 20 genes and a further 15 loci have been shown to be involved! A very similar story applies to autosomal recessive retinitis pigmentosa, and there are now six distinct loci for primary autosomal recessive microcephaly.

Disorders with the same phenotype due to different genetic loci are known as genocopies, while the same phenotype being the result of environmental causes is known as a *phenocopy*.

### Mutational heterogeneity

Heterogeneity can also occur at the allelic level. In the majority of single-gene disorders, e.g. β thalassemia, a large number of different mutations have been identified as being responsible (p. 152). There are individuals who have two different mutations at the same locus and are known as *compound heterozygotes*, constituting what is known as allelic or *mutational heterogeneity*. Most individuals affected with an autosomal recessive disorder are probably, in fact, compound heterozygotes rather than true homozygotes, unless their parents are related, when they are likely to be homozygous for the same mutation by descent, having inherited the same mutation from a common ancestor.

## SEX-LINKED INHERITANCE

Sex-linked inheritance refers to the pattern of inheritance shown by genes that are located on either of the sex chromosomes. Genes carried on the X chromosome are referred to as being X-linked, while genes carried on the Y chromosome are referred to as exhibiting *Y-linked* or *holandric inheritance*.

### X-linked recessive inheritance

An X-linked recessive trait is one determined by a gene carried on the X chromosome and usually only manifests in males. A male with a mutant allele on his single X chromosome is said to be hemizygous for that allele. Diseases inherited in an X-linked manner are transmitted by healthy heterozygous female carriers to affected males, as well as by affected males to their obligate carrier daughters, with a consequent risk to male grandchildren through these daughters (Fig. 7.10). This type of pedigree is sometimes said to show 'diagonal' or a 'knight's move' pattern of transmission.

The mode of inheritance whereby only males are affected by a disease that is transmitted by normal females was appreciated by the Jews nearly 2000 years ago. They excused from circumcision the sons of all the sisters of a mother who had sons with the 'bleeding disease', in other words, hemophilia (p. 310). The sons of the father's siblings were not excused. Queen Victoria was a carrier of hemophilia and her carrier daughters, who were perfectly healthy, introduced the gene into the Russian and Spanish royal families. Fortunately for the British royal family, Queen Victoria's son, Edward VII, did not inherit the gene, and so could not transmit it to his descendants.

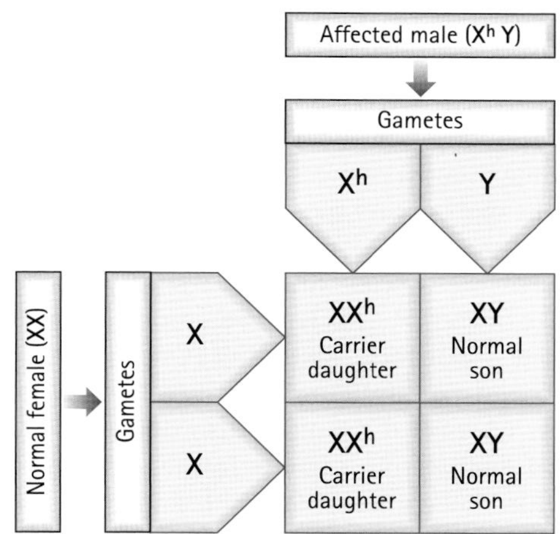


**Fig. 7.11**
Punnett's square showing possible gamete combinations for the offspring of a male affected by an X-linked recessive disorder ($X^h$ represents a mutation for an X-linked gene).

Carrier female ($X^h$ X)

| Normal male (XY) gametes | $X^h$ | X |
|---|---|---|
| X | $X^h$ X Carrier daughter | XX Normal daughter |
| Y | $X^h$ Y Affected son | XY Normal son |

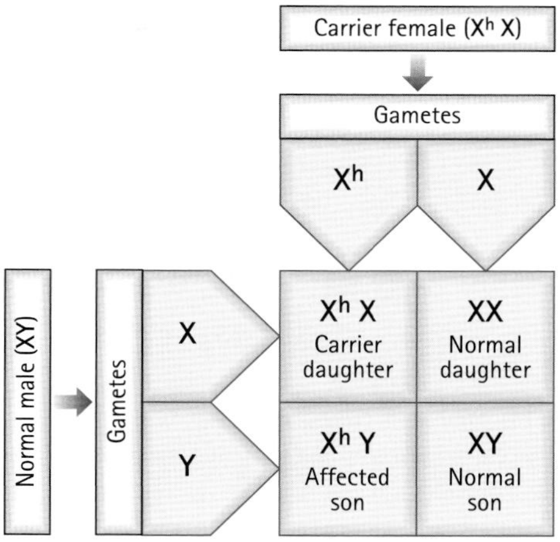

**Fig. 7.12**
A Punnett's square showing possible gamete combinations for the offspring of a female carrier of an X-linked recessive disorder ($X^h$ represents a mutation for an X-linked gene).

### *Genetic risks*

A male transmits his X chromosome to each of his daughters and his Y chromosome to each of his sons. If a male affected with hemophilia has children with a normal female, then all his daughters will be *obligate carriers* but none of his sons will be affected (Fig. 7.11). A male cannot transmit an X-linked trait to his son, with the very rare exception of uniparental heterodisomy (p. 117).

For a carrier female of an X-linked recessive disorder having children with a normal male, each son has a 1 in 2 (50%) chance of being affected and each daughter has a 1 in 2 (50%) chance of being a carrier (Fig. 7.12).

Some X-linked disorders are not compatible with survival to reproductive age and are not, therefore, transmitted by affected males. Duchenne muscular dystrophy is the commonest muscular dystrophy and is a severe disease (p. 308). The first signs are a waddling gait, difficulty in climbing stairs unaided, and a tendency to fall over easily. By about the age of 10 years affected boys usually need to use a wheelchair. The muscle weakness gradually progresses and affected males ultimately become confined to bed and will often die in their late teenage years or early 20s (Fig. 7.13). Since affected boys do not usually survive to reproduce, the disease is transmitted almost entirely by healthy female carriers (Fig. 7.14).

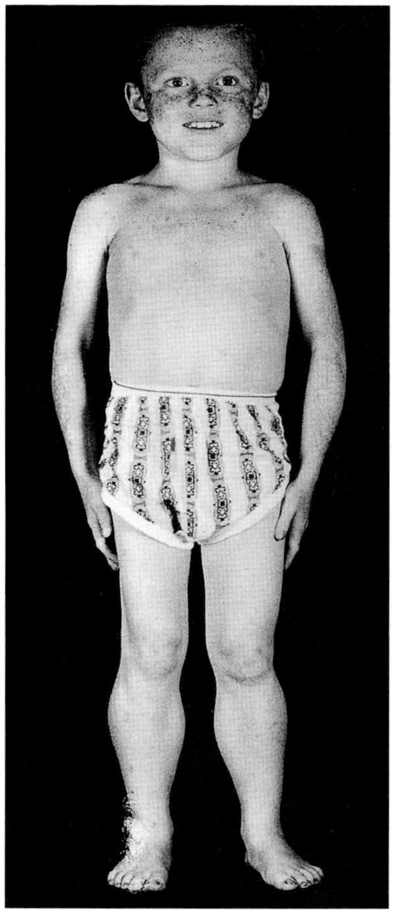

**Fig. 7.13**
Boy with Duchenne muscular dystrophy; note the enlarged calves and wasting of the thigh muscles.

### *Variable expression in heterozygous females*

In humans, several X-linked disorders are known in which heterozygous females have a mosaic phenotype with a mixture of features of the normal and mutant alleles. In X-linked ocular albinism the iris and ocular fundus

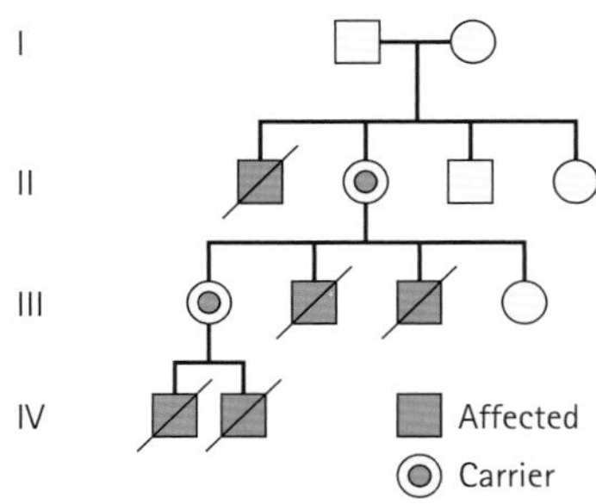


Fig. 7.14
Family tree of Duchenne muscular dystrophy with the disorder being transmitted by carrier females and affecting males who do not survive to transmit the disorder.

of affected males lack pigment. Careful examination of the ocular fundus in females heterozygous for ocular albinism reveals a mosaic pattern of pigmentation (Fig. 6.21, p. 100). This mosaic pattern of involvement can be explained through the random process of X-inactivation (p. 99). In the pigmented areas the normal gene is on the active X chromosome while in the depigmented areas the mutant allele is on the active X chromosome.

## Females affected with X-linked recessive disorders

Occasionally a woman might manifest features of an X-linked recessive trait. There are several explanations for how this can happen.

**Homozygosity for X-linked recessive disorders**

A common X-linked recessive trait is red–green color blindness – the inability to distinguish between the colors red and green. About 8% of males are red–green color blind and, although it is unusual, because of the high frequency of this allele in the population, about 1 in 150 women are red–green colour blind by virtue of both parents having the allele on the X chromosome. Therefore, a female can be affected with an X-linked recessive disorder as a result of homozygosity for an X-linked allele but the rarity of most X-linked conditions means that the phenomenon is uncommon. A female could also be homozygous if her father was affected and her mother was normal but a new mutation occurred on the X chromosome transmitted to the daughter; or alternatively if her mother was a carrier and her father was normal but a new mutation occurred on the X chromosome he transmitted to his daughter – but these scenarios are rare.

**Skewed X-inactivation**

The process of X-inactivation usually occurs randomly, there being an equal chance of either of the two X chromosomes in a heterozygous female being inactivated in any one cell. Following X-inactivation in embryogenesis, therefore, in roughly half the cells one of the X chromosomes is active, whilst in the other half it is the other X which is active. Sometimes this process is not random, allowing for the possibility that the active X chromosome in most of the cells of a heterozygous female carrier is the one bearing the mutant allele. If this happens, a carrier female would exhibit some of the symptoms and signs of the disease and be a so-called *manifesting heterozygote* or *carrier*. This has been reported in a number of X-linked disorders, including Duchenne muscular dystrophy and hemophilia A (p. 312). In addition, there are reports of several X-linked disorders in which there are several manifesting carriers in the same family, consistent with the coincidental inheritance of an abnormality of X-inactivation (p. 99).

**Numerical X chromosome abnormalities**

A female could manifest an X-linked recessive disorder through being a carrier of an X-linked recesssive mutation and having only a single X chromosome, i.e. Turner syndrome (p. 282). Women with Turner syndrome and hemophilia A or Duchenne muscular dystrophy have been reported.

**X-autosome translocations**

Females with a translocation involving one of the X chromosomes and an autosome can be affected with an X-linked recessive disorder. If the break-point of the translocation disrupts a gene on the X chromosome, then a female can be affected. This is because the X chromosome involved in the translocation survives preferentially so as to maintain functional disomy of the autosomal genes (Fig. 7.15). The observation of females affected with Duchenne muscular dystrophy with X-autosome translocations involving the same region of the short arm of the X chromosome helped to map the Duchenne muscular dystrophy gene (p. 309). This type of observation has been vital in the positional cloning of a number of genes in humans (p. 78).

## X-linked dominant inheritance

Although uncommon, there are disorders that are manifest in the heterozygous female as well as in the male who has the mutant allele on his single X chromosome. This is known as X-linked dominant inheritance (Fig. 7.16). X-linked dominant inheritance superficially resembles that of an autosomal dominant trait because both the daughters and sons of an affected female have a 1 in 2 (50%) chance of being affected. There is, however, an important difference. With an X-linked dominant trait an affected male transmits the trait to all his daughters but to none of his sons. Therefore, in families with an X-linked dominant disorder there is an excess of affected females and direct male-to-male transmission cannot occur.

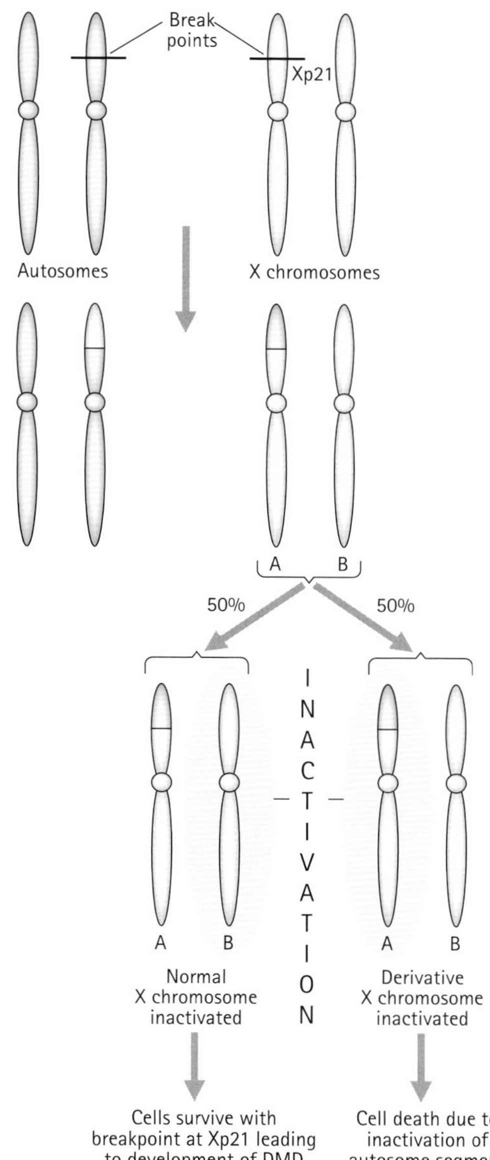


**Fig. 7.15**
Shows the generation of an X-autosome translocation with break-point in a female and how this results in the development of Duchenne muscular dystrophy.

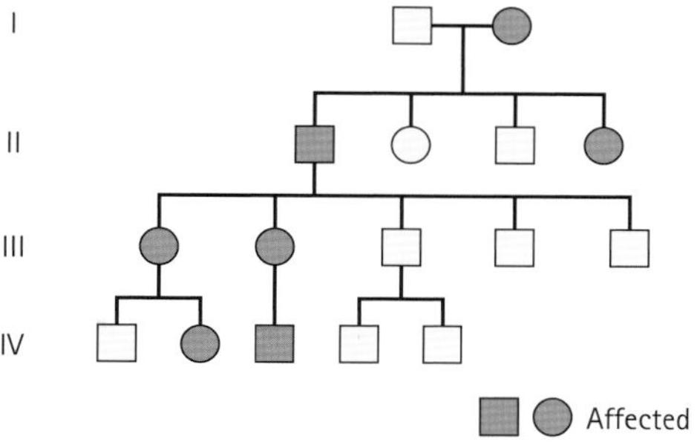


**Fig. 7.16**
Family tree of an X-linked dominant trait.

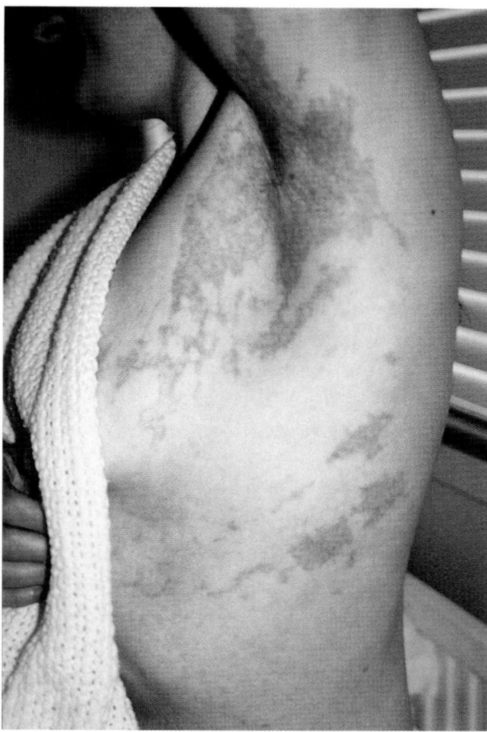

**Fig. 7.17**
Mosaic pattern of skin pigmentation in a female with the X-linked dominant disorder incontinentia pigmenti. She has a mutation in a gene on one of her X chromosomes and the pigmented areas indicate tissue in which the normal X chromosome has been inactivated. This developmental pattern follows Blaschko's lines (see Ch. 18, p. 281).

An example of an X-linked dominant trait is vitamin D-resistant rickets. Rickets can be due to a dietary deficiency of vitamin D, but in vitamin D-resistant rickets the disorder occurs even when there is an adequate dietary intake of vitamin D. In the X-linked dominant form of vitamin D-resistant rickets both males and females are affected, although the females usually have less severe skeletal changes than the males. The X-linked form of Charcot–Marie–Tooth disease (hereditary motor and sensory neuropathy) is another example.

A mosaic pattern of involvement can be demonstrated in females heterozygous for some X-linked dominant disorders. An example is the mosaic pattern of abnormal pigmentation of the skin that follows developmental lines seen in females heterozygous for the X-linked dominant disorder incontinentia pigmenti (Fig. 7.17). This is also an example of a disorder that is usually lethal for male embryos that inherit the mutated allele. Others include the neurological conditions Rett syndrome and periventricular nodular heterotopia.

### Y-linked inheritance

*Y-linked* or *holandric inheritance* implies that only males are affected. An affected male transmits Y-linked traits to all his sons but to none of his daughters. In the past it has been suggested that bizarre sounding conditions such as porcupine skin, hairy ears and webbed toes are Y-linked traits. With the possible exception of hairy ears, these claims of holandric inheritance have not stood up to more careful study. Evidence clearly indicates, however, that the H-Y histocompatibility antigen (p. 194) and genes involved in spermatogenesis are carried on the Y chromosome and, therefore, manifest holandric inheritance. The latter, if deleted, lead to infertility due to azoospermia (absence of the sperm in semen) in males. The recent advent of techniques of assisted reproduction, particularly the technique of intracytoplasmic sperm injection (ICSI), means that if a pregnancy with a male conceptus results after the use of this technique, the child will also necessarily be infertile!

### Partial sex-linkage

*Partial sex-linkage* has been used in the past for certain disorders that appear to exhibit autosomal dominant inheritance in some families and X-linked inheritance in others. This is now known to be likely to be because of genes carried on that portion of the X chromosome sharing homology with the Y chromosome, and which escapes X-inactivation. During meiosis pairing occurs between the homologous distal parts of the short arms of the X and Y chromosomes, the so-called *pseudoautosomal region*. As a result of a cross-over, a gene could be transferred from the X to the Y chromosome, or vice versa, allowing the possibility of male-to-male transmission. The latter instances would be consistent with autosomal dominant inheritance. A rare skeletal dysplasia Leri–Weil dyschondrosteosis, in which affected individuals have short stature and a characteristic wrist deformity (Madelung deformity), has been reported to show both autosomal dominant and X-linked inheritance. The disorder has been shown to be due to deletions of, or mutations in, the short stature homeobox (*SHOX*) gene (p. 282), which is located in the pseudoautosomal region.

### Sex influence

Some autosomal traits are expressed more frequently in one sex than another, so-called *sex influence*. Gout and presenile baldness are examples of sex-influenced autosomal dominant traits, males being predominantly affected in both cases. The influence of sex in these two examples is probably through the effect of male hormones. Gout, for example, is very rare in women before the menopause but the frequency increases in later life. Baldness does not occur in males who have been castrated. In hemochromatosis (p. 242), the most common autosomal recessive disorder in Western society, homozygous females are much less likely than homozygous males to develop iron overload and associated symptoms; the explanation usually given is that women have a form of natural blood loss through menstruation.

### Sex limitation

*Sex limitation* refers to the appearance of certain features in individuals of only one sex. Examples include virilization of female infants affected with the autosomal recessive endocrine disorder, congenital adrenal hyperplasia (p. 168).

## ESTABLISHING THE MODE OF INHERITANCE OF A GENETIC DISORDER

In experimental animals it is possible to arrange specific types of mating to establish the mode of inheritance of a trait or disorder. In humans, when a disorder is newly recognized the geneticist approaches the problem indirectly by fitting likely models of inheritance to the observed outcome in the offspring. Certain features are necessary to support a particular mode of inheritance. Formally establishing the mode of inheritance is not usually possible with a single family and normally requires study of a number of families (Table 7.1).

**Table 7.1 Features that support the single-gene or Mendelian patterns of inheritance**

**Autosomal dominant**
- Males and females affected in equal proportions
- Affected individuals in multiple generations
- Transmission by individuals of both sexes, i.e. male to male, female to female, male to female and female to male

**Autosomal recessive**
- Males and females affected in equal proportions
- Affected individuals usually only in a single generation
- Parents can be related, i.e. consanguineous

**X-linked recessive**
- Males usually only affected
- Transmitted through unaffected females
- Males cannot transmit the disorder to their sons, i.e. no male-to-male transmission

**X-linked dominant**
- Males and females affected but often with an excess of females
- Females less severely affected than males
- Affected males can transmit the disorder to their daughters but not sons

**Y-linked inheritance**
- Affected males only
- Affected males must transmit it to their sons

### Autosomal dominant inheritance

In order to determine whether a trait or disorder is inherited in an autosomal dominant manner, there are three specific features which need to be observed. Firstly, it should affect both males and females in equal proportions. Secondly, it is transmitted from one generation to the next. Thirdly, all forms of transmission between the sexes are observed, i.e. male to male, female to female, male to female and the converse. Male-to-male transmission excludes the possibility of the gene being on the X chromosome. In the case of sporadically occurring disorders, increased paternal age may suggest a new autosomal dominant mutation.

### Autosomal recessive inheritance

There are three features which suggest the possibility of autosomal recessive inheritance. Firstly, the disorder affects males and females in equal proportions. Secondly, it usually only affects individuals in one generation in a single sibship, i.e. brothers and sisters, and does not occur in previous and subsequent generations. Thirdly, consanguinity in the parents provides further support for autosomal recessive inheritance.

### X-linked recessive inheritance

There are three main features necessary to establish X-linked recessive inheritance. Firstly, the trait or disorder should affect males almost exclusively. Secondly, X-linked recessive disorders are transmitted through unaffected carrier females to their sons. Affected males, if they survive to reproduce, can have affected grandsons through their daughters who are obligate carriers. Thirdly, male-to-male transmission is not observed, i.e. affected males cannot transmit the disorder to their sons.

### X-linked dominant inheritance

There are three features necessary to establish X-linked dominant inheritance. Firstly, males and females are affected but affected females are more frequent than affected males. Secondly, females are usually less severely affected than males. Thirdly, while affected females can transmit the disorder to both male and female offspring, affected males can only transmit the disorder to their daughters (except in partial sex-linkage – see p. 114), all of whom will be affected. In the case of X-linked dominant disorders that are lethal in male embryos, only females will be affected and families may show an excess of females over males as well as a number of miscarriages that are the affected male pregnancies.

### Y-linked inheritance

There are two features necessary to establish a Y-linked pattern of inheritance. Firstly, it affects males only. Secondly, affected males must transmit the disorder to their sons, e.g. male infertility by ICSI (p. 337).

## MULTIPLE ALLELES AND COMPLEX TRAITS

So far, each of the traits we have considered has involved only two alleles, the normal and the mutant. However, some traits and diseases are neither *monogenic* nor *polygenic*. Some genes have more than two allelic forms, i.e. multiple alleles. Multiple alleles are the result of a normal gene having mutated to produce various different alleles, some of which can be dominant and others recessive to the normal allele. In the case of the ABO blood group system (p. 198), there are at least four alleles ($A_1$, $A_2$, B and O). An individual can possess any two of these alleles, which can be the same or different (AO, $A_2$B, OO, and so on). Alleles are carried on homologous chromosomes and therefore a person transmits only one allele for a certain trait to any particular offspring. For example, if a person has the genotype AB, he will transmit to any particular offspring either the A allele or the B allele, but never both or neither (Table 7.2). This relates only to genes located on the autosomes and does not apply to alleles on the X chromosome. In this instance a woman would have two, either of which could be transmitted to offspring, whereas a man only has one to transmit.

The dramatic advances in genome scanning using multiple DNA probes has made it possible to begin investigating so called *complex traits*, i.e. conditions which are usually much more common than Mendelian

**Table 7.2 Possible genotypes, phenotypes and gametes formed from the four alleles $A_1$, $A_2$, B and O at the ABO locus**

| Genotype | Phenotype | Gametes |
|---|---|---|
| $A_1A_1$ | $A_1$ | $A_1$ |
| $A_2A_2$ | $A_2$ | $A_2$ |
| BB | B | B |
| OO | O | O |
| $A_1A_2$ | $A_1$ | $A_1$ or $A_2$ |
| $A_1$B | $A_1$B | $A_1$ or B |
| $A_1$O | $A_1$ | $A_1$ or O |
| $A_2$B | $A_2$B | $A_2$ or B |
| $A_2$O | $A_2$ | $A_2$ or O |
| BO | B | B or O |

disorders and likely to be due to the interaction of more than one gene. The effects may be additive, one may be rate-limiting over the action of another, or one may enhance or multiply the effect of another. This is considered in more detail in Chapter 15. The possibility of a small number of gene loci being implicated in some disorders has given rise to the concept of *oligogenic* inheritance, examples of which include the following.

### *Digenic inheritance*

This refers to the situation where a disorder has been shown to be due to the additive effects of heterozygous mutations at two different gene loci, a concept referred to as *digenic inheritance*. This is seen in certain transgenic mice. Mice that are homozygotes for *rv* or *Dll1* manifest abnormal phenotypes whereas their respective heterozygotes are normal. However, mice that are *double heterozygotes* for *rv* (rib-vertebrae) and *Dll1* (Delta-like 1) show vertebral defects. In man one form of retinitis pigmentosa, a disorder of progressive visual impairment, is caused by double heterozygosity for mutations in two unlinked genes, *ROM1* and *peripherin*, which both encode proteins present in photoreceptors. Individuals with only one of these mutations are not affected.

### *Triallelic inheritance*

Bardet–Biedl syndrome is a rare dysmorphic condition – though relatively more common in some inbred communities – with obesity, polydactyly, renal abnormalities, retinal pigmentation and learning disability. Seven different gene loci have been identified and, until recently, it was believed to follow straightforward autosomal recessive inheritance. However, it is now known that one form only occurs when an individual who is homozygous for mutations at one locus *is also* heterozygous for mutation at another Bardet–Biedl locus; this is referred to as *triallelic inheritance*.

Other patterns of inheritance that are not classically Mendelian are also recognized and explain some unusual phenomena.

## ANTICIPATION

In some autosomal dominant traits or disorders, such as myotonic dystrophy, the onset of the disease occurs at an earlier age in the offspring than in the parents, or the disease occurs with increasing severity in subsequent generations. This phenomenon is called *anticipation*. It used to be believed that this effect was the result of a bias of ascertainment, because of the way in which the families were collected. It was argued that this arose because persons in whom the disease begins earlier or is more severe are more likely to be ascertained and only those individuals who are less severely affected tend to have children. In addition, it was felt that because the observer is in the same generation as the affected presenting probands, many individuals who at present are unaffected would, by necessity, develop the disease later in life.

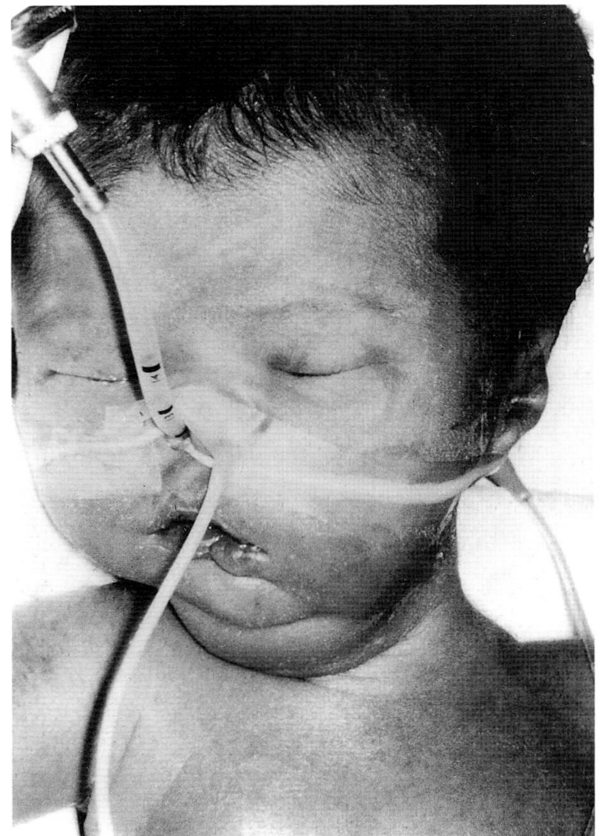

Fig. 7.18
Newborn baby with severe hypotonia requiring ventilation as a result of having inherited myotonic dystrophy from his mother.

Recent studies, however, have shown that in a number of disorders, including Huntington disease and myotonic dystrophy, anticipation is, in fact, a real biological phenomenon occurring as a result of the expansion of unstable triplet repeat sequences (p. 24). An expansion of the CTG triplet repeat in the 3′ untranslated end of the myotonic dystrophy gene, occurring predominantly in maternal meiosis, appears to be the explanation for the severe neonatal form of myotonic dystrophy that usually only occurs when the gene is transmitted by the mother (Fig. 7.18). A similar expansion in the CAG expansion in the 5′ end of the Huntington disease gene (Fig. 7.19) in paternal meiosis appears to account for the increased risk of juvenile Huntington disease when the gene is transmitted by the father. Fragile X syndrome and the

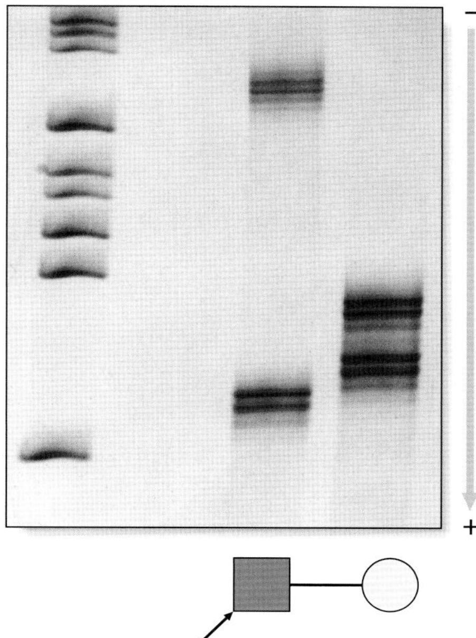


**Fig. 7.19**
Silver staining of a 5% denaturing gel of the PCR products of the CAG triplet in the 5′ untranslated end of the Huntington disease gene from an affected male and his wife showing her to have two similar sized repeats in the normal range (20 and 24 copies) and him to have one normal sized triplet repeat (18 copies) and an expanded triplet repeat (44 copies). The bands in the left lane are standard markers to allow sizing of the CAG repeat. (Courtesy of Alan Dodge, Regional DNA Laboratory, St Mary's Hospital, Manchester.)

inherited spinocerebellar ataxia group of conditions are other examples.

## MOSAICISM

An individual, or a particular tissue of the body, can consist of more than one cell type or line, through an error occurring during mitosis at any stage after conception. This is known as *mosaicism* (p. 54). Mosaicism of either somatic or germ cells can account for some instances of unusual patterns of inheritance or phenotypic features in an affected individual.

### Somatic mosaicism

The possibility of somatic mosaicism is suggested by the features of a single-gene disorder being less severe in an individual than usual or by being confined to a particular part of the body in a segmental distribution, e.g. as occasionally occurs in neurofibromatosis type I (p. 298). Depending on when a mutation arises in development, it may or may not be transmitted to the next generation with full expression depending on whether the mutation is also present in all or some of the germ line cells.

### Gonadal mosaicism

There have been many reports of families with autosomal dominant disorders, such as achondroplasia and osteogenesis imperfecta, and X-linked recessive disorders, such as Duchenne muscular dystrophy and hemophilia, in which the parents are phenotypically normal and the results of investigations or genetic tests have also all been normal, but in which more than one of their children has been affected. The most favored explanation for these observations is gonadal or germ line mosaicism in one of the parents, i.e. the mutation being present in a proportion of the gonadal cells. An elegant example of this was provided by the demonstration of a mutation in the collagen gene responsible for osteogenesis imperfecta in a proportion of individual sperm from a clinically normal father who had two affected infants with different partners. It is important to keep germ line mosaicism in mind when providing recurrence risks in genetic counseling for apparently new autosomal dominant and X-linked recessive mutations (p. 346).

## UNIPARENTAL DISOMY

An individual normally inherits one of a pair of homologous chromosomes from each parent (p. 43). Over the last decade, with the advent of DNA technology, some individuals have been shown to have inherited both homologs of a chromosome pair from only one of their parents, so-called *uniparental disomy*. If an individual inherits two copies of the same homolog from one parent, through an error in meiosis II (p. 45), this is called *uniparental isodisomy* (Fig. 7.20). If, however, the individual inherits the two different homologs from one parent through an error in meiosis I (p. 43), this is termed *uniparental heterodisomy*. In either instance it is presumed that the conceptus would originally be trisomic, with early loss of a chromosome leading to the 'normal' disomic state. One-third of such chromosome losses, if they occurred with equal frequency, would result in uniparental disomy. Alternatively, it is postulated that uniparental disomy could arise as a result of a gamete from one parent that does not contain a particular chromosome homolog, or what is termed *nullisomic*, being 'rescued' by fertilization with a gamete that, through a second separate chance error in meiosis, is disomic.

Using DNA techniques, uniparental disomy has been shown to be the cause of a father with hemophilia having an affected son and of a child with cystic fibrosis being born to a couple in which only the mother was a carrier (with proven paternity!). Uniparental paternal disomy for chromosome 11 has also been shown in a proportion of cases of the rare overgrowth syndrome known as the Beckwith–Wiedemann syndrome.

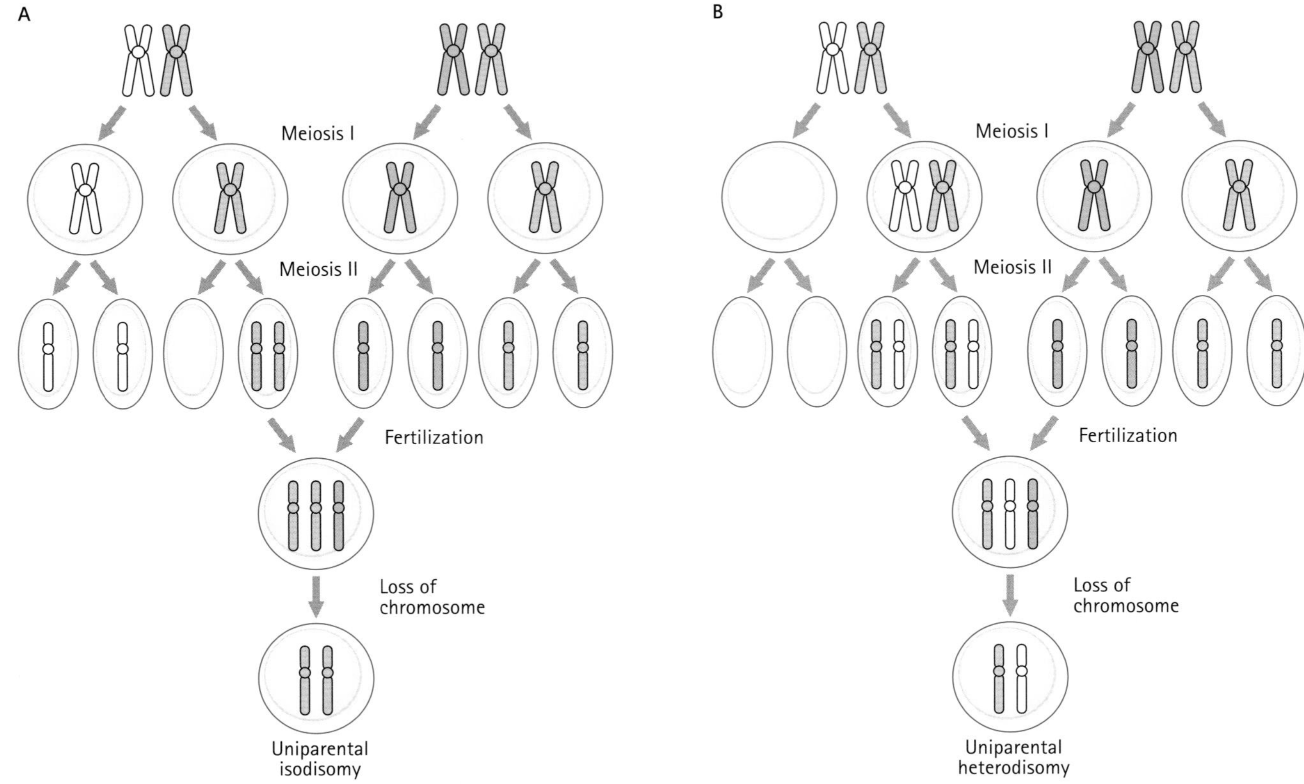


**Fig. 7.20**
Mechanism of origin of uniparental disomy. (A) Uniparental isodisomy occurring through a disomic gamete arising from non-disjunction in meiosis II fertilizing a monosomic gamete with loss of the chromosome from the parent contributing the single homolog. (B) Uniparental heterodisomy occurring through a disomic gamete arising from non-disjunction in meiosis I fertilizing a monosomic gamete with loss of the chromosome from the parent contributing the single homolog.

## GENOMIC IMPRINTING

Although it was originally believed that genes on homologous chromosomes were expressed equally, it is now recognized that different clinical features can result, depending on whether a gene is inherited from the father or from the mother. This 'parent of origin' effect is referred to as *genomic imprinting* and *methylation of DNA* is thought to be the main mechanism by which expression is modified. Methylation is therefore thought to be the *imprint* applied to certain DNA sequences in their passage through gametogenesis, though only a small proportion of the human genome is in fact subjected to this process.

Evidence of genomic imprinting has been observed in two dysmorphic syndromes associated with learning difficulties known as the Prader–Willi and Angelman syndromes.

### The Prader–Willi syndrome

Prader–Willi syndrome (p. 276) is characterized by short stature, obesity, hypogonadism and learning difficulty (Fig. 7.21). Approximately 50–60% of individuals with Prader–Willi syndrome can be shown to have an interstitial deletion of the proximal portion of the long arm of chromosome 15 visible by conventional cytogenetic means, and in a further 15% a submicroscopic deletion can be demonstrated by FISH (p. 35) or molecular means. DNA analysis has revealed that the chromosome deleted is almost always the paternally derived homolog. Most of the remaining 25% of individuals with Prader–Willi syndrome found not to have a chromosome deletion, have been shown to have maternal uniparental disomy. This is functionally the equivalent of a deletion in the paternally derived chromosome 15.

It is now known that only the paternally inherited allele of a critical region of the proximal portion of chromosome 15, which includes the gene for the small nuclear ribonucleoprotein polypeptide N (*SNRPN*), is expressed, i.e. the *SNRPN* gene and adjacent genes are maternally imprinted. These findings are consistent with the hypothesis that expression of a functional *SNRPN* gene product or closely adjacent genes is lacking in Prader–Willi syndrome, and its deficiency could lead, in part, to the features of the disorder.

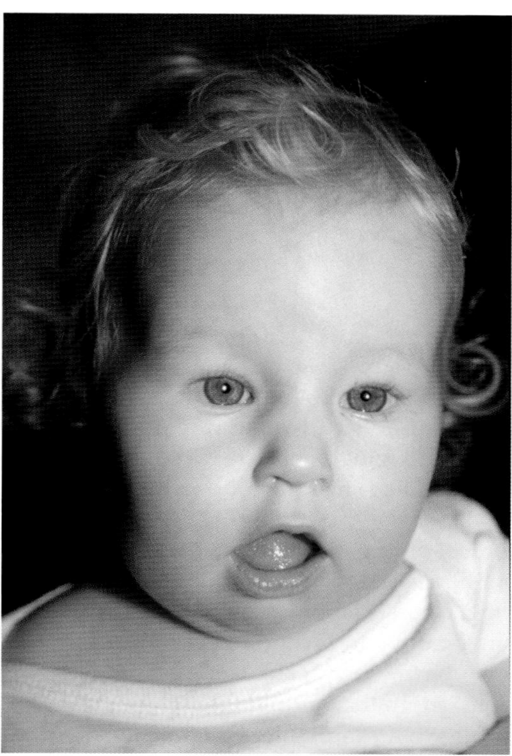

Fig. 7.21
Female child with Prader–Willi syndrome.

## The Angelman syndrome

Angelman syndrome (p. 276) is characterized by epilepsy, severe learning difficulties, an unsteady or ataxic gait and a happy affect (Fig. 7.22A, B). Interestingly, 70% of individuals with Angelman syndrome have been shown to have an interstitial deletion of the same region of chromosome 15 as that involved in Prader–Willi syndrome, but in this case on the maternally derived homolog. In a further 2–3% of individuals with Angelman syndrome, it can be shown to have arisen through paternal uniparental disomy. In up to 10% of individuals with Angelman syndrome, mutations have been identified in *UBE3A*, one of the ubiquitin genes, which appears to be preferentially or exclusively expressed from the maternally derived chromosome 15 in brain. How mutations in *UBE3A* lead to the features seen in persons with Angelman syndrome is not clear, but could involve ubiquitin-mediated destruction of proteins in the central nervous system in development, particularly where *UBE3A* is expressed most strongly, namely the hippocampus and Purkinje cells of the cerebellum.

About 2% of individuals with Prader–Willi syndrome and approximately 5% of individuals with Angelman syndrome have abnormalities of the imprinting process itself. This last group, unlike the other three, is associated with a risk of recurrence. In the case of Angelman

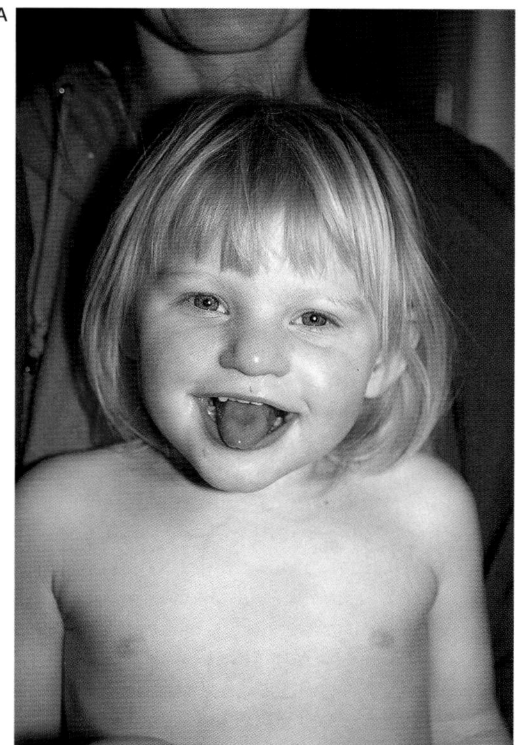

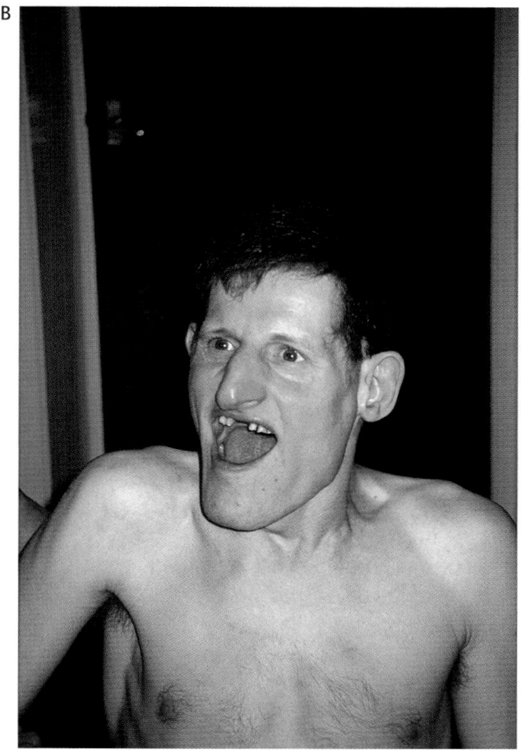

Fig. 7.22
(A) Female child with Angelman syndrome. (B) An adult male with Angelman syndrome.

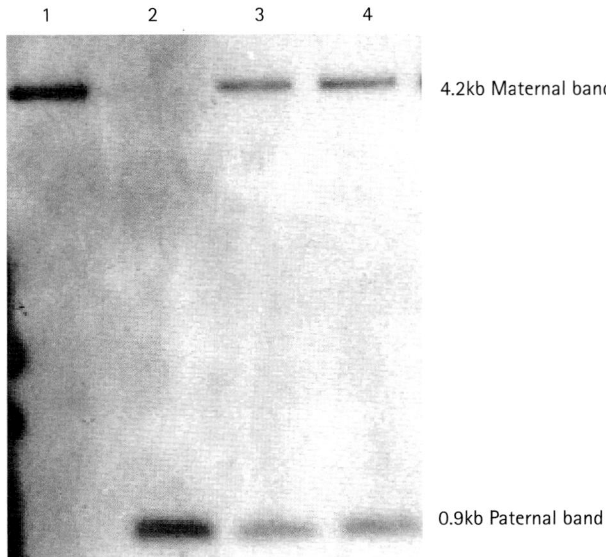


**Fig. 7.23**
Southern blot to detect methylations of *SNRPN*. DNA digested with *Xba I* and *Not I* was probed with KB17, which hybridizes to a CpG island within exon α of *SNRPN*. Patient 1 has Prader–Willi syndrome, patient 2 has Angelman syndrome and patients 3 and 4 are unaffected. (Courtesy of A. Gardner, Department of Molecular Genetics, Southmead Hospital, Bristol.)

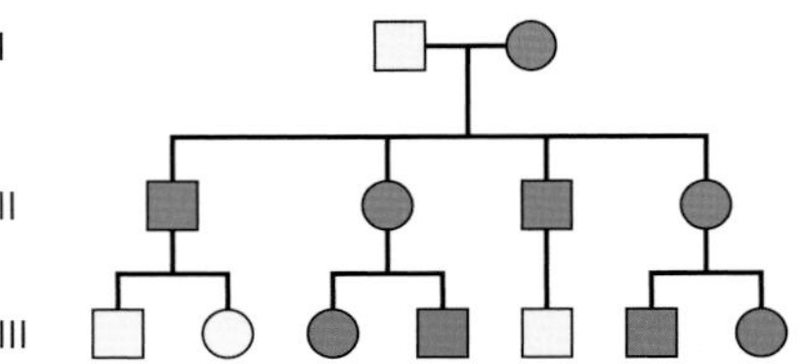


**Fig. 7.24**
Family tree consistent with mitochondrial inheritance.

syndrome, if the *mother* carries the same mutation as the child the recurrence risk is 50% – but even if she tests negative for the mutation there is an appreciable recurrence risk due to gonadal mosaicism.

Rare families have been reported in which a translocation of the proximal portion of the long arm of chromosome 15 involved in these two syndromes is segregating. Depending on whether the translocation is transmitted by the father or mother, the affected offspring within the family have had either Prader–Willi syndrome or Angelman syndrome!

In many genetics service laboratories a simple DNA test is used to diagnose both Prader–Willi syndrome and Angelman syndrome, exploiting the differential DNA methylation characteristics at the 15q locus (Fig. 7.23).

## MITOCHONDRIAL INHERITANCE

Each cell contains thousands of copies of mitochondrial DNA with more being found in cells that have high energy requirements, such as brain and muscle. Mitochondria, and therefore their DNA, are inherited almost exclusively from the mother through the oocyte (p. 19). Mitochondrial DNA has a higher rate of spontaneous mutation than nuclear DNA and the accumulation of mutations in mitochondrial DNA has been proposed as being responsible for some of the somatic effects seen with aging.

In humans, *cytoplasmic* or *mitochondrial inheritance* has been proposed as a possible explanation for the pattern of inheritance observed in some rare disorders that affect both males and females but are transmitted only through females, so-called maternal or matrilineal inheritance (Fig. 7.24).

A number of rare disorders with unusual combinations of neurological and myopathic features, sometimes occurring in association with other conditions such as cardiomyopathy and conduction defects, diabetes or deafness, have been characterized as being due to mutations in mitochondrial genes (p. 178). As mitochondria have an important role in cellular metabolism through oxidative phosphorylation, it is not surprising that the organs most susceptible to mitochondrial mutations are the central nervous system, skeletal muscle and heart.

In most persons the mitochondrial DNA from different mitochondria is identical, or shows what is termed *homoplasmy*. If a mutation occurs in the mitochondrial DNA of an individual, initially there will be two populations of mitochondrial DNA, so-called *heteroplasmy*. The proportion of mitochondria with a mutation in their DNA varies between cells and tissues and this, together with mutational heterogeneity, is a possible explanation for the range of phenotypic severity seen in persons affected with mitochondrially inherited disorders (Fig. 7.25).

Whilst matrilineal inheritance applies to disorders that are directly due to mutations in mitochondrial DNA, it is also very important to be aware that mitochondrial *proteins* are mainly encoded by nuclear genes. Mutations in these genes can have a devastating impact on respiratory chain functions within mitochondria. Examples include genes encoding proteins within the cytochrome-c (COX) system, which follow autosomal recessive inheritance, and the *G4.5* (*TAZ*) gene that is X-linked and causes Barth syndrome (endocardial fibroelastosis) in males (p. 179). There is even a mitochondrial myopathy following autosomal dominant inheritance where multiple mitochondrial DNA deletions can be detected, though the gene(s) mutated in this condition are as yet unknown. Further space is devoted to mitochondrial disorders in Chapter 11 (p. 178).

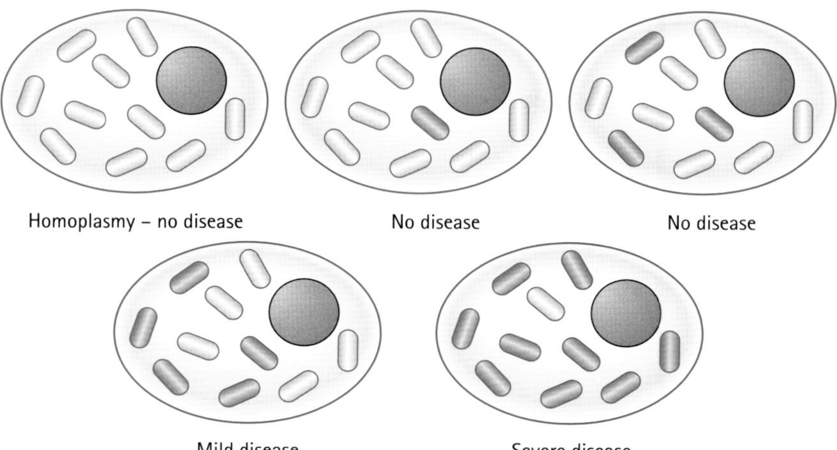


**Fig. 7.25**
The progressive effects of heteroplasmy on the clinical severity of disease due to mutations in the mitochondrial genome. Low proportions of mutant mitochondria are tolerated well, but as the proportion increases different thresholds for cellular, and hence tissue, dysfunction are breached (gray circle represents the cell nucleus).

## FURTHER READING

Bateson W, Saunders E R 1902 Experimental studies in the physiology of heredity. Royal Society Reports to the Evolution Committee, pp. 132–134
*Early observations on Mendelian inheritance.*
Bennet R L, Steinhaus K A, Uhrich S B, et al 1995 Recommendations for standardized human pedigree nomenclature. Am J Hum Genet 56: 745–752
Hall J G 1988 Somatic mosaicism: observations related to clinical genetics. Am J Hum Genet 43: 355–363
*Good review of findings arising from somatic mosaicism in clinical genetics.*
Hall J G 1990 Genomic imprinting: review and relevance to human diseases. Am J Hum Genet 46: 857–873
*Extensive review of examples of imprinting in inherited diseases in humans.*
Heinig R M 2000 The monk in the garden: the lost and found genius of Gregor Mendel. Houghton Mifflin, London
*The life and work of Gregor Mendel as the history of the birth of genetics.*
Kingston H M 1994 An ABC of clinical genetics, 2nd edn. British Medical Association, London
*A simple outline primer of the basic principles of clinical genetics.*
Reik W, Surami A (eds) 1997 Genomic imprinting (Frontiers in Molecular Biology), IRL Press, London
*Detailed discussion of examples and mechanisms of genomic imprinting.*
Vogel F, Motulsky A G 1996 Human genetics, 3nd edn. Springer-Verlag, Berlin
*This text has detailed explanations of many of the concepts in human genetics outlined in this chapter.*

## ELEMENTS

1. Family studies are often necessary to determine the mode of inheritance of a trait or disorder and to give appropriate genetic counseling. A standard shorthand convention exists for pedigree documentation of the family history.

2. Mendelian, or single-gene, disorders can be inherited in five ways: autosomal dominant, autosomal recessive, X-linked dominant, X-linked recessive and Y-linked inheritance.

3. Autosomal dominant alleles are manifest in the heterozygous state and are usually transmitted from one generation to the next but can occasionally arise as a new mutation. They usually affect both males and females equally. Each offspring of a parent with an autosomal dominant gene has a 1 in 2 chance of inheriting it from the affected parent. Autosomal dominant alleles can exhibit reduced penetrance, variable expressivity and sex limitation.

4. Autosomal recessive disorders are only manifest in the homozygous state and normally only affect individuals in one generation, usually in one sibship in a family. They affect both males and females equally. Offspring of parents who are heterozygous for the same autosomal recessive allele have a 1 in 4 chance of being homozygous for that allele. The less common an autosomal recessive allele, the greater the likelihood that the parents of a homozygote are consanguineous.

5. X-linked recessive alleles are normally only manifest in males. Offspring of females heterozygous for an X-linked recessive allele have a 1 in 2 chance of inheriting the allele from their mother. Daughters of males with an X-linked recessive allele are obligate heterozygotes but sons cannot inherit the allele. Rarely, females manifest an X-linked recessive trait because they are homozygous for the allele, have a single X chromosome, have a structural rearrangement of one of their X chromosomes, or are heterozygous but show skewed or non-random X-inactivation.

6. There are only a few disorders known to be inherited in an X-linked dominant manner. In X-linked dominant disorders hemizygous males are more severely affected than heterozygous females.

7. Unusual features in single-gene patterns of inheritance can be explained by phenomena such as genetic heterogeneity, mosaicism, anticipation, imprinting, uniparental disomy and mitochondrial inheritance.

CHAPTER

# 8 Mathematical and population genetics

*"Do not worry about your difficulties in mathematics. I can assure you mine are still greater."*

Albert Einstein

In this chapter some of the more mathematical aspects of the ways in which genes are inherited will be considered, together with how genes are distributed and maintained at particular frequencies in populations. This subject constitutes what is known as *population genetics*. By its very nature genetics lends itself to a numerical approach with many of the most influential pioneering figures in human genetics having come from a mathematical background. They were particularly attracted by the challenges of trying to determine the frequencies of genes in populations and the rates at which they mutate. Much of this early work impinges on the specialty of medical genetics, and in particular on genetic counseling, and by the end of this chapter it is hoped that the reader will have gained an understanding of the following:

1. Why a dominant trait does not increase in a population at the expense of a recessive one.
2. How the carrier frequency and mutation rate can be determined, knowing the disease incidence.
3. Why a particular genetic disorder can be more common in one population or community than in another.
4. How it can be confirmed that a genetic disorder shows a particular pattern of inheritance.
5. The concept of genetic linkage and how this differs from linkage disequilibrium.
6. The effects of medical intervention.

## ALLELE FREQUENCIES IN POPULATIONS

On first reflection it would be reasonable to predict that dominant genes and traits in a population would tend to increase at the expense of recessive ones. After all, on average three-quarters of the offspring of two heterozygotes will manifest the dominant trait, but only one-quarter will have the recessive trait. It might be concluded therefore that eventually almost everyone in the population would have the dominant trait. However, it can be shown that in a large randomly mating population, in which there is no disturbance by outside influences, dominant traits do not increase at the expense of recessive ones. In fact, in such a population, the relative proportions of the different genotypes (and phenotypes) remain constant from one generation to another. This is known as the *Hardy–Weinberg principle*, as it was proposed, independently, by an English mathematician, G. H. Hardy, and a German physician, W. Weinberg, in 1908. This is one of the most important fundamental principles in human genetics.

### THE HARDY–WEINBERG PRINCIPLE

Consider an 'ideal' population in which there is an autosomal locus with two alleles A and a, which have frequencies of p and q, respectively. These are the only alleles found at this locus, so that p + q = 100% or 1. The frequency of each genotype in the population can be determined by construction of a Punnett's square, which shows how the different genes can combine (Fig. 8.1).

From Figure 8.1 it can be seen that the frequencies of the different genotypes are:

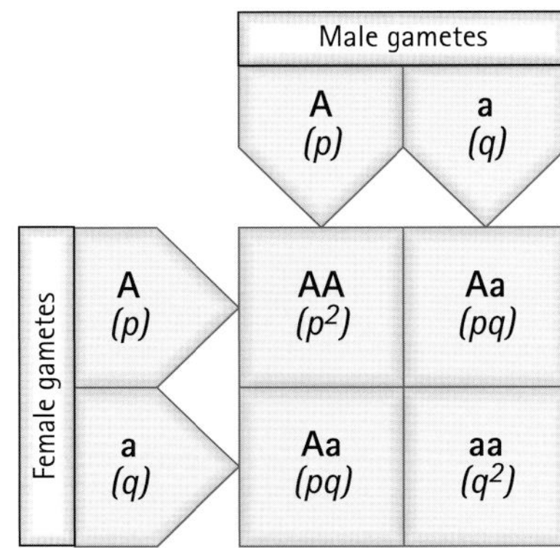


**Fig. 8.1**
Punnett's square showing the allele frequencies and resulting genotype frequencies for a two-allele system in the first generation.

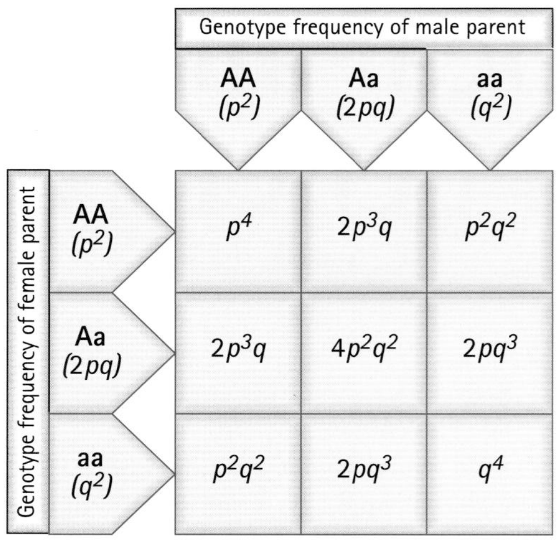


**Fig. 8.2**
Punnett's square showing the frequencies of the different matings in the second generation.

| Genotype | Phenotype | Frequency |
|---|---|---|
| AA | A | $p^2$ |
| Aa | A | 2pq |
| aa | a | $q^2$ |

We have now established that if there is random mating of sperm and ova the frequencies of the different genotypes in the first generation will be as shown above. Next consider that these individuals mate with each other to produce a second generation. Once again a Punnett's square is used to show the different matings and their frequencies (Fig. 8.2).

From Figure 8.2 a table can be drawn up to calculate the total frequency for each genotype in the second generation (Table 8.1). This reveals that the relative frequency or proportion of each genotype is the same in the second generation as in the first. In fact, it can be shown that no matter how many generations are studied the relative frequencies will remain constant. The actual numbers of individuals with each genotype will change as the population size increases or decreases, but their relative frequencies or proportions remain constant. This is the fundamental tenet of the Hardy–Weinberg principle. When studies confirm that the relative proportions of each genotype are indeed remaining constant with frequencies of $p^2$, 2pq and $q^2$, then that population is said to be in a state of *Hardy–Weinberg equilibrium* for that particular genotype.

## FACTORS THAT CAN DISTURB HARDY–WEINBERG EQUILIBRIUM

The discussion above relates to an 'ideal' population. By definition such a population is large and shows random mating with no new mutations and no selection for or against any particular genotype. For some human characteristics, such as neutral genes for blood groups or enzyme variants, these criteria can be fullfilled. However, in genetic disorders, several factors can disturb the Hardy–Weinberg equilibrium, either by influencing the distribution of genes in the population or by altering the gene frequencies. These factors include:

1. Non-random mating
2. Mutation
3. Selection
4. Small population size
5. Gene flow (migration).

### Non-random mating

*Random mating*, or *panmixis*, refers to the selection of a partner regardless of that partner's genotype. Non-random mating can lead to an increase in the frequency of affected homozygotes by two mechanisms, either assortative mating or consanguinity.

**Table 8.1 Shows the frequency of the various types of offspring from the matings shown in Figure 8.2**

| | Frequency of offspring | | | |
|---|---|---|---|---|
| **Mating type** | **Frequency** | **AA** | **Aa** | **aa** |
| AA × AA | $p^4$ | $p^4$ | — | — |
| AA × Aa | $4p^3q$ | $2p^3q$ | $2p^3q$ | — |
| Aa × Aa | $4p^2q^2$ | $p^2q^2$ | $2p^2q^2$ | $p^2q^2$ |
| AA × aa | $2p^2q^2$ | — | $2p^2q^2$ | — |
| Aa × aa | $4pq^3$ | — | $2pq^3$ | $2pq^3$ |
| aa × aa | $q^4$ | — | — | $q^4$ |
| Total | | $p^2(p^2+2pq+q^2)$ | $2pq(p^2+2pq+q^2)$ | $q^2(p^2+2pq+q^2)$ |
| Relative frequency | | $p^2$ | $2pq$ | $q^2$ |

### *Assortative mating*

*Assortative mating* is the tendency for human beings to choose partners who share characteristics such as height, intelligence and racial origin. If assortative mating extends to conditions such as autosomal recessive deafness, which accounts for a large proportion of all congenital hearing loss, then this will lead to a small increase in the relative frequency of affected homozygotes.

### *Consanguinity*

Consanguinity is the term used to describe marriage between blood relatives who have at least one common ancestor no more remote than a great-great-grandparent. Widespread consanguinity in a community will lead to a relative increase in the frequency of affected homozygotes and a relative decrease in the frequency of heterozygotes.

### Mutation

The validity of the Hardy–Weinberg principle is based on the assumption that no new mutations occur. If a particular locus shows a high mutation rate then there will be a steady increase in the proportion of mutant alleles in a population. In practice mutations do occur at almost all loci, albeit at different rates, but the effect of their introduction is usually balanced by the loss of mutant alleles due to reduced fitness of affected individuals. If a population is found to be in Hardy–Weinberg equilibrium, it is generally assumed that these two opposing factors have roughly equal effects. This is discussed further in the section that follows on the estimation of mutation rates.

### Selection

In the 'ideal' population there is no selection for or against any particular genotype. In reality for deleterious characteristics there is likely to be negative selection, with affected individuals having reduced reproductive (= biological = 'genetic') fitness. This implies that they do not have as many offspring as unaffected control members of the same population. In the absence of new mutations this reduction in fitness will lead to a gradual reduction in the frequency of the mutant gene and disturbance of Hardy–Weinberg equilibrium.

Selection can act in the opposite direction by increasing fitness. For some autosomal recessive disorders there is evidence that heterozygotes show a slight increase in biological fitness compared to unaffected homozygotes. This is referred to as *heterozygote advantage*. The best, understood example is sickle-cell disease, in which affected homozygotes have severe anemia and often show persistent ill-health (p. 154). However, heterozygotes are relatively immune to infection with *Plasmodium falciparum* malaria because if their red blood cells are invaded by the parasite they undergo sickling and are rapidly destroyed. In areas in which this form of malaria is endemic, carriers of sickle-cell anemia, who are described as having sickle-cell trait, are at a biological advantage compared to unaffected homozygotes. Therefore, in these communities there will be a tendency for the proportion of heterozygotes to increase relative to the proportions of normal and affected homozygotes. Once again this will result in a disturbance of Hardy–Weinberg equilibrium.

### Small population size

In a large population the numbers of children produced by individuals with different genotypes, assuming no alteration in fitness for any particular genotype, will tend to balance out, so that gene frequencies will remain stable. However, in a small population it is possible that by random statistical fluctuation one allele could be transmitted to a high proportion of offspring by chance, resulting in marked changes in allele frequency from one generation to the next, so that Hardy–Weinberg equilibrium is disturbed. This phenomenon is referred to as *random genetic drift*. If one allele is lost altogether then it is said to be extinguished and the other allele is described as having become fixed (Fig. 8.3).

### Gene flow (migration)

If new alleles are introduced into a population as a consequence of migration with subsequent intermarriage, this will lead to a change in the relevant allele frequencies. This slow diffusion of alleles across a racial or geographical boundary is known as *gene flow*. The most widely quoted example is the gradient shown by the incidence of the B blood group allele throughout the world (Fig. 8.4). This allele is thought to have originated in Asia and spread slowly westward as a result of admixture through invasion.

## VALIDITY OF HARDY–WEINBERG EQUILIBRIUM

It is relatively simple to establish whether a population is in Hardy–Weinberg equilibrium for a particular trait if all possible genotypes can be identified. Consider a system with two alleles A and a, with three resulting genotypes AA, Aa/aA and aa. Amongst 1000 individuals selected at random, the following genotype distributions are observed:

| | |
|---|---|
| AA | 800 |
| Aa/aA | 185 |
| aa | 15 |

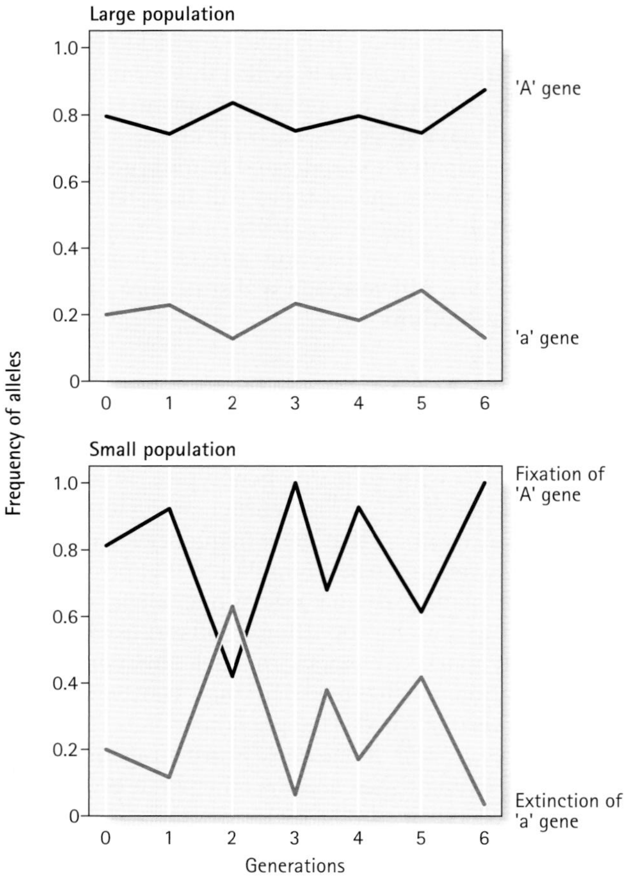


**Fig. 8.3**
The possible effects of random genetic drift in large and small populations.

From these figures the incidence of the A allele (p) equals [(2 × 800) + 185]/2000 = 0.8925 and the incidence of the a allele (q) equals [185 + (2 × 15)]/2000 = 0.1075.

Now consider what the expected genotype frequencies would be if the population is in Hardy–Weinberg equilibrium and compare these with the observed values.

| Genotype | Observed | Expected |
|---|---|---|
| AA | 800 | 796.5 ($p^2 \times 1000$) |
| Aa/aA | 185 | 192 ($2pq \times 1000$) |
| aa | 15 | 11.5 ($q^2 \times 1000$) |

These observed and expected values correspond closely and formal statistical analysis with a $\chi^2$ test would confirm that the observed values do not differ significantly from those expected if the population is in equilibrium.

Next consider a different system with two alleles B and b. Amongst 1000 randomly selected individuals the observed genotype distributions are:

| | |
|---|---|
| BB | 430 |
| Bb/bB | 540 |
| bb | 30 |



From these figures the incidence of the B allele (p) equals [(2 × 430) + 540]/2000 = 0.7 and the incidence of the b allele (q) equals [540 + (2 × 30)]/2000 = 0.3.

Using these values for p and q the observed and expected genotype distributions can be compared.

| Genotype | Observed | Expected |
|---|---|---|
| BB | 430 | 490 ($p^2 \times 1000$) |
| Bb/bB | 540 | 420 ($2pq \times 1000$) |
| bb | 30 | 90 ($q^2 \times 1000$) |

These values differ considerably, with an increased number of heterozygotes at the expense of homozygotes. Deviation such as this from Hardy–Weinberg equilibrium should prompt a search for factors that could result in increased numbers of heterozygotes, such as heterozygote advantage or negative assortative mating, i.e. the attraction of opposites!

Unless there is strong evidence to the contrary it is usually assumed that most populations are in equilibrium for most genetic traits, despite the number of factors that can disturb this equilibrium, as it is very unusual to find a population in which genotype frequencies show significant deviation from those that would be expected.

## APPLICATIONS OF HARDY–WEINBERG EQUILIBRIUM

### Estimation of carrier frequencies

If the incidence of an autosomal recessive disorder is known, then it is possible to calculate the carrier frequency using some relatively simple algebra. If, for example, the disease incidence equals 1 in 10000, then $q^2 = \frac{1}{10\,000}$ and $q = \frac{1}{100}$. As $p + q = 1$, therefore $p = \frac{99}{100}$. The carrier frequency can then be calculated as $2 \times \frac{99}{100} \times \frac{1}{100}$, i.e. 2pq, which approximates to 1 in 50. Thus a rough approximation of the carrier frequency can be obtained by doubling the square root of the disease incidence. Approximate values for gene frequency and carrier frequency derived from the disease incidence can be extremely useful when calculating risks for genetic counseling (p. 344) (Table 8.2). Note that if the disease incidence includes cases resulting from consanguineous relationships, then it is not valid to use the Hardy–Weinberg principle to calculate heterozygote frequences as a relatively high incidence of consanguinity disturbs the equilibrium by leading to a relative increase in the proportion of affected homozygotes.

For an X-linked disorder the frequency of affected males equals the frequency of the mutant allele, q. Thus for a trait such as red–green color blindness, which affects approximately 1 in 12 male Western European caucasians, q equals $\frac{1}{12}$ and p equals $\frac{11}{12}$. This means that the frequency of affected females ($q^2$) and carrier females (2pq) equals $\frac{1}{144}$ and $\frac{22}{144}$ respectively.

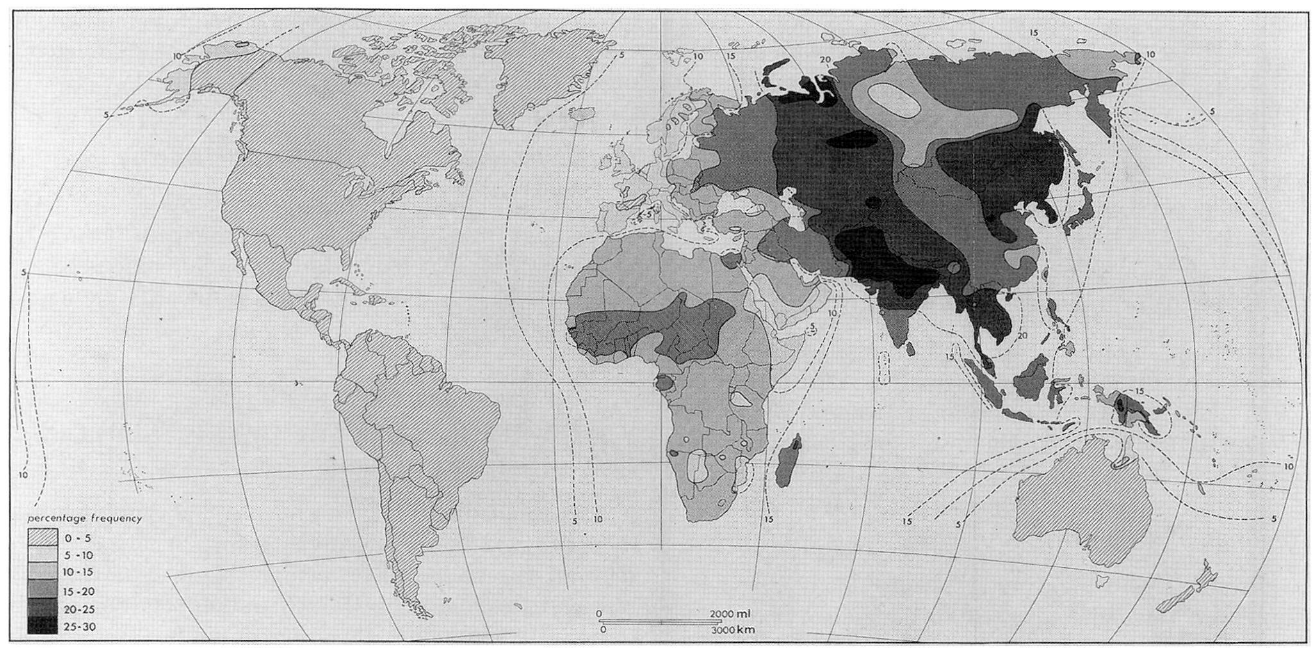


**Fig. 8.4**
Distribution of blood group B throughout the world. (From Mourant, Kopéc and Domianiewska-Sobczaz 1976 The distribution of the human blood groups and other polymorphisms, 2nd edn. Oxford University Press, with permission.)

**Table 8.2 Approximate values for gene frequency and carrier frequency calculated from the disease incidence assuming Hardy–Weinberg equilibrium**

| Disease incidence (q2) | Gene frequency (q) | Carrier frequency (2pq) |
|---|---|---|
| $\frac{1}{1000}$ | $\frac{1}{32}$ | $\frac{1}{16}$ |
| $\frac{1}{2000}$ | $\frac{1}{45}$ | $\frac{1}{23}$ |
| $\frac{1}{5000}$ | $\frac{1}{71}$ | $\frac{1}{36}$ |
| $\frac{1}{10\,000}$ | $\frac{1}{100}$ | $\frac{1}{50}$ |
| $\frac{1}{50\,000}$ | $\frac{1}{224}$ | $\frac{1}{112}$ |
| $\frac{1}{100\,000}$ | $\frac{1}{316}$ | $\frac{1}{158}$ |

## Estimation of mutation rates

### *Direct method*

If an autosomal dominant disorder shows full penetrance and is therefore always expressed in heterozygotes, an estimate of its mutation rate can be made relatively easily by counting the number of new cases in a defined number of births. Consider a sample of 100 000 children, 12 of whom have a particular autosomal dominant disorder such as achondroplasia (p. 92). Only two of these children have an affected parent, so that the remaining 10 must have acquired their disorder as a result of new mutations. Therefore 10 new mutations have occurred among the 200 000 genes inherited by these children (each child inherits two genes), giving a mutation rate of 1 per 20 000 gametes per generation. In fact, all new mutations in achondroplasia occur on the paternally derived chromosome 4, so that the mutation rate is 1 per 10 000 in spermatogenesis and, as far as we know, zero in oogenesis.

### *Indirect method*

For an autosomal dominant disorder with reproductive fitness (f) equal to zero, all cases must result from new mutations. If the incidence of a disorder is denoted as I and the mutation rate as $\mu$, then as each child inherits two alleles, either of which can mutate to cause the disorder, the incidence equals twice the mutation rate, i.e. $I = 2\mu$.

If fitness is greater than zero, and the disorder is in Hardy–Weinberg equilibrium, then genes lost through reduced fitness must be counterbalanced by new mutations. Therefore, $2\mu = I\,(1\text{-}f)$ or $\mu = [I\,(1\text{-}f)]/2$.

Thus if an estimate of genetic fitness can be made by comparing the average number of offspring born to affected parents compared with controls such as their unaffected siblings, it will be possible to calculate the mutation rate.

A similar approach can be used to estimate mutation rates for autosomal recessive and sex-linked recessive disorders. With an autosomal recessive condition, two genes will be lost for each homozygote who fails to reproduce. These will be balanced by new mutations. Therefore, $2\mu = I(1\text{-}f) \times 2$ or $\mu = I(1\text{-}f)$.

For a sex-linked recessive condition with incidence in males equal to $I^M$, three X chromosomes are transmitted per couple per generation. Therefore, $3\mu = I^M(1\text{-}f)$ or $\mu = [I^M(1\text{-}f)]/3$.

### Why is it helpful to know mutation rates?

At first sight it might seem that knowledge of these formulae linking mutation rates with disease incidence and fitness is of little practical value. However, there are several ways in which this information can be useful.

#### *Estimation of gene size*

If a disorder has a high mutation rate this could yield information about the structure of the gene that would help expedite its isolation and characterization. For example, the gene could contain a high proportion of GC residues which are thought to be particularly prone to copy error (p. 24), or it could contain a high proportion of repeat sequences (p. 18) that could predispose to misalignment in meiosis resulting in deletion and duplication, or it could simply be that the gene is very large.

#### *Determination of mutagenic potential*

If valuable information is to be gained about the potential mutagenic effects of nuclear accidents such as Chernobyl (p. 28), it will be necessary to have accurate methods for determining mutation rates and how these are related to observed changes in disease incidence (p. 28).

#### *Consequences of treatment of genetic disease*

Knowledge of the relationship between disease incidence, fitness and mutation rate is necessary to determine the possible effects of improved treatment for serious genetic disorders. This is discussed further towards the end of this chapter.

## WHY ARE SOME GENETIC DISORDERS MORE COMMON THAN OTHERS?

It is axiomatic that if a gene shows a high mutation rate, then this will usually result in a high incidence of the relevant disease. However, factors other than the mutation rate and the fitness of affected individuals can also be involved. Mention has already been made of some of the mechanisms that can account for a high gene frequency of a particular disorder in a specific population. These will now be considered in the context of population size.

### Small populations

Several rare autosomal recessive disorders show a relatively high incidence in certain populations and communities (Table 8.3). The most likely explanation for most of these observations is that the high allele frequency has resulted from a combination of a *founder effect* coupled

**Table 8.3 Rare recessive disorders which are relatively common in certain groups of people**

| Group | Disorder | Clinical features |
|---|---|---|
| Finns | Congenital nephrotic syndrome | Oedema, proteinuria, susceptibility to infection |
| | Aspartylglycosaminuria | Progressive mental and motor deterioration, coarse features |
| | MULIBREY–nanism | MUscle, LIver, BRain and EYe involvement |
| | Congenital chloride diarrhoea | Reduced Cl– absorption, diarrhoea |
| | Diastrophic dysplasia | Progressive epiphyseal dysplasia with dwarfism and scoliosis |
| Amish | Cartilage–hair hypoplasia | Dwarfism, fine, light-coloured and sparse hair |
| | Ellis–van Creveld syndrome | Dwarfism, polydactyly, congenital heart disease |
| | Glutaric aciduria type 1 | Episodic encephalopathy and cerebral palsy-like dystonia |
| Hopi and San Blas Indians | Albinism | Lack of pigmentation |
| Ashkenazi Jews | Tay–Sachs disease | Progressive mental and motor deterioration, blindness |
| | Gaucher disease | Hepatosplenomegaly, bone lesions, skin pigmentation |
| | Dysautonomia | Indifference to pain, emotional lability, lack of tears, hyperhidrosis |
| Karaite Jews | Werdnig–Hoffmann disease | Infantile spinal muscular atrophy |
| Afrikaners syndactyly | Sclerosteosis | Tall stature, overgrowth of craniofacial bones with cranial nerve palsies, |
| | Lipoid proteinosis | Thickening of skin and mucous membranes |
| Ryukyan islands (off Japan) | 'Ryukyan' spinal muscular atrophy | Muscle weakness, club foot, scoliosis |

with social, religious or geographical isolation of the relevant group. Such groups are referred to as genetic isolates. In some of the smaller populations genetic drift could also have played a role.

For example, several otherwise very rare autosomal recessive disorders have been found to occur at a relatively high frequency in the Old Order Amish living in Pennsylvania – Christians originating from the Anabaptist movement who fled Europe during religious persecution in the eighteenth century. Presumably, by chance, one or two original founders of the group carried abnormal alleles that became established at relatively high frequency because of the restricted number of partners available to members of the community.

A founder effect can also be observed for autosomal dominant disorders. Variegate porphyria, which is characterized by photosensitivity and drug-induced neurovisceral disturbance, has a much higher incidence in the Afrikaner population of South Africa than in any other country or race. This is thought to be due to one of the early Dutch settlers having the condition and transmitting it to a large number of his or her descendants (p. 105).

One particularly novel explanation for a high gene frequency in a small population is provided by the Hopi Indians of Arizona, who show a high incidence of albinism. Affected males were protected from outdoor farming activity because of their susceptibility to bright sunlight and it seems that this provided them with opportunity for reproductive activity in the absence of their unaffected peers. It is worth noting that several famous historical figures were affected with albinism: these include the Reverend William Spooner, who was famous for transposing the initial letters of words – hence 'Spoonerism'.

## Large populations

When a serious autosomal recessive disorder, which results in reduced fitness in affected homozygotes, has a high incidence in a large population, the explanation must lie in either a very high mutation rate or in heterozygote advantage. The latter explanation is the more probable for most autosomal recessive disorders (Table 8.4).

### *Heterozygote advantage*

For sickle-cell anemia (p. 154) and thalassemia (p. 155) there is good evidence that heterozygote advantage results from reduced susceptibility to *Plasmodium falciparum* malaria. The mechanism by which this is thought to occur is that the red cells of heterozygotes for sickle-cell can more effectively express malarial or altered self antigens that will result in more rapid removal of parasitized cells from the circulation. Americans of Afro-Caribbean origin are no longer exposed to malaria, so it would be expected that the frequency of the sickle-cell allele amongst these individuals would gradually decline. However, the predicted rate of decline is so slow that it will be many generations before it is detectable.

For several autosomal recessive disorders the mechanisms proposed for heterozygote advantage are largely speculative (Table 8.4). The recent discovery of the cystic fibrosis gene, with the subsequent elucidation of the role of its protein product in membrane permeability (p. 303), supports the hypothesis of selective advantage through increased resistance to the effects of gastrointestinal infections such as cholera and dysentery in the heterozygote. This relative resistance could result from reduced loss of fluid and electrolytes. It is likely that this selective

**Table 8.4 Presumed increased resistance in heterozygotes which could account for the maintenance of various genetic disorders in certain populations**

| Disorder | Genetics | Region/population | Resistance or advantage |
|---|---|---|---|
| Sickle-cell disease | AR | Tropical Africa | Falciparum malaria |
| α and β thalassaemia | AR | South-east Asia and Mediterranean | Falciparum malaria |
| G6PD deficiency | XR | Mediterranean | Falciparum malaria |
| Cystic fibrosis | AR | Western Europe | Tuberculosis?<br>The plague?<br>Cholera? |
| Tay–Sachs disease | AR | Eastern European Jews | Tuberculosis? |
| Congenital adrenal hyperplasia | AR | Yupik Eskimos | Influenza B |
| Non-insulin dependent diabetes | AD | Pima Indians and others | Periodic starvation |
| Phenylketonuria | AR | Western Europe | Spontaneous abortion rate lower? |

AR: autosomal recessive; XR: X-linked recessive; AD: autosomal dominant advantage was of greatest value several hundred years ago when these infections were endemic in Western Europe. If so, a gradual decline in the incidence of cystic fibrosis would be expected. However, if this theory is correct one has to ask why cystic fibrosis has not become relatively common in other parts of the world where gastrointestinal infections are endemic, particularly the tropics; in fact, the opposite is the case, for cystic fibrosis is rare in these regions.

An alternative and entirely speculative mechanism for the high incidence of a condition such as cystic fibrosis is that the mutant allele is preferentially transmitted at meiosis. This type of segregation distortion, whereby an allele at a particular locus is transmitted more often than would be expected by chance, i.e. in more than 50% of gametes, is referred to as *meiotic drive*. Firm evidence for this phenomenon in cystic fibrosis is lacking although it has been demonstrated in the autosomal dominant disorder myotonic dystrophy (p. 295).

A major practical problem when studying heterozygote advantage is that even a tiny increase in heterozygote fitness compared with the fitness of unaffected homozygotes can be sufficient to sustain a high allele frequency. For example in cystic fibrosis, with an allele frequency of approximately 1 in 50, a heterozygote advantage of between 2% and 3% would be sufficient to account for this high allele frequency.

## GENETIC POLYMORPHISM

*Polymorphism* is the occurrence in a population of two or more genetically determined forms (alleles, sequence variants) in such frequencies that the rarest of them could not be maintained by mutation alone. By convention, a polymorphic locus is one at which there are at least two alleles each with frequencies greater than 1%. Alleles with frequencies of less than 1% are referred to as rare variants.

Studies of enzyme and protein variability have shown that in humans at least 30% of structural gene loci are polymorphic, with each individual being heterozygous at between 10% and 20% of all structural loci. Known polymorphic protein systems include the ABO blood groups (p. 198) and many serum proteins. A large number of enzymes exhibit polymorphic electrophoretic differences or what are known as *isozymes*.

Polymorphism at the DNA level has proved particularly valuable in the positional cloning studies that have led to the isolation of many disease genes (p. 78). Polymorphic DNA markers are also of use in gene tracking (p. 73), which can be used in presymptomatic diagnosis, prenatal diagnosis and carrier detection for a large number of single-gene disorders. The value of a particular polymorphic system is assessed by determining its *polymorphic information content* (PIC). The higher the PIC value, the more likely it is that a polymorphic marker will be of value in linkage analysis and gene tracking.

Finally, mention should be made of the distinction between *balanced* and *transient polymorphisms*. In a balanced polymorphism, two or more different forms are maintained by a balance between the selective advantage of the heterozygote and the reduced fitness of the affected homozygote. Thus the high incidence of the sickle-cell allele in areas where malaria is endemic is an example of a balanced polymorphism. However, as has already been discussed, the incidence of the sickle-cell allele is likely to decline in populations that are no longer exposed to malaria, so that in these situations the polymorphism can be considered as transient.

## SEGREGATION ANALYSIS

*Segregation analysis* refers to the study of the way in which a disorder is transmitted in families so as to establish the underlying mode of inheritance. The mathematical aspects of segregation analysis are extremely complex and fall far beyond the scope of this book and most doctors! However, it is important that those who encounter families with genetic disease have some understanding of the principles involved in segregation analysis as well as an awareness of some of the pitfalls and problems.

### AUTOSOMAL DOMINANT INHERITANCE

For an autosomal dominant disorder the simplest approach is to compare the observed numbers of affected offspring born to affected parents with what would be expected based on the disease penetrance, i.e. 50% if penetrance is complete. A $\chi^2$ test can be used to see if the observed and expected numbers differ significantly. Care must be taken to ensure that a bias is not introduced by excluding parents who were ascertained through an affected child.

### AUTOSOMAL RECESSIVE INHERITANCE

For disorders believed to show autosomal recessive inheritance, formal segregation analysis is much more difficult. This is because some couples who are both carriers will by chance not have any affected children. Usually such couples and their healthy offspring will not be ascertained. To illustrate this consider 64 possible sibships of size 3 in which both parents are carriers, drawn from a large hypothetical population (Table 8.5). The sibship structure shown in Table 8.5 is that which would be expected on average, assuming that the birth of

**Table 8.5 Shows the expected sibship structure in a hypothetical population that contains 64 sibships each of size 3, in which both parents are carriers of an autosomal recessive disorder. If no allowance is made for truncate ascertainment, in that the 27 sibships with no affected cases will not be ascertained, then a falsely high segregation ratio of 48/111 (= 0.43) will be obtained**

| No. of affected in sibship | Structure of sibship | No. of sibships | No. of affected | Total no. of sibs |
|---|---|---|---|---|
| 3 | ■■■ | 1 | 3 | 3 |
| 2 | ■■□ | 3 | 6 | 9 |
| | □■■ | 3 | 6 | 9 |
| | ■□■ | 3 | 6 | 9 |
| 1 | ■□□ | 9 | 9 | 27 |
| | □■□ | 9 | 9 | 27 |
| | □□■ | 9 | 9 | 27 |
| 0 | □□□ | 27 | 0 | 81 |
| Total | | 64 | 48 | 192 |

an affected child does not deter the parents from having further children.

In this population, on average, 27 of the 64 sibships will not contain any affected individuals. This can be calculated simply by cubing $\frac{3}{4}$, i.e. $\frac{3}{4} \times \frac{3}{4} \times \frac{3}{4} = \frac{27}{64}$. Therefore when the families are analyzed these 27 sibships containing only healthy individuals will not be ascertained. This is referred to as *truncate* or *incomplete ascertainment*. If this is not taken into account, a falsely high segregation ratio of 0.43 will be obtained instead of the correct figure of 0.25.

Mathematical methods have been devised to cater for truncate ascertainment, but analysis is usually further complicated by the problems associated with achieving full or complete ascertainment. In practice it can actually be very difficult to 'prove' that a disorder shows autosomal recessive inheritance unless accurate molecular or biochemical methods are available for carrier detection. A high incidence of parental consanguinity provides strong supportive evidence for autosomal recessive inheritance, a point first noted by Bateson and Garrod as long ago as 1902 (pp. 7, 109).

## GENETIC LINKAGE

Mendel's third law, the principle of independent assortment, states that members of different gene pairs assort to gametes independently of one another (p. 5). Stated more simply, the alleles of genes at different loci segregate independently. While this is true of genes on different chromosomes, it is not always true for genes that are located on the same chromosome, i.e. *syntenic*.

If two loci are positioned close together on the same chromosome, so that alleles at these loci are inherited together more often than not, then these loci are said to be *linked*. In effect the two loci are sufficiently close together for it to be unlikely that they will be separated by a cross-over or recombination in meiosis I (Fig. 8.5).

Alleles at linked loci on the same chromosome are said to be in *coupling*, whereas those on opposite homologous chromosomes are described as being in *repulsion*. This is known as the *linkage phase*. Thus in Fig 8.5C, in the parental chromosomes, A and B, as well as a and b, are in coupling, whereas A and b, as well as a and B, are in repulsion.

### RECOMBINATION FRACTION

The *recombination fraction*, which is usually designated as θ (Greek theta), is a measure of the distance separating two loci, or more precisely an indication of the likelihood that a cross-over will occur between them. If two loci are not linked then θ equals 0.5 as, on average, genes at unlinked loci will segregate together during 50% of all meioses. If θ equals 0.05, this means that on average the syntenic alleles will segregate together 19 times out of 20, i.e. a cross-over will occur between them during, on average, only 1 in 20 meioses.

### CENTIMORGANS

The unit of measurement for genetic linkage is known as a *map unit* or *centiMorgan* (cM). If two loci are 1 cM apart, then a cross-over occurs between them during on average only 1 in every 100 meioses, i.e. θ = 0.01. CentiMorgans are a measure of the *genetic* or *linkage* distance between two loci. This is *not* the same as physical distance, which is measured in base pairs (kb – kilobases: 1000 base pairs: Mb – megabases: 1000 000 base pairs).

The human genome has been estimated by recombination studies to be about 3000 cM in length in males. As the physical length of the haploid human genome is approximately $3 \times 10^9$ bp, 1 cM corresponds to approximately $10^6$ bp (1 Mb or 1000 kb). However, the relationship between linkage map units and physical length is not linear. Some chromosome regions appear to be particularly prone to recombination, so-called 'hot spots', and for reasons that are not understood, recombination tends to occur less often during meiosis in males than in females, in whom the genome 'linkage' length has been estimated to be 4200 cM. Generally in humans there are one or two recombination events between each pair of homologous chromosomes in meiosis I with a total of around 40 across

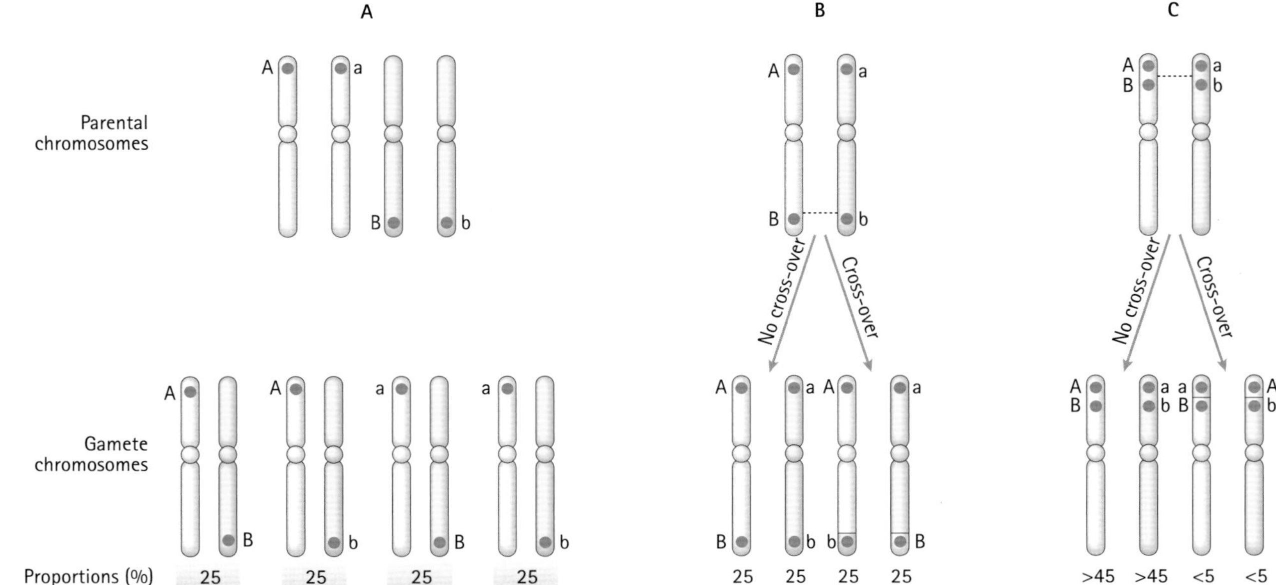


Fig. 8.5
Segregation at meiosis of alleles at two loci. In (A) the loci are on different chromosomes and in (B) they are on the same chromosome but widely separated. Hence these loci are not linked and there is independent assortment. In (C) the loci are closely adjacent so that separation by a cross-over is unlikely, i.e. the loci are linked.

the entire genome. Recombination events are rare close to the centromeres and relatively common in telomeric regions.

## LINKAGE ANALYSIS

Linkage analysis has proved to be an extremely valuable tool for mapping genes (p. 78). The basic methodology involves study of the segregation of the disease in large families with polymorphic markers from each chromosome. Eventually a marker will be identified which cosegregates with the disease more often than would be expected by chance, i.e. the marker and disease loci are linked. The mathematical analysis tends to be very complex, particularly if lots of closely adjacent markers are being used, as in *multipoint linkage analysis*. However, the underlying principle is relatively straightforward and involves the use of likelihood ratios, the logarithms of which are known as LOD scores (Logarithm of the ODds).

## LOD SCORES

When studying the segregation of alleles at two loci which could be linked, a series of likelihood ratios is calculated for different values of the recombination fraction (θ), ranging from $\theta = 0$ to $\theta = 0.5$. The likelihood ratio at a given value of θ equals the likelihood of the observed data if the loci are linked at recombination value of θ divided by the likelihood of the observed data if the loci are not linked ($\theta = 0.5$). The logarithm to the base 10 of this ratio is known as the LOD score (Z), i.e. LOD (θ) = $\log_{10}$ [Lθ/L(0.5)]. Logarithms are used because they allow results from different families to be added together.

For example, when a research paper reports that linkage of a disease with a DNA marker has been identified with a LOD score (Z) of 4 at recombination fraction (θ) 0.05, this means that in the families that have been studied the results indicate that it is 10 000 ($10^4$) times more likely that the disease and marker loci are closely linked (i.e. 5 cM apart) than that they are not linked. It is generally agreed that a LOD score of +3 or greater is confirmation of linkage. This would yield a ratio of 1000 to 1 in favor of linkage, but because there is a prior probability of only 1 in 50 that any two given loci are linked, a LOD score of +3 means that the overall probability that the loci are linked is approximately 20 to 1, i.e. [$1000 \times \frac{1}{50}$]:1. The importance of taking prior probabilities into account in probability theory is discussed in the section on Bayes' theorem (p. 341).

### A 'simple' example

Consider a three-generation family in which several members have an autosomal dominant disorder (Fig. 8.6). A and B are alleles at a locus which is being tested for linkage to the disease locus.

To establish whether it is likely that these two loci are linked, the LOD score is calculated for various values of

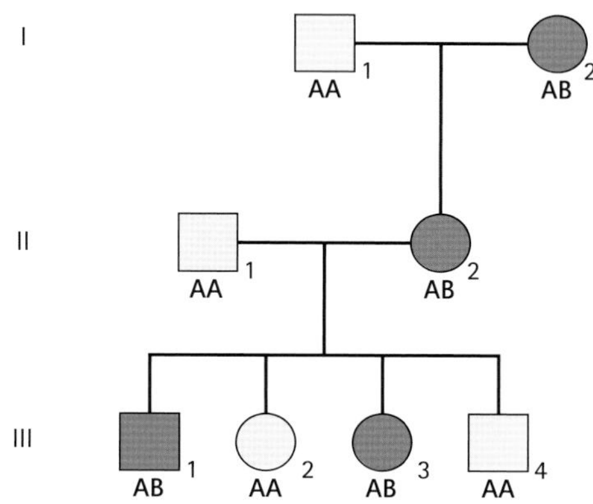


Fig. 8.6
A three-generation pedigree showing segregation of an autosomal dominant disorder and alleles (A and B) at a locus which may or may not be linked to the disease locus.

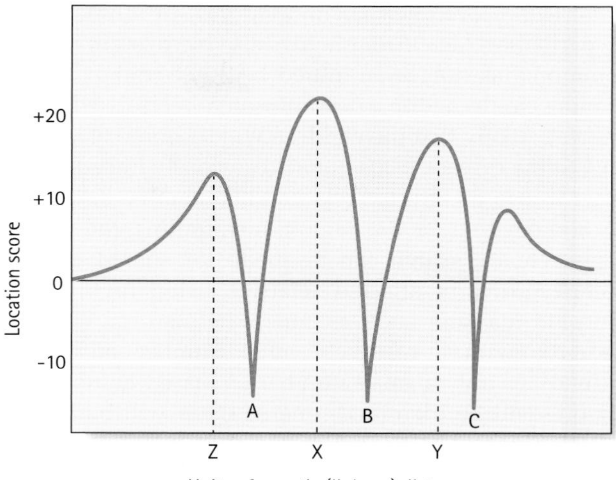


Fig. 8.7
Multipoint linkage analysis. A, B and C represent the known linkage relationships of three polymorphic marker loci. X, Y and Z represent in descending order of likelihood the probable position of the disease locus.

θ. The value of θ that gives the highest LOD score is taken as the best estimate of the recombination fraction. This is known as a maximum likelihood method.

To demonstrate the underlying principle, the LOD score will be calculated for a value of θ equal to 0.05. If θ equals 0.05 then the loci are linked, in which case the disease gene and the B marker must be on the same chromosome in II2, as both of these characteristics have been inherited from the mother. Thus in II2 the linkage phase is known – the disease allele and the B allele are in coupling. Therefore the probability that III1 would be affected and would also inherit the B marker equals 0.95, i.e. 1-θ. A similar result is obtained for the remaining three members of the sibship in generation III, giving a value for the numerator of $(0.95)^4$. If the loci are not linked, then the likelihood of observing both the disease and marker B in III1 equals 0.5. A similar result is obtained for his three siblings, giving a value for the denominator of $(0.5)^4$.

Therefore the LOD score for this family given a value of $\theta = 0.05$ equals $\log_{10} 0.95^4/0.5^4 = \log_{10} 13.032 = 1.12$. For a value of $\theta = 0$ the LOD score equals $\log_{10} 1^4/0.5^4 = \log_{10} 16 = 1.20$. For a value of $\theta = 0.1$ the LOD score equals $\log_{10} 0.9^4/0.5^4 = \log_{10} 10.498 = 1.02$. The highest LOD score is obtained for a value of θ equals 0, which is consistent with the fact that if the disease and marker loci are linked then there have been no recombinations between the two loci in members of generation III.

To confirm linkage other families would have to be studied by pooling all the results until a LOD score of +3 or greater is obtained. A LOD score of –2 or less is taken as proof that the loci are not linked. This less stringent requirement for proof of non-linkage, i.e. a LOD score of –2 compared with +3 for proof of linkage, is due to the high prior probability of $\frac{49}{50}$ that any two loci are not being linked.

## MULTIPOINT LINKAGE ANALYSIS

Two-point linkage analysis is often used to map a disease locus to a specific chromosome region. This gives a rather rough or 'coarse' indication of the location of the disease locus. The next step often involves multipoint linkage analysis using a series of polymorphic markers that are known to map to the disease region. This process allows 'fine' tuning of the probable position of the disease locus within the narrow interval defined by the small number of previously ordered polymorphic marker loci.

Using this approach the results of linkage studies with the various markers are analyzed using a computer program that calculates the overall likelihood of the position of the disease locus in relation to the marker loci. The results are presented in the form of a likelihood ratio known as a *location score*. This is calculated for different positions of the disease locus and a graph is drawn up of location score against map distance (Fig. 8.7). On this graph the peaks represent possible positions of the disease locus, with the tallest peak being the most probable location. The troughs represent the positions of the polymorphic marker loci.

Multipoint linkage analysis is used to define the smallest possible interval in which a disease locus is located, so that physical mapping methods can then be applied to isolate the disease gene (p. 76).

## AUTOZYGOSITY MAPPING

This is an ingenious form of linkage analysis that has been used to map many rare autosomal recessive disorders.

*Autozygosity* occurs when individuals are homozygous at particular loci through identity by descent from a common ancestor. In an inbred pedigree containing two or more children with a rare autosomal recessive disorder it is very likely that the children will be homozygous not only at the disease locus but also at closely linked loci. In other words, all affected relatives in an inbred family will be homozygous at the region surrounding the disease locus. Thus a search can be made for shared areas of homozygosity in affected relatives using highly polymorphic markers such as microsatellites (p. 18). In a pedigree with a relatively large number of affected individuals only a small number of shared homozygous regions will be identified; one of these will harbor the relevant disease locus, which can then be isolated using physical mapping strategies.

Autozygosity mapping can be applied in both small inbred families and in genetic isolates (p. 129) with a shared common genetic ancestry, e.g. the Old Order Amish. It is a particularly powerful technique in large inbred families where more than one branch has affected individuals. Several of the genes that cause autosomal recessive sensorineural hearing loss have been mapped in this way, besides a number of skeletal dysplasias and primary microcephalies.

## LINKAGE DISEQUILIBRIUM

*Linkage disequilibrium* is defined formally as the association of two alleles at linked loci more frequently than would be expected by chance, and is also referred to as *allelic association*. The concept and the term relate to the study of diseases in *populations* rather than families. In the latter, an association between specific alleles and the disease in question only holds true within an individual family, and in a separate affected family a different pattern of alleles, or markers, at the same locus may show association with the disease – because the alleles themselves are *polymorphic*. The rationale for studying allelic association in populations is based on the assumption that a mutation occurred in a *founder* case some generations previously and is still causative of the disease. If this is true then the pattern of markers in a small region close to the mutation will have been maintained and thus constitute what is termed the *founder haplotype*. The underlying principles used in mapping are the same as for linkage analysis in families, the difference being in the degree of relatedness of the individuals under study. In the pedigree shown in Figure 8.6 support was obtained for linkage of the disease gene with the B marker allele. Assume that further studies confirm linkage of these loci and that the A and B alleles have an equal frequency of 0.5. It would be reasonable to expect that the disease gene would be in coupling with allele A in approximately 50% of families and with allele B in the remaining 50%. If, however, the disease allele was found to be in coupling almost exclusively with one particular marker allele this would be an example of linkage disequilibrium.

The demonstration of linkage disequilibrium in a particular disease suggests that the mutation causing the disease has occurred relatively recently and that the marker locus studied is very closely linked to the disease locus. For example, one of the very small number of the original mutations for sickle-cell disease occurred in a β-globin gene that was closely adjacent to a very rare syntenic RFLP. Selection for this sickle-cell mutation, with only very rare recombination having occurred between it and the adjacent tightly linked locus, has resulted in a very high proportion of present-day, sickle-cell alleles being in coupling with this otherwise rare RFLP. There may be pitfalls, however, in interpreting haplotype data that suggest linkage disequilibrium. Other possible reasons for linkage disequilibrium include the rapid growth of genetically isolated populations leading to large regions of allelic association throughout the genome, selection – where particular alleles enhance or diminish reproductive fitness – and population admixture, where population subgroups with different patterns of allele frequencies are combined into a single study. Allowance for the latter problem can be made by using family-based controls and analyzing the transmission of alleles using a method called the *transmission/disequilibrium test* (TDT) (p. 145). This uses the fact that transmitted and non-transmitted alleles from a given parent are paired observations, and examines the preferential transmission of one allele over the other in all heterozygous parents. The technique has been applied, among others, to studies based on sibling pairs that are discordant for the disease or condition under study.

## MEDICAL AND SOCIETAL INTERVENTION

Recent developments in molecular biology, such as the human genome project (Ch. 23) and pilot studies using gene therapy (p. 358), have reawakened concern that future generations could have to cope with an ever increasing burden of genetic disease. The term eugenics was first used by Charles Darwin's cousin, Francis Galton, to refer to the improvement of a population by selective breeding. The notion that this should be applied to human populations became popular during the early years of the twentieth century, culminating in the horrifying and totally unacceptable practices of Nazi Germany. Ensuing revulsion led to the total abandonment of eugenic programs in humans, with universal condemnation and agreement that these have no place in modern medical practice.

Nevertheless, doctors who care for patients and families with hereditary disease are faced with a dilemma. On the one hand, by helping patients with serious genetic disease to survive and reproduce they are indeed increasing the numbers of 'bad genes' in society, thereby potentially adding to humanity's future genetic load. Such behavior could be interpreted as dysgenic. On the other hand, most medical practitioners would argue that their responsibility to an individual patient far outweighs their obligation to either contemporary society or future generations.

Before returning to this ethical debate it is worth considering the possible long-term effects of artificial selection for or against genetic disorders.

## AUTOSOMAL DOMINANT DISORDERS

If everyone with an autosomal dominant disorder was successfully encouraged not to reproduce, then the incidence of that disorder would decline rapidly, with all future cases only being the result of new mutations. This would have a particularly striking effect on the incidence of relatively mild conditions such as familial hypercholesterolemia, in which genetic fitness is close to 1.

Alternatively, if successful treatment became available for all patients with a serious autosomal dominant disorder that at present is associated with a marked reduction in genetic fitness, then there would be an immediate increase in the frequency of the disease gene followed by a more gradual leveling off at a new equilibrium level. If, at one time, all those with a serious autosomal dominant disorder died in childhood (f = 0) then the incidence of affected individuals would be 2μ. If treatment raised the fitness from 0 to 0.9, then the incidence of affected children in the next generation would rise to 2μ due to new mutations plus 1.8μ inherited, which equals 3.8μ. Eventually a new equilibrium would be reached, by which time the disease incidence would have risen tenfold to 20μ. This can be calculated relatively easily using the formula $\mu = [I(1\text{-}f)]/2$ (p. 127), which can be expressed alternatively as $I = 2\mu/(1\text{-}f)$. The net result would be that the proportion of affected children who die would be less (100% down to 10%), but the total number affected would be much greater, although the actual number who die from the disease would remain unchanged at 2μ.

## AUTOSOMAL RECESSIVE DISORDERS

In contrast to an autosomal dominant disorder, artificial selection against an autosomal recessive condition will have only a very slow effect.

The reason for this difference is that in autosomal recessive conditions most of the genes in a population are present in healthy heterozygotes who would not be affected by eugenic measures. It can be shown that if there is complete selection against an autosomal recessive disorder so that no homozygotes reproduce, then the number of generations (n) required to change the allele frequency from $q_o$ to $q_n$ equals $1/q_n\text{-}1/q_o$. Therefore, for a condition with an incidence of approximately 1 in 2000 and an allele frequency of roughly 1 in 45, if all affected patients refrained from reproduction then it would take over 500 years (18 generations) to reduce the disease incidence by half and over 1200 years (45 generations) to reduce the gene frequency by half, assuming an average generation time of 27 years.

Now consider the opposite situation, where selection operating against a serious autosomal recessive disorder is relaxed because of improvement in medical treatment. More affected individuals will reach adult life and transmit the mutant allele to their offspring. The result will be that the frequency of the mutant allele will increase until a new equilibrium is reached. Using the formula $\mu = I(1\text{-}f)$ (p. 127), it can be shown that when the new equilibrium is eventually reached, an increase in fitness from 0 to 0.9 will have resulted in a tenfold increase in the disease incidence.

## SEX-LINKED RECESSIVE DISORDERS

When considering the effects of selection against these disorders, it is necessary to take into account the fact that a large proportion of the relevant genes are present in entirely healthy female carriers, who are often unaware of their carrier status. For a very serious condition, such as Duchenne muscular dystrophy (p. 308), with fitness equal to 0 in affected males, selection will have no effect unless female carriers choose to limit their families. If all female carriers opted not to have any children, then the incidence would be reduced by two-thirds, i.e. from 3μ to μ.

A much more plausible possibility is that effective treatment will be forthcoming for these disorders. This will result in a steady increase in the disease incidence. For example, an increase in fitness from 0 to 0.5 will lead to a doubling of the disease incidence by the time a new equilibrium has been established. This can be calculated using the formula $\mu = [I^M)\ (1\text{-}f)]/3$ (p. 127).

## CONCLUSION

In reality it is extremely difficult to predict the long-term impact of medical intervention on the incidence and burden of genetic disease. Non-directive genetic counseling could lead to a reduction in the number of affected children being born, but it is quite likely that many of these children will be 'replaced' by carrier siblings, either by such couples compensating by having large families, or through the use of prenatal diagnosis, so that the overall effects on gene frequency are almost impossible to determine. While it is true that improvements in medical treatment could result in an increase in genetic load in future generations, it is equally possible that successful gene therapy will have eased the overall burden of these disorders in terms of human suffering. Some of these arguments could have been made many years ago for other major medical developments, such as the discovery of insulin and antibiotics, which have had overwhelming financial implications in terms of burgeoning pharmaceutical costs and an increasingly aging population. Ultimately it can reasonably be argued that it is how a society copes with these challenges that gives a true measure of the validity of its claim to be civilized.

## FURTHER READING


Allison A C 1954 Protection afforded by sickle-cell trait against subtertian malarial infection. BMJ i: 290–294
*A landmark paper providing clear evidence that the sickle-cell trait provides protection against parasitemia by falciparum malaria.*

Emery A E H 1986 Methodology in medical genetics, 2nd edn. Churchill Livingstone, Edinburgh
*A useful handbook of basic population genetics and mathematical methods for analyzing the results of genetic studies.*

Francomano A, Biesecker L G (eds) 2003 Medical genetic studies in the Amish. Am J Med Genet (Seminars in Medical Genetics) 121C.[1]

Haldane J B S 1935 The rate of spontaneous mutation of a human gene. J Genet 31: 317–326
*The first estimate of the mutation rate for hemophilia using an indirect method.*

Hardy G H 1908 Mendelian proportions in a mixed population. Science 28: 49–50
*A short letter in which Hardy pointed out that in a large randomly mating population dominant 'characters' would not increase at the expense of recessives.*

Khoury M J, Beaty T H, Cohen B H 1993 Fundamentals of genetic epidemiology. Oxford University Press, New York
*A comprehensive textbook of population genetics and its areas of overlap with epidemiology.*

Ott J 1991 Analysis of human genetic linkage. Johns Hopkins University Press, Baltimore
*A detailed mathematical explanation of linkage analysis.*

Vogel F, Motulsky A G 1997 Human genetics, problems and approaches, 3rd edn. Springer-Verlag, Berlin
*The definitive textbook of human genetics with extensive coverage of mathematical aspects.*


## ELEMENTS

1. According to the Hardy–Weinberg principle the relative proportions of the possible genotypes at a particular locus remain constant from one generation to the next.

2. Factors which may disturb Hardy–Weinberg equilibrium are non-random mating, mutation, selection for or against a particular genotype, small population size, and migration.

3. If an autosomal recessive disorder is in Hardy–Weinberg equilibrium the carrier frequency can be estimated by doubling the square root of the disease incidence.

4. The mutation rate for an autosomal dominant disorder can be measured directly by estimating the proportion of new mutations among all members of one generation. Indirect estimates of mutation rates can be made using the formula:
   = $[I(1\text{-}f)]/2$ for autosomal dominant inheritance
   = $I(1\text{-}f)$ for autosomal recessive inheritance
   = $[I^M(1\text{-}f)]/3$ for sex-linked recessive inheritance.

5. Otherwise rare single-gene disorders can show a high incidence in a small population because of a founder effect coupled with genetic isolation.

6. When a serious autosomal recessive disorder has a relatively high incidence in a large population this is likely to be due to heterozygote advantage.

7. Closely adjacent loci on the same chromosome are said to be linked if genes at these loci segregate together during more than 50% of meioses. The recombination fraction (θ) indicates how often two such genes will be separated (recombine) at meiosis.

8. The LOD score is a mathematical indication of the relative likelihood that two loci are linked. A LOD score of +3 or greater is taken as confirmation of linkage. Two-point linkage analysis is used to map a disease locus to a chromosome region. Then multipoint linkage analysis can be used to determine the probable order of polymorphic loci within that region and to narrow down the size of the interval to be studied by physical mapping.

CHAPTER

# 9 Polygenic and multifactorial inheritance

Many disorders demonstrate familial clustering that does not conform to any recognized pattern of Mendelian inheritance. Examples include several of the most common congenital malformations and many of the common acquired diseases of childhood and adult life (Table 9.1). These conditions show a definite familial tendency but the incidence in close relatives of affected individuals is usually around 2–4%, instead of the much higher figures that would be seen if these conditions were caused by mutations in single genes.

As it is likely that many factors, both genetic and environmental, are involved in causing these disorders, they are generally referred to as showing *multifactorial* inheritance. This does not mean that the underlying genetic mechanisms are well understood – in fact they are not! The prevailing view until recently has been that in multifactorial inheritance environmental factors interact with many genes to generate a normally distributed susceptibility. According to this theory individuals are affected if they lie at the wrong end of the distribution curve. This concept of a normal distribution generated by many genes, known as *polygenes*, each acting in an additive fashion, is plausible for physiological characteristics such as height and possibly blood pressure. However, for disease states such as insulin-dependent diabetes mellitus (T1DM) recent research has shown that the genetic contribution is not straightforward and probably involves many loci, some of which play a much more important role than others.

**Table 9.1 Disorders which show multifactorial inheritance**

**Congenital malformations**
Cleft lip/palate
Congenital dislocation of the hip
Congenital heart defects
Neural tube defects
Pyloric stenosis
Talipes

**Acquired diseases of childhood and adult life**
Asthma
Autism
Diabetes mellitus
Epilepsy
Glaucoma
Hypertension
Inflammatory bowel disease (Crohn disease and ulcerative colitis)
Ischaemic heart disease
Ischaemic stroke
Manic depression
Multiple sclerosis
Parkinson disease
Psoriasis
Rheumatoid arthritis
Schizophrenia

## POLYGENIC INHERITANCE AND THE NORMAL DISTRIBUTION

Before considering the impact of recent research in detail, it is necessary to outline briefly the scientific basis of what is known as *polygenic* or *quantitative* inheritance. This involves the inheritance and expression of a phenotype being determined by many genes at different loci, with each gene exerting a small additive effect. Additive implies that the effects of the genes are cumulative, i.e. no one gene is dominant or recessive to another.

Several human characteristics (Table 9.2) show a continuous distribution in the general population, which closely resembles a normal distribution. This takes the form of a symmetrical bell-shaped curve distributed evenly about a mean (Fig. 9.1). The spread of the distribution about the mean is determined by the standard deviation. Approximately 68%, 95% and 99.7% of observations fall

**Table 9.2 Human characteristics that show a continuous normal distribution**

Blood pressure
Dermatoglyphics (ridge count)
Head circumference
Height
Intelligence
Skin color

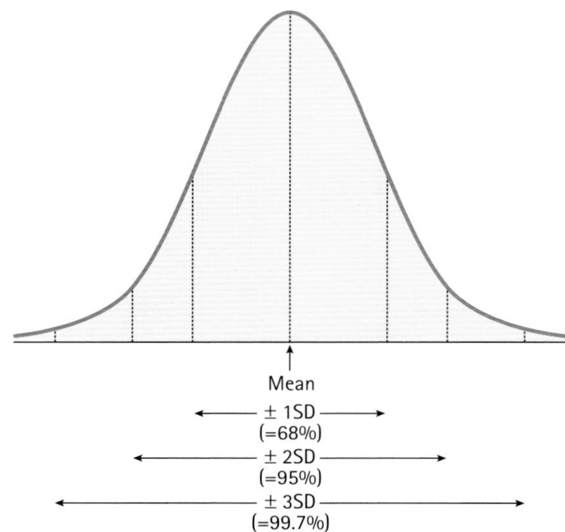


**Fig. 9.1**
The normal (gaussian) distribution.

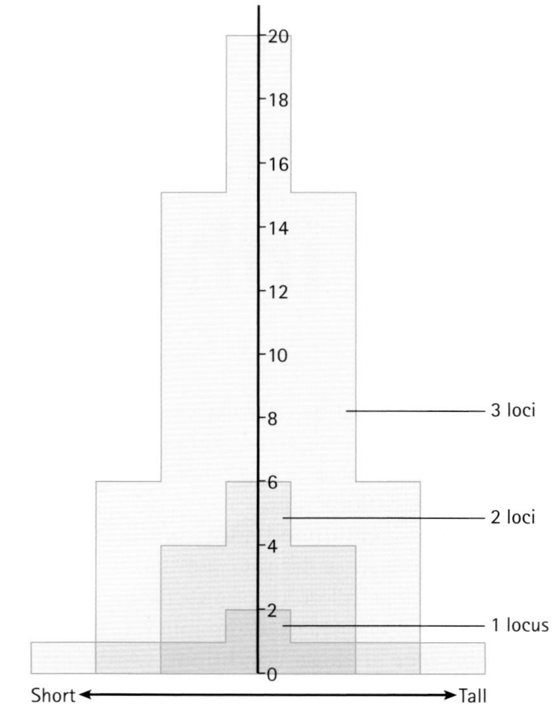


**Fig. 9.2**
Shows the distribution of genotypes for a characteristic such as height with 1, 2 and 3 loci each with two alleles of equal frequency. The values for each genotype can be obtained from the binomial expansion $(p+q)^{(2n)}$, where p = q = 1/2 and n equals the number of loci.

within the mean plus or minus one, two or three standard deviations respectively.

It is possible to show that a phenotype with a normal distribution in the general population can be generated by polygenic inheritance involving the action of many genes at different loci, each of which exerts an equal additive effect. This can be illustrated by considering a trait such as height. If height were to be determined by two equally frequent alleles, a (tall) and b (short), at a single locus, then this would result in a discontinuous phenotype with three groups in a ratio of 1 (tall-aa) to 2 (average-ab/ba) to 1 (short-bb). If the same trait were to be determined by two alleles at each of two loci interacting in a simple additive way, then this would lead to a phenotypic distribution of five groups in a ratio of 1 (4 tall genes) to 4 (3 tall + 1 short) to 6 (2 tall + 2 short) to 4 (1 tall + 3 short) to 1 (4 short). For a system with three loci each with two alleles the phenotypic ratio would be 1-6-15-20-15-6-1 (Fig. 9.2).

It can be seen that as the number of loci increases, the distribution increasingly comes to resemble a normal curve, thereby lending support to the concept that characteristics such as height are determined by the additive effects of many genes at different loci. Further support for this concept comes from the study of familial correlations for characteristics such as height and, to a lesser extent, intelligence. *Correlation* is a statistical measure of the degree of association of variable phenomena, or in more simple terms a measure of the degree of resemblance or relationship between two parameters. As first-degree relatives share on average 50% of their genes (Table 9.3), it would be reasonable to predict that, if a parameter such as height is polygenic, then the correlation between first-degree relatives such as siblings should be 0.5. Several studies have shown that the sib–sib correlation for height is indeed close to 0.5.

**Table 9.3 Degrees of relationship**

| Relationship | Proportion of genes shared |
|---|---|
| **First degree**<br>Parents<br>Siblings<br>Children | {1/2} |
| **Second degree**<br>Uncles and aunts<br>Nephews and nieces<br>Grandparents<br>Grandchildren<br>Half-siblings | {1/4} |
| **Third degree**<br>First cousins<br>Great-grandparents<br>Great-grandchildren | {1/8} |

In reality, human characteristics such as height and intelligence are also influenced by environment, and possibly also by genes that are not additive in that they exert a dominant effect. These factors probably account for the observed tendency of offspring to show what is known as 'regression to the mean'. This is demonstrated by tall or intelligent parents (the two are not mutually exclusive!) having children whose average height or intelligence is slightly lower than the average or mid-parental value.

Similarly, parents who are very short or of low intelligence tend to have children whose average height or intelligence is lower than the general population average, but higher than the average value of the parents. If a trait was to show true polygenic inheritance with no external influences then the measurements in offspring would be distributed evenly around the mean of their parents' values.

## MULTIFACTORIAL INHERITANCE – THE LIABILITY/THRESHOLD MODEL

Efforts have been made to extend the polygenic theory for the inheritance of quantitative or continuous traits to try to account for *discontinuous* multifactorial disorders. According to the *liability/threshold* model, all of the factors which influence the development of a multifactorial disorder, whether genetic or environmental, can be considered as a single entity known as liability. The liabilities of all individuals in a population form a continuous variable, which has a normal distribution in both the general population and in relatives of affected individuals. However, the curves for these relatives will be shifted to the right, with the extent to which they are shifted being directly related to the closeness of their relationship to the affected index case (Fig. 9.3).

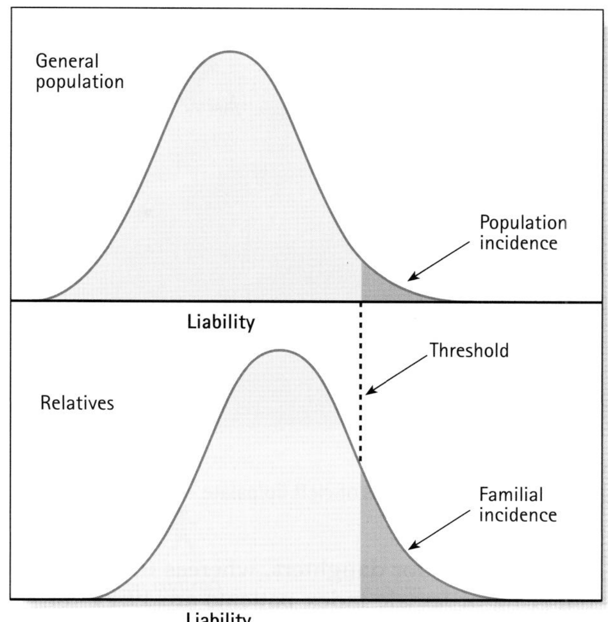


**Fig. 9.3**
Hypothetical liability curves in the general population and in relatives for a hereditary disorder in which the genetic predisposition is multifactorial.

To account for a discontinuous phenotype (i.e. affected or not affected) with an underlying continuous distribution, it is proposed that a threshold exists above which the abnormal phenotype is expressed. In the general population the proportion beyond the threshold is the population incidence, and among relatives the proportion beyond the threshold is the familial incidence.

It is important to emphasize once again that liability includes all factors that contribute to the cause of the condition. Looked at very simply, a deleterious liability can be viewed as consisting of a combination of several 'bad' genes and adverse environmental factors. Liability cannot be measured but the mean liability of a group can be determined from the incidence of the disease in that group using statistics of the normal distribution. The units of measurement are standard deviations and these can be used to estimate the correlation between relatives.

## CONSEQUENCES OF THE LIABILITY/THRESHOLD MODEL

Part of the attraction of this model, and it should be emphasized once again that this is a hypothesis rather than proven fact, is that it provides a simple explanation for the observed patterns of familial risks in conditions such as cleft lip/palate, pyloric stenosis and spina bifida. For example:

1. The incidence of the condition is greatest among relatives of the most severely affected patients, presumably because they are the most extreme deviants along the liability curve. For example, in cleft lip/palate the proportion of affected first-degree relatives (parents, siblings and offspring) is 6% if the index patient has bilateral cleft lip and palate, but only 2% if the index patient has a unilateral cleft lip (Fig. 9.4).
2. The risk is greatest among close relatives of the index case and decreases rapidly in more distant relatives. For example, in spina bifida the risks to first-, second- and third-degree relatives of the index case are approximately 4%, 1% and less than 0.5%, respectively.
3. If there is more than one affected close relative then the risks for other relatives are increased. In spina bifida, if two siblings are affected, the risk to a subsequent sibling is approximately 10%.
4. If the condition is more common in individuals of one particular sex, then relatives of an affected individual of the less frequently affected sex will be at higher risk than relatives of an affected individual of the more frequently affected sex. This is illustrated by the condition pyloric stenosis. Pyloric stenosis shows a male to female ratio of 5 to 1. The proportions of affected offspring of male index patients are 5.5% for

of this progress is discussed in the following sections on autism and diabetes, and further examples are given in Chapter 14 on the 'common diseases'. It has been recognized for some time that one of the best approaches would be to undertake disease association studies and linkage analysis utilizing a so-called 'ideal' population. Such a population would be relatively large yet historically isolated and therefore genetically homogeneous, with extensive medical records dating back many generations, a large tissue bank, good medical services and a co-operative willing citizenship. The 270 000 citizens of Iceland have been deemed to represent such an ideal population and a genomics company, known as DeCODE Genetics, has been granted a licence to set up a national medical database and undertake genetic research. While on the one hand this initiative has raised serious concern about the issue of informed consent (p. 370), on the other hand it could lead to the relatively rapid isolation of genes that make a significant contribution to human morbidity and mortality.

### Affected sibling-pair analysis

Standard linkage analysis requires information regarding the mode of inheritance, gene frequencies and penetrance. For multifactorial disorders this information is not usually available. One solution to this problem is to use a model-free method of linkage analysis that seeks to identify alleles or chromosome regions shared by affected individuals. A common approach is to look for regions of the genome that are *'identical by descent'* (IBD) in affected sibling pairs. If affected siblings inherit a particular allele more or less often than would be expected by chance, this indicates that the allele or its locus is involved in some way in causing the disease.

Consider a set of parents with alleles AB (father) and CD (mother) at a particular locus. The probability that any two of their children will have both alleles in common is 1 in 4 (Fig. 9.6). The probability that they will have one allele in common is 1 in 2 and the probability that they will have no alleles in common equals 1 in 4. If siblings who are affected with a particular disease show deviation from this 1:2:1 ratio for a particular variant, this implies that there is a causal relationship between the locus and the disease.

Many genome-wide scans (p. 78) have been performed for various disorders and although a number of loci have been mapped, the number of disease susceptibility genes identified by this approach is disappointingly small. One reason is probably the complex nature of multifactorial disease, with numerous genes of modest effect interacting with each other and the environment. Some studies are simply underpowered and recent effort has concentrated on large collections of carefully phenotyped affected sibling pairs.

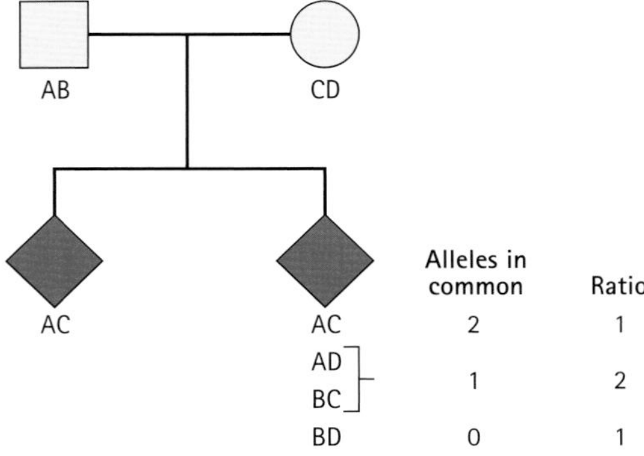


**Fig. 9.6**
The probability that siblings will have 2, 1 or 0 parental alleles in common. Significant deviation from the 1:2:1 ratio indicates that the locus is causally related to the disease.

### Linkage disequilibrium mapping

Once a chromosome region which appears to confer susceptibility has been identified, the next step is to reduce the genetic interval by 'fine mapping'. The most powerful method uses *linkage disequilibrium* (LD) (p. 134) mapping to construct haplotypes by genotyping SNPs within the region. Historical cross-over points reduce the genetic interval by defining LD 'blocks'. Candidate genes within the region are then sequenced to find variants which can be tested for association with the disease.

## ASSOCIATION STUDIES

The study of disease associations is undertaken by comparing the incidence of a particular variant in affected patients with the incidence in a carefully matched control group. This approach is often described as a 'case–control' study. If the incidences in the two groups differ significantly, this provides evidence for a positive or negative association.

The polymorphic system which has been studied most often is the HLA histocompatibility complex on chromosome 6 (p. 194). One of the strongest known HLA associations is that between ankylosing spondylitis and the B27 allele. This is present in approximately 90% of all patients and in only 5% of controls. The strength of an HLA association is indicated by the ratio of the risk of developing the disease in those with the antigen to the risk of developing the disease in those without the antigen (Table 9.5). This is known as the *odds ratio* and it gives an indication of how much more frequently the disease occurs in individuals with a specific marker than in those without that marker.

One of the major difficulties with disease associations is to establish how they should best be interpreted. In particular it is important to try to rule out a chance or

**Table 9.5 Calculation of odds ratio for a disease association**

| | Allele 1 | Allele 2 |
|---|---|---|
| Patients | a | b |
| Controls | c | d |
| Odds ratio | = {a/c} ÷ {b/d}<br>= {ad/bc} | |

spurious observation by ensuring as far as possible that the proposed association is biologically plausible and that the patient and control groups are closely matched. If evidence for a strong association is forthcoming this suggests that the allele encoded by the marker locus is directly involved in causing the disease (i.e. a susceptibility locus) or that the marker locus is in linkage disequilibrium (p. 134) with a closely linked susceptibility locus. When considering disease associations it is important to remember that the identification of a susceptibility locus does not mean that the definitive disease gene has been identified. This is illustrated by the association of HLA B27 with ankylosing spondylitis. Although this is one of the strongest disease associations known, only 1% of all HLA B27 individuals develop ankylosing spondylitis, so that many other factors, genetic and environmental, must be involved in causing this condition.

Positive results from association studies require replication in other cohorts. A common reason for false-positive association is population stratification, where the population contains a number of subsets and both the disease and the allele happen to be common within that subset. A famous example was reported in a study by Lander and Schork which showed that in a San Francisco population HLA-A1 is associated with the ability to eat with chopsticks. This association is explained by the fact that HLA-A1 is more common amongst Chinese than Caucasians.

### Transmission disequilibrium test

One way to overcome population stratification problems is to use family-based controls. The *transmission disequilibrium* test (TDT) requires a collection of trios which consist of an affected proband and both parents (regardless of affection status). Parents who are heterozygous for the marker allele in question are selected and the number of times this allele is transmitted to their affected offspring is compared to the number of times the other allele is transmitted. Overtransmission of the marker allele strengthens the evidence for association, but definitive evidence that a variant is a predisposing allele usually requires functional studies.

## DISEASE MODELS FOR MULTIFACTORIAL INHERITANCE

The search for susceptibility loci and polygenes, sometimes also referred to as *quantitative trait loci*, in human multifactorial disorders has met with some success, and it is hoped that knowledge gained from the Human Genome Project (p. 351) together with developments in SNP genotyping technology, will accelerate the rate of progress. Recent research in four conditions will be considered to illustrate the extent of the challenges that lie ahead.

## AUTISM

Autism is a severe neurodevelopmental disorder that affects between 4 and 10 individuals per 10 000, with onset during the first 3 years of life. The incidence is 3–4 times higher in boys than girls and the diagnostic features are severe impairment in the development of social responsivenesss, very poor verbal and non-verbal communication, and repetitive, stereotypic behavior and interests. Many affected children show significant developmental delay and, conversely, many children with developmental delay can show autistic features. For example, autistic behavior is well recognized in children with tuberous sclerosis and various forms of chromosome imbalance, as well as in boys with the Fragile X syndrome (p. 283). Autism is part of a spectrum that includes Asperger syndrome and, overall, the 'autistic spectrum disorders' have a much higher prevalence of up to 60 per 10 000 individuals.

The cause of autism in isolation (non-syndromal) is not clear, but there is increasing evidence that genetic factors play an important role. This is based on the results of twin studies, which for autistic spectrum disorders yield concordance rates of up to 80% and 20% in monozygotic and dizygotic twins, respectively, depending on the diagnostic criteria used. On the evidence of familial aggregation, the empiric recurrence risk for siblings is between 2 and 6%, very much greater than the 0.04–0.1% in the general population. Autism and autistic spectrum disorders are therefore highly heritable.

In an attempt to clarify the genetic contribution to autism, large genome-wide screening studies have been performed using several hundred families with more than one affected member. Using complex computer-based statistical analysis the most consistent finding is for a susceptibility locus on chromosome 7q, but in addition there is evidence for linkage to chromosomes 17q (close to a serotonin transporter locus), 5p, 11, 4 and 9. Many additional loci have been implicated in different studies, indicating that a full understanding of the genetic contribution to autism and genetically based therapeutic strategies are likely to be a long way off.

Falconer D S 1965 The inheritance of liability to certain diseases estimated from the incidence among relatives. Ann Hum Genet 29: 51–76

*The original exposition of the liability/threshold model and how correlations between relatives can be used to calculate heritability.*

Fraser F C 1980 Evolution of a palatable multifactorial threshold model. Am J Hum Genet 32: 796–813

*An amusing and 'reader-friendly' account of models proposed to explain multifactorial inheritance.*

Gloyn AL, Weedon MN, Owen KR et al 2003 Large-scale association studies of variants in genes encoding the pancreatic beta-cell KATP channel subunits Kir6.2 (KCNJ11) and SUR1 (ABCC8) confirm that the KCNJ11 E23K variant is associated with type 2 diabetes. Diabetes 52: 568–572

*The results of a large-scale association study and meta-analysis of previous studies to confirm that E23K increases risk of type 2 diabetes.*

Hugot JP, Chamaillard M, Zouali H et al 2001 Association of NOD2 leucine-rich repeat variants with susceptibility to Crohn disease. Nature 411: 599–603

*Description of the positional cloning strategy which led to the identification of the NOD2/CARD15 susceptibility gene for Crohn disease.*

King R A, Rotter J I, Motulsky A G (eds) 1992 The genetic basis of common diseases. Oxford University Press, Oxford

*A lengthy and detailed review of the genetic aspects of common adult onset disorders.*

Lernmark A, Ott J 1998 Sometimes it's hot, sometimes it's not. Nature Genet 19: 213–214

*A brief account of possible explanations for the conflicting results obtained in studies to identify susceptibility loci in IDDM.*

Ogura Y, Bonen DK, Inohara N et al 2001 A frameshift mutation in NOD2 is associated with Crohn disease.

*Description of the positional cloning strategy that led to the identifcation of the NOD2/CARD15 susceptibility gene for Crohn disease.*

Risch N, Spiker D, Lotspeich L et al 1999 A genomic screen of autism: evidence for a multilocus etiology. Am J Hum Genet 65: 493–507

*The results of multilocus sibling pair analysis in 139 sibships with autism.*

## ELEMENTS

1. The concept of multifactorial inheritance has been proposed to account for the common congenital malformations and acquired disorders that show non-Mendelian familial aggregation. These disorders are thought to result from the interaction of genetic and environmental factors.

2. Human characteristics such as height and intelligence, which show a normally distributed continuous distribution in the general population, are probably caused by the additive effects of many genes, i.e. polygenic inheritance.

3. According to the liability/threshold model for multifactorial inheritance the population's genetic and environmental susceptibility, which is known as liability, is normally distributed. Individuals are affected if their liability exceeds a threshold superimposed on the liability curve.

4. Recurrence risks to relatives for multifactorial disorders are influenced by the disease severity, the degree of relationship to the index case, the number of affected close relatives and, if there is a higher incidence in one particular sex, the sex of the index case.

5. Heritability is a measure of the proportion of the total variance of a character or disease that is due to the genetic variance.

6. Loci that contribute to susceptibility for multifactorial disorders can be identified by (a) a search for disease associations and (b) linkage analysis looking for example for chromosomal regions which are identical by descent in affected sibling pairs. These approaches have led to the identification of one major and 10–20 minor susceptibility loci for type 1 diabetes mellitus. Recent successes include the identification of variants in at least five genes that confer susceptibility to type 2 diabetes, and three gene variants that are associated with Crohn disease.

SECTION B

# GENETICS IN MEDICINE

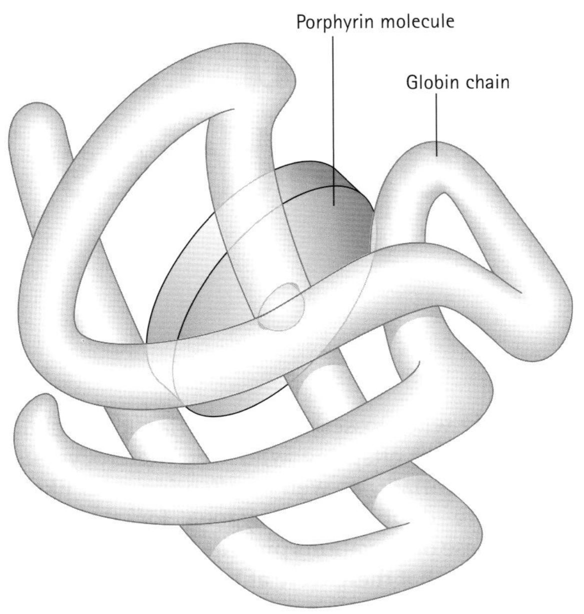


Fig. 10.1
Diagrammatic representation of one of the globin chains and associated porphyrin molecule of human hemoglobin.

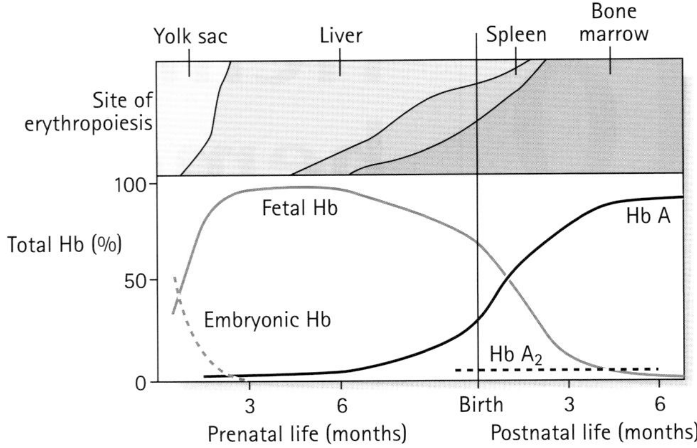


Fig. 10.2
Hemoglobin synthesis during prenatal and postnatal development. There are several embryonic hemoglobins. (After Huehns E R, Shooter E M 1965 Human haemoglobins. J Med Genet 2: 48–90, with permission.)

sequence resembled the β-globin chain and which were designated gamma (γ). Hb F makes up somewhere in the region of 0.5% of hemoglobin in the blood of normal adults.

Analysis of Hb from embryos earlier in gestation reveals there to be a developmental or ontological succession of different embryonic Hbs, Hb Gower I and II, and Hb Portland, which are produced in varying amounts at different times of gestation. Subsequent analysis has revealed that these various Hbs, which are transiently expressed in development, are in fact tetramers of various combinations of α or α-like zeta (ζ) chains with β or β-like γ- and epsilon (ε)-globin chains (Table 10.1). Apart from the transient expression of the ζ chain early in embryonic life, the α-globin chain gene is expressed throughout development. Similarly, ε-globin chain expression occurs early in embryonic life, with γ chain expression occurring throughout fetal life followed by increasing levels of expression of the β-globin chain towards the end of fetal life. The ordered expression of these chains results in the various Hb tetramers seen during development (Fig. 10.2).

**Table 10.1 Human hemoglobins**

| Stage in development | Hemoglobin | Structure | Proportion in normal adult (%) |
|---|---|---|---|
| Embryonic | Gower I | $\zeta_2\varepsilon_2$ | — |
| | Gower II | $\alpha_2\varepsilon_2$ | — |
| | Portland I | $\zeta_2\gamma_2$ | — |
| Fetal | F | $\alpha_2\gamma_2$ | <1 |
| Adult | A | $\alpha_2\beta_2$ | 97–98 |
| | $A_2$ | $\alpha_2\delta_2$ | 2–3 |

## GLOBIN CHAIN STRUCTURE

The analysis of the structure of the individual globin chains was initially carried out at the protein level.

### PROTEIN STUDIES

Amino-acid sequencing of the various globin polypeptides, carried out in the 1960s by a number of different investigators, showed that the α-globin chain was 141 amino acids long while the β chain contained 146 amino acids. The α and β chains were found to have a similar sequence of amino acids but were by no means identical. Analysis of the amino acid sequence of the δ chain showed it to differ from the β-globin chain by 10 amino acids. Similar analysis of the γ-globin chain showed that it also most closely resembled the β-globin chain, differing by 39 amino acids. In addition, it was found that there were two types of fetal Hb in which the γ chain contained either the amino acid glycine or alanine at position 136, which were consequently named (G)γ and (A)γ, respectively. More recently, partial sequence analyses of the ζ and ε chains of embryonic Hb suggest that ζ is similar in amino acid sequence to the α chain, while ε resembles the β chain.

Thus, it appeared that there are two groups of globin chains, the α-like and β-like, all of which seem to be derived from an ancestral primordial Hb gene, which has undergone a number of gene duplications, and diverged during the course of evolution.

## GLOBIN GENE MAPPING

The first evidence for the arrangement of the various globin structural genes on the human chromosomes was provided by analysis of the Hb electrophoretic variant, Hb Lepore. Comparison of trypsin digests of Hb Lepore with Hb from normal persons revealed that the α chains were normal, whereas the non-α chains appeared to consist of an amino-terminal δ-globin-like sequence and a carboxy-terminal β-globin-like sequence.

It was therefore proposed that Hb Lepore could represent a 'fusion' globin chain that had arisen as a result of a cross-over coincidental with mispairing of the δ- and β-globin genes during meiosis as a result of the sequence similarity of the two genes and the close proximity of the δ- and β-globin genes on the same chromosome (Fig. 10.3). If this hypothesis was correct, it was argued that there should also be an 'anti-Lepore' Hb, i.e. a β-δ-globin fusion product in which the non-α-globin chains contained β chain residues at the amino-terminal end and δ chain residues at the carboxy-terminal end. In the late 1960s, a new Hb electrophoretic variant, Hb Miyada, was identified by investigators in Japan in which analysis of trypsin digests did, indeed, show it to contain β-globin sequence at the amino-terminal end and δ-globin sequence at the carboxy-terminal end, as predicted.

Further evidence at the protein level for the physical mapping of the human globin genes was provided by the report of another Hb electrophoretic variant, Hb Kenya. Amino-acid sequence analysis of this variant suggested that it was a γ-β fusion product with a cross-over having occurred somewhere between amino acids 81 and 86 in the two globin chains. It was suggested that, in order for this fusion polypeptide to have occurred, the γ-globin structural gene must also be in close physical proximity to the β-globin gene.

Little evidence was forthcoming from protein studies about the mapping of the α-globin genes. The presence of normal Hb A in individuals who, by family studies, should have been homozygous for a particular α-globin chain variant or obligate compound heterozygotes (p. 110) suggested that there could be more than one α-globin gene. In addition, the proportion of the total Hb made up by the α-globin chain variant, in persons heterozygous for those variants, was consistently lower (less than 20%) than that seen with the β-globin chain variants (usually more than 30%), suggesting that there could be more than one α-globin structural gene.

## GLOBIN GENE STRUCTURE

Detailed information on the structure of the globin genes has been made possible by DNA techniques (p. 59). Immature red blood cells, reticulocytes, provide a rich source of globin mRNA for the synthesis of cDNA because they synthesize little else! Use of β-globin cDNA for restriction mapping studies of DNA from normal persons revealed that the non-α, or β-like, globin genes are located in a 50 kb stretch on the short arm of chromosome 11 (Fig. 10.4). The whole of this 50 kb stretch has been cloned and the nucleotide sequence of each of the various globin structural genes is known. Of particular interest are regions with sequences similar to the globin structural genes but which are non-functional and do not produce an identifiable message or protein product, that is, pseudogenes (p. 17).

Similar studies of the α-globin structural genes have shown that there are, in fact, two α-globin structural genes, α1 and α2, located on the short arm of chromosome 16 (Fig. 10.4). DNA sequence analysis has revealed nucleotide sequence differences between these two structural genes even though the α-globin chains produced have an identical amino-acid sequence, evidence of the 'degeneracy' of the genetic code. In addition, there are pseudo-α, pseudo-ζ and ζ genes to the 5′ side of the α-globin genes as well as a recently discovered theta (θ)-globin gene to the 3′ side of the α1-globin gene. This latter gene,

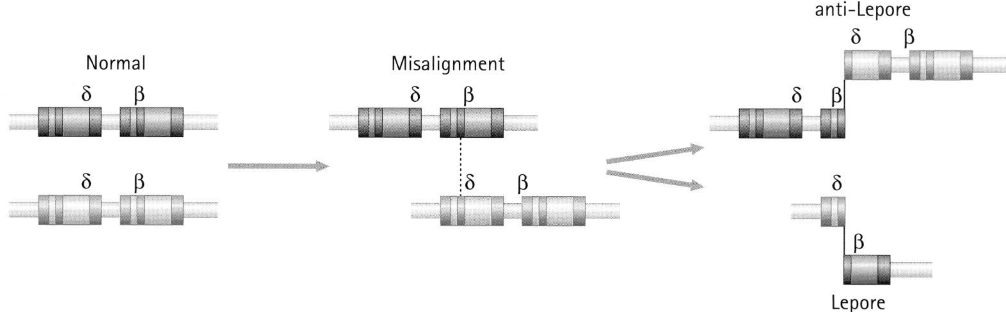


**Fig. 10.3**
Mechanism of unequal crossing over which generates Hb Lepore and anti-Lepore. (Adapted from Weatherall D J, Clegg J B 1981 The thalassaemia syndromes. Blackwell, Oxford.)

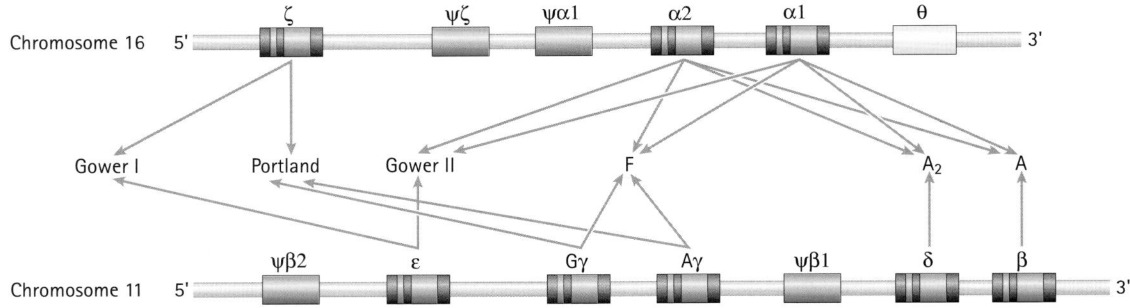


Fig. 10.4
The α- and β-globin regions on chromosomes 16 and 11 showing the structural genes and pseudogenes (ψ) and the various hemoglobins produced. (Adapted from Carrell R W, Lehman H 1985 The haemoglobinopathies. In: Dawson A M, Besser G, Compston N (eds) Recent advances in medicine 19. Churchill Livingstone, Edinburgh, pp. 223–225.)

whose function is unknown, is of interest because, unlike the globin pseudogenes, which are not expressed, its structure is compatible with expression. It has been suggested that it could be expressed in very early erythroid tissue such as the fetal liver and yolk sac.

## SYNTHESIS AND CONTROL OF HEMOGLOBIN EXPRESSION

From in-vitro translation studies with reticulocyte mRNA from normal persons it is known that α- and β-globin chains are synthesized in roughly equal proportions. In-vitro studies of globin chain synthesis have shown, however, that β-globin mRNA is slightly more efficient in protein synthesis than α-globin mRNA, and that this difference is compensated for in the red blood cell precursors by a relative excess of α-globin mRNA. It seems that the most important level of regulation of expression of the globin genes, like other eukaryotic genes, is likely to occur at the level of transcription (pp. 19–22).

DNA studies of the β-globin genes and flanking regions have revealed that, in addition to promoter sequences in the 5′ flanking regions of the various globin genes, there are sequences 6–20 kb 5′ to the ε-globin gene necessary for the expression of the various β-like globin genes. This region has been called the *locus control region* or *lcr*, and is involved in the timing and tissue specificity of expression or *switching* of the β-like globin genes in development. There is a similar region 5′ to the α-globin genes involved in the control of their expression. Both are involved in the binding of proteins and transcription factors involved in the control of expression of the globin genes.

## DISORDERS OF HEMOGLOBIN

The disorders of human Hb can be divided into two main groups, structural globin chain variants such as sickle-cell disease, and disorders of synthesis of the globin chains, the thalassemias.

## STRUCTURAL VARIANTS/DISORDERS

In 1975, Ingram demonstrated that the difference between Hb A and Hb S lay in the substitution of valine for glutamic acid in the β-globin chain. Since then more than 300 Hb electrophoretic variants have been described due to a variety of types of mutation (Table 10.2). Some 200 of these electrophoretic variants are single amino-acid substitutions resulting from a point mutation. The majority of these are rare and not associated with clinical disease. A few are associated with disease and relatively prevalent in certain populations.

### Types of mutation

#### *Point mutation*

A point mutation which results in substitution of one amino acid for another can lead to an altered hemoglobin, such as Hb S, C or E, which are missense mutations (p. 25).

#### *Deletion*

There are a number of Hb variants in which one or more amino acids of one of the globin chains is missing or deleted (p. 24), e.g. Hb Freiburg.

#### *Insertion*

Conversely, there are variants in which the globin chains are longer than normal because of insertions (p. 24), such as Hb Grady.

#### *Frameshift mutation*

Frameshift mutations involve disruption of the normal triplet reading frame, i.e. addition or removal of a number of bases that are not a multiple of three (p. 26). In this

**Table 10.2 Structural variants of hemoglobin**

| Type of mutation | Examples | Chain/residue(s)/alteration |
|---|---|---|
| Point (over 200 variants) | Hb S<br>Hb C<br>Hb E | β, 6 glu to val<br>β, 6 glu to lys<br>β, 26 glu to lys |
| Deletion (shortened chain) | Hb Freiburg<br>Hb Lyon<br>Hb Leiden<br>Hb Gun Hill | β, 23 to 0<br>β, 17–18 to 0<br>β, 6 or 7 to 0<br>β, 92–96 or 93–97 to 0 |
| Insertion (elongated chain) | Hb Grady | α, 116–118 (glu, phe, thr) duplicated |
| Frameshift (insertion/ deletion of other than multiples of three base pairs) | Hb Tak, Hb Cranston | *β, + 11 residues, loss of termination codon, insertion of 2 base pairs in codon 146/147 |
| | Hb Wayne | *α, + 5 residues, due to loss of termination codon by single base pair deletion in codon 138/139 |
| | Hb McKees Rock | *β, –2 residues, point mutation in 145, generating premature termination codon |
| Chain termination | Hb Constant Spring | *α, + 31 residues, point mutation in termination codon |
| Fusion chain (unequal crossing over) | Hb Lepore/ anti-Lepore<br>Hb Kenya/ anti-Kenya | non-α, δ-like residues at N-terminal end and β-like residues at C-terminal end and vice versa, respectively<br>non-α, γ-like residues at N-terminal end and β-like residues at C-terminal end and vice versa, respectively |

*Residues are either added (+) or lost (–)

instance, translation of the mRNA continues until a termination codon is read 'in frame'. These variants can result in either an elongated or a shortened globin chain.

### Chain termination

A mutation in the termination codon itself can lead to an elongated globin chain, e.g. Hb Constant Spring.

### Fusion polypeptides

The last type of structural variant are the *fusion polypeptides*, Hbs Lepore and Kenya, which result from unequal cross-over events in meiosis, as previously detailed (p. 152).

## Clinical aspects

Some of the hemoglobin variants are associated with disease, but many are harmless and do not interfere with normal function, having been identified only in the course of population surveys of Hb electrophoretic variants. A number, however, do interfere in a variety of ways with the normal function of Hb (Table 10.3).

**Table 10.3 Functional abnormalities of structural variants of hemoglobin**

| Clinical features | Examples |
|---|---|
| **Hemolytic anemia** | |
| Sickling disorders | Hb S<br>Hb C<br>Hb E |
| Unstable hemoglobin | Hb Köln<br>Hb Gun Hill<br>Hb Bristol |
| **Cyanosis** | |
| Hemoglobin M (methemoglobinemia) | Hb M (Boston)<br>Hb M (Hyde Park) |
| Low $O_2$ affinity | Hb Kansas |
| **Polycythemia** | |
| High $O_2$ affinity | Hb Chesapeake<br>Hb Heathrow |

If the mutation is on the inside of the globin subunits, in close proximity to the heme pockets or at the interchain contact areas, this can produce an unstable Hb molecule which precipitates in the red blood cell, damaging the membrane and resulting in hemolysis of the cell. Alternatively, mutations can interfere with the normal oxygen transport function of Hb, leading either to an enhanced or a reduced oxygen affinity or to an Hb which is stable in its reduced form, so-called *methemoglobin*.

The structural variants of Hb identified by electrophoretic techniques probably represent a minority of the total number of variants that exist, since it is predicted that only one-third of the possible Hb mutations which could occur will produce an altered charge in the Hb molecule and thereby be detectable by electrophoresis (Fig. 10.5).

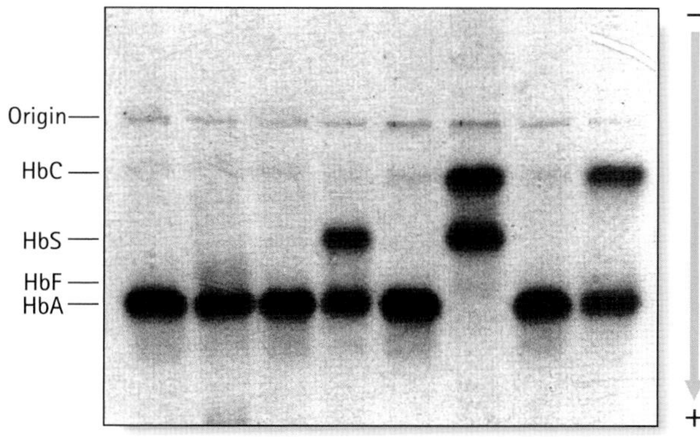


**Fig. 10.5**
Hemoglobin electrophoresis showing hemoglobins A, C and S. (Courtesy of Dr D. Norfolk, General Infirmary, Leeds.)

## SICKLE-CELL DISEASE

Although the severe hereditary hemolytic anemia *sickle-cell disease* was first recognized early in the twentieth century, it was only in 1940 that the red blood cells from persons with sickle-cell disease were noted to appear birefringent when viewed in polarized light under the microscope, reflecting polymerization of the sickle hemoglobin, leading to distortion in the shape of the red blood cells under deoxygenated conditions, so-called *sickling* (Fig. 10.6). Pauling, in 1949, analysing Hb from patients with sickle-cell disease by electrophoresis, demonstrated that it had a different mobility from Hb A, and called it Hb S for sickle.

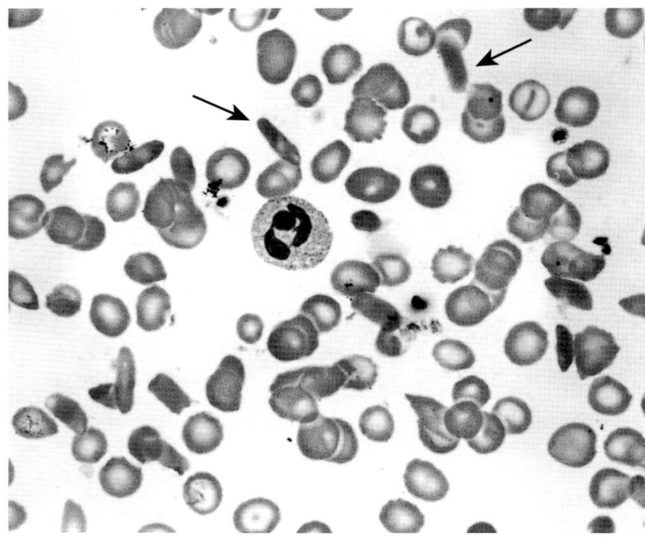

Fig. 10.6
Blood film showing sickling of red cells in sickle-cell disease. Sickled cells are arrowed. (Courtesy of Dr D. Norfolk, General Infirmary, Leeds.)

### Clinical aspects of sickle-cell disease

Sickle-cell disease, an autosomal recessive condition, is the most common hemoglobinopathy and the clinical manifestations are manifold, including cerebral symptoms, kidney failure, 'pneumonia', heart failure, weakness and lassitude. All of these are a manifestation of the mutant allele. Hb S is less soluble than normal hemoglobin and tends to polymerize, causing the sickle-shaped deformation of the red cells. A proportion of sickle cells become irreversibly sickled because of damage to the red cell membrane and are taken up by the reticuloendothelial system. The shorter red cell survival time leads to a more rapid red cell turnover, with consequent anemia. In addition the sickle cells have a reduced deformability, tending to obstruct small arteries, resulting in an inadequate oxygen supply to the tissues (Fig. 10.7).

Persons with sickle-cell disease can present acutely unwell with a sudden onset of chest, back, or limb pain, fever and dark urine, the latter due to the presence of free hemoglobin in the urine, a so-called *sickle-cell crisis*.

When compared to the general population, persons with sickle-cell disease have an increased risk of early death; earlier recognition and treatment of the known complications of sickle-cell disease have resulted in improved life expectancy. Some simple measures, such as prophylactic penicillin to prevent the risk of overwhelming sepsis due to splenic infarction, have met with limited success in treating specific complications. It is fair to state that although there has been an understanding of the

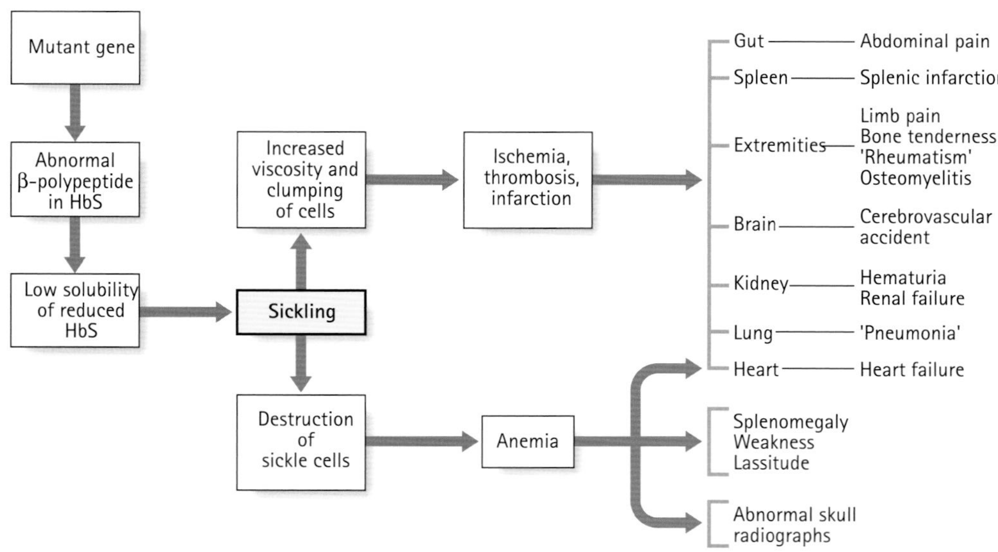


Fig. 10.7
The pleiotropic effects of the gene for sickle-cell disease.

molecular basis of sickle-cell disease for over 30 years, the therapeutic approaches available to date to prevent the sickling process have had limited benefit.

### Sickle-cell trait

The heterozygous or carrier state for the sickle-cell allele is known as *sickle-cell trait* and is not thought, in general, to be associated with any significant risk to health. There are, however, reports suggesting a small increased risk of sudden death associated with strenuous exercise. In addition, there is continuing controversy about whether there are risks from hypoxia in persons with sickle-cell trait on airplane flights.

### Mutational basis of sickle-cell disease

In sickle-cell disease, knowledge of the genetic code (pp. 20–21) suggested that the substitution of valine at the sixth position of the β-globin chain was due to an alteration in the second base of the triplet coding for glutamic acid, i.e. GAG to GTG. Using the restriction enzyme *Mst* II, the nucleotide recognition sequence of which is abolished by the point mutation in Hb S, it is possible to demonstrate a difference between persons with sickle-cell disease and normal persons in the restriction fragments when hybridized with a radioactively labeled β-globin probe.

Use of a mutation-specific RFLP is possible with Hb E using the restriction enzymes *Hph*I or *Mn*II. Family studies using linked polymorphic DNA sequence variants are needed for carrier testing and prenatal diagnosis for the other hemoglobinopathies.

## DISORDERS OF HEMOGLOBIN SYNTHESIS

The *thalassemias* are the commonest single group of inherited disorders in humans, occurring in persons from the Mediterranean area, the Middle East, the Indian subcontinent and South-East Asia. They are a heterogeneous group of disorders and are classified according to the particular globin chain or chains synthesized in reduced amounts, e.g. α, β, δβ thalassemia.

The pathophysiology is similar in all forms of thalassemia. An imbalance of globin chain production results in the accumulation of free globin chains in the red blood cell precursors, which, being insoluble, precipitate, resulting in hemolysis of the red blood cells, i.e. a hemolytic anemia, with consequent compensatory hyperplasia of the bone marrow.

### α Thalassemia

α Thalassemia results from an underproduction of the α-globin chains. It occurs most commonly in persons from South-East Asia. There are two main types of α thalassemia that differ in their severity: the severe form, in which no α-globin chains are produced, is associated with death of the fetus in utero, as a result of massive edema because of heart failure from the severe in utero anemia, so-called *hydrops fetalis* (Fig. 10.8).

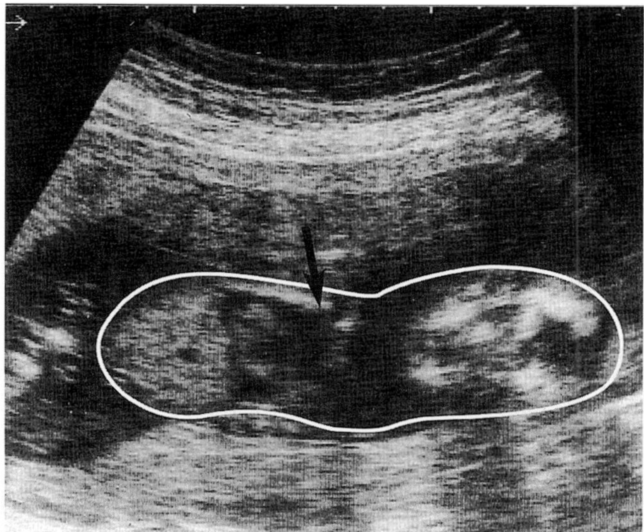

Fig. 10.8
Longitudinal ultrasound scan of a coronal section of the head (to the right) and thorax of a fetus with hydrops fetalis due to the severe form of a thalassemia, Hb Barts, showing a large pleural effusion (arrowed). (Courtesy Mr J. Campbell, St James's Hospital, Leeds.)

Analysis of the Hb present in fetuses with hydrops fetalis reveals it to be a tetramer of γ-globin chains, which used to be called Hb Barts. In the milder forms of α thalassemia compatible with survival, although some α-globin chains are produced, there is still a relative excess of β-globin chains that results in the production of the β-globin tetramer Hb H, or what is known as Hb H disease. Both the Hb Barts and Hb H globin tetramers have an oxygen affinity similar to that of myoglobin and do not release oxygen normally in the peripheral tissues. In addition, Hb H is unstable and precipitates, resulting in hemolysis of the red blood cells.

### *Mutational basis of α Thalassemia*

In-vitro translation studies using mRNA from reticulocytes from fetuses with hydrops fetalis show no synthesis of α-globin. However, when mRNA from reticulocytes of persons with the milder form of α thalassemia, Hb H disease, is used, α-globin is produced but in reduced amounts when compared to mRNA from reticulocytes from normal persons. Studies comparing the quantitative hybridization of radioactively labeled α-globin cDNA

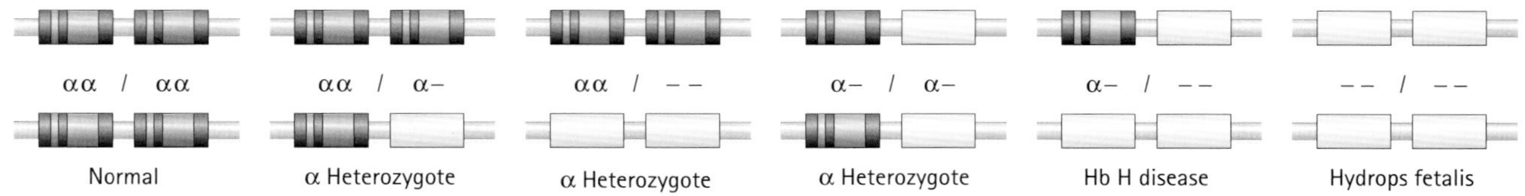


**Fig. 10.9**
The structure of the normal and deleted α-globin structural genes in the various forms of α thalassemia. (Adapted from Emery A E H 1984 An introduction to recombinant DNA. John Wiley, Chichester.)

to DNA from fetuses with hydrops fetalis, persons with Hb H disease and normal persons are consistent with α thalassemia being due to deletions of the α-globin genes.

Restriction mapping studies of the α-globin region of chromosome 16 reveal that there are two α-globin structural genes on the short arm of chromosome 16. The various forms of α thalassemia have been shown to be mostly due to deletions of one or more of these structural genes (Fig. 10.9).

Deletions of the α-globin genes in α thalassemia are believed to have arisen as a result of unequal cross-over events in meiosis which are thought to be more likely to occur where genes with homologous sequences are in close proximity. Support for this hypothesis comes from the finding of the other product of such an event, i.e. persons with three α-globin structural genes located on one chromosome.

These observations resulted in the recognition of two other milder forms of α thalassemia that are not associated with anemia and can only be detected by the transient presence in the immediate newborn period of Hb Barts. The results of the DNA mapping studies of the α-globin genes have shown that these milder forms of α thalassemia are due to the deletion of one or two of the α-globin genes. Less commonly, non-deletion mutations that include point mutations in the α-globin genes and mutations in the 5′ region involved in the control of their transcription have been found to cause α thalassemia.

An exception to this classification of the α thalassemias is the Hb variant Constant Spring, named after the town in the USA where the original patient came from. This was detected as an electrophoretic variant in a person with Hb H disease, i.e. α thalassemia. Hb Constant Spring is due to an abnormally long α chain that is the result of a mutation in the normal termination codon at position 142 in the α-globin gene. Translation of this α-globin mRNA continues until the occurrence of another termination codon, resulting in an abnormally long α-globin chain variant. In addition, this abnormal α-globin mRNA molecule is unstable, with a consequent relative deficiency of α-globin chains, resulting in the presence of the β-globin tetramer, Hb H.

## β Thalassemia

β Thalassemia is caused by underproduction of the β-globin chain of hemoglobin. In-vitro translation studies using mRNA from persons with β thalassemia due to these different types of mutation show either reduced or absent production of β-globin chains, β(+) and $\beta^0$, respectively. Persons homozygous for $\beta^0$ thalassemia mutations have a severe transfusion-dependent anemia.

### *Mutational basis of β thalassemia*

Restriction mapping studies have shown that β thalassemia is rarely due to a deletion, and DNA sequencing has often been necessary to reveal the molecular pathology. In excess of 100 different mutations have been shown to cause β thalassemia. These involve a wide variety of different types of mutation, including point mutations, insertions and deletions of one or more bases. These occur at a number of places, within both the coding and non-coding portions of the β-globin genes as well as in the 5′ flanking promoter region, the 5′ capping sequences (p. 19) and the 3′ polyadenylation sequences (p. 19) (Fig. 10.10).

The various types of mutation causing β thalassemia are often unique to certain population groups and can be considered to fall into six main functional types.

#### Transcription mutations

Mutations in the 5′ flanking TATA box or the promoter region of the β-globin gene can result in reduced transcription levels of the β-globin mRNA.

#### mRNA splicing mutations

Mutations involving the invariant 5′GT or 3′AG dinucleotides of the introns in the β-globin gene or the consensus donor or acceptor sequences (p. 20) result in abnormal splicing with consequent reduced levels of β-globin mRNA. In the most common β thalassemia mutation in persons from the Mediterranean region, the mutation leads to the creation of a new acceptor AG dinucleotide splice site sequence in the first intron of the β-globin gene, creating a so-called cryptic splice site (p. 26).

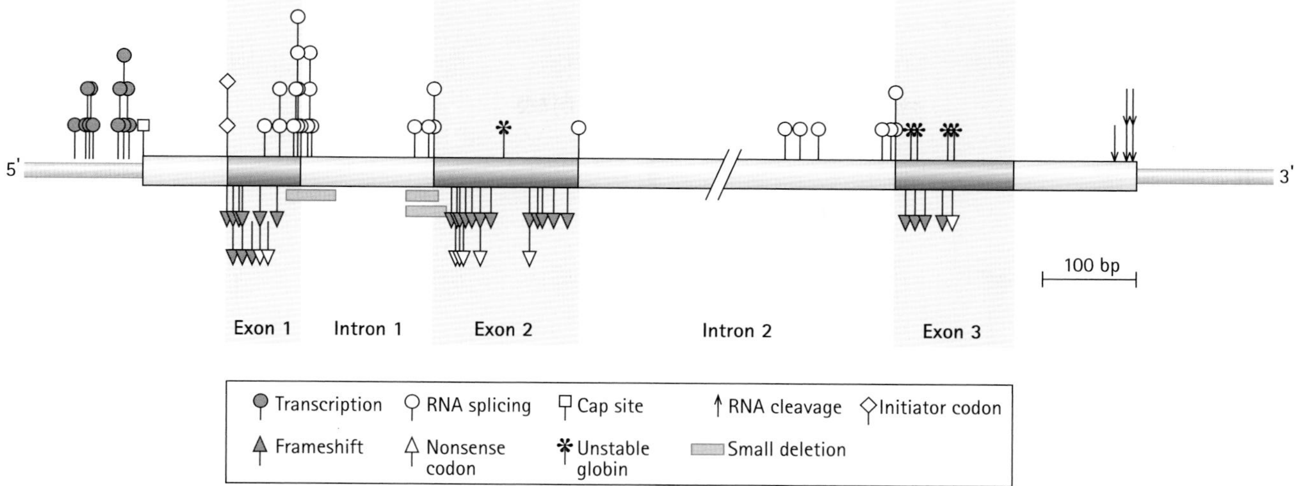


**Fig. 10.10**
Location and some of the types of mutation in the β-globin gene and flanking region which result in β thalassemia. (Adapted from Orkin S H, Kazazian H H 1984 The mutation and polymorphism of the human β-globin gene and its surrounding DNA. In: Roman H L, Campbell A, Sandler L M (eds) Annu Rev Genet 18: 131–171.)

The cryptic splice site competes with the normal splice site, leading to reduced levels of the normal β-globin mRNA. Mutations in the coding regions of the β-globin region can also lead to cryptic splice sites.

### Polyadenylation signal mutations

Mutations in the 3′ end of the untranslated region of the β-globin gene can lead to loss of the signal for cleavage and polyadenylation of the β-globin gene transcript.

### RNA modification mutations

Mutations in the 5′ and 3′ DNA sequences, involved respectively in the capping (p. 19) and polyadenylation (p. 19) of the mRNA, can result in abnormal processing and transportation of the β-globin mRNA to the cytoplasm, with consequent reduced levels of translation.

### Chain termination mutations

Insertions, deletions and point mutations can all generate a nonsense or chain termination codon, resulting in the premature termination of translation of the β-globin mRNA. This will result in the majority of instances in a shortened β-globin mRNA that is often unstable and more rapidly degraded, with consequent reduced levels of translation of an abnormal β-globin.

### Missense mutations

Missense mutations which lead to a β-globin that is highly unstable can rarely result in β thalassemia. An example is Hb Indianapolis.

### *Clinical aspects of β thalassemia*

Children affected with thalassemia major, or Cooley's anemia as it was originally known, usually present in the first year of life with a severe transfusion-dependent anemia. Unless the child is adequately transfused compensatory expansion of the bone marrow results in an unusually shaped face and skull (Fig. 10.11). Although persons with thalassemia major used to die in their late teens or early 20s as a result of complications due to iron overload from repeated transfusions, the regular daily use of iron-chelating drugs, such as desferrioxamine, has improved their long-term survival.

Individuals heterozygous for β thalassemia, *thalassemia trait* or *thalassemia minor*, usually have no symptoms or signs. They do, however, have a mild hypochromic, microcytic anemia, which can often be confused with iron deficiency anemia.

### δβ Thalassemia

In *δβ thalassemia* there is underproduction of both the δ- and β-globin chains. Persons homozygous for δβ thalassemia produce no δ- or β-globin chains. Although one would expect such persons to have a fairly profound illness, they are only mildly anemic because of increased production of γ-globin chains, with Hb F levels being much higher than the mild compensatory increase seen in homozygotes for β thalassemia.

### *Mutational basis of δβ thalassemia*

δβ Thalassemia has been shown to be caused by extensive deletions in the β-globin region involving the δ- and

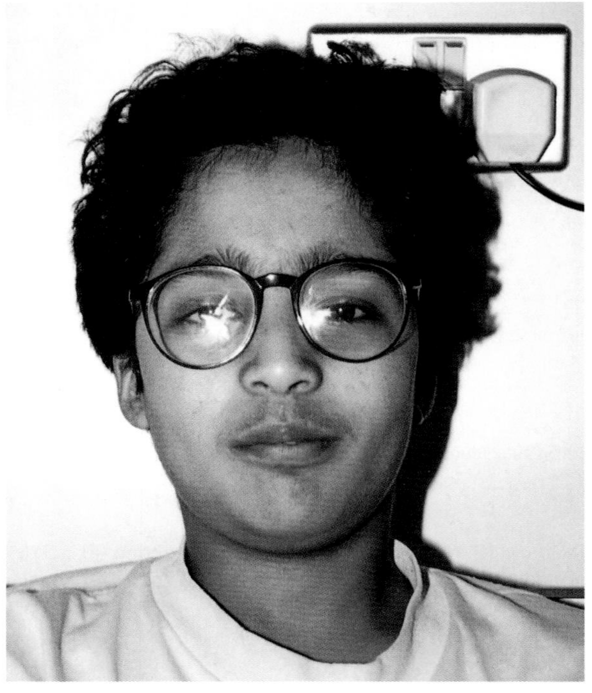

Fig. 10.11
Facies of a child with $\beta$ thalassemia showing prominence of the forehead through changes in skull shape as a result of bone marrow hypertrophy. (Courtesy of Dr D. Norfolk, General Infirmary, Leeds.)

$\beta$-globin structural genes (Fig. 10.12). Some deletions extend to include the A$\gamma$-globin gene so that only the G$\gamma$-globin chain is synthesized.

### Hereditary persistence of fetal hemoglobin

Hereditary persistence of fetal Hb, or HPFH, in which there is persistence of the production of fetal Hb into childhood and adult life, is included in the thalassemias. Most forms of HPFH are, in fact, a form of $\delta\beta$ thalassemia in which continued $\gamma$ chain synthesis compensates for the lack of production of $\delta$- and $\beta$-globin chains. Persons with hereditary persistence of fetal Hb continue to produce significant amounts of fetal Hb after birth, accounting for 20–30% of total Hb in heterozygotes and 100% in homozygotes. This is not associated with any symptoms and was originally considered more of a scientific curiosity than a medical problem.

#### *Mutational basis of HPFH*

Some forms of HPFH have been shown to be due to deletions of the $\delta$- and $\beta$-globin genes. Analysis of the non-deletion forms of HPFH has shown point mutations in the 5′ flanking promoter region of either the G$\gamma$ or A$\gamma$ globin genes near the CAAT box sequences (p. 20) involved in the control of expression of the hemoglobin genes.

## CLINICAL VARIATION OF THE HEMOGLOBINOPATHIES

The marked mutational heterogeneity of $\beta$ thalassemia means that affected individuals are often compound heterozygotes (p. 110), i.e. they have different mutations in their $\beta$-globin genes, leading to a broad spectrum of severity in the disorder. One form of $\beta$ thalassemia of intermediate severity, known as thalassemia intermedia, requires less frequent transfusions.

In certain populations many of the hemoglobinopathies are relatively 'common' and, not unexpectedly, persons are reported who have two different disorders of Hb. Understandably, in the past, recognition of such individuals was

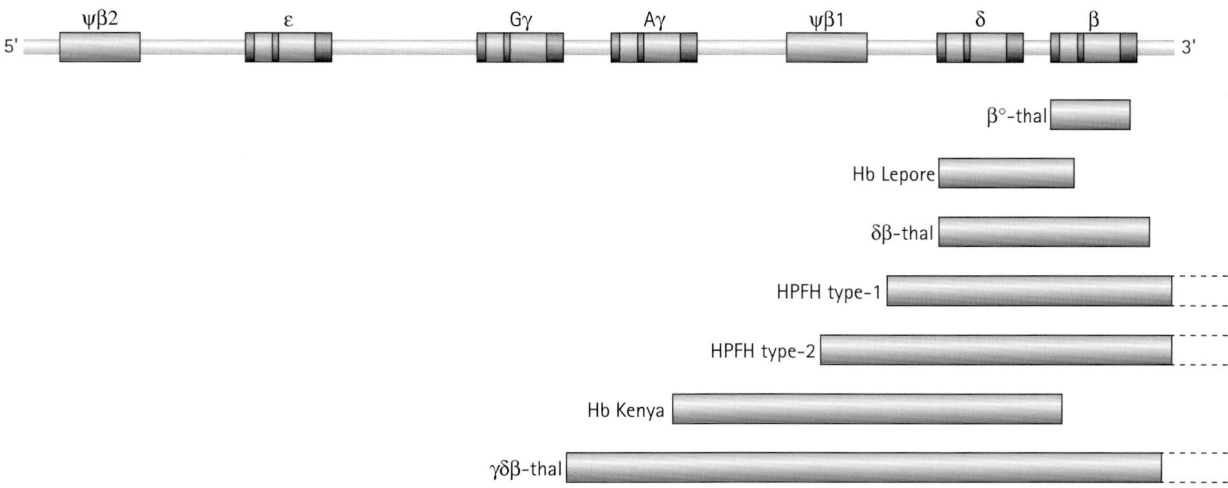


Fig. 10.12
Some of the deletions in the $\beta$-globin region which result in some forms of thalassemia and hereditary persistence of fetal hemoglobin.

often quite difficult. Because of the high prevalence in certain populations of some of the structural variants of hemoglobin, such as Hb S, individuals can present with severe anemia who are found to be heterozygous for both Hb S and β thalassemia, i.e. are compound heterozygotes (p. 110).

Finally, certain combinations of hemoglobinopathies can also result in a previously unexplained mild form of what is normally thought to be an invariably severe hemoglobinopathy. For example, deletion of one or two of the α-globin genes in a person homozygous for $\beta^+$ thalassemia results in a milder illness because there is less of an imbalance in globin chain production. Similarly, the presence of one of the forms of HPFH in a person homozygous for β thalassemia or sickle-cell disease can contribute to amelioration of the disease as the increased production of γ-globin chains compensates for the deficient β-globin chain production. This finding has been exploited therapeutically by the use of drugs, such as hydroxyurea and butyrate, which have been found to be associated with increased Hb F levels. Recent developments in gene therapy (see Ch. 24) for the hemoglobinopathies in a mouse model for sickle-cell disease, in which the introduction of the fetal Hb gene resulted in increased Hb F levels, led to a reduction in the sickling phenomenon. This approach holds great promise for a reduction in the morbidity and mortality associated with this disorder.

## FURTHER READING

Cay J C, Phillips J A, Kazazian H H 1996 Haemoglobinopathies and thalassemias. In: Rimoin D L, Connor J M, Pyeritz R E (eds) Principles and practice of medical genetics, 3rd edn. Churchill Livingstone, Edinburgh, pp. 1599–1626

*A useful up-to-date concise summary of the hemoglobinopathies.*

Cooley T B, Lee P 1925 A series of cases of splenomegaly in children with anemia and peculiar bone changes. Trans Am Pediatr Soc 37: 29–40

*The original description of β thalassemia.*

Pauling L, Itano H A, Singer S J, Wells I C 1949 Sickle-cell anaemia, a molecular disease. Science 110: 543–548

*The first genetic disease in which a molecular basis was described, leading to a Nobel Prize.*

Serjeant G R 1992 Sickle cell disease, 2nd edn. Oxford University Press, Oxford

*Excellent comprehensive text covering all aspects of this important disorder.*

Weatherall D J, Clegg J B, Higgs D R, Woods W G 1995 The hemoglobinopathies. In: Scriver C R, Beaudet A L, Sly W S, Valle D (eds) The metabolic and molecular basis of inherited disease, 7th edn. McGraw Hill, New York, pp. 3417–3484

*A very comprehensive detailed account of hemoglobin and the hemoglobinopathies.*

## ELEMENTS

1. Hb, the protein present in red blood cells responsible for oxygen transport, is a tetramer made up of two dissimilar pairs of polypeptide chains and the iron-containing molecule heme.

2. Human Hb is heterogeneous. During development it comprises a succession of different globin chains that are differentially expressed during embryonic, fetal and adult life, i.e. $\alpha_2\varepsilon_2$, $\alpha_2\gamma_2$, $\alpha_2\delta_2$, $\alpha_2\beta_2$, etc.

3. The disorders of Hb – the hemoglobinopathies – can be divided into two main groups: the structural disorders, e.g. sickle-cell Hb or Hb S, and disorders of synthesis, the thalassemias. The former can be subdivided by the way in which they interfere with the normal function of Hb and/or the red blood cell, e.g. abnormal oxygen affinity or hemolytic anemia. The latter can be subdivided according to which globin chain is synthesized abnormally, i.e. α, β or δβ thalassemia.

4. Family studies of the various disorders of human Hb and analysis of the mutations responsible for these at the protein and DNA levels have led to an understanding of the normal structure, function and synthesis of Hb. This has allowed demonstration of the molecular pathology of these disorders, and prenatal diagnosis of a number of the inherited disorders of human Hb is possible.

CHAPTER 11

# Biochemical genetics

In this chapter we shall consider single-gene biochemical or metabolic diseases, including mitochondrial disorders. The range of known disorders is vast, so only an overview is possible, but it is hoped that the reader will gain a flavor of this fascinating area of medicine. At the beginning of the twentieth century Garrod introduced the concept of 'chemical individuality', leading in turn to the concept of the *inborn error of metabolism*. Beadle and Tatum later developed the idea that metabolic processes, whether in humans or any other organism, proceed by steps. They proposed that each step was controlled by a particular enzyme and that this, in turn, was the product of a particular gene. This was referred to as the 'one gene–one enzyme (or protein) concept'.

## INBORN ERRORS OF METABOLISM

In excess of 200 inborn errors of metabolism are known which can be grouped either by the metabolite, metabolic pathway, function of the enzyme or cellular organelle involved (Table 11.1). Most inborn errors of metabolism are inherited in an autosomal recessive or X-linked manner with only a few being inherited in an autosomal dominant manner. This is because the defective protein in most inborn errors is an enzyme which is diffusible, and there is usually sufficient residual activity in the heterozygous state (i.e. loss-of-function mutation, p. 26) for the enzyme to function normally in most situations. If, however, the reaction catalysed by an enzyme is rate limiting (i.e. haploinsufficiency mutation, p. 26) or the gene product is part of a multimeric complex (i.e. dominant-negative mutation, p. 27), the disorder can manifest in the heterozygous state, i.e. be dominantly inherited (p. 105).

## DISORDERS OF AMINO-ACID METABOLISM

There are a number of disorders of amino-acid metabolism, the best known of which is phenylketonuria.

### PHENYLKETONURIA

Children with phenylketonuria (PKU), if untreated, are severely mentally retarded and often have convulsions. In PKU, the particular enzyme necessary for the conversion of phenylalanine to tyrosine, phenylalanine hydroxylase (PAH), is deficient. In other words there is a 'genetic block' in the metabolic pathway (Fig. 11.1).

PKU was, in fact, the first genetic disorder in humans shown to be caused by a specific enzyme deficiency, by Jervis in 1953. As a result of the enzyme defect, phenylalanine accumulates and is converted into phenylpyruvic acid and other metabolites that are excreted in the urine. The enzyme block leads to a deficiency of tyrosine, with a consequent reduction in melanin formation. Affected children therefore often have blond hair and blue eyes (Fig. 11.2). In addition, areas of the brain that are usually pigmented, e.g. the substantia nigra, can also lack pigment.

#### Treatment of PKU

An obvious method of treating children with PKU would be to replace the missing enzyme, but this cannot be done simply by any conventional means of treatment (p. 356). Bickel, only 1 year after the enzyme deficiency had been identified, suggested that PKU could be treated by removal of phenylalanine from the diet. This has proved to be an effective treatment. If PKU is detected early enough in infancy, mental retardation can be prevented by giving a diet containing a restricted amount of phenylalanine. Phenylalanine is an essential amino acid and therefore cannot be entirely removed from the diet. By monitoring the level of phenylalanine in the blood, it is possible to supply sufficient amounts to meet normal requirements and avoid levels that would result in mental retardation. Once brain development is complete dietary restriction can be relaxed – from adolescence onwards.

The mental retardation seen in children with phenylketonuria is most likely the result of an elevation of phenylalanine and/or its metabolites to toxic levels rather

**Table 11.1 Characteristics of some inborn errors of metabolism**

| Type of defect | Genetics | Deficiency | Main clinical features |
|---|---|---|---|
| **Amino-acid metabolism** | | | |
| Phenylketonuria | AR | Phenyalanine hydroxylase | Mental retardation, fair skin, eczema, epilepsy |
| Alkaptonuria | AR | Homogentisic acid oxidase | Arthritis |
| Oculocutaneous albinism | AR | Tyrosinase | Lack of skin and hair pigment, eye defects |
| Homocystinuria | AR | Cystathione β-synthetase | Mental retardation, dislocation of lens, thrombosis, skeletal abnormalities |
| Maple syrup urine disease | AR | Branched chain α-ketoacid decarboxylase | Mental retardation |
| **Urea cycle disorders** | | | |
| Carbamyl synthetase deficiency | AR | Carbamyl synthetase | Hyperammonemia, coma, death |
| Ornithine carbamyl transferase | XD | Ornithine carbamyl transferase deficiency | Hyperammonemia, death in early infancy |
| Citrullinemia | AR | Argininosuccinic acid synthetase | Variable clinical course |
| Argininosuccinic aciduria | AR | Argininosuccinic acid lyase | Hyperammonemia, mild mental retardation, protein intolerance |
| Hyperargininaemia | AR | Arginase | Hyperammonemia, progressive spasticity, intellectual deterioration |
| **Carbohydrate metabolism** | | | |
| **Monosaccharide metabolism** | | | |
| Galactosemia | AR | Galactose-1-phosphate uridyl transferase | Cataracts, mental retardation, cirrhosis |
| Hereditary fructose intolerance | AR | Fructose-1-phosphate aldolase | Failure to thrive, vomiting, jaundice, convulsions |
| **Glycogen storage diseases** | | | |
| ***Primarily affecting liver*** | | | |
| von Gierke disease (GSD I) | AR | Glucose-6-phosphatase | Hepatomegaly, hypoglycemia |
| Cori disease (GSD III) | AR | Amylo-1,6-glucosidase | Hepatomegaly, hypoglycemia |
| Anderson's disease (GSD IV) | AR | Glycogen brancher enzyme | Abnormal liver function/failure |
| Hepatic phosphorylase deficiency (GSD VI) | AR/ X-linked | Hepatic phosphorylase | Hepatomegaly, hypoglycemia, failure to thrive |
| ***Primarily affecting muscle*** | | | |
| McArdle disease (GSD V) | AR | Muscle phosphorylase | Muscle cramps |
| Pompe disease (GSD II) | AR | Lysosomal α-1,4-glucosidase | Heart failure, muscle weakness |
| **Steroid metabolism** | | | |
| Congenital adrenal hyperplasia | AR | 21-hydroxylase, 11β-hydroxylase, 3β-dehydrogenase | Virilization, salt losing |
| Androgen insensitivity | XR | Androgen receptor | Female external genitalia, testes, male chromosomes |
| **Lipid metabolism** | | | |
| Familial hypercholesterolemia | AD | Low-density lipoprotein receptor | Early coronary artery disease |
| Lysosomal storage diseases | | | |
| **Mucopolysaccharidoses** | | | |
| Hurler syndrome (MPS I) | AR | α-L-iduronidase | Mental retardation, skeletal abnormalities, hepatosplenomegaly, corneal clouding |
| Hunter syndrome (MPS II) | XR | Iduronate sulphate sulphatase | Mental retardation, skeletal abnormalities, hepatosplenomegaly |
| Sanfilippo syndrome (MPS III) | AR | Heparan-S-sulphaminidase (MPS III A), N-ac-α-D-glucosaminidase (MPS III B), Ac-CoA-α-glucosaminidase, N-acetyltransferase (MPS III C), N-ac-glucosaminine-6-sulphate sulphatase (MPS III D) | Behavioral problems, dementia, fits |
| Morquio syndrome (MPS IV) | AR | Galactosamine-6-sulphatase (MPS IV A), β-galactosidase (MPS IV B) | Corneal opacities, short stature, skeletal abnormalities |

**Table 11.1 Characteristics of some inborn errors of metabolism (*cont'd*)**

| Type of defect | Genetics | Deficiency | Main clinical features |
|---|---|---|---|
| MPS V (formerly Scheie — now known to be a mild allelic form of MPS I) | | | |
| Maroteaux–Lamy syndrome (MPS VI) | AR | Arylsulphatase B, *N*-acetyl-galactosamine, α-4-sulphate sulphatase | Corneal clouding, skeletal abnormalities, cardiac abnormalities |
| Sly syndrome (MPS VII) | AR | β-glucuronidase | Variable presentation, skeletal and cardiac abnormalities, hepatosplenomegaly, corneal clouding, mental retardation |
| **Sphingolipidoses** | | | |
| Tay–Sachs disease | AR | Hexosaminidase-A | Developmental regression, blindness, cherry-red spot, deafness |
| Gaucher disease | AR | Glucosylceramide β-glucosidase | Type I — joint and limb pains, splenomegaly<br>Type II — spasticity, fits, death |
| Niemann–Pick disease | AR | Sphingomyelinase | Failure to thrive, hepatomegaly, cherry red spot, developmental regression |
| **Purine/pyrimidine metabolism** | | | |
| Lesch–Nyhan disease | XR | Hypoxanthine guanine phosphoribosyltransferase | Mental retardation, uncontrolled movements, self-mutilation |
| Adenosine deaminase deficiency | AR | Adenosine deaminase | Severe combined immunodeficiency |
| Purine nucleoside phosphorylase | AR | Purine nucleoside phosphorylase | Severe viral infections due to impaired T-cell function |
| Hereditary orotic aciduria | AR | Orotate phosphoribosyltransferase, orotidine 5(-phosphate decarboxylase | Megaloblastic anemia, failure to thrive, developmental delay |
| **Porphyrin metabolism** | | | |
| **Hepatic porphyrias** | | | |
| Acute intermittent porphyria (AIP) | AD | Uroporphyrinogen I synthetase | Abdominal pain, CNS effects |
| Hereditary coproporphyria | AD | Coproporphyrinogen oxidase | As for AIP, photosensitivity |
| Porphyria variegata | AD | Protoporphyrinogen oxidase | Photosensitivity, as for AIP |
| **Erythropoietic porphyrias** | | | |
| Congenital erythropoietic porphyria | AR | Uroporphyrinogen III synthase | Hemolytic anemia, photosensitivity |
| Erythropoietic protoporphyria | AD | Ferrochelatase | Photosensitivity, liver disease |
| **Organic acid disorders** | | | |
| Methylmalonic acidemia | AR | Methylmalonyl-CoA mutase | Hypotonia, poor feeding, acidosis, developmental delay |
| Propionic acidemia | AR | Propionyl-CoA carboxylase | Poor feeding, failure to thrive, vomiting, acidosis, hypoglycemia |
| **Copper metabolism** | | | |
| Wilson disease | AR | ATPase membrane copper | Spasticity, rigidity, dysphagia, cirrhosis transport protein |
| Menkes disease | XR | ATPase membrane copper | Failure to thrive, neurological deterioration transport protein |
| **Peroxisomal disorders** | | | |
| **Peroxisomal biogenesis disorders** | | | |
| Zellweger syndrome | AR | All peroxisomal enzymes | Dysmorphic features, hypotonia, large liver, renal cysts |
| **Isolated peroxisomal enzyme deficiency** | | | |
| Adrenoleukodystrophy | XR | Very long-chain fatty acid-CoA synthetase | Mental deterioration, fits, behavioral changes, adrenal failure |

**Table 11.1 Characteristics of some inborn errors of metabolism (*cont'd*)**

| Type of defect | Genetics | Deficiency | Main clinical features |
|---|---|---|---|
| **Disorders involving mitochondria** | | | |
| MERFF | Mt | Mutation in lysine tRNA G>A 8344 substitution T>C 8356 substitution | Myoclonus, seizures, optic atrophy, hearing impairment, dementia, myopathy |
| MELAS | Mt | Mutation in leucine (UUR) tRNA – 3243G mutation | Encephalomyopathy, stroke-like episodes, seizures, dementia, migraine, lactic acidosis |
| Leigh disease | Mt | Mutation in subunit 6 of ATPase (usually T>G 8993 substitution –'NARP' mutation) | Hypotonia, psychomotor regression, ataxia, spastic quadriparesis |
| Leber hereditary optic neuropathy | Mt | Mutations in ND1, ND4, ND6, 11778A mutation | Retinal degeneration, occasional cardiac conduction defects |
| Barth syndrome | XR | Uncertain. Deficient mitochondrial cardiolipins and raised urinary3-methylglutaconic acid | Cardioskeletal myopathy, growth retardation, neutropenia |
| **Fatty-acid oxidation disorders** | | | |
| MCAD | AR | Medium-chain Acyl-CoA | Episodic hypoketotic hypoglycemia dehydrogenase |
| Glutaric aciduria type I | AR | Glutaryl-CoA dehydrogenase | Episodic encephalopathy, cerebral palsy-like dystonia |
| Glutaric aciduria type II | AR | Multiple acyl-CoA dehydrogenase | Hypotonia, hepatomegaly, acidosis, hypoglycemia |

AR = autosomal recessive; AD = autosomal dominant; XR = X-linked recessive; XD = X-linked dominant; MT = mitochondrial.

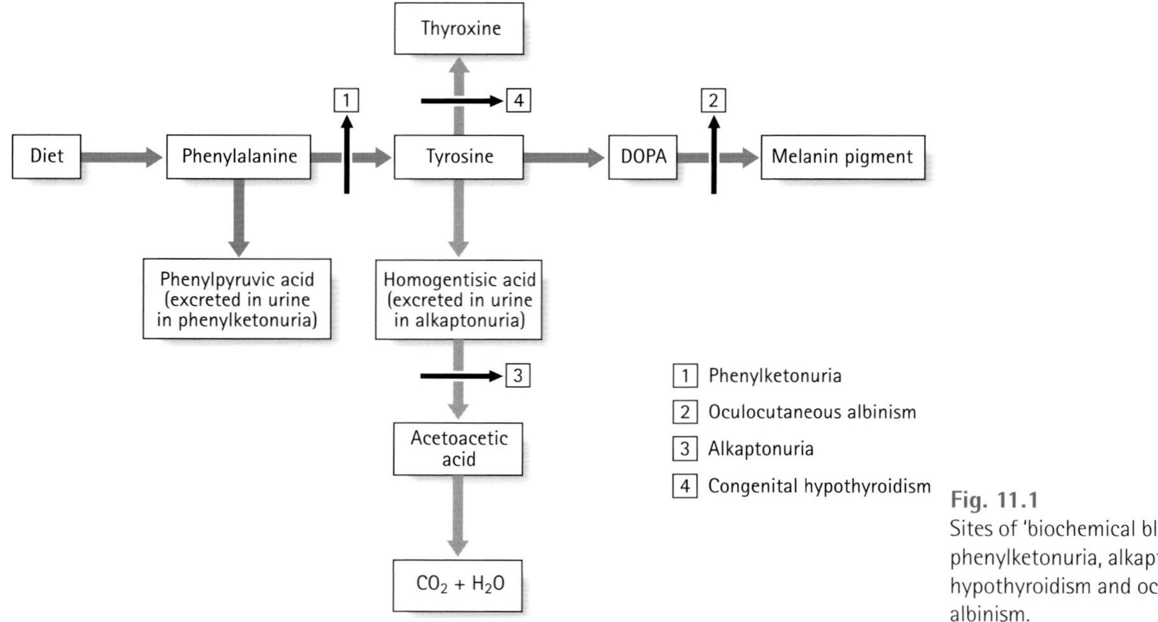


**Fig. 11.1**
Sites of 'biochemical block' in phenylketonuria, alkaptonuria, congenital hypothyroidism and oculocutaneous albinism.

than a deficiency of tyrosine, since an adequate amount of the latter amino acid is usually available in a normal diet. It could well be that there are both prenatal as well as postnatal factors responsible for the mental retardation in persons with untreated PKU.

## Diagnosis of PKU

Although PKU only affects approximately 1 in 10 000 persons of Western European origin, PKU was the first inborn error routinely screened for in newborns. This can be done by tests that detect the presence of the metabolite of phenylalanine, phenylpyruvic acid, in the urine by its reaction with ferric chloride or through elevated levels of phenylalanine in the blood. The latter test, known as the Guthrie test, involves taking blood samples from children in the first week of life and comparing the amount of growth induced by the sample with standards in a strain of the bacterium *Bacillus subtilis,* which requires phenylalanine for growth. This technique has been replaced by

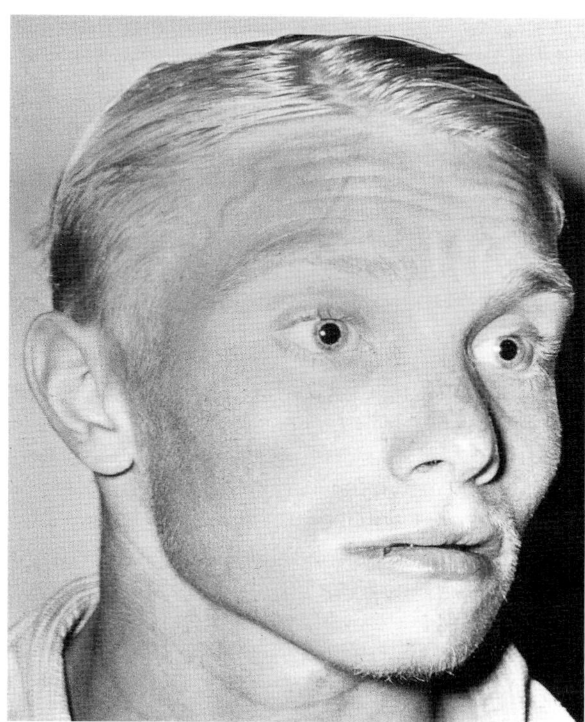

Fig. 11.2
Facies of a male with phenylketonuria; note the fair complexion.

the use of a variety of biochemical assays of phenylalanine levels.

### Heterogeneity of hyperphenylalaninemia

Elevated phenylalanine levels in the newborn period can be the result of causes other than PKU. A small proportion of newborn infants have a condition called benign hyperphenylalaninemia, caused by a transient immaturity of liver cells to metabolize phenylalanine; they do not require treatment as they are not at risk of developing mental retardation. There are, however, two other rare causes of hyperphenylalanemia with serious consequences: in these two disorders the enzyme phenylalanine hydroxylase is normal but there is a deficiency of either dihydropteridine reductase or dihydrobiopterin synthetase. These two enzymes are involved in the synthesis of tetrahydrobiopterin, a cofactor necessary for normal activity of phenylalanine hydroxylase. Both disorders are more serious than classic PKU because there is a high likelihood of mental handicap despite satisfactory management of phenylalanine levels.

### Mutational basis of PKU

Although all cases of classic PKU arise from a deficiency of phenylalanine hydroxylase, more than 450 different mutations in the *PAH* gene have now been identified. Certain mutations are more common in persons with PKU from specific population groups. In addition, in persons of Western European origin with PKU, the mutations occur on a limited number of DNA haplotypes. Interestingly, however, a variety of different individual mutations have been found in association with some of these haplotypes.

### Maternal phenylketonuria

Children born to mothers with phenylketonuria have an increased risk of mental retardation even when their mothers are on closely controlled dietary restriction (p. 161). It has been suggested that the reduced ability of the mother with PKU to deliver an appropriate amount of tyrosine to her fetus in utero could result in reduced fetal brain growth.

## ALKAPTONURIA

Alkaptonuria was the original autosomal recessive inborn error of metabolism described by Garrod (p. 7). In alkaptonuria there is a block in the breakdown of homogentisic acid, a metabolite of tyrosine, through a deficiency of the enzyme homogentisic acid oxidase (Fig. 11.1). As a consequence, homogentisic acid accumulates and is excreted in the urine, to which it imparts a dark color on exposure to air. Dark pigment is also deposited in certain tissues, such as the ear wax, cartilage and joints, where it is known as ochronosis, which in the latter location can lead to arthritis later in life.

## OCULOCUTANEOUS ALBINISM

Oculocutaneous albinism (OCA) is an autosomal recessive disorder due to deficiency of the enzyme tyrosinase, which is necessary for the formation of melanin from tyrosine (see Fig. 11.1). In persons with OCA there is a lack of pigment in the skin, hair, iris and ocular fundus (Fig. 11.3). The lack of pigment in the eye results in poor visual acuity and typical uncontrolled pendular eye movement (nystagmus). The reduced pigmentation appears to lead to underdevelopment of the part of retina for fine vision, the fovea, and abnormal projection of the visual pathways to the optic cortex.

### Heterogeneity of oculocutaneous albinism

OCA is genetically and biochemically heterogeneous. Cells from persons with classic albinism have no measurable tyrosinase activity, the so-called *tyrosinase-negative* form. However, cells from some persons with albinism show reduced but residual tyrosinase activity and are termed *tyrosinase positive*. This is usually reflected clinically by variable development of pigmentation of their hair and

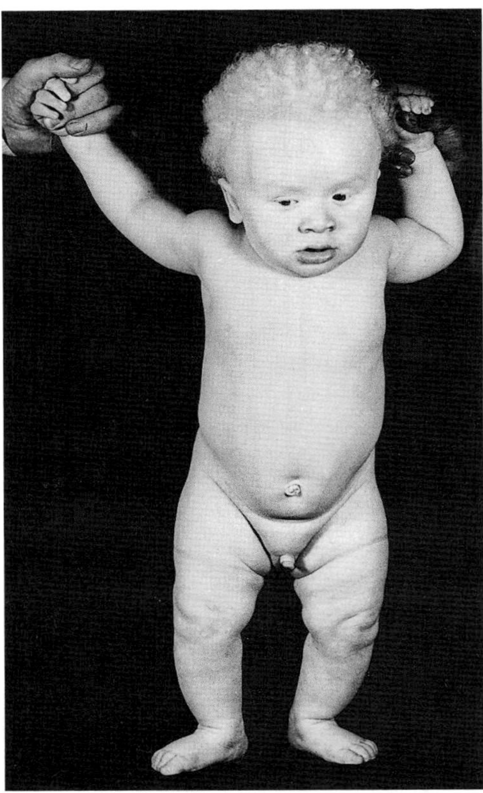

Fig. 11.3
Oculocutaneous albinism in a child of Afro-Caribbean origin. (Courtesy of Dr V. A. McKusick.)

skin with age. Both types are known as tyrosinase gene-related oculocutaneous albininism type 1, or OCA 1.

DNA studies have revealed classic tyrosinase-negative and some tyrosinase-positive families with oculocutaneous albinism to be due to mutations in the tyrosinase gene on the long arm of chromosome 11. Linkage studies in some of the families with tyrosinase-positive oculocutaneous albinism, however, have excluded the tyrosinase gene as being responsible. A number of these families, interestingly, have a mutation in the P gene, the human homolog of a gene in the mouse called *pink-eyed dilution*, or pink-eye for short, located on the long arm of chromosome 15. This has been termed oculocutaneous albinism type 2, or OCA 2. In addition, in a proportion of families with oculocutaneous albinism linkage to both of these two loci has been excluded, consistent with the existence of a third locus responsible for OCA.

### HOMOCYSTINURIA

Homocystinuria is a recessively inherited inborn error of sulphur amino-acid metabolism characterized by mental retardation, fits, thromboembolic episodes, osteoporosis and a tendency to dislocation of the lenses. This last feature, along with a tendency to develop a curvature of the spine (scoliosis), together with a pectus excavatum, and long fingers and toes (arachnodactyly), can lead to confusion with the autosomal dominant disorder Marfan syndrome (p. 301).

Homocystinuria is caused by a deficiency of the enzyme cystathionine β-synthetase and can be screened for by means of a positive cyanide nitroprusside test which detects the presence of increased levels of homocystine in the urine. The diagnosis is confirmed by elevated plasma homocystine levels. Treatment involves a low-methionine diet with cystine supplementation. A proportion of individuals with homocystinuria are responsive to the enzyme cofactor pyridoxine, what is known as the pyridoxine-responsive form. A small proportion of affected individuals have mutations in genes leading to deficiencies of enzymes involved in the synthesis of cofactors for cystathionine β-synthetase.

## DISORDERS OF BRANCHED CHAIN AMINO-ACID METABOLISM

The essential branched chain amino acids leucine, isoleucine and valine have a part of their metabolic pathways in common. Deficiency of the enzyme involved results in maple syrup urine disease.

### MAPLE SYRUP URINE DISEASE

Newborn infants with this autosomal recessive disorder present in the first week of life with vomiting, then alternating decreased and increased tone, proceeding to death within a few weeks if left untreated. There is a characteristic odor of the urine likened to that of maple syrup. The disorder is caused by a deficiency of the branched-chain ketoacid decarboxylase producing increased excretion of the branched-chain amino acids valine, leucine and isoleucine in the urine, the presence of which suggest the diagnosis that is confirmed by the presence of the three essential branched-chain amino acids in blood. Treatment involves a diet limiting the intake of the three branched-chain amino acids to the amount necessary for growth. Affected individuals are particularly susceptible to deterioration, in association with intercurrent illnesses resulting from the catabolic degradation of proteins.

## UREA CYCLE DISORDERS

The urea cycle is a five-step metabolic pathway that takes place primarily in liver cells for the removal of waste

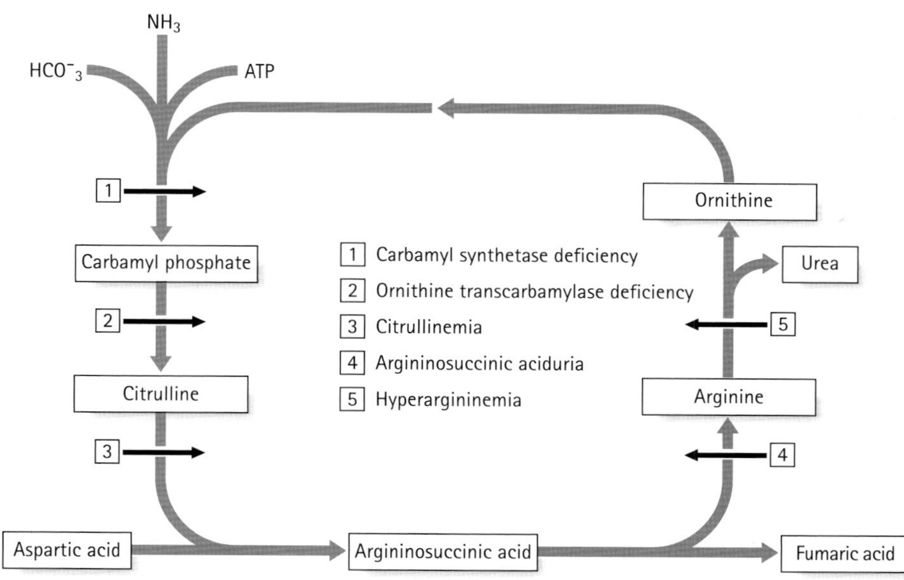


**Fig. 11.4**
Diagram indicating the position of the various inborn errors of the urea cycle.

nitrogen from the amino groups of amino acids arising from the normal turnover of protein. It converts two molecules of ammonia and one of bicarbonate into urea (Fig. 11.4). Deficiencies of enzymes in the urea cycle result in intolerance to protein due to the accumulation of ammonia in the body, or what is known as hyperammonemia. Elevated ammonia levels are toxic to the central nervous system and can lead to coma and, with some of the urea cycle disorders, if left untreated, death. The various disorders of the urea cycle are collectively rare and individually very rare. They are all inherited as autosomal recessive disorders except ornithine transcarbamylase deficiency which is X-linked.

## DISORDERS OF CARBOHYDRATE METABOLISM

The inborn errors of carbohydrate metabolism can be considered in two main groups, disorders of monosaccharide metabolism and the glycogen storage disorders.

### DISORDERS OF MONOSACCHARIDE METABOLISM

Two examples of disorders of monosaccharide metabolism are galactosemia and hereditary fructose intolerance.

#### Galactosemia

Galactosemia is an autosomal recessive disorder due to deficiency of the enzyme galactose-1-phosphate uridyl transferase, which is necessary for the metabolism of the dietary sugar galactose. Newborn infants with galactosemia present with vomiting, lethargy, failure to thrive and jaundice in the second week of life. If untreated, they go on to develop complications that include mental retardation, cataracts and cirrhosis of the liver. Galactosemia can be screened for by the presence of reducing substances in the urine with specific testing for galactose. The complications of galactosemia can be prevented by early diagnosis and feeding of affected infants with milk substitutes that do not contain galactose or lactose, the sugar found in milk, which is broken down into galactose. Early diagnosis and treatment are essential if the severe complications are to be prevented.

#### Hereditary fructose intolerance

Hereditary fructose intolerance is an autosomal recessive disorder due to deficiency of the enzyme fructose-1-phosphate aldolase. Dietary fructose is present in honey, fruit and certain vegetables, and in combination with glucose in the disaccharide sucrose in cane sugar. Individuals with hereditary fructose intolerance present at different ages, depending on when fructose is introduced into the diet. Symptoms can be minimal but might also be as severe as those seen in galactosemia which include failure to thrive, vomiting, jaundice and convulsions. The diagnosis is confirmed by the presence of fructose in the urine and enzyme assay on an intestinal mucosal or a liver biopsy sample. Dietary restriction of fructose is associated with a good long-term prognosis.

### GLYCOGEN STORAGE DISEASES

Glycogen is the form in which the sugar glucose is stored in muscle and liver as a polymer, acting as a reserve energy source. In the glycogen storage diseases (GSDs) glycogen accumulates in excessive amounts in skeletal muscle, cardiac muscle and/or liver due to a variety of inborn errors of the enzymes involved in synthesis and degradation of glycogen. In addition, because of the metabolic block, glycogen is unavailable as a normal glucose source. This can result in hypoglycemia, impairment of liver function and neurological abnormalities.

In each of the six major types of GSD there is a specific enzyme defect involving one of the steps in the metabolic pathways of glycogen synthesis or degradation. The various types can be grouped according to whether they affect primarily the liver or muscle. All six types are inherited as autosomal recessive disorders, although there are variants of the hepatic phosphorylase which are X-linked.

### Glycogen storage diseases that primarily affect liver

#### *von Gierke disease (GSD I)*

Von Gierke disease was the first described disorder of glycogen metabolism and is due to deficiency of the enzyme glucose-6-phosphatase, which is responsible for degradation of liver glycogen to release glucose. Affected infants present with an enlarged liver (hepatomegaly) and/or sweating and a fast heart rate due to hypoglycemia, which can occur after fasting of only 3–4 h duration. Treatment is simple: frequent feeding and the avoidance of fasting to maintain the blood sugar.

#### *Cori disease (GSD III)*

Cori disease is caused by deficiency of the enzyme amylo-1,6-glucosidase, which is also known as the debrancher enzyme. Deficiency of the enzyme results in glycogen accumulation in the liver and other tissues resulting from the inability to cleave the 'branching' links of the glycogen polymer. Affected infants can present with hepatomegaly because of glycogen accumulation and/or muscle weakness. Treatment involves avoiding hypoglycemia by frequent feeding and avoiding prolonged periods of fasting.

#### *Anderson disease (GSD IV)*

Anderson disease results from deficiency of glycogen brancher enzyme which leads to formation of abnormal glycogen consisting of long chains with few branches which cannot be broken down by the enzymes normally responsible for glycogen degradation. Affected infants present with hypotonia and abnormal liver function in the first year of life, the latter progressing rapidly to liver failure. No effective treatment is available apart from the possibility of a liver transplant.



#### *Hepatic phosphorylase deficiency (GSD VI)*

Hepatic phosphorylase is a multimeric enzyme complex with subunits coded for by both autosomal and X-linked genes. Deficiency of hepatic phosphorylase obstructs glycogen degradation, which results in children presenting in the first 2 years of life with hepatomegaly, hypoglycemia and failure to thrive. Treatment is with carbohydrate supplements that improve growth.

### Glycogen storage diseases that primarily affect muscle

#### *Pompe disease (GSD II)*

Infants with Pompe disease usually present in the first few months of life with floppiness (hypotonia) and delay in the gross motor milestones because of muscle weakness. They then develop an enlarged heart and die of cardiac failure in the first or second year. Voluntary and cardiac muscle accumulates glycogen due to the deficiency of the lysosomal enzyme $\alpha$-1,4-glucosidase that is needed to break down glycogen. The diagnosis can be confirmed by enzyme assay on white blood cells or fibroblasts. Early reports of enzyme replacement therapy appear promising.

#### *McArdle disease (GSD V)*

Persons with McArdle disease present with muscle cramps on exercise in the teenage years. It is caused by a deficiency of muscle phosphorylase, which is necessary for degradation of muscle glycogen. There is no effective form of treatment, although in some affected individuals the muscle cramps tend to decline if exercise is continued, probably as a result of other energy sources becoming available from alternative metabolic pathways.

## DISORDERS OF STEROID METABOLISM

The disorders of steroid metabolism include a number of autosomal recessive inborn errors of the biosynthetic pathways of cortisol. These can result in the virilization of a female fetus along with an associated salt loss in both affected male and female infants due to deficiency of the hormone aldosterone. In addition, defects of the androgen receptor result in lack of virilization of chromosomally male individuals (Fig. 11.5).

### CONGENITAL ADRENAL HYPERPLASIA (ADRENOGENITAL SYNDROME)

The diagnosis of congenital adrenal hyperplasia (CAH) should be considered in any newborn female infant presenting with virilization of the external genitalia, as this is the commonest cause of ambiguous genitalia in female

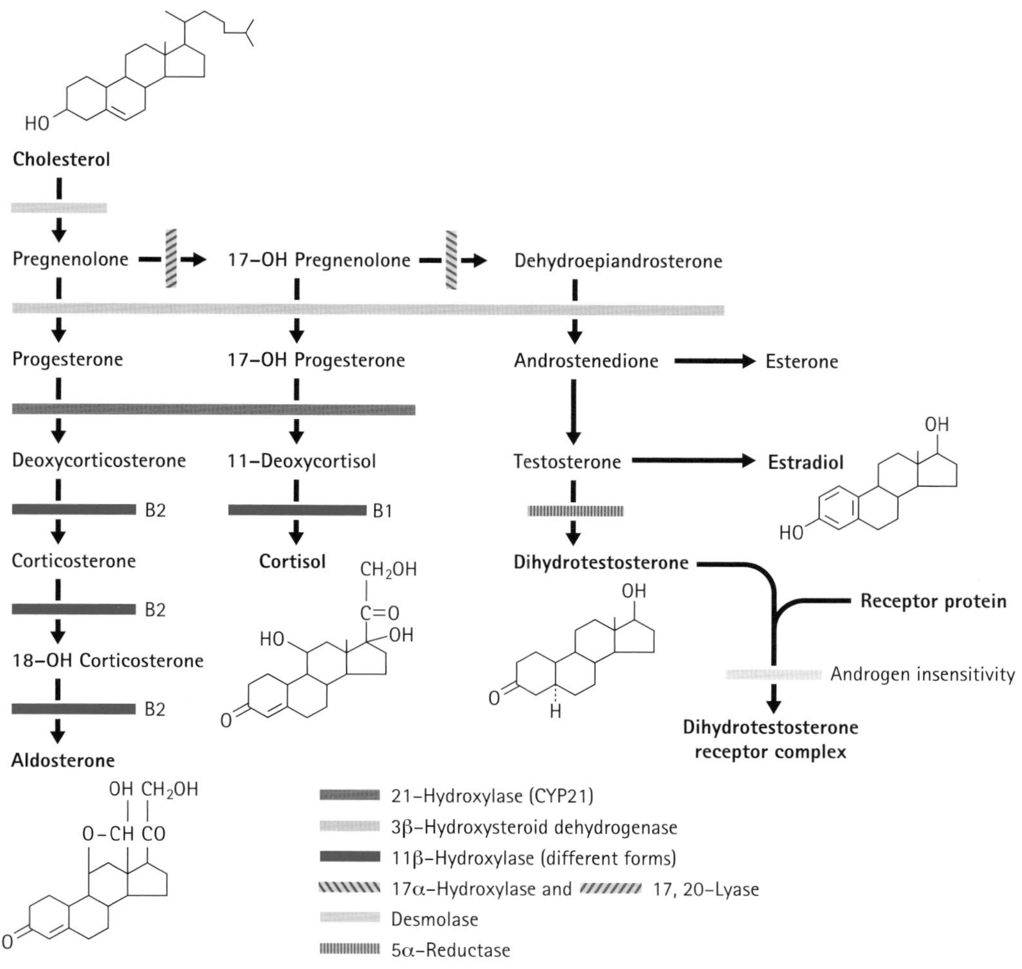


**Fig. 11.5**
Steroid biosynthesis indicating the site of the common inborn errors of steroid biosynthesis.

newborns (p. 287) (Fig. 11.6). 21-Hydroxylase deficiency accounts for over 90% of cases. About one-quarter of affected infants will have the salt-losing form, presenting in the second or third week of life with circulatory collapse, hyponatremia and hyperkalemia. Less commonly CAH is due to deficiency of the enzymes 11β-hydroxylase or 3β-dehydrogenase, and very rarely occurs as a result of deficiencies of enzymes 17α-hydroxylase and 17,20-lyase. Desmolase deficiency is also very rare, with all the pathways blocked. The phenotype is reversed with ambiguous genitalia in males, and severe addisonian crises may occur. Males with the rare 5α-reductase deficiency are significantly undermasculinized but do not suffer other metabolic problems and are likely to be raised as females. At puberty, however, the surge in androgen production is sufficient to stimulate growth of the phallus, making gender identity and assignment problematic.

Affected females with virilizing (classic) CAH have normal müllerian-derived internal genitalia, the virilization of the external genitalia being caused by an accumulation of the adrenocortical steroids proximal to the enzyme block in the steroid biosynthetic pathway, many of which have testosterone-like activity (Fig. 11.5). The possibility of CAH should not be forgotten, of course, in male infants presenting with circulatory collapse in the first few weeks of life.

Affected infants, in addition to requiring urgent correct assignment of gender, are treated with replacement cortisol, along with fludrocortisone if they have the salt-losing form. Virilized females may require plastic surgery in due course. Steroid replacement is lifelong and needs to be increased during intercurrent illness or times of stress, e.g. surgery. Menarche in girls with salt-losing CAH is late, menstruation irregular, and they are sub-fertile.

## ANDROGEN INSENSITIVITY SYNDROME

Individuals with the androgen insensitivity syndrome (AIS) have female external genitalia, and undergo breast development in puberty (p. 286). They classically present

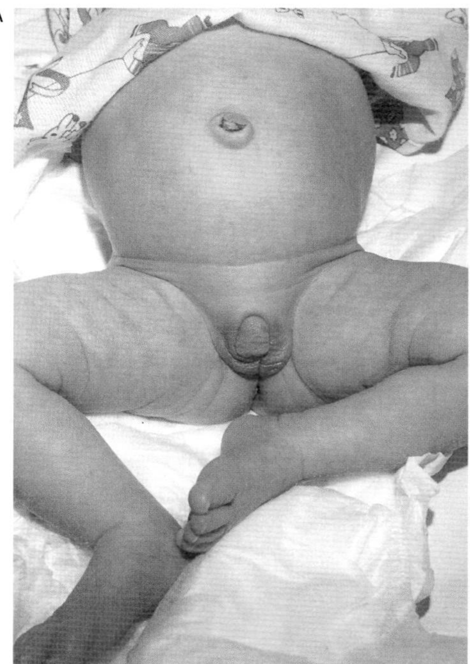

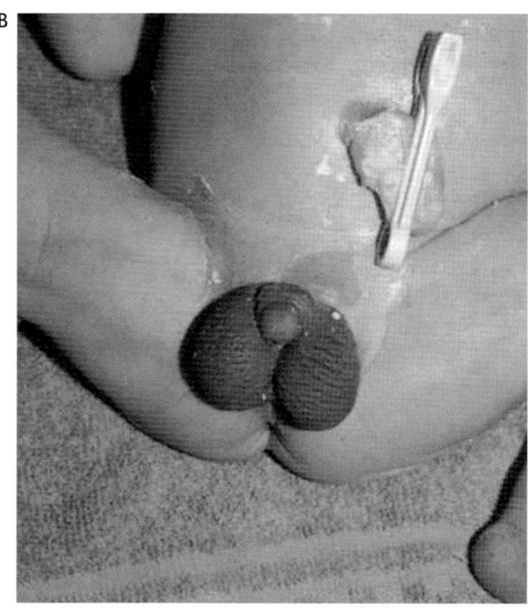

Fig. 11.6
(A) Virilized external genitalia in a female with congenital adrenal hyperplasia, (B) A male baby with hypospadias who clearly has testes in the scrotal sacs.

either with primary amenorrhea, which is the lack of onset of menstrual periods, or with an inguinal hernia containing a gonad that turns out to be a testis. Inguinal hernia is uncommon in girls and if present, especially bilaterally, the possibility of AIS should be considered. There is often scanty secondary sexual hair and investigation of the internal genitalia reveals an absent uterus and fallopian tubes with a blind-ending vagina. Chromosome analysis reveals a normal male karyotype, 46,XY.

Androgen production by the testes is normal in affected individuals but they do not bind androgen normally because of an abnormal androgen receptor (Fig. 11.5) – a mutation is present in the androgen receptor gene on the X chromosome. This can be functionally assayed in skin fibroblasts. Some individuals have incomplete or partial androgen insensitivity and undergo variable virilization. Affected individuals usually have a female sexual orientation but obviously will be sterile. They require removal of their testes because of an increased risk of developing a testicular malignancy, and should be placed on estrogen for secondary sexual development and to prevent osteoporosis in the longer term.

## DISORDERS OF LIPID METABOLISM

Familial hypercholesterolemia is the commonest autosomal dominant single-gene disorder in Western society and is associated with a high morbidity and mortality through premature coronary artery disease (p. 234).

### FAMILIAL HYPERCHOLESTEROLEMIA

Persons with familial hypercholesterolemia (FH) have elevated cholesterol levels with a significant risk of developing early coronary artery disease (p. 234). They can present in childhood or adolescence with subcutaneous deposition of lipid, known as xanthomata (Fig. 11.7). Starting with families who presented with early coronary artery disease, Brown and Goldstein unraveled the biology of the low-density lipoprotein (LDL) receptor (p. 234) and the pathological basis of FH.

Cells normally derive their cholesterol from either endogenous cholesterol synthesis or by uptake of dietary cholesterol from LDL receptors on the cell surface. Intracellular cholesterol levels are maintained by a feedback system, with free cholesterol inhibiting LDL receptor synthesis as well as reducing the level of de novo endogenous cholesterol synthesis.

The high cholesterol levels in persons with FH are due to deficient or defective function of the LDL receptors leading to increased levels of endogenous cholesterol synthesis. Four main functional types or classes of mutation in the LDL receptor have been identified: reduced or defective biosynthesis of the receptor; reduced or defective transport of the receptor from the endoplasmic reticulum to the Golgi apparatus; abnormal binding of

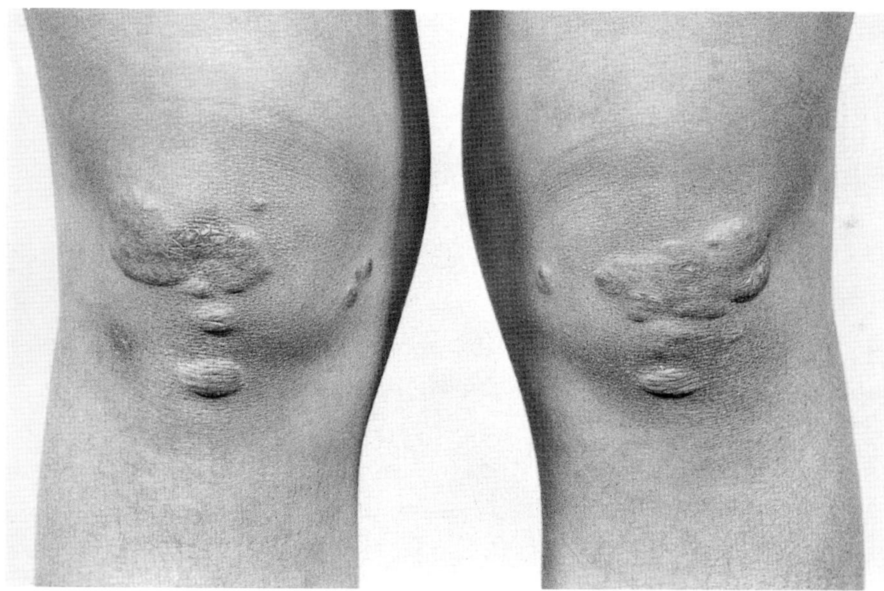

**Fig. 11.7**
Legs of a person homozygous for familial hypercholesterolemia, showing multiple xanthomata. (Courtesy of Dr E. Wraith, Royal Manchester Children's Hospital, Manchester.)

the LDL by the receptor; and abnormal internalization of the LDL by the receptor (Fig. 11.8). Specific mutations are found more commonly in persons with FH from certain ethnic groups, as a result of founder effects (p. 128).

Dietary restriction of cholesterol intake and drug treatment with agents such as cholestyramine, which sequesters cholesterol from the enterohepatic circulation, can lower cholesterol levels and, in part, reduce the risk of coronary artery disease. The recent detailed elucidation of the metabolic and biosynthetic pathways of cholesterol has enabled further therapeutic measures through the development of drugs that inhibit the endogenous synthesis of cholesterol by inhibiting the enzyme HMG CoA reductase. These are proving to be more effective in preventing long-term complications.

## LYSOSOMAL STORAGE DISORDERS

In addition to the inborn errors of metabolism, in which an enzyme defect leads to deficiency of an essential metabolite and accumulation of intermediate metabolic precursors, there are a number of disorders in which a deficiency of a lysosomal enzyme involved in the degradation of complex macromolecules leads to their accumulation. This accumulation occurs because macromolecules are normally in a constant state of flux, with a delicate balance between their rates of synthesis and breakdown. Children born with lysosomal storage diseases are usually normal at birth but with the passage of time commence a downhill course of differing duration to owing the accumulation of one or more of a variety or type of macromolecules.

### MUCOPOLYSACCHARIDOSES

Children with one of the mucopolysaccharidoses (MPSs) present with skeletal, vascular or central nervous system findings along with coarsening of the facial features. These features are due to progressive accumulation of sulfated polysaccharides (also known as glycosaminoglycans) caused by defective degradation of the carbohydrate side-chain of acid mucopolysaccharide.

Six different MPSs are recognized, based on clinical and genetic differences. Each specific MPS type has a characteristic pattern of excretion in the urine of the glycosaminoglycans, dermatan, heparan, keratan and chondroitin sulfate. Subsequent biochemical investigation has revealed the various types to be due to deficiency of different individual enzymes. All but Hunter syndrome, which is X-linked, are inherited as autosomal recessive disorders.

#### Hurler syndrome (MPS I)

Hurler syndrome is the most severe of the mucopolysaccharidoses. Affected infants present in the first year with corneal clouding, a characteristic curvature of the lower spine and subsequent poor growth. They develop hearing loss, coarse facial features, an enlarged liver and spleen, joint stiffness and vertebral changes in the second year. There is progression of these features along with mental deterioration and eventually death by the mid-teens

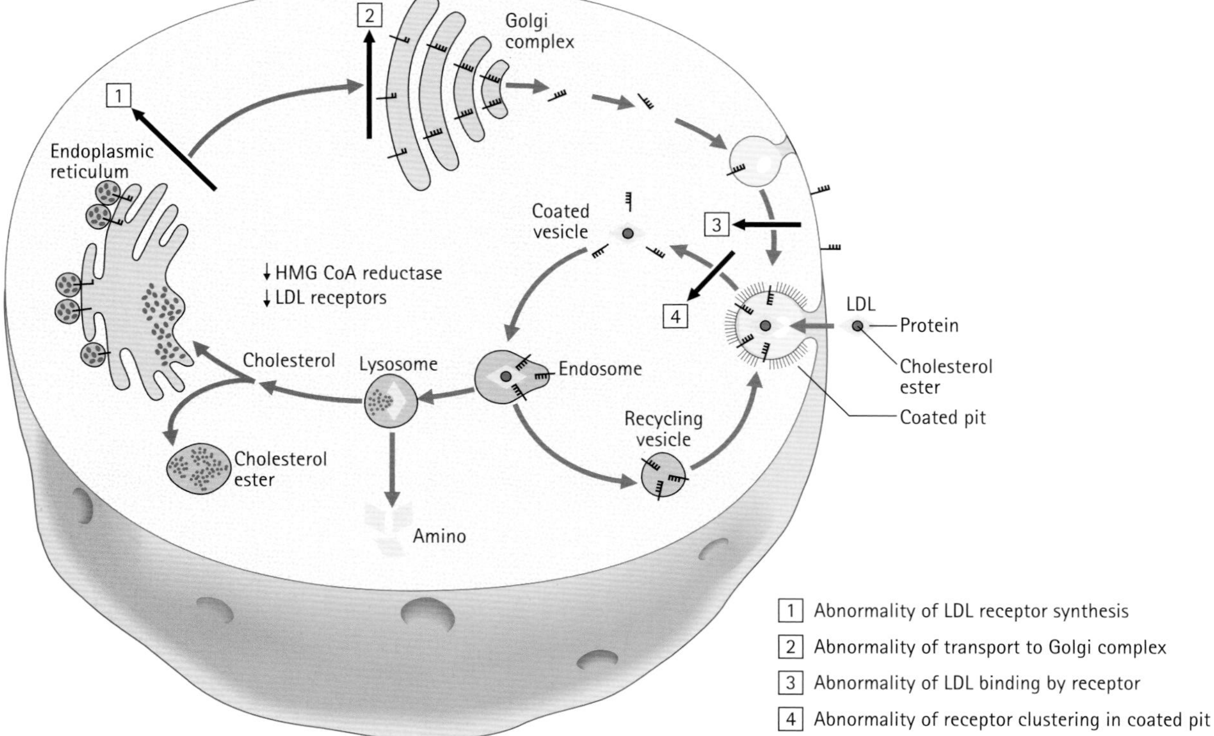


**Fig. 11.8**
Stages in cholesterol biosynthesis and in the metabolism of low-density lipoprotein receptors, indicating the types of mutation in familial hypercholesterolemia. (Adapted from Brown M S, Goldstein J L 1986 A receptor-mediated pathway for cholesterol homeostasis. Science 232: 34–47.)

from a combination of cardiac failure and respiratory infections.

The diagnosis of Hurler syndrome was initially made by demonstration of the presence of metachromatic granules in the cells, i.e. lysosomes distended by the storage material that is primarily dermatan sulfate. Increased urinary excretion of dermatan and heparan sulfate is commonly used as a screening test, but confirmation of the diagnosis involves demonstration of reduced activity of the lysosomal hydrolase, α-L-iduronidase. Less severe allelic forms of Hurler syndrome, caused by varying levels of residual α-L-iduronidase activity, were previously classified separately as Scheie disease (MPSIS) and Hurler/Scheie disease (MPS I H/S).

## Hunter syndrome (MPS II)

Males with Hunter syndrome usually present between the ages of 2 and 5 years with hearing loss, a history of recurrent infection, diarrhea and poor growth. Examination reveals a characteristic coarsening of their facial features (Fig. 11.9), along with enlargement of their liver and spleen and stiffness of their joints. X-rays of the spine reveal abnormalities in the shape of the vertebrae. There is progressive physical and mental deterioration, with death usually in the teenage years.

The diagnosis is confirmed by the presence of excess amounts of dermatan and heparan sulfate in the urine and deficient or decreased activity of the enzyme iduronate sulfate sulfatase in serum or white blood cells.

## Sanfilippo syndrome (MPS III)

Sanfilippo syndrome is the most common MPS. Affected individuals present in their second year with mild coarsening of features, skeletal changes and progressive intellectual loss with behavioral problems, proceeding to convulsions and death in early adult life. The diagnosis is confirmed by the presence of increased urinary heparan and chondroitin sulfate excretion and deficiency of one of four enzymes involved in the degradation of heparan sulfate: sulphaminidase (MPS III A), *N*-acetyl-α-D-glucosaminidase (MPS III B), acetyl-CoA-α-glucosaminidase-*N*-acetyltransferase (MPS III C) or *N*-acetyl-glucosamine-6-sulphate sulphatase (MPS III D).

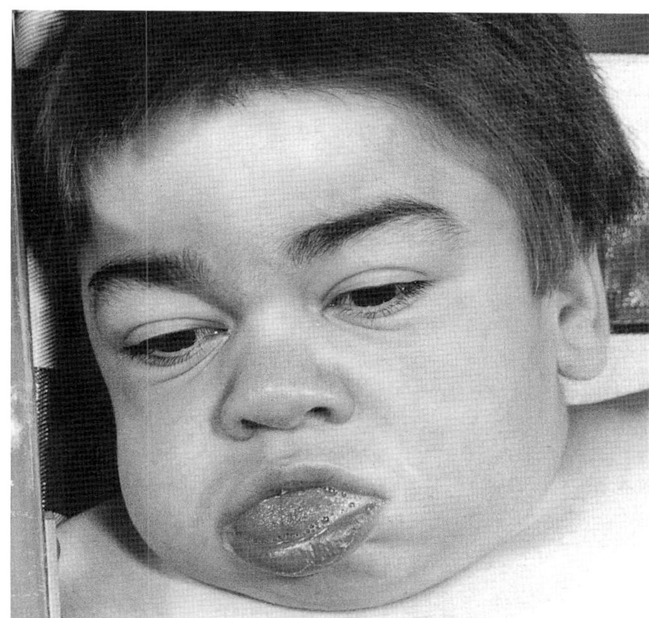

Fig. 11.9
Facies of a male with the mucopolysaccharidosis, Hunter syndrome. (Courtesy of Dr E. Wraith, Royal Manchester Children's Hospital, Manchester.)

Individuals with these different enzyme deficiencies cannot be distinguished clinically.

### Morquio syndrome (MPS IV)

Children with Morquio syndrome present in the second or third year of life with skeletal abnormalities that include short stature, thoracic deformity and curvature of the spine (kyphoscoliosis). Intelligence is normal and survival is long term, although there is a risk of spinal-cord compression due to progression of the skeletal involvement. The diagnosis is confirmed by the presence of keratan sulfate in the urine and deficiency of either galactosamine-6-sulphatase (MPS IV A) or β-galactosidase (MPS IV B).

### Maroteaux–Lamy syndrome (MPS VI)

Individuals affected with the Maroteaux–Lamy syndrome present with Hurler-like features in early childhood. These include coarse facial features, short stature with thoracic deformity, kyphosis and restriction of joint mobility. In addition they develop corneal clouding and cardiac valve abnormalities but retain normal intelligence. A less severe form presents later with survival into late adulthood, in contrast to the more severe form in which survival is usually only until the third decade. The diagnosis is confirmed by the presence of increased urinary dermatan sulfate excretion and arylsulfatase B deficiency in white blood cells or fibroblasts.

### Sly syndrome (MPS VII)

Sly syndrome shows marked variability in the severity of presentation. This ranges from skeletal features that include mild kyphoscoliosis and hip dysplasia to coarse facial features, hepatosplenomegaly, corneal clouding, cardiac abnormalities and mental retardation, with death in childhood or adolescence. Increased urinary glycosaminoglycans excretion and β-glucuronidase deficiency in serum, white blood cells or fibroblasts confirm the diagnosis.

### Treatment of the mucopolysaccharidoses

Treatment of the mucopolysaccharidoses has been attempted by enzyme replacement but there are a number of practical difficulties that have been responsible for its lack of success (p. 356). More recently, however, treatment by bone marrow transplantation has been attempted, with varying reports of success, biochemically and clinically, in the skeletal and cerebral features.

## SPHINGOLIPIDOSES (LIPID STORAGE DISEASES)

In the sphingolipidoses there is an inability to degrade sphingolipid, resulting in the progressive deposition of lipid or glycolipid primarily in the brain, liver and spleen. Central nervous system involvement results in progressive mental deterioration, often with fits, usually resulting in death in childhood. There are at least 10 different types with specific enzyme deficiencies: Tay–Sachs, Gaucher and Niemann–Pick diseases are the most common.

### Tay–Sachs disease

This is the best known sphingolipidosis and affects approximately 1 in 3600 persons of Ashkenazi Jewish ancestry (p. 128). Affected infants usually present by 6 months of age with poor feeding, lethargy and floppiness. Loss of developmental milestones or developmental regression will usually become apparent in the second half of the first year. Feeding becomes increasingly difficult and the infant progressively deteriorates, with deafness, visual impairment and spasticity, which progresses to rigidity. Death usually occurs by the age of 3 years as a result of respiratory infection. Less severe juvenile, adult and chronic forms are also reported.

The diagnosis of Tay–Sachs disease is further supported clinically by the presence of a 'cherry-red' spot in the centre of the macula of the fundus. Biochemical confirmation of Tay–Sachs disease is by demonstration of reduced hexosaminidase A levels in serum, white blood cells or cultured fibroblasts. Reduced hexosaminidase A activity is due to deficiency of the $\alpha$ subunit of the enzyme $\beta$-hexosaminidase that leads to accumulation of the sphingolipid, $GM_2$ ganglioside. Deficiency of the $\beta$ subunit of $\beta$-hexosaminidase leads to reduced activity of the isozyme, hexosaminidase B, causing the other $GM_2$ gangliosidosis, Sandhoff disease, in which affected individuals present with similar clinical features.

### Gaucher disease

This is the commonest sphingolipidosis, and like Tay–Sachs disease, it occurs with an increased frequency among persons of Ashkenazi Jewish ancestry. There are two main types based on the age of onset. In type I, or the adult type, which is the most common form of Gaucher disease, affected persons present with febrile episodes and limb, joint or trunk pain and a tendency to pathologic fractures. Clinical examination usually reveals an enlarged spleen and liver. Affected persons often show mild anemia and X-ray changes in the vertebral bodies and proximal femora. The central nervous system is spared.

In type II, or infantile Gaucher disease, central nervous involvement is a major feature. Affected infants usually present between 3 and 6 months of age with failure to thrive and hepatosplenomegaly. By 6 months of age they begin to show developmental regression and neurological deterioration, with spasticity and fits leading on to recurrent pulmonary infection and death in the second year.

The diagnosis of Gaucher disease is confirmed by reduced activity of the enzyme glucosylceramide $\beta$-glucosidase in white blood cells or cultured fibroblasts.

Treatment of individuals with the adult type of Gaucher disease involves symptomatic relief of pain. In addition, it is often necessary to remove the enlarged spleen because it causes a secondary anemia due to premature sequestering of red blood cells, a condition known as hypersplenism.

The lack of central nervous system involvement in type I Gaucher disease meant that it was an obvious candidate for enzyme replacement therapy since it was not necessary for the enzyme to cross the blood–brain barrier (p. 326). Initial attempts to treat adults with Gaucher disease by enzyme replacement therapy met with little success because of difficulty in obtaining sufficient quantities of enzyme and in targeting the appropriate sites. However, modification of $\beta$-glucosidase by the addition of mannose-6-phosphate, which targets the enzyme to macrophage lysosomes, has led to dramatic alleviation of symptoms and regression of the organomegaly in affected persons. The treatment is, however, expensive and regimens using lower doses and alternative methods to target the enzyme more efficiently are being assessed.

### Niemann–Pick disease

Infants with Niemann–Pick disease present with failure to thrive and hepatomegaly and can be found to have a cherry-red spot on their macula. Developmental regression rapidly progresses by the end of the first year, with death by the age of 4 years. A characteristic finding is the presence of what are called foam cells in the bone marrow due to sphingomyelin accumulation. Confirmation of the diagnosis is by demonstration of deficiency of the enzyme sphingomyelinase. A less severe form without neurological involvement has been reported. Niemann–Pick disease, like Tay–Sachs and Gaucher diseases, occurs more commonly in Jews of Ashkenazi Eastern European ancestry.

## DISORDERS OF PURINE/PYRIMIDINE METABOLISM

Gout is the disorder in humans that is classically associated with abnormalities of purine metabolism. Joint pain, swelling and tenderness are a result of the inflammatory response of the body to deposits of crystals of a salt of uric acid. In fact, only a minority of persons who present with gout are found to have an inborn error of metabolism. The cause in most instances results from a combination of genetic and environmental factors; it is, however, always important to consider disorders that can result in an increased turnover of purines (e.g. a malignancy such as leukemia) or reduced secretion of the metabolites (e.g. renal impairment) as a possible underlying precipitating cause.

## LESCH–NYHAN SYNDROME

A particularly disabling disorder of purine metabolism is the Lesch–Nyhan syndrome. This X-linked disorder is due to the deficiency of the enzyme hypoxanthine guanine phosphoribosyltransferase that results in increased levels of phosphoribosylpyrophosphate. The latter is normally a rate-limiting chemical in the synthesis of purines. Its excess leads to an increased rate of purine synthesis which results in an accumulation of excessive amounts of uric acid and some of its metabolic precursors. The main effect is on the central nervous system, resulting in uncontrolled movements, spasticity, mental retardation and compulsive self-mutilation. Although drugs such as allopurinol, which inhibit uric acid formation, can lower uric acid levels, none yet offers any satisfactory treatment for the debilitating central nervous system effects.

## IMMUNODEFICIENCY DISEASES CAUSED BY DEFECTS IN PURINE METABOLISM

Two inherited immunodeficiency disorders (p. 197), somewhat surprisingly, are inborn errors of purine metabolism.

### Adenosine deaminase deficiency

About a half of all children with the autosomal recessive form of severe combined immunodeficiency with impaired B and T cell function (p. 197) have deficiency of the enzyme adenosine deaminase. Affected children present in the first year of life with recurrent viral and bacterial infections and, if untreated, will die of overwhelming infection in the first year. The diagnosis is confirmed by deficient red blood cell adenosine deaminase activity. Correction of the immunodeficiency by transfusion of irradiated red blood cells has been reported. More recently bone marrow transplantation has been successfully carried out, even antenatally in utero!

### Purine nucleoside phosphorylase deficiency

A proportion of children susceptible to severe, recurrent and potentially lethal viral infections with isolated impaired T-cell function have been shown to have a deficiency of the enzyme purine nucleoside phosphorylase. Treatment with irradiated red blood cells has been reported to result in a temporary improvement in immune function.

## HEREDITARY OROTIC ACIDURIA

Children with hereditary orotic aciduria present in the first year of life with a megaloblastic anemia, failure to thrive and developmental delay. They have deficiency of one of two enzymes, orotate phosphoribosyltransferase or orotidine-5′-phosphate decarboxylase, both of which are necessary for the synthesis of pyrimidines, resulting in excretion of large quantities of orotic acid in the urine. Treatment with the pyrimidine uridine has been reported to reduce urinary orotic acid excretion, correct the anemia and restore growth.

# DISORDERS OF PORPHYRIN METABOLISM

There are several different disorders of porphyrin metabolism which are due to deficiency of enzymes in the biosynthetic pathway of the iron-containing group in hemoglobin, heme (p. 149). They are all inherited as autosomal dominant disorders, except for congenital erythropoietic porphyria, which is an autosomal recessive disorder. This is because the enzymes are rate limiting (p. 26), so that haploinsufficiency results in clinical disease.

The different types of porphyria are variably associated with neurological or visceral involvement and cutaneous photosensitivity due to accumulation of the different porphyrin precursors in those organs. The porphyrias are divided into two types depending on whether the excess production of porphyrins occurs predominantly in the liver or in the erythropoietic system.

## HEPATIC PORPHYRIAS

These include acute intermittent porphyria, hereditary coproporphyria and porphyria variegata.

### Acute intermittent porphyria

Acute intermittent porphyria (AIP) is characterized by attacks of abdominal pain, weakness, vomiting and mental disturbance in the form of confusion, emotional upset or hallucinations. Coma can even occur and women are more severely affected than men, with symptoms sometimes associated with the menstrual cycle. Attacks can also be precipitated by the administration of certain drugs, such as exogenous steroids, anticonvulsants and barbiturates. It is caused by a partial deficiency of the enzyme uroporphyrinogen I synthetase leading to increased excretion of the porphyrin precursors porphobilinogen and δ-aminolevulinic acid in urine.

### Hereditary coproporphyria

In hereditary coproporphyria, a related condition also inherited as a dominant trait, there is partial deficiency of the enzyme coproporphyrinogen oxidase. The disorder is clinically indistinguishable from acute intermittent porphyria, although approximately one-third of affected persons also have photosensitivity of their skin.

### Porphyria variegata

Persons with this form of porphyria, which is particularly prevalent in those of Afrikaaner origin in South Africa (p. 107), have variable skin photosensitivity with neurological and visceral findings that can also be triggered by drugs. Increased fecal excretion of the porphyrin precursors protoporphyrin and coproporphyrin can be demonstrated and the disorder has been shown to be due to deficiency of the enzyme protoporphyrinogen oxidase.

## ERYTHROPOIETIC PORPHYRIAS

The erythropoietic porphyrias include congential erythropoietic porphyria and erythropoietic protoporphyria.

### Congenital erythropoietic porphyria

The main feature of congenital erythropoietic porphyria (CEP) is an extreme photosensitivity with blistering of the skin leading to extensive scarring, to the extent that most affected persons are unable to go out in normal daylight. In addition, many have a hemolytic anemia requiring regular blood transfusion and frequently splenectomy. Affected individuals have red-brown discoloration of their teeth, which show red fluorescence under ultraviolet light. Congential erythropoietic porphyria is due to deficiency of the enzyme uroporphyrinogen III synthase.

### Erythropoietic protoporphyria

Erythropoietic protoporphyria (EPP) is due to deficiency of the enzyme ferrochelatase, which is responsible for the insertion of ferrous iron into the porphyrin precursor to form heme. Affected persons have photosensitivity and can sometimes develop chronic liver disease. Successful treatment of the photosensitivity has been reported with β-carotene.

## ORGANIC-ACID DISORDERS

Children affected with one of the organic-acid disorders present with periodic episodes of poor feeding, vomiting and lethargy in association with a severe metabolic acidosis, low white cell (neutropenia) and platelet (thrombocytopenia) counts, low blood sugar (hypoglycemia) and high blood ammonia levels (hyperammonemia). These episodes are often precipitated by intercurrent illness or increased protein intake, and after such an episode affected children can lose developmental skills. Analysis of blood from children at the time of these episodes reveals high levels of glycine, i.e. hyperglycinemia. It was subsequently found that the acidosis in these episodes was due to increased levels of the organic acids, either propionic or methylmalonic acid.

The two autosomal recessive organic-acid disorders methylmalonic acidemia (MMA) and propionic acidemia (PPA) are caused by deficiency of the enzymes methylmalonyl-CoA mutase and proprionyl-CoA carboxylase, respectively. The enzyme deficiency results in accumulation of the toxic organic-acid metabolites derived from deamination of certain amino acids, specific long-chain fatty acids and cholesterol side-chains. Therapy of the acute episode involves treatment of any infection, fluid replacement, correction of the metabolic acidosis and cessation of protein intake. Long-term prophylactic treatment involves restriction of protein intake and rapid recognition and management of any intercurrent illness. A proportion of individuals affected with propionic acidemia are responsive to biotin, while some persons with methylmalonic acidemia are sensitive to vitamin $B_{12}$.

## DISORDERS OF COPPER METABOLISM

There are two inborn errors of copper metabolism, Menkes' disease and Wilson disease.

### MENKES DISEASE

Menkes disease is an X-linked disorder in which affected males presenting in the first few months of life with feeding difficulties, vomiting and poor weight gain. Subsequently floppinesss (hypotonia), fits and progressive neurological deterioration ensue, with death due to recurrent respiratory infection usually occurring by the age of 3 years. A characteristic feature is the hair, which lacks pigment and is kinky and brittle and breaks easily. This was noted to resemble the wool of sheep suffering from copper deficiency. Serum copper and ceruloplasmin levels are very low. Cloning of the gene for Menkes disease was facilitated through an affected female with an X;autosome translocation (p. 78) and revealed it to code for an ATPase cation transport protein for copper. Treatment regimens with different exogenous copper sources have had limited benefit to date.

### WILSON DISEASE

Persons affected with the autosomal recessive disorder Wilson disease commonly present in childhood or the early teenage years with fits and abnormal neurological findings. These can include deterioration of coordination, involuntary movements, abnormal tone, dysarthria (difficulty in speaking), dysphagia (difficulty with swallowing) and changes in behavior or frank pyschiatric disturbance. Clinical examination can reveal the presence of what is called a Kayser–Fleischer ring, which is a golden brown or greenish collarette at the corneal margin. Investigation can reveal the presence of abnormal liver function, which can progress to cirrhosis.

High copper levels in the liver, decreased serum concentrations of the copper transport protein ceruloplasmin, and abnormal copper loading tests are suggestive of the diagnosis. The gene for Wilson disease was cloned on the basis of anticipated homology to the Menkes gene and the gene product has been shown to be an ATPase cation transport protein involved in copper transfer from the hepatocytes to the biliary collecting system.

There are dramatic reports of striking improvement of the neurological features in persons with Wilson disease using the chelating agents D-penicillamine and trientine, although these can cause side-effects.

## PEROXISOMAL DISORDERS

The peroxisomes are subcellular organelles bound by a single trilayer lipid membrane present in all cells; they are especially abundant in liver and renal parenchymal cells. The organelle matrix contains more than 40 enzymes that carry out a number of reactions involved in fatty-acid oxidation and cholesterol biosynthesis interacting with metabolic pathways outside the peroxisomes. The enzymes of the peroxisomal matrix are synthesized on the polyribosomes, enter the cytosol and are transferred into the peroxisomes.

There are two main categories of peroxisomal disorder, disorders of peroxisome biogenesis, such as Zellweger syndrome, in which there are severely reduced numbers of peroxisomes in all cells, and single isolated peroxisomal enzyme deficiencies, such as X-linked adrenoleukodystrophy.

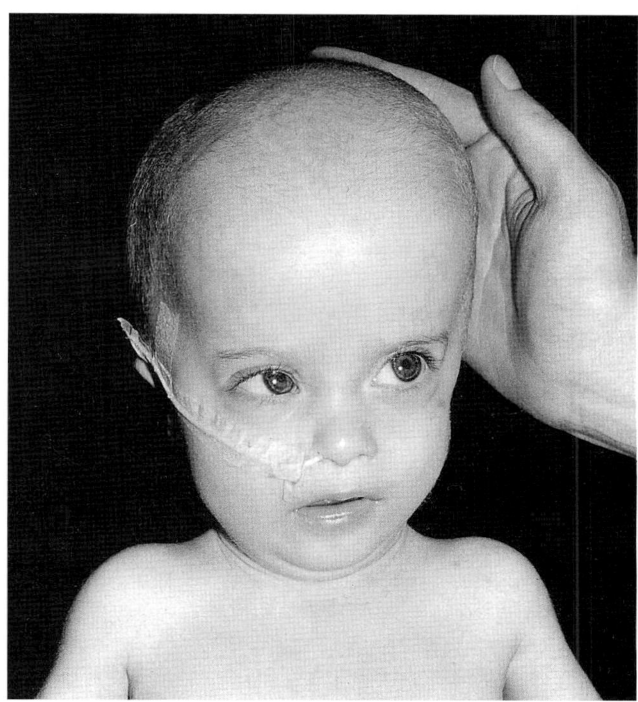

**Fig. 11.10**
Facies of an infant with Zellweger syndrome showing a prominent forehead.

### ZELLWEGER SYNDROME

Newborn infants with Zellweger syndrome present with hypotonia and weakness and have mildly dysmorphic facial features (Fig. 11.10) consisting of a prominent forehead and a large anterior fontanelle ('soft spot'). They may also have cataracts and an enlarged liver. They generally go on to have fits with developmental regression and usually die by 1 year of age. Investigations can reveal renal cysts and abnormal calcification in the cartilaginous growing ends of the long bones (Fig. 11.11). There is a range of severity of this disorder, with different clinical diagnoses being given to the less severe types. The diagnosis can be confirmed by elevated levels of plasma long-chain fatty acids. The gene for Zellweger syndrome encodes a protein involved in the peroxisome assembly.

It is unusual for inborn errors of metabolism to be associated with a dysmorphic syndrome (p. 250). In addition to Zellweger syndrome, the Smith–Lemli–Opitz syndrome has recently been found to be caused by an inborn error of cholesterol biosynthesis.

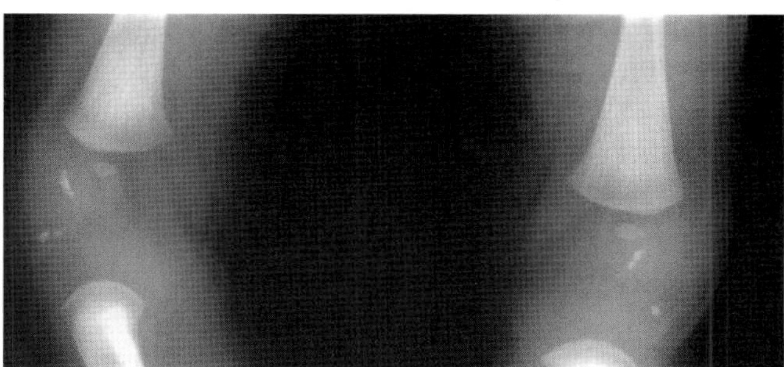

**Fig. 11.11**
Radiograph of the knee of a newborn infant with Zellweger syndrome showing abnormal punctate calcification of the distal femoral epiphyses.

### ADRENOLEUKODYSTROPHY

Males with the X-linked disorder adrenoleukodystrophy (ALD) classically present in late childhood with deteriorating school performance, although affected males can present at any age and even, on occasion, be asymptomatic. A proportion of affected males can also present in adult life with less severe neurological features and adrenal insufficiency, or what is termed adrenomyeloneuropathy. ALD has been shown to be associated with a deficiency of the enzyme very long-chain fatty acid (VLCFA) CoA synthetase, but is secondary to deficiency of a peroxisomal membrane protein.

Treatment of ALD is being undertaken with a diet that uses as a source of fat an oil that has low levels of the very long-chain fatty acids. This has been popularly called 'Lorenzo's oil' after a film of that name made about a child with adrenoleukodystrophy. The efficacy of this diet has, however, been disappointing.

## DISORDERS AFFECTING MITOCHONDRIAL FUNCTION

Mitochondrial disease was first identified in 1962 in a patient whose mitochondria showed structural abnormalities and there was loss of coupling between oxidation and phosphorylation, though it was not until the late 1970s and early 1980s that the relevance of mutated mitochondrial DNA (mtDNA) to human disease began to be appreciated. The small circular double-stranded mtDNA (Fig. 2.7, p. 19) contains genes coding for ribosomal RNA production and various transfer RNAs (tRNA) required for mitochondrial protein biosynthesis as well as some of the proteins involved in electron transport. There are 5523 codons and a total of 37 gene products. Guanine and cytosine nucleotides are asymmetrically distributed between the two mtDNA strands – the guanine-rich strand being called the heavy (H) strand and the cytosine-rich the light (L) strand. Replication and transcription is controlled by a 1122-bp sequence of mtDNA known as the displacement loop (D-loop). Oxidative phosphorylation (OXPHOS) is the biochemical process responsible for generating much of the ATP required for cellular energy. The process is mediated by five intramitochondrial enzyme complexes, referred to as complexes I to V, and the mtDNA encodes 13 OXPHOS subunits, 22 tRNAs and 2 rRNAs.

The 'complexes' are aptly named! Analysis of complex I, for example, has revealed approximately 41 different subunits, of which seven are polypeptides encoded by mtDNA genes known as ND1, ND2, ND3, NDL4, ND4, ND5 and ND6, with the remaining 34 subunits encoded by nuclear DNA genes. Complex V comprises 12 or 13 subunits of which two, ATPase 6 and 8, are encoded by mtDNA. Maximal activity of complex V appears to require tight linking with cardiolipin (see Barth syndrome, p. 179), encoded by nuclear DNA.

As most mitochondrial proteins, including subunits involved in electron transport, are encoded by nuclear genes, these most often follow autosomal recessive inheritance. As with other metabolic autosomal recessive diseases, disorders resulting from mutations in these genes tend to breed true. However, the disorders due to mutations in mtDNA are extremely variable owing to the phenomenon of heteroplasmy (Fig. 7.25, p. 120). The clinical features are mainly a combination of neurological signs – encephalopathy, dementia, ataxia, dystonia, neuropathy and seizures, and myopathic signs – hypotonia, weakness and cardiomyopathy with conduction defects. Other symptoms and signs may include deafness, diabetes mellitus and retinal pigmentation, and acidosis may be a feature. So variable can be the clinical manifestations that a mitochondrial cytopathy should be considered as a possibility at any age when the presenting illness has a neurological or myopathic component. A number of distinct clinical entities have been determined and, although some of them overlap considerably, there is a degree of genotype–phenotype correlation.

### MYOCLONIC EPILEPSY AND RAGGED RED FIBER DISEASE (MERRF)

Myoclonic epilepsy and ragged red fiber (MERRF) disease was first described in 1973 and so called because Gomori-trichrome staining of muscle revealed abnormal deposits of mitochondria as 'ragged red'; in 1988 it was appreciated that the condition was maternally inherited. The classic picture is of progressive myoclonic epilepsy, myopathy and slowly progressive dementia. Optic atrophy is frequently present and the EEG is characteristically abnormal. Postmortem brain examination reveals widespread neurodegeneration. In 1990 it was reported that MERRF results from a point mutation in the gene for lysine transfer RNA-tRNA(lysine).

### MITOCHONDRIAL ENCEPHALOMYOPATHY, LACTICE ACIDOSIS AND STROKE-LIKE EPISODES (MELAS)

First delineated in 1984, this extremely variable condition is now recognized as one of the commonest mitochondrial disorders. Short stature may be a feature, but it is stroke-like episodes that mark out this particular mitochondrial disorder, though these episodes do not necessarily occur in all affected family members. When they do occur, they may manifest as vomiting, headache, or visual disturbance, and sometimes lead to transient hemiplegia or hemianopia. A common presenting feature of MELAS is type 2 diabetes mellitus, and a sensorineural hearing hearing loss may also occur (described as maternally inherited diabetes and deafness [MIDD]). These latter clinical features are associated with the most common mutation, which is an A>G substitution at position 3243, which affects tRNA leucine$^{UUR}$. This is found in about 80% of patients, followed by a T>C transition at position 3271, also affecting tRNA leucine$^{UUR}$.

### NEURODEGENERATION, ATAXIA AND RETINITIS PIGMENTOSA (NARP)

The early presenting feature is night blindness, which may be followed years later by neurological symptoms. Dementia may occur in older patients, but seizures can present at almost any age and younger patients show developmental delay. The majority of cases are due to a single mutation – the T>G substitution at position 8993, which occurs in the coding region of subunit 6 of ATPase. This change is often referred to as the NARP mutation.

## LEIGH DISEASE

This condition is characterized by its neuropathology, consisting of typical spongiform lesions of the basal ganglia, thalamus, substantia nigra and tegmental brainstem. In its severe form death occurs in infancy or early childhood, and it was in such a patient that the 8993 NARP mutation was first identified. In effect, therefore, one form of Leigh disease is simply a severe form of NARP, and higher proportions of mutant mtDNA have been reported in these cases. However, variability is again sometimes marked and the author knows one family where a mother, whose daughter died in early childhood, was found to have low levels of the 8993 mutation and her only symptom was slow recovery from a general anesthetic.

The same or very similar pathology, and a similar clinical course, has now been described in patients with different molecular defects. Cytochrome-c deficiency has been reported in a number of patients and some of these have been shown to have mutations in *SURF1*, a nuclear gene. These cases follow autosomal recessive inheritance. Leigh disease is therefore genetically heterogeneous.

## LEBER HEREDITARY OPTIC NEUROPATHY

Leber hereditary optic neuropathy (LHON) was the first human disease shown to result from a mtDNA point mutation, and about a dozen different mutations are now described. The most common mutation occurs at position 11,778 (*ND4* gene), accounting for up to 70% of cases in Europe and over 90% of cases in Japan. It presents with acute, or subacute, loss of central visual acuity without pain, which typically occurs between 12 and 30 years of age. Males in affected pedigrees are much more likely to develop visual loss than are females. In some LHON pedigrees additional neurological problems occur.

## BARTH SYNDROME

Also known as X-linked cardioskeletal myopathy, this is characterized by congenital dilated cardiomyopathy (including endocardial fibroelastosis), a generalized myopathy and growth retardation. Abnormal mitochondria are found in many tissues, deficient in cardiolipin, and skeletal muscle shows increased lipid levels. A variable and sometimes fluctuating increase in urinary levels of 3-methylglutaconic acid may be useful in achieving a diagnosis, and mutations have been identified in the *G4.5* (*TAZ*) gene, but the enzyme defect leading to 3-methylglutaconic aciduria is currently unknown.

## DISORDERS OF MITOCHONDRIAL FATTY-ACID OXIDATION

In the 1970s the first reports appeared of patients with skeletal muscle weakness and abnormal muscle fatty-acid metabolism associated with decreased muscle carnitine. The carnitine cycle is a biochemical pathway required for the transport of long-chain fatty acids into the mitochondrial matrix, and those less than 10 carbons in length are then activated to form acyl-CoA esters. The carnitine cycle is one part of the pathway of mitochondrial β-oxidation that plays a major role in energy production, especially during periods of fasting. Carnitine deficiency is a secondary feature of the β-oxidation disorders, with the exception of the carnitine transport defect where it is primary, and this rare condition responds dramatically to carnitine replacement. The more common fatty-acid oxidation disorders are outlined.

### Medium-chain acyl-CoA dehydrogenase deficiency

Medium-chain acyl-CoA dehydrogenase (MCAD) deficiency is the commonest of this group of disorders, presenting most frequently as episodic hypoketotic hypoglycemia provoked by fasting. The onset is often in the first 2 years of life and, tragically, is occasionally fatal, resembling sudden infant death syndrome. Management rests on maintaining adequate caloric intake and avoidance of fasting, which can be challenging in young children with intercurrent illnesses. Inherited as an autosomal recessive disorder, 90% of alleles result from a single-point mutation, which has led to discussion that this could be a candidate disease for neonatal population screening.

### Long-chain (LCAD) and short chain acyl-CoA (SCAD) and long-chain 3-hydroxyacyl-CoA dehydrogenase (LCHAD) deficiencies

These rare conditions all show autosomal recessive inheritance and present early in life with a variable combination of skeletal and cardiomyopathy, hepatocellular dysfunction with hepatomegaly, and encephalopathy. Treatment revolves around nutritional maintenance and avoidance of fasting, but is not very rewarding in SCAD.

## GLUTARIC ACIDURIAS

Glutaric acidurias types I (glutaryl-CoA dehydrogenase deficiency) and II (multiple acyl-CoA dehydrogenase deficiency) are included as examples of organic acidurias that are intermediate in fatty-acid oxidation, and both show autosomal recessive inheritance. In type I macrocephaly is present at birth and infants suffer episodes of encephalopathy with spasticity, dystonia, seizures and developmental delay. Treatment is by dietary restriction of glutarigenic amino acids – lysine, tryptophan and hydroxylysine. Common among the Old Order Amish of Pennsylvania, neonatal screening has been introduced in the area.

Type II glutaric aciduria is variable, with two severe forms having neonatal onset, one of these including urogenital anomalies. In both of these severe types hypotonia, hepatomegaly, metabolic acidosis and hypoketotic hypoglycemia occur. The late-onset form may present in early childhood, rather than the neonatal period, with failure to thrive, metabolic acidosis, hypoglycemia and encephalopathy. Treatment of the severe forms is supportive only, but in the milder form riboflavin, carnitine, and diets low in protein and fat have been more successful.

## PRENATAL DIAGNOSIS OF INBORN ERRORS OF METABOLISM

For the majority of inborn errors of metabolism in which an abnormal or deficient gene product can be identified, prenatal diagnosis is possible. Biochemical analysis of cultured amniocytes obtained at mid-trimester amniocentesis is possible but has largely given way to earlier testing using direct or cultured chorionic villi (CV), which allows a diagnosis to be made by 12–14 weeks gestation (p. 328). For many conditions a biochemical analysis on cultured CV tissue is the appropriate test but, increasingly, direct mutation analysis is possible. This avoids the inherent delay of culturing CV tissue and is of particular value for inborn errors for which the biochemical basis is not clearly identified, or where the enzyme is not expressed in amniocytes or chorionic villi.

Prenatal diagnosis of mitochondrial disorders due to mtDNA mutations presents particular difficulties because of the problem of heteroplasmy and the inability to predict the outcome for any result obtained, whether positive or negative for the mutation in question. This presents challenging counseling issues and also raises consideration of other reproductive options, such as ovum donati and, perhaps in the future, nuclear transfer technology to circumvent maternal mtDNA.

## FURTHER READING

Benson P F, Fensom A H 1985 Genetic biochemical disorders. Oxford University Press, Oxford
*A good reference source for detailed basic further information on the inborn errors of metabolism.*

Clarke J T R 1996 A clinical guide to inherited metabolic diseases. Cambridge University Press, Cambridge
*A good basic text, problem based and clinically oriented.*

Cohn R M, Roth K S 1983 Metabolic disease: a guide to early recognition. WB Saunders, Philadelphia
*Useful text as it considers the inborn errors from their mode of presentation rather than starting from the diagnosis.*

Garrod A E 1908 Inborn errors of metabolism. Lancet ii: 1–7, 73–79, 142–148, 214–220
*Reports of the first inborn errors of metabolism.*

Nyhan W L, Ozand P T 1998 Atlas of metabolic diseases. Chapman & Hall, London
*A detailed text but very readable and full of excellent illustrations and clinical images.*

Rimoin D L, Connor J M, Pyeritz R E, Korf B R (eds) 2001 Principles and practice of medical genetics, 4th edn. Churchill Livingstone, Edinburgh
*The section on metabolic disorders includes 13 chapters covering in succinct detail the various groups of metabolic disorders.*

Scriver C R, Beaudet A L, Sly W S, Valle D (eds) 2000 The metabolic basis of inherited disease, 8th edn. McGraw Hill, New York
*A huge multi-author three volume comprehensive detailed text on biochemical genetics with an exhaustive reference list and, with this edition, a CD-ROM.*

## ELEMENTS

1. Metabolic processes in all species occur in steps, each being controlled by a particular enzyme which is the product of a specific gene, leading to the one gene–one enzyme concept.

2. A block in a metabolic pathway results in the accumulation of metabolic intermediates and/or a deficiency of the end-product of the particular metabolic pathway concerned, a so-called inborn error of metabolism.

3. The majority of the inborn errors of metabolism are inherited as autosomal recessive or X-linked recessive traits. A few are inherited as autosomal dominant disorders involving rate-limiting enzymes, cell surface receptors or multimeric enzymes, through haploinsufficiency or dominant negative mutations.

4. A number of the inborn errors of metabolism can be screened for in the newborn period and successfully treated by dietary restriction or supplementation.

5. Prenatal diagnosis of many of the inborn errors of metabolism is possible either by conventional biochemical methods, the use of linked DNA markers or by direct mutation detection.

CHAPTER 12

# Pharmacogenetics

*"If it were not for the great variability among individuals medicine might as well be a science and not an art."*
Sir William Osler (1892)

## DEFINITION

Some individuals can be especially sensitive to the effects of a particular drug, whereas others can be quite resistant. Such individual variation can be the result of factors which are not genetic. For example, both the young and the elderly are very sensitive to morphine and its derivatives, as are persons with liver disease. Individual differences in response to drugs in humans are, however, often genetically determined.

The term *pharmacogenetics* was introduced by Vogel in 1959 for the study of genetically determined variations that are revealed solely by the effects of drugs. Such a definition would strictly exclude those hereditary disorders in which symptoms are usually only precipitated or aggravated by drugs. Many investigators, however, also include these latter disorders within the sphere of pharmacogenetics.

Pharmacogenetics is an important branch of genetics because adverse drug reactions are a major cause of morbidity and mortality. It is also likely to be of increasing importance in the future, particularly as a result of the development of new drugs from information that becomes available from the Human Genome Project (Ch. 23), or what has been termed *pharmacogenomics*. In addition, these developments will extend our understanding of the inherited differences that lead to susceptibility for the common diseases that are the consequence of interaction with environmental or occupational exposures, or what is termed *ecogenetics*.

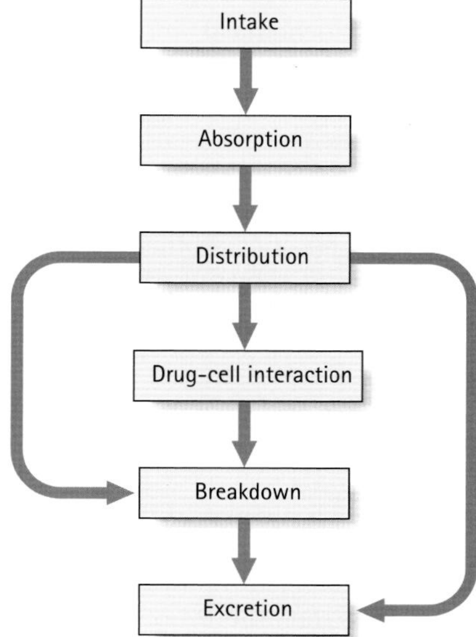


**Fig. 12.1**
Stages of metabolism of a drug.

## DRUG METABOLISM

The metabolism of a drug usually follows a common sequence of events (Fig. 12.1). A drug is first absorbed from the gut, passes into the bloodstream, and so becomes distributed and partitioned in the various tissues and tissue fluids. Only a small proportion of the total dose of a drug will be responsible for producing a specific pharmacological effect, most of it being broken down or excreted unchanged.

## BIOCHEMICAL MODIFICATION

The actual breakdown process, which usually takes place in the liver, varies with different drugs. Some are completely oxidized to carbon dioxide, which is exhaled through the lungs. Others are excreted in modified forms either via the kidneys into the urine, or by the liver into the bile and thence the feces. Many drugs undergo biochemical modifications that increase their solubility, resulting in their being more readily excreted.

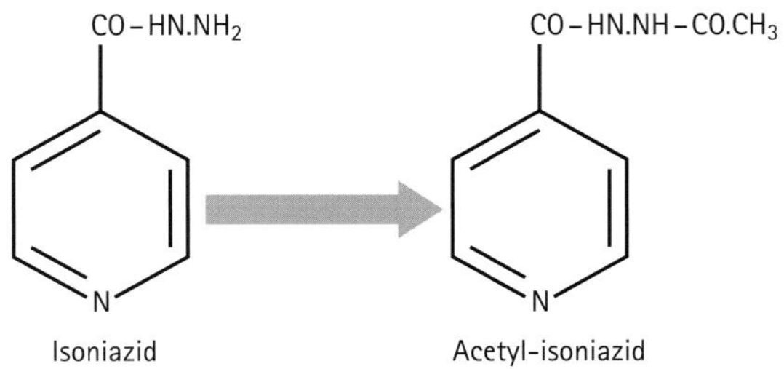


**Fig. 12.2**
Acetylation of the antituberculosis drug isoniazid.

One important biochemical modification of many drugs is conjugation, which involves union with the carbohydrate glucuronic acid. Glucuronide conjugation occurs primarily in the liver. The elimination of morphine and its derivatives, such as codeine, is almost entirely dependent on this process. Isoniazid, used in the treatment of tuberculosis, and a number of other drugs, including the sulfonamides, are modified by the introduction of an acetyl group into the molecule, a process known as acetylation (Fig. 12.2).

## KINETICS OF DRUG METABOLISM

The study of the metabolism and effects of a particular drug usually involves giving a standard dose of the drug and then after a suitable time interval determining the response, measuring the amount of the drug circulating in the blood or determining the rate at which it is metabolized. Such studies show that there is considerable variation in the way different individuals respond to certain drugs. This variability in response can be continuous or discontinuous.

If a dose–response test is carried out on a large number of subjects, their results can be plotted. A number of different possible responses can be seen (Fig. 12.3). In continuous variation the results form a bell-shaped or unimodal distribution. With discontinuous variation the curve is bimodal or sometimes even trimodal. A discontinuous response suggests that the metabolism of the drug is under monogenic control. For example, if the normal metabolism of a drug is controlled by a dominant gene, R, and if some people are unable to metabolize the drug because they are homozygous for a recessive gene, r, there will be three classes of individual: RR, Rr and rr. If the responses of RR and Rr are indistinguishable, then a bimodal distribution will result. If RR and Rr are distinguishable, then a trimodal distribution will result, each peak or mode representing a different genotype. A unimodal distribution implies that the metabolism of the drug in question is under the control of many genes, i.e. is polygenic (p. 139).

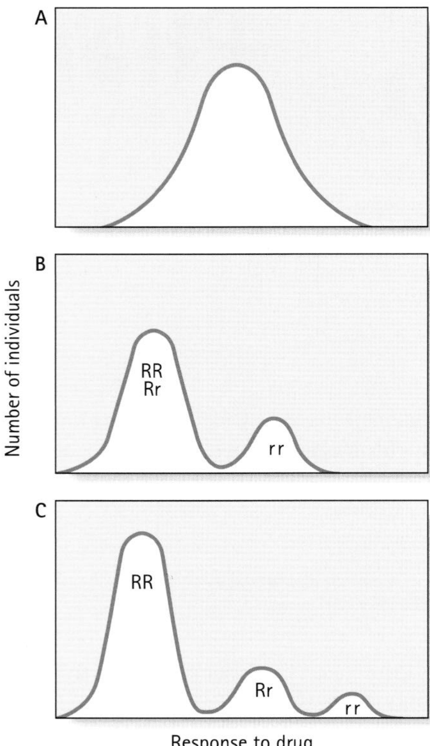


**Fig. 12.3**
Various types of response to different drugs consistent with polygenic and monogenic control of drug metabolism. (A) Continuous variation, multifactorial control of drug metabolism, (B) discontinuous bimodal variation, (C) discontinuous trimodal variation.

## GENETIC VARIATIONS REVEALED SOLELY BY THE EFFECTS OF DRUGS

Among the best-known examples of drugs that have been responsible for revealing genetic variation in response are isoniazid, succinylcholine, primaquine, coumarin anticoagulants, certain anesthetic agents, the thiopurines, phenylbutazone, debrisoquine and alcohol.

### *N*-ACETYLTRANSFERASE ACTIVITY

Isoniazid is one of the drugs used in the treatment of tuberculosis. It has been shown that it is rapidly absorbed from the gut, resulting in an initial high blood level that is slowly reduced as the drug is inactivated and excreted. The metabolism of isoniazid allows two groups to be distinguished: rapid and slow inactivators. In the former, blood levels of the drug fall rapidly after an oral dose; in the latter, blood levels remain high for some time. Family studies have shown that slow inactivators of isoniazid are homozygous for an autosomal recessive allele of the liver enzyme *N*-acetyltransferase, with lower activity levels.

*N*-acetyltransferase activity varies in different populations. In the USA and Western Europe about 50% of the population are slow inactivators, in contrast to the Japanese, who are predominately rapid inactivators.

In some individuals, isoniazid can cause side-effects such as polyneuritis, a systemic lupus erythematosus-like disorder, or liver damage. Blood levels of isoniazid remain higher for longer periods in slow inactivators than in rapid inactivators on equivalent doses. Slow inactivators have a significantly greater risk of developing side-effects on doses that rapid inactivators require to ensure adequate blood levels for successful treatment of tuberculosis. Conversely, rapid inactivators have an increased risk of liver damage due to isoniazid. A number of other drugs are also metabolized by *N*-acetyltransferase, and therefore slow inactivators of isoniazid are also more likely to exhibit side-effects. These drugs include hydralazine, which is an antihypertensive, and sulfasalazine, which is a sulfonamide derivative used to treat Crohn disease.

### DNA studies

Studies in other animal species led to the cloning of the genes responsible for *N*-acetyltransferase activity in humans. This has revealed that there are three genes, one of which is not expressed and represents a pseudogene (*NATP*), one that does not exhibit differences in activity between individuals (*NAT1*), and a third (*NAT2*), mutations in which are responsible for the inherited polymorphic variation. These inherited variations in *NAT2* have been reported to modify the risk of developing a number of cancers that include bladder, colorectal, breast and lung cancer. This is thought to be through differences in acetylation of aromatic and heterocyclic amine carcinogens.

## SUCCINYLCHOLINE SENSITIVITY

Curare is a plant extract used in hunting by certain South American Indian tribes, which produces profound muscular paralysis. Medically, curare is used in surgical operations because of the muscular relaxation it produces. Succinylcholine, also known as suxamethonium, is another drug that produces muscular relaxation, though by a different mechanism from curare. Suxamethonium has the advantage over curare that the relaxation of skeletal and respiratory muscles and the consequent apnea (cessation of breathing) it induces is only short lived. Therefore, it is most often used in the induction phase of an anesthetic for intubation. The anesthetist, therefore, needs to maintain respiration by artificial means for only 2–3 min before it returns spontaneously. However, about one patient in every 2000 has a period of apnea that can last 1 h or more after the use of suxamethonium. It was found that the apnea in such instances can be corrected by transfusion of blood or plasma from a normal person. The anesthetist, if a suxamethonium-induced apnea occurs, has to maintain respiration until the effects of the drug have worn off.

Succinylcholine is normally destroyed in the body by the plasma enzyme pseudocholinesterase. In patients who are highly sensitive to succinylcholine, the plasma pseudocholinesterase in their blood destroys the drug at a markedly slower rate than normal, or in some very rare cases is entirely deficient. Family studies have shown that succinylcholine sensitivity is inherited as an autosomal recessive trait.

A refined method of studying plasma pseudocholinesterase activity in the blood involves determining the percentage inhibition of the enzyme by the local anesthetic dibucaine (syn: cinchocaine). The result is termed the dibucaine number. The frequency distribution of dibucaine number values in families with succinylcholine-sensitive individuals gives a trimodal curve. The three modes represent the normal homozygotes, the heterozygotes and the affected homozygotes.

Suxamethonium sensitivity is now known to be determined by the inheritance of mutations of the *CHE1* gene, and genetic testing may be offered to the relatives of a patient in whom a genetic predisposition has been identified.

## GLUCOSE-6-PHOSPHATE DEHYDROGENASE VARIANTS

For many years, quinine was the drug of choice in the treatment of malaria. Although it has been very effective in acute attacks, it is not very effective in preventing relapses. In 1926 primaquine was introduced and proved to be much better than quinine in preventing relapses. However, it was not long after primaquine was introduced that some people were found to be sensitive to the drug. The drug could be taken for a few days with no apparent ill effects, and then suddenly some individuals would begin to pass very dark, often black, urine. Jaundice developed and the red cell count and hemoglobin concentration gradually fell as a consequence of hemolysis of the red blood cells. Affected individuals usually recovered from such a hemolytic episode, but occasionally the destruction of the red cells was extensive enough to be fatal. The cause of such cases of primaquine sensitivity was subsequently shown to be a deficiency in the red cell enzyme glucose-6-phosphate dehydrogenase (G6PD).

Family studies have shown that G6PD deficiency is inherited as an X-linked recessive trait (p. 110). G6PD deficiency is rare in most Caucasians but affects about 10% of Afro-Caribbean males and is also relatively common in males of Mediterranean origin. G6PD deficiency is thought to be relatively common in these populations as a result of conferring increased resistance to the malarial parasite. The red cell G6PD levels in persons of Mediterranean extraction with G6PD deficiency are very much lower than in persons of Afro-Caribbean origin with G6PD deficiency.

Persons with G6PD deficiency are sensitive not only to primaquine but also to many other compounds, including phenacetin, nitrofurantoin and certain sulfonamides. These drugs should be used with caution in males of Afro-Caribbean and Mediterranean origin if their G6PD status is unknown, and in a person known to be G6PD-deficient such drugs are absolutely contraindicated. Drug-induced hemolysis is uncommon and, in fact, the main risk of G6PD deficiency is favism, in which a hemolytic crisis occurs after eating fava beans. This is thought to be the first recognized pharmacogenetic disorder, having been described by Pythagoras around 500 BC!

## COUMARIN METABOLISM

Coumarin anticoagulant drugs, such as warfarin, are used in the treatment of a number of different disorders to prevent the blood from clotting, e.g. after a deep venous thrombosis. Warfarin is metabolized by the cytochrome P450 enzyme encoded by the *CYP2C9* gene, and two variants (CYP2C9*2 and CYP2C9*3) result in decreased metabolism. Consequently these patients require a lower warfarin dose to maintain their target INR range and may be at increased risk of bleeding.

## MALIGNANT HYPERTHERMIA

Malignant hyperthermia (MH) is a rare complication of anesthesia. Susceptible individuals develop muscle rigidity as well as an increased temperature (hyperthermia), often as high as 42.3°C (108°F) during anesthesia. This usually occurs when halothane is used as the anesthetic agent, particularly when succinylcholine is used as the muscle relaxant for intubation. If it is not recognized rapidly and treated with vigorous cooling, the affected individual will die.

MH susceptibility is inherited as an autosomal dominant trait affecting approximately 1 in 10 000 persons. Susceptible individuals occasionally have a raised serum creatine kinase level but this cannnot be used as a reliable screening test for at-risk family members. The most reliable prediction of an individual's susceptibility status requires a muscle biopsy with in-vitro muscle contracture testing in response to exposure to halothane and caffeine.

A person known to be or suspected of being susceptible to MH can undergo a general anesthetic provided that recognized precipitating anesthetic agents are avoided. Should hyperthermia develop during surgery, it is treated by cooling and intravenous procaine or procainamide, but most effectively with dantrolene.

Malignant hyperthermia is genetically heterogeneous but the most common cause is a mutation in the ryanodine receptor (*RYR1*) gene. Seven other candidate genes have been identified and variants in these genes may influence susceptibility within individual families. This observation may explain the discordant results of the in vitro contracture test and genotype in members of some families that segregate *RYR1* mutations.

## THIOPURINE METHYLTRANSFERASE

A group of potentially toxic substances known as the thiopurines, which include 6-mercaptopurine, 6-thioguanine and azathioprine, are used extensively in the treatment of leukemia, to suppress the immune response in patients with autoimmune disorders such as systemic lupus erythematosus and to prevent rejection of organ transplants. They are very effective drugs clinically but have serious side-effects, such as leukopenia and severe liver damage. Azathiopurine is reported to cause toxicity in 10–15% of patients and it may be possible to predict those patients susceptible to side-effects by analyzing genetic variation within the thiopurine methyltransferase (*TPMT*) gene. This gene encodes an enzyme responsible for methylation of thiopurines and approximately two-thirds of patients who experience toxicity have one or more variant alleles.

## PHENYLBUTAZONE METABOLISM

Phenylbutazone is used in the treatment of the more severe forms of arthritis. The metabolism of this drug differs from the examples discussed so far in that it appears to be under polygenic control. Individuals who are relatively slow in metabolizing phenylbutazone are more likely to develop drug-associated side-effects such as hypoplastic anemia.

## DEBRISOQUINE METABOLISM

Debrisoquine is a drug that was frequently used in the past for the treatment of hypertension. There is a bimodal distribution in the response to the drug in the general population. Approximately 5–10% of persons of European origin are poor metabolizers, being homozygotes for an autosomal recessive gene with reduced hydroxylation activity. Such individuals are more prone to overreact to the drug and develop hypotension with treatment. They are also more susceptible to adverse reactions to several other drugs, such as the β-blockers propranolol and metoprolol, the antidepressants amitryptiline and imipramine, and the antipsychotics thioridazine and haloperidol.

### DNA studies

Molecular studies have revealed that the gene involved in debrisoquine metabolism is one of the P450 family of genes on chromosome 22, known as *CYP2D6*. The mutations responsible for the poor metabolizer phenotype are heterogeneous; 18 different variants have been described to date. It is postulated that these enzymes could have evolved in the past to metabolize dietary toxic plant alkaloids.

## DIHYDROPYRIMIDINE DEHYDROGENASE

Dihydropyrimidine dehydrogenase (DPYD) is the initial and rate-limiting enzyme in the catabolism of the chemotherapeutic drug 5-fluorouracil (5FU). Deficiency of DPYD is recognized as an important pharmacogenetic factor in the etiology of severe 5FU-associated toxicity. Measurement of DPYD activity in peripheral blood mononuclear cells or genetic testing for the most common *DPYD* gene mutation (a splice site mutation, IVS14+1G>A, which results in the deletion of exon 14) may be warranted in cancer patients prior to the administration of 5-fluorouracil.

## ALCOHOL METABOLISM

Under the heading of pharmacogenetics we can also include alcoholism and alcoholic cirrhosis, which in terms of their frequency and social implications dwarf all others, although some persons would debate whether alcohol should really be considered a drug. Alcoholism is clearly related to the amount consumed as well as to dietary and various social and economic factors. Nevertheless, evidence is gradually emerging which clearly indicates that genetic factors can also be involved. Some of this evidence is based on twin studies, which have shown high concordance rates (p. 228), and family studies, which have shown a high prevalence of alcohol-related problems among relatives of alcoholics. Clearly, however, behavior patterns within families could artificially inflate what would appear to be genetic factors. Similarly, apparent racial or ethnic differences in the incidence of alcoholism, such as the high incidence among certain American Indians and Eskimos, could well be affected by social factors.

Perhaps the most convincing evidence for the possible role of genetic factors in alcoholism comes from the study of the enzymes involved in alcohol metabolism. Alcohol is metabolized in the liver by alcohol dehydrogenase (ADH) to acetaldehyde, and then further degraded by acetaldehyde dehydrogenase (ALDH). Human ADH consists of dimers of various combinations of subunits of three different polypeptide units coded for by three loci, *ADH1* coding for the α subunit, *ADH2* for the β subunit and *ADH3* for the γ subunit. *ADH1* is primarily expressed in early fetal life, while *ADH2* is expressed in adult life.

Persons of Far East Asian origin tolerate alcohol less well than persons of Caucasian origin and often exhibit an acute flushing reaction to it. This sensitivity is due to differences in the rate of metabolism of acetaldehyde. There are two major acetaldehyde dehydrogenase variants or isozymes, ALDH1 which is present in the cytosol and ALDH2 which is present in the mitochondria. The acute flushing reaction to alcohol in Far East Asians has been shown, in fact, to be due to absent ALDH2 activity. It has been suggested that this unpleasant reaction could account for the reported lower incidence of alcoholism and alcohol-related liver disease in that population.

## HEREDITARY DISORDERS WITH ALTERED DRUG RESPONSE

Not all investigators include hereditary disorders with altered drug response within the sphere of pharmacogenetics. However, this is of immense importance in medical practice.

### PORPHYRIA VARIEGATA

Porphyria variegata, one of the types of porphyria (p. 175), is inherited as an autosomal dominant trait. Some affected individuals develop skin lesions particularly on sun-exposed surfaces. Others have attacks of severe abdominal pain, muscular paralysis or mental disturbance. During an acute attack the patient can die. Clinical expression of the disease occurs in response to an increase in the concentration of heme in the liver. This occurs upon administration of drugs which induce the heme-containing cytochrome P450 proteins, such as barbiturates, steroid hormones and numerous others.

### HEMOGLOBINOPATHIES

Sulfonamides can cause severe hemolysis in individuals with certain hemoglobinopathies. Examples include hemoglobin H, a hemoglobin which consists entirely of β-globin chains, and hemoglobin Zurich, which was first described in members of a Swiss family in 1962. These hemoglobinopathies are, however, very rare.

### GOUT AND CHLOROTHIAZIDE

The treatment of congestive heart failure often involves the use of diuretics. These drugs increase the excretion of water and consequently reduce the amount of edema. One of the most widely used diuretics is chlorothiazide. Not long after it was first used, it was realized that chlorothiazide diuretics could cause problems in persons who suffer from gout. In genetically predisposed individuals attacks often follow dietary excesses which lead to an elevation in serum uric acid. Chlorothiazide has a similar effect by raising the serum level of uric acid in genetically predisposed individuals.

## CRIGLER–NAJJAR SYNDROME

The Crigler–Najjar syndrome is characterized by a severe non-hemolytic jaundice, appearing on the first or second day after birth, and can result in deposition of unconjugated bilirubin in the central nervous system, leading to neurological sequelae. Affected children often die in infancy. The condition is inherited as an autosomal recessive trait, heterozygotes being perfectly healthy. Patients with type I Crigler–Najjar syndrome have a complete deficiency of the UDP-glucuronosyltransferase gene (*UGT1A1*), whereas those with the less severe type II form show partial deficiency. This results in an inability of the liver to conjugate bilirubin with glucuronides, and affected individuals are unable to conjugate certain drugs such as salicylates.

## MATURITY-ONSET DIABETES OF THE YOUNG

Maturity-onset diabetes of the young (MODY) is a monogenic form of diabetes characterized by young age of onset (often before 25 years), dominant inheritance and β-cell dysfunction (p. 230). Patients with mutations in the *HNF-1α* gene (MODY3) are sensitive to sulfonylureas and may experience episodes of hypoglycemia on standard doses. However, this sensitivity is advantageous at lower doses, and sulfonylureas are the recommended oral treatment in this genetic subgroup.

## EVOLUTIONARY ORIGIN OF VARIATION IN DRUG RESPONSE

What is the evolutionary significance of genetic variations in response to certain drugs in particular ethnic groups (Table 12.1)? Man has been exposed to these drugs for no more than a few decades, yet there is no doubt that mutations in genes conferring abnormal responses to these drugs arose, in many instances, many thousands of years ago. There is evidence in the case of G6PD deficiency that it can confer some protection against malaria. With most hereditary variation in response to drugs we have very little idea of how or why it arose. A mutation could have conferred selective advantage under certain past dietary or environmental conditions, or have conferred resistance to particular infections.

**Table 12.1 Ethnic variations in some pharmacogenetic disorders**

| Disorder | Ethnic group | Frequency (%) |
|---|---|---|
| Slow acetylation | Europeans<br>Orientals | 50<br>10 |
| Pseudocholinesterase variants | Europeans<br>Eskimos | <1<br>1–2 |
| G6PD deficiency | N. Europeans<br>S. Europeans<br>Afro-Caribbeans | <1<br>up to 25<br>10 |
| Atypical ADH | Europeans<br>Orientals | 5<br>85 |

## PHARMACOGENOMICS

*Pharmacogenomics* is defined as the study of the interaction of an individual's genetic makeup and response to a drug. The key distinction between pharmacogenetics and pharmacogenomics is that the former describes the study of variability in drug responses attributed to individual genes and the latter describes the study of the entire genome related to drug response. The expectation is that inherited variation at the DNA level results in functional variation in the gene products which will play an essential role in determining the variability in responses, both therapeutic and adverse, to a drug. If polymorphic DNA sequence variation occurs in the coding portion or regulatory regions of genes, it is likely to result in variation in the gene product through alteration of function, activity or level of expression. Automated analysis of genome-wide SNPs (p. 70) allows the possibility of identifying genes involved in drug metabolism, transport and receptors, which are likely to play a role in determining the variability in efficacy, side-effects and toxicity of a drug.

The availability of whole-genome SNP maps will enable an SNP profile to be created for patients who experience adverse events or who respond clinically to the drug (efficacy). An individual's whole-genome SNP type has been described as an 'SNP print'. However, this raises issues pertaining to the disclosure of information of uncertain significance that is later shown to be associated with an adverse outcome unrelated to the reason for the original test. An example is ApoE genotyping, where ApoE ε4 was first reported to be associated with variation in cholesterol levels but later with age of onset of Alzheimer disease.

## ADVERSE EVENTS

The objective of adverse-event pharmacogenetics is to identify a genetic profile that characterizes patients who are more likely to suffer the adverse event. An example is abacavir, a reverse transcriptase inhibitor used to treat HIV. Approximately 5% of patients show potentially fatal hypersensitivity to abacavir and this limits its use. A strong association with an HLA haplotype defined as B*5701, DR7 and DQ3 has been reported, but the actual gene responsible for this effect has not yet been identified.

The anti-epileptic drug felbamate is a second example of a drug whose use has been limited because of adverse reactions that probably resulted from inter-individual variation in metabolism of the drug. Felbamate is rapidly metabolized in the liver to highly toxic metabolites that are usually rapidly detoxified by conjugation with glutathione. Both overproduction of the toxic metabolites and inadequate conjugation might cause adverse reactions in genetically susceptible individuals.

### EFFICACY

There is no doubt that the cost-effectiveness of drugs is improved if they are only prescribed to those patients likely to respond to them. The drug herceptin is an antibody which targets overexpression of HER2/neu protein observed in approximately one third of patients with breast cancer. Consequently patients are only prescribed herceptin if their tumor has been shown to overexpress HER2/neu.

## ECOGENETICS

An extension of pharmacogenetics is the study of genetically determined differences in susceptibility to the action of physical, chemical and infectious agents in the environment. This has been referred to as *ecogenetics*, a term first coined by Brewer in 1971. Such differences in susceptibility can be either unifactorial or multifactorial in causation (Table 12.2).

**Table 12.2 Ecogenetics: genetic variation in susceptibility to environmental agents**

| Environmental agent | Genetic susceptibility | Disease |
|---|---|---|
| **UV light** | Fair complexion | Skin cancer |
| **Drugs (see text)** | | |
| **Foods** | | |
| Fats | Hypercholesterolemia | Atherosclerosis |
| Fava beans | G6PD deficiency | Favism |
| Gluten | Gluten sensitivity | Celiac disease |
| Salt | Na–K pump defective | Hypertension |
| Milk | Lactase deficiency | Lactose intolerance |
| Alcohol | Atypical ADH | Alcoholism |
| Oxalates | Hyperoxaluria | Renal stones |
| Fortified flour | Hemochromatosis | Iron overload |
| **Inhalants** | | |
| Dust | $\alpha_1$-antitrypsin deficiency | Emphysema |
| Allergens | Atopy | Asthma |
| **Infections** | Defective immunity | Diabetes mellitus? Spondylitis? |

### ORGANOPHOSPHATE METABOLISM

Paraoxonase is an enzyme that catalyzes the breakdown of organophosphates that are widely used as insecticides in agriculture. Individuals can have different enzyme activity levels that result from a two-allele polymorphic system. Those who are homozygous for the low-activity allele are likely to be particularly sensitive to accidental or occupational exposure to organophosphates. Reports of individuals experiencing either acute or chronic neurological or psychiatric symptoms through exposure to organophosphates could be the result of these inherited differences in paraoxonase activity.

### DISEASE SUSCEPTIBILITY

An extension of ecogenetics which will be particularly important is the identification of individuals at high risk of developing diseases after environmental exposures, e.g. particular cancers after exposure to mutagens or carcinogens (p. 28).

There are reports of an increased risk of bladder cancer in persons who are slow acetylators and who have had occupational exposure to aromatic amines that are used as industrial dyes. There is also the possibility of an increased risk of bladder cancer for slow acetylators in the general population in which no specific hazardous exposure has been recognized. Conversely, there are recent reports suggesting the possibility of an increased risk of colorectal cancer in rapid acetylators.

Recent studies have suggested that poor debrisoquine metabolizer status is less common than would be expected in persons with cancer of the lung. This is in contrast to another polymorphism for the enzyme glutathione S-transferase (GSTM1), which shows an increase in the incidence of the null phenotype, i.e. no activity, in persons with adenocarcinoma of the lung when compared to the general population. This enzyme is involved in the conjugation of glutathione with electrophilic compounds, including carcinogens such as benzopyrene, and could have a protective role against the development of cancer.

This susceptibility to disease is not just limited to cancer. Many of the common diseases in humans could be due to genetically determined differences in response to environmental agents or susceptibilities (p. 227). There are reports of a possible increased risk of developing Parkinson disease because of differences in the detoxification of potential neurotoxins in association with a poor metabolizer phenotype in the hepatic cytochrome P450 *CYP2D6* gene.

The ability to screen large numbers of persons for SNPs (p. 70) should allow identification of genes involved in determining the inherited contribution for many of the common diseases. As well as identifying individuals at high risk of developing a common disease, this will allow a better understanding of the disease pathways involved, which holds the promise of directly linking possible therapeutic interventions for those individuals. The major international/multinational pharmaceutical and biotechnology companies, not surprisingly, are investing heavily in these developments. While there is the prospect of reducing the likelihood of individuals developing many of the common diseases, this raises many social and ethical problems when the knowledge of genetic variation and susceptibility is translated into public policy with vested commercial interests (p. 377).

Genetic profiling is a step towards personalized medicine. This information can be used to select the appropriate treatment at the correct dose and to avoid adverse drug reactions.

## FURTHER READING

Beutler E 1991 Glucose-6-phosphate dehydrogenase deficiency. N Engl J Med 324: 169–174
*Review of an important ethnic pharmacogenetic polymorphism.*

Goldstein D B, Tate S K and Sisodiya S M 2003 Pharmacogenetics goes genomic. Nature Genet Rev 4: 937–947
*Recent review of pharmacogenetics/genomics.*

Nebert D W 1999 Pharmacogenetics and pharmacogenomics: why is this relevant to the clinical geneticist? Clin Genet 56: 247–258
*A good summary of the two areas.*

Neumann D A, Kimmel C A 1998 Human variability in response in chemical exposures: measures, modelling, and risk assessment. CRC Press, London
*A detailed discussion of the inherited human variability to exposure to the toxic effects of environmental chemicals.*

Roses AD 2001 Pharmacogenetics. Hum Mol Genet 10: 2261–2267
*A recent review of pharmacogenetics and pharmacogenomics.*

Vogel F, Buselmaier W, Reichert W, Kellerman G, Berg P (eds) 1978 Human genetic variation in response to medical and environmental agents: pharmacogenetics and ecogenetics. Springer-Verlag, Berlin
*One of the early definitive outlines of the field of pharmacogenetics.*

Wendell W 1997 Pharmacogenetics (Oxford Monographs on Medical Genetics, 32). Oxford University Press, Oxford
*A detailed comprehensive text on pharmacogenetics.*

## ELEMENTS

1. Pharmacogenetics is defined as the study of genetically determined variations revealed solely by the effects of drugs. Hereditary disorders in which symptoms can occur spontaneously or can be exacerbated or precipitated by drugs are often also included.

2. The metabolism of many drugs involves biochemical modification, often by conjugation with another molecule, which usually takes place in the liver. This biochemical transformation facilitates the excretion of the drug.

3. The ways in which many drugs are metabolized vary from person to person and can be genetically determined. In some instances, the biochemical basis is understood. For example, persons differ in the rate at which they inactivate the antituberculosis drug isoniazid by acetylation in the liver, being either rapid or slow inactivators. Slow inactivators have an increased risk of toxic side-effects associated with isoniazid therapy. Other examples include sensitivity to the muscle relaxant succinylcholine because of abnormal or reduced plasma pseudocholinesterase activity, and the development of a severe hemolytic anemia when given the antimalarial drug primaquine (or a number of other drugs) due to deficiency of the enzyme glucose-6-phosphate dehydrogenase in red blood cells.

4. In some instances, genetic variation can be revealed exclusively by exposure to drugs. One such example is malignant hyperthermia. This rare disorder is associated with the use of certain anesthetic agents and muscle relaxants in general anesthesia.

5. A number of hereditary disorders, such as porphyria variegata and some of the hemoglobinopathies, are associated with altered response to certain drugs. With disorders such as diabetes and gout, where the etiology is complex, biochemical evidence of variation in response to drugs suggests a genetic contribution.

6. The information from the Human Genome Project allows the possibility of the development of new drugs, or what is called pharmacogenomics, as well as the prospect of identifying the genes that result in an increased susceptibility for developing the common diseases.

7. Ecogenetics is the term used for the study of genetically determined differences between persons in their susceptibility to the action of physical, chemical and infectious agents in the environment.

CHAPTER 13

# Immunogenetics

*"Medicinal discovery,*
*It moves in mighty leaps,*
*It leapt straight past the common cold*
*And gave it us for keeps."*

Pam Ayers

## IMMUNITY

Microorganisms, insects and other infectious agents are far more numerous than members of the human race and without effective defense mechanisms against their activity humankind would rapidly succumb. The immune system in all its forms is mankind's defense mechanism, and in order to understand the inherited disorders of immunity, we must first understand the fundamentals of the genetic basis of immunity.

Immune defence mechanisms can be divided into two main types: *innate immunity*, which includes a number of non-specific systems which do not require or involve prior contact with the infectious agent, and *specific acquired* or *adaptive immunity*, which involves a tailor-made immune response that occurs after exposure to an infectious agent. Both types can involve either *humoral immunity*, which combats extracellular infections, or *cell-mediated immunity*, which fights intracellular infections.

## INNATE IMMUNITY

The first simple type of defense against infection is a mechanical barrier. The skin functions most of the time as an impermeable barrier but, in addition, the acidic pH of sweat is inhibitory to bacterial growth. The membranes lining the respiratory and gastrointestinal tracts are protected by mucus. In the case of the respiratory tract further protection is provided by ciliary movement, while other bodily fluids contain a variety of bactericidal agents, e.g. lysozymes in tears. If an organism succeeds in invading the body, phagocytosis and bactericidal agents come into effect.

## HUMORAL INNATE IMMUNITY

A number of soluble factors are involved in innate immunity by helping to minimize tissue injury by limiting the spread of infectious microorganisms. These are often called the *acute phase proteins* and include C-reactive protein, mannose binding protein and serum amyloid P component. The first two act by facilitating the attachment of one of the components of complement, C3b, to the surface of the microorganism, which becomes opsonized (made ready) for adherence to phagocytes, while the latter binds lysosomal enzymes to connective tissues. In addition, cells when infected by a virus synthesize and secrete *interferon*, which interferes with viral replication through reducing mRNA stability and interfering with translation.

### Complement

*Complement* is a complex series of 20 or so interacting plasma proteins that can be activated by the cell membranes of invading microorganisms, in what is termed the *alternative pathway*. The various components of complement interact in a specific cascade sequence, resulting in a localized acute inflammatory response through the action of mediators released from mast cells and tissue macrophages. These result in increased vascular permeability and the attraction of phagocytes in the process known as *chemotaxis*. In addition, the later components of the complement cascade generate a membrane attack complex that induces defects in the cell membrane, resulting in the lysis of microorganisms (Fig. 13.1).

Complement can also be activated through the *classic pathway*, by the binding of antibody with antigen (see below, p. 190).

## CELL-MEDIATED INNATE IMMUNITY

### Phagocytosis

Microorganisms are engulfed and digested by two major types of cell, either polymorphonuclear neutrophils or macrophages. Polymorphonuclear neutrophils are found mainly in the bloodstream, while macrophages occur primarily in tissues around the basement membrane of

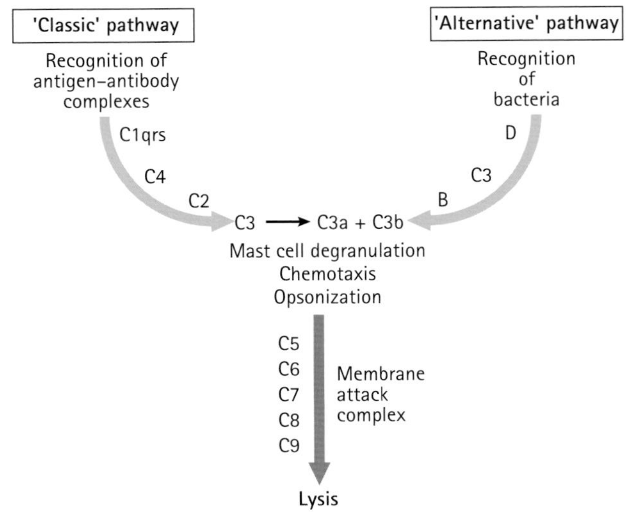


Fig. 13.1
Classic and alternative pathways of complement activation. (Adapted from Paul W E (ed) 1993 Fundamental immunology. Raven Press, New York.)

blood vessels in connective tissue, lung, liver and in the lining of the sinusoids of the spleen and the medullary sinuses of the lymph nodes. Surface antigens on microorganisms result in their being engulfed and fusing with the granules of the phagocyte, subjecting them to the action of the bactericidal agents of the intracellular granules which contain hydrogen peroxide, hydroxyl radicals and nitrous oxide, which leads to their destruction.

### Extracellular killing

Virally infected cells can be killed by large granular lymphocytes, known as *natural killer cells*. These have carbohydrate binding receptors on their cell surface which recognize high molecular weight glycoproteins expressed on the surface of the infected cell as a result of the virus taking over the cellular replicative functions. Attachment of the natural killer cells to the infected cells results in the release of a number of agents, which in turn results in damage to the membrane of the infected cell, leading to cell death.

## SPECIFIC ACQUIRED IMMUNITY

Many infective microorganisms have, through mutation and selective pressures, developed strategies to overcome or evade the mechanisms associated with innate immunity. There is the need, therefore, to be able to generate specific acquired or adaptive immunity. This can, like innate immunity, be separated into both humoral and cell-mediated processes.

## HUMORAL SPECIFIC ACQUIRED IMMUNITY

The main mediators of humoral specific acquired immunity are immunoglobulins or antibodies. Antibodies are able to recognize and bind to antigens of infecting microorganisms, leading to the activation of phagocytes and the initiation of the *classic pathway* of complement, resulting in the generation of the membrane attack complex (Fig.13.1). Exposure to a specific antigen results in the clonal proliferation of a small lymphocyte derived from the bone marrow, hence 'B' lymphocytes, resulting in mature antibody-producing cells or *plasma cells*.

Lymphocytes capable of producing antibodies express on their surface copies of the immunoglobulin for which they code, which acts as a surface receptor for antigen. Binding of the antigen results, in conjunction with other membrane-associated proteins, in signal transduction leading to the clonal expansion and production of antibody. This results in the first instance in the *primary response* with production of IgM and subsequently IgG. Re-exposure to the same antigen results in enhanced antibody levels in a shorter period of time, known as the *secondary response*, reflecting what is known as antigen-specific *immunological memory*.

### Immunoglobulins

The immunoglobulins (Ig), or antibodies, are one of the major classes of serum protein. Their function, both in the recognition of antigenic variability and in effector activities, was initially revealed by protein, and more recently by DNA, studies of their structure.

#### *Immunoglobulin structure*

Papaine, a proteolytic enzyme, splits the immunoglobulin molecule into three fragments. Two of the fragments are similar, each containing an antibody site capable of combining with a specific antigen and therefore referred to as the *antigen-binding fragment* or *Fab*. The third fragment can be crystallized and was therefore called Fc. The Fc fragment determines the secondary biological functions of antibody molecules, binding complement and Fc receptors on a number of different cell types involved in the immune response.

The immunoglobulin molecule is made up of four polypeptide chains: two 'light' (L) and two 'heavy' (H) chains of approximately 220 and 440 amino acids in length. They are held together in a Y-shape by disulfide bonds and non-covalent interactions. Each Fab fragment is composed of L chains linked to the amino-terminal portion of the H chains, whereas each Fc fragment is composed only of the carboxy-terminal portion of the H chains (Fig. 13.2).

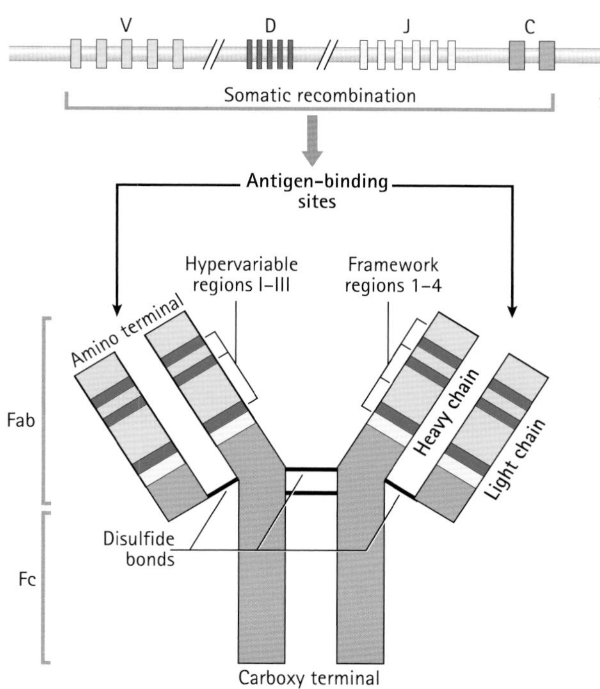


Fig. 13.2
Model of antibody molecule structure.

### Immunoglobulin isotypes, subclasses and idiotypes

There are five different types of heavy chain, designated respectively as γ, μ, α, δ and ε, one each respectively for the five major antibody classes, or what are known as *isotypes*, IgG, IgM, IgA, IgD and IgE. Further analysis has revealed that the L chains are one of two types, either kappa (κ) or lambda (λ), the two types of L chain occurring in all five classes of antibody, but with only one type of light chain occurring in each individual antibody. Thus the molecular formula for IgG will be $\lambda_2\gamma_2$ or $\kappa_2\gamma_2$. The characteristics of the various classes of antibody are outlined in brief in Table 13.1. In addition, there are four IgG subclasses, IgG1, IgG2, IgG3 and IgG4, and two IgA subclasses, IgA1 and IgA2, which differ in their amino acid sequence and interchain disulfide bonds. Individual antibody molecules which recognize specific antigens are known as idiotypes.

### Immunoglobulin allotypes

The five classes of immunoglobulin occur in all normal individuals, but allelic variants or what are known as antibody *allotypes* of these classes have also been identified. These are the *Gm* system associated with the heavy chain of IgG, the *Am* system associated with the IgA heavy chain, the *Km* and *Inv* systems associated with the κ light chain, the *Oz* system for the λ light chain and the *Em* allotype for the IgE heavy chain. The Gm and Km systems are independent of each other and are polymorphic (p. 130), the frequencies of the different alleles varying in different ethnic groups.

### The generation of antibody diversity

It could seem paradoxical for a single protein molecule to exhibit sufficient structural heterogeneity to have specificity for a large number of different antigens. Different combinations of heavy and light chains could, to some extent, account for this diversity. It would, however, require thousands of structural genes for each chain type to provide sufficient variability for the large number of antibodies produced in response to the equally large number of antigens to which individuals can be exposed. Our initial understanding of how this could occur came from persons with a malignancy of antibody-producing cells, or what is known as *multiple myeloma*.

### Multiple myeloma

Persons with *multiple myeloma* make a single or monoclonal antibody species in large abundance, which is excreted in large quantities in their urine. This protein, known as *Bence Jones protein*, consists of antibody light chains. Comparisons of this protein from different myeloma patients revealed the amino-terminal ends of the molecule to be quite variable in their amino-acid sequence whereas the carboxy-terminal ends were relatively constant. These are called the *variable*, or *V*, and *constant*, or *C*, regions, respectively. Further detailed analysis of the amino acid sequence of the V regions of different myeloma proteins showed four regions that vary little from one

**Table 13.1 Classes of human immunoglobulin**

| Class | Mol. wt | Serum concentration (mg/ml) | Antibody activity | Complement fixation | Placental transfer |
|---|---|---|---|---|---|
| IgG | 150 000 | 8–16 | Binds to microorganisms and neutralizes bacterial toxins | + | + |
| IgM | 900 000 | 0.5–2 | Produced in early immune response, especially in bacteremia | + | – |
| IgA | 160 000 | 1.4–4 | Guards mucosal surfaces | + | – |
| IgD | 185 000 | 0–0.4 | On lymphocyte cell surface, involved in control of activation and suppression | – | – |
| IgE | 200 000 | trace | In parasitic and allergic reactions | – | – |

antibody to another, known as *framework regions* (FR 1–4), and three markedly variable regions interspersed between these, known as *hypervariable regions* (HV I–III) (Fig. 13.2).

### DNA studies of antibody diversity

As long ago as 1965, Dreyer and Bennett proposed that an antibody could be encoded by separate 'genes' in germ line cells which undergo rearrangement, or, as they termed it, 'scrambling', in lymphocyte development. Comparison of the restriction maps of the DNA segments coding for the C and V regions of the immunoglobulin λ light chains in embryonic and antibody-producing cells revealed that they were far apart in the former but close together in the latter. More detailed analysis revealed that the DNA segments coding for the V and C regions of the light chain are separated by some 1500 bp in antibody-producing cells. The intervening DNA segment was found to code for a *joining*, or *J*, region immediately adjacent to the V region of the light chain. The κ light chain was shown to have the same structure. Cloning and DNA sequencing of heavy chain genes in germ line cells have revealed that they have a fourth region, called *diversity*, or D, between the V and J regions.

There are estimated to be some 60 different DNA segments coding for the V region of the heavy chain, approximately 40 DNA segments coding for the V region of the κ light chain and 30 DNA segments coding for the λ light chain V region. Six functional DNA segments code for the J region of the heavy chain, five for the J region of the κ light chain and four for the J region of the λ light chain. A single DNA segment codes for the C region of the κ light chain, seven DNA segments code for the C region of the λ light chain and 11 functional DNA segments code for the C region of the different classes of heavy chain. There are also 27 functional DNA segments coding for the D region of the heavy chain (Fig. 13.3).

Estimation of the number of DNA segments coding for these various portions of the antibody molecule is confounded by the presence of a large number of unexpressed DNA sequences or pseudogenes (p. 17). While the coding DNA segments for the various regions of the antibody molecule can be referred to as genes, use of this term in regard to antibodies has deliberately been avoided because they could be considered to be an exception to the general rule of 'one gene–one enzyme (or protein)' (p. 161).

### Antibody gene rearrangement

The genes for the κ and λ light chains and the heavy chains in humans have been assigned to chromosomes 2, 22 and 14, respectively. Only one of each of the relevant types of DNA segments is expressed in any single antibody molecule. The DNA coding segments for the various portions of the antibody chains on these chromosomes

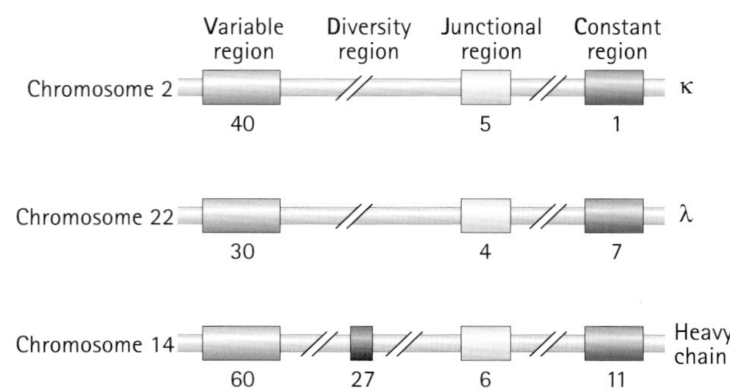


**Fig. 13.3**
Estimated number of the various DNA segments coding for the κ, λ and various heavy chains.

are separated by DNA that is non-coding. Somatic recombinational events involved in antibody production involve short conserved recombination signal sequences that flank each germline DNA segment (Fig. 13.4). Further diversity occurs by variable mRNA splicing at the V–J junction in RNA processing and by somatic mutation of the antibody genes. These mechanisms can easily account for the antibody diversity seen in nature. Although this probably involves some form of clonal selection, it is still not entirely clear how particular DNA segments are selected to produce an antibody to a specific antigen. 'Gene shuffling' of this form is also known to account for the marked variability seen in the surface antigens of the trypanosome parasite and the different mating types in yeast.

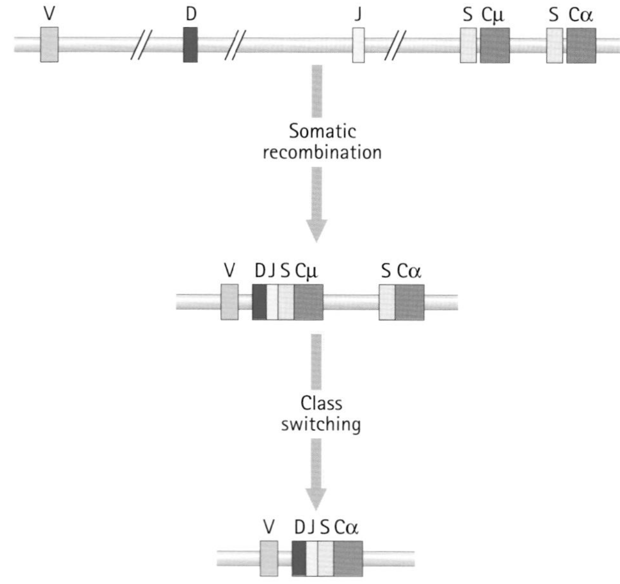


**Fig. 13.4**
Immunoglobulin heavy-chain gene rearrangement and class switching.

### Class switching of antibodies

There is a normal switch of antibody class produced by B cells on continued or further exposure to antigen, from IgM which is the initial class of antibody produced in response to exposure to an antigen, to IgA or IgG. This process, known as *class switching*, involves retention of the specificity of the antibody to the same antigen. Analysis of class switching in a population of cells derived from a single B cell has shown that both classes of antibody have the same antigen binding sites, having the same V region, differing only in their C region. Class switching occurs by a somatic recombination event that involves DNA segments designated S (for switching) that lead to looping out and deletion of the intervening DNA. The result is to eliminate the DNA segment coding for the C region of the heavy chain of the IgM molecule and to bring the gene segment encoding the C region of the new class of heavy chain adjacent to the segment encoding the V region (Fig.13.4).

### The immunoglobulin gene superfamily

Studies of the structure of other molecules involved in the immune response have shown a number to have structural and DNA sequence homology to the immunoglobulins. This involves a 110 amino-acid sequence characterized by a centrally placed disulfide bridge that stabilizes a series of antiparallel β strands into what is called an antibody fold. This group of molecules with similar structure has been called the *immunoglobulin superfamily* (p. 17). It consists of eight multigene families that, in addition to the κ and λ light chains and different classes of heavy chain, include the chains of the T-cell receptor (p. 18), the class I and II major histocompatibility complex (MHC), or human leukocyte (HLA) antigens (p. 194), and $\beta_2$-microglobulin (p. 193). The latter is a receptor for transporting certain classes of immunoglobulin across mucosal membranes. A series of other molecules show homology to the Ig superfamily. These include the T-cell CD4 and CD8 cell surface receptor molecules that cooperate with T-cell receptors in antigen recognition and the intercellular adhesion molecules, ICAM-1, 2 and 3, which are involved in the interaction of lymphocytes with antigen-presenting cells.

### Antibody engineering

The techniques of genetic engineering have led to the prospect of reshaping or designing human antibodies for specific therapeutic or diagnostic purposes. These are what are known as monoclonal antibodies. Recombinant antibodies can be constructed using the human variable region framework, the human constant regions of the heavy and light chains and the antigen binding site of a mouse antibody. Persons treated with these 'engineered' antibodies do not mount an immune response to them, a problem met with in the use of rodent hybridoma-derived monoclonal antibodies. It is hoped that the use of human-derived myeloma cells for expression of these recombinant antibodies could overcome this difficulty.

## CELL-MEDIATED SPECIFIC ACQUIRED IMMUNITY

Certain microorganisms, viruses and parasites, live inside host cells. As a result, a separate form of specific acquired immunity has evolved to combat intracellular infections involving lymphocytes differentiated in the thymus, hence *T cells*. T lymphocytes have specialized receptors on the cell surface, known as *T-cell surface antigen receptors*, which in conjunction with the *major histocompatibility complex* on the cell surface of the infected cell result in the involvement of *T helper cells* and *cytotoxic T cells* to combat intracellular infections by leading to the death of the infected cell.

### T-cell surface antigen receptor

T cells express on their surface an antigen receptor. This consists of two different polypeptide chains, linked by a disulfide bridge, which both contain two immunoglobulin-like domains, one that is relatively invariant in structure, the other highly variable like the Fab portion of an immunoglobulin. The diversity in T-cell receptors required for recognition of the range of antigenic variation that can occur is generated by a similar process as seen with immunoglobulins. Rearrangement of variable (V), diversity (D), junctional (J) and constant (C) DNA segments during T-cell maturation, through a similar recombination mechanism as occurs in B cells, results in a contiguous VDJ sequence. Binding of antigen to the T-cell receptor, in conjunction with an associated complex of transmembrane peptides, results in signaling the cell to differentiate and divide.

### The major histocompatibility complex

The major histocompatibility complex (MHC) plays a central role in the immune system. Association of an antigen with the MHC molecule on the surface of the cells is required for recognition of the antigen by the T-cell receptor that, in conjunction with the closely associated protein $\beta_2$-microglobulin, results in the recruitment of cytotoxic and helper T cells in the immune response. MHC molecules occur in three classes: class I molecules occurring on virtually all cells and which are responsible for recruiting cytotoxic T cells; class II molecules that occur on B cells and macrophages and are involved in signaling T helper cells to recruit further B cells and macrophages; the non-classic class III molecules that include a number of other proteins with a variety of other immunological functions. The latter include inflammatory mediators such as the tumor necrosis factor, heat shock proteins and the various components of complement (p. 189).

Structural analysis of the class I and II MHC molecules reveals them to be heterodimers with homology to immunoglobulin. The genes coding for the class I (A, B, C, E, F and G), class II (DR, DQ and DP) and class III MHC molecules, or what is also known as the *human leukocyte antigen* (HLA) system, are located on chromosome 6.

## Transplantation genetics

Replacement of diseased organs by transplantation has become routine in clinical medicine. Except for corneal and bone grafts, the success of such transplants depends on the degree of antigenic similarity between the donor and recipient. The closer the similarity, the greater the likelihood that the transplanted organ or tissue, which is known as a *homograft*, will be accepted rather than rejected. Homograft rejection does not occur between identical twins or between non-identical twins where there has been mixing of the placental circulations before birth (p. 56). In all other instances, the antigenic similarity of donor and recipient has to be assessed by testing them with suitable antisera or monoclonal antibodies for antigens on donor and recipient tissues. These were originally known as transplantation antigens and are now known to be a result of the major histocompatibility complex. As a general rule, a recipient will reject a graft from any person who has antigens the recipient lacks. HLA typing of an individual is carried out using PCR-based molecular techniques (p. 62).

The HLA system is highly polymorphic (Table 13.2). A virtually infinite number of phenotypes resulting from different combinations of the various alleles at these loci are theoretically possible. Two unrelated individuals are therefore very unlikely to have identical HLA phenotypes. The close linkage of the HLA loci means that they tend to be inherited en bloc, the term *haplotype* being used to indicate the particular HLA alleles that an individual carries on each of his two number 6 chromosomes. Thus any individual will have a 25% chance of having identical HLA antigens with a sibling, as there are only four possible combinations of the two paternal haplotypes (say P and Q) and the two maternal haplotypes (say R and S), i.e. PR, PS, QR and QS. The siblings of a particular recipient are more likely to be antigenically similar than either of his/her parents, and the latter more than an unrelated person. For this reason, a brother or sister is frequently selected as a potential donor for organ or tissue transplantation.

Although crossing over does occur within the HLA region, certain alleles tend to occur together more frequently than would be expected by chance, i.e. they tend to exhibit linkage disequilibrium (p. 134). An example is the association of the HLA antigens A1 and B8 in populations of Western European origin.

**Table 13.2 Alleles at the HLA loci**

| HLA locus | Number of alleles |
|---|---|
| A | 57 |
| B | 111 |
| C | 34 |
| D | 228 |

### H-Y antigen

In a number of different animal species it was noted that tissue grafts from males were rejected by females of the same inbred strain. These incompatibilities were found to be due to a histocompatibility antigen, known as the H-Y antigen. The H-Y antigen seems, however, to play little part in transplantation in humans. Although the H-Y antigen seems to be important for testicular differentiation and function, its expression does not necessarily correlate with the presence or absence of testicular tissue. A separate sex-determining region of the Y chromosome (*SRY*) has been isolated which is now known to be the testis-determining gene (p. 97).

## HLA polymorphisms and disease associations

A finding which helps to throw light on the pathogenesis of certain diseases is the demonstration of their association with certain HLA types (Table 13.3). The best documented is that between ankylosing spondylitis and HLA B27. In the case of narcolepsy, a condition of unknown etiology characterized by a periodic uncontrollable tendency to fall asleep, almost all affected individuals are HLA DR2. The possession of a particular HLA antigen does not

**Table 13.3 Some HLA-associated diseases**

| Disease | HLA |
|---|---|
| Ankylosing spondylitis | B27 |
| Celiac disease | DR4 |
| 21-hydroxylase deficiency | A3/Bw47/DR7 |
| Hemochromatosis | A3 |
| Insulin-dependent diabetes (type 1) | DR3/4 |
| Myasthenia gravis | B8 |
| Narcolepsy | DR2 |
| Rheumatoid arthritis | DR4 |
| Systemic lupus erythematosus | DR2/DR3 |
| Thyrotoxicosis (Graves' disease) | DR3 |

mean that an individual will necessarily develop the associated disease, merely that he or she has a greater *relative* risk of being affected than the general population (p. 141). In a family, the risks to first-degree relatives of those affected is low, usually no more than 5%.

Explanations for the various HLA-associated disease susceptibilities include close linkage to a susceptibility gene near the HLA complex, cross-reactivity of antibodies to environmental antigens or pathogens with specific HLA antigens, and abnormal recognition of 'self' antigens through defects in T-cell receptors or antigen processing. These conditions are known as *autoimmune diseases*. An example of close linkage is congenital adrenal hyperplasia (CAH) due to 21-hydroxylase deficiency (p. 169). The *CYP21* gene (mutated in CAH) lies within the HLA major histocompatibility locus on chromosome 6p21.3. There is a strong association between salt-losing 21-hydroxylase deficiency and HLA A3/Bw47/DR7 in Northern European populations. Non-classic 21-hydroxylase deficiency is associated with HLA B14/DR1, and HLA A1/B8/DR3 is *negatively* associated with 21-hydroxylase deficiency. In general, the mechanisms involved in most HLA disease associations are not well understood.

## INHERITED IMMUNODEFICIENCY DISORDERS

Inherited immunodeficiency disorders are uncommon and are usually associated with severe morbidity and mortality. They can occur as a primary isolated abnormality or can be a secondary or associated finding. The presentation is variable but is usually in early childhood after the benefits of maternal transplacental immunity have declined. Investigation of immune function should be considered in children with unexplained failure to thrive and diarrhea, recurrent bacterial, chronic and opportunistic infections. Unexplained hepatosplenomegaly may also be a feature.

## PRIMARY INHERITED DISORDERS OF IMMUNITY

The manifestations of at least some of the primary immunological deficiency diseases in humans (Table 13.4) can be understood by considering whether they are disorders of innate immunity or of specific acquired immunity. Abnormalities of humoral immunity are associated with reduced resistance to bacterial infections that can lead to death in infancy. Abnormalities of specific acquired immunity that are cell mediated are associated with increased susceptibility to virus infections and are manifest experimentally in animals by prolonged survival of skin homografts.

### Disorders of innate immunity

Primary disorders of innate immunity involving humoral and cell-mediated immunity have been described.

### *Disorders of innate humoral immunity*

There are a variety of defects of complement that can lead to disordered innate immunity.

**Disorders of complement**

Defects of the third component of complement, C3, lead to abnormalities of opsonization of bacteria, resulting in difficulties in combating pyogenic infections. Defects in the later components of complement involved in the formation of the membrane attack complex also result in susceptibility to a particular bacterial species, primarily *Neisseria*.

Deficiency of the C1 inhibitor results in inappropriate activation of the classic pathway of complement, leading to uncontrolled production of C2a, which is vasoactive, resulting in fluid accumulation in soft tissue and the airways, sometimes leading to life-threatening laryngeal edema. This is known as hereditary angioneurotic edema, which is inherited as an autosomal dominant

**Table 13.4 Some immunological deficiency diseases and their features**

| Disorder | Thymus gland | Lymphocytes | Cell-mediated | Plasma cells | Ig synthesis | Genetics | Treatment |
|---|---|---|---|---|---|---|---|
| Severe combined immunodeficiency | Vestigial | ↓ | ↓ | ↓ | ↓ | AR/XR | BMT, enzyme replacement for ADA deficiency |
| DiGeorge/ Sedláčková syndrome | Absent (parathyroids absent as well) | + | ↓ | + | N | Deletion | Transplantation of fetal thymus |
| Bruton-type | + | + | N | ↓ | ↓ | XR | Ig injections agammaglobulinemia and antibiotics |

AR: autosomal recessive; XR: X-linked recessive; BMT: bone marrow transplant; ADA: adenosine deaminase; N: normal; ÿ: reduced; +: present

Until the advent of bone marrow transplantation, the majority of affected boys died by mid-adolescence from hemorrhage or B-cell malignancies.

### Carrier tests for X-linked immunodeficiencies

Before the identification of the genes responsible for the Wiskott–Aldrich syndrome, Bruton-type hypogammaglobulinemia and X-linked SCID, the availability of closely linked DNA markers allowed carrier testing by studies of the pattern of X-inactivation (p. 99) in the lymphocytes of females at risk. A non-random pattern of X-inactivation in the T-lymphocyte population, in a female relative of a sporadically affected male with an X-linked immunodeficiency demonstrating that all her peripheral blood T lymphocytes have the same chromosome inactivated, would confirm her to be a carrier (Fig. 13.6).

The carrier (C) and non-carrier (NC) are both heterozygous for an *Hpa*II/*Msp*I restriction site polymorphism. *Hpa*II and *Msp*I recognize the same nucleotide recognition sequence but *Msp*I cuts double-stranded DNA whether it is methylated or not, while *Hpa*II will only cut unmethylated DNA, i.e. only the active X chromosome. In the carrier female the mutation in the SCID gene is on the X chromosome on which the *Hpa*II/*Msp*I restriction site is present. *Eco*RI/*Msp*I double digests of T lymphocytes result in 6, 4 and 2 kb DNA fragments on gel analysis of the restriction fragments for both the carrier and non-carrier females. *Eco*RI/*Hpa*II double digests of T lymphocyte DNA result, however, in a single 6 kb fragment in the carrier female. This is because in a carrier the only T cells to survive will be those in which the normal gene is on the active unmethylated X chromosome. Thus in a carrier inactivation appears non-random, although strictly speaking it is cell population survival that is non-random.

A mixed pattern of X-inactivation in the lymphocytes of the mother of a sporadically affected male is consistent with the disorder, either having arisen as a new X-linked mutation or being due to the autosomal recessive form. Similar X-inactivation studies of the peripheral blood B-lymphocyte population can be used to determine the carrier status of women at risk for Bruton-type agammaglobulinemia and the Wiskott–Aldrich syndrome. This technique is being replaced by direct identification of mutations in the genes responsible.

## BLOOD GROUPS

Blood groups reflect the antigenic determinants on red cells and were one of the first areas in which an understanding of basic biology led to significant advances in clinical medicine. Our knowledge of the ABO and rhesus blood groups has resulted in safe blood transfusion and the prevention of rhesus hemolytic disease of the newborn.

### THE ABO BLOOD GROUPS

The ABO blood groups were discovered by Landsteiner just after the turn of the twentieth century. The transfusion of red blood cells from certain persons to others, in some instances, resulted in rapid hemolysis; in other words, their blood was incompatible. Studies revealed there to be four major ABO blood groups: A, B, AB and O. Persons who are blood group A possess the antigen A on the surface of their red blood cells, persons of blood group B have antigen B, persons who are AB have both A and B antigens, while persons who are blood group O have neither. Persons of blood group A have naturally occurring anti-B antibodies in their blood, persons of blood group B have anti-A, and persons of blood group O have both. The alleles at the ABO blood group locus for antigens A and B are inherited in a codominant manner but are both dominant to the gene

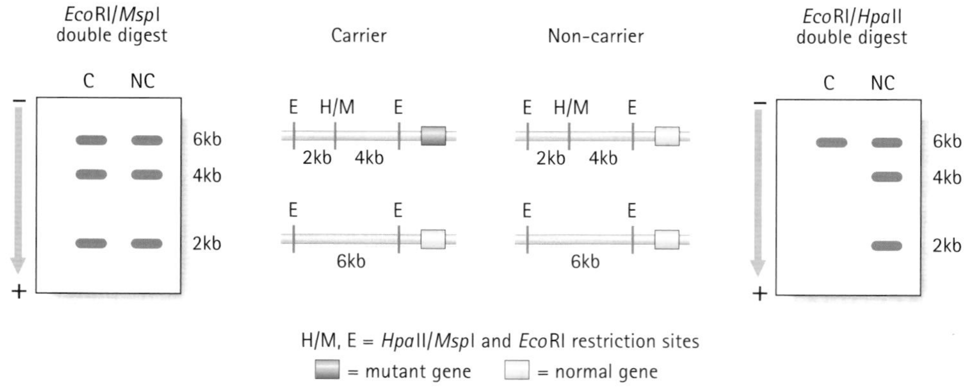


Fig. 13.6
Non-random inactivation in T lymphocytes for carrier testing in X-linked SCID.

**Table 13.5 ABO blood group phenotypes and genotypes**

| Red blood cells Phenotype | Genotype | React with antiserum Antibodies | Anti-A | Anti-B |
|---|---|---|---|---|
| O | OO | anti-A,B | – | – |
| A | AA, AO | anti-B | + | – |
| B | BB, BO | anti-A | – | + |
| AB | AB | – | + | + |

for the O antigen (p. 115). There are, therefore, six possible genotypes. The homozygous and heterozygous states for antigens A and B (i.e. AA, AO, BB, BO) can only be determined by family studies (Table 13.5).

Since individuals of blood group AB do not produce A or B antibodies they can receive a blood transfusion from individuals of all other ABO blood groups and are therefore referred to as *universal recipients*. On the other hand, since individuals of group O do not express either A or B antigens on their red cells they are referred to as *universal donors*. Antisera can differentiate two subgroups of blood groups A, A1 and A2, but this is of little practical importance as far as blood transfusions are concerned.

### Molecular basis of ABO blood groups

Individuals with blood groups A, B and AB possess enzymes with glycosyltransferase activity that convert the basic blood group, which is known as the H antigen, into A or B antigens. The alleles for blood groups A and B differ in seven single base substitutions that result in different A and B transferase activities, the A allele being associated with the addition of *N*-acetylgalactosaminyl groups and the B allele with the addition of D-galactosyl groups. The O allele results from a critical single base pair deletion that results in an inactive protein incapable of modifying the H antigen.

### Secretor status

In the majority of persons the ABO blood group antigens, in addition to being expressed on red blood cells, are secreted in various body fluids, including saliva. This is controlled by two alleles at the so-called *secretor locus*, persons being either *secretor positive* or *secretor negative*, the former being dominant to the latter. *Secretor status* has been associated with a predisposition to peptic ulcers. The secretor locus has also been shown to be linked to the locus for myotonic dystrophy. Before the advent of DNA markers, family studies of secretor status were used to predict whether an asymptomatic person had inherited the gene for this disorder (p. 275).

## RHESUS BLOOD GROUP

The rhesus (Rh) blood group system involves three sets of closely linked antigens, Cc, Dd and Ee. D is very strongly antigenic and persons are, for practical purposes, either Rh positive (possessing the D antigen) or Rh negative (lacking the D antigen).

### Rhesus hemolytic disease of the newborn

A proportion of women who are Rh negative have an increased chance of having a child who will either die in utero or be born severely anemic because of hemolysis unless transfused in utero. This occurs for the following reason. If Rh-positive blood is given to persons who are Rh negative, the majority will develop anti-Rh antibodies. Such sensitization occurs with exposure to very small quantities of blood and, once a person is sensitized, further exposure results in the production of very high antibody titers.

In the case of an Rh-negative mother carrying an Rh positive fetus, red cells of fetal origin can enter the mother's circulation, for example after a miscarriage or at the time of delivery. This can induce the formation of Rh antibodies in the mother. In a subsequent pregnancy these antibodies can cross the placenta and enter the fetal circulation. This leads to hemolysis of the fetal red blood cells if the fetus is Rh negative, which can result either in fetal death, which is known as *erythroblastosis fetalis*, or a severe hemolytic anemia of newborn infants that is called *hemolytic disease of the newborn*. Once a woman is sensitized there is a significantly greater risk that a child in a subsequent pregnancy, if Rh positive, will be more severely affected.

To avoid sensitizing an Rh negative woman, Rh-compatible blood must always be used in any blood transfusion. Furthermore, the development of sensitization and therefore Rh incompatibility after delivery can be prevented by giving the mother an injection of Rh antibodies, so-called anti-D, so that any fetal cells that have found their way into the maternal circulation are destroyed before the mother can become sensitized.

It is routine to screen all Rh-negative women during pregnancy for the development of Rh antibodies. Despite these measures, a small proportion of women do become sensitized. If Rh antibodies appear, tests are then carried out to see if the fetus is affected. If so, then there is a delicate balance between early delivery, with the risks of prematurity and exchange transfusion, and treating the fetus in utero with blood transfusions.

### Molecular basis of the rhesus blood group

Recent biochemical evidence has shown there to be two types of Rh red cell membrane polypeptide. One corresponds to the D antigen and the other to the C and E

# CHAPTER 14 Cancer genetics

*"All cancer is genetic, but some cancers are more genetic than others."*

Paraphrased from *Animal Farm*, by **George Orwell**

Cell biology and molecular genetics have revolutionized our understanding of cancer in recent years; all cancer is a genetic disease of *somatic* cells because of aberrant cell division or loss of normal programmed cell death, but a small proportion is strongly predisposed by inherited *germ line* mutations behaving as Mendelian traits. However, this does not contradict our traditional understanding that for many cancers environmental factors are of primary etiological importance, whilst heredity seems to play little or no part. The latter is certainly true of the 'industrial cancers', which result from prolonged exposure to carcinogenic chemicals. Examples include cancer of the skin in tar workers, cancer of the bladder in aniline dye workers, angiosarcoma of the liver in process workers making polyvinyl chloride (PVC), and cancer of the lung in asbestos workers. Even so, for those who have been exposed to these substances and are unfortunate enough to suffer, it is possible that a significant proportion may have a genetic predisposition to the activity of the carcinogen. The link between cigarette smoking and lung cancer (as well as some other cancers) has been recognized for nearly half a century, but not all smokers develop a tobacco-related malignancy. Recent studies have shown that smokers with short chromosome telomeres (p. 32) appear to be at substantially greater risk for tobacco-related cancers than people with short telomeres who never smoked, or smokers who have long telomeres. The recognition that a number of rare cancer-predisposing syndromes, as well as a small but significant proportion of common cancers having a hereditary basis, has led over the last 25 years to an explosion in our understanding of the genetic basis and cellular biology of cancer in humans. As a general principle it is now clear that cancers arise as the end result of an accumulation of both inherited and somatic mutations in proto-oncogenes and tumor suppressor genes. A third class of genes – the DNA mismatch repair genes – are also important because their inactivation is believed to contribute to the genesis of mutations in other genes directly affecting the survival and proliferation of cells.

## DIFFERENTIATION BETWEEN GENETIC AND ENVIRONMENTAL FACTORS IN CANCER

In many cancers the differentiation between genetic and environmental etiological factors is not always obvious. In the majority of cancers in humans there is no clear-cut mode of inheritance nor is there any clearly defined environmental cause. In certain of the common cancers, such as breast and bowel, genetic factors play an important, but not exclusive, role in the etiology. Evidence to help differentiate environmental and genetic factors can come from a combination of epidemiologic, family and twin studies, disease associations, biochemical factors and animal studies.

### EPIDEMIOLOGIC STUDIES

Breast cancer is the most common cancer in women. Reproductive and menstrual histories are well-recognized risk factors. Women who have had children have a lower risk of developing breast cancer than nulliparous women. In addition, the younger the age at which a woman has her first pregnancy, the lower her risk of developing breast cancer. Also, the later the age of onset of menstrual periods, the lower the risk of developing breast cancer.

The incidence of breast cancer varies greatly between different populations, being highest in women in North America and Western Europe and up to eight times lower in women of Japanese and Chinese origin. While these differences could be attributed to genetic differences between these population groups, study of immigrant populations moving from an area with a low incidence to one with a high incidence has shown that the risk of developing breast cancer rises with time to that of the native population, supporting the view that breast cancer has a significant environmental component.

It has long been recognized that persons from the less well-off socioeconomic groups have an increased risk of developing gastric cancer. Specific dietary irritants, such as salts and preservatives, or potential environmental agents, such as nitrates, have been suggested as being possible carcinogens. Gastric cancer also shows variations in incidence in different populations, being up to eight times more common in Japanese and Chinese populations than in persons of Western European origin. Migration studies have shown that the risk of gastric cancer for immigrants from high-risk populations does not fall to that of the native low-risk population for two or three generations. It has been suggested previously that this could be due to exposure to environmental factors at an early critical age. There is a substantial body of evidence accumulating that early infection with *Helicobacter pylori*, which causes chronic gastric inflammation, is associated with a five- to sixfold increased risk of developing gastric cancer.

## FAMILY STUDIES

The frequency with which other family members develop the same cancer can provide evidence supporting a genetic contribution. The risk of developing breast cancer for a woman who lives until her mid-70s in Western Europe is at least 1 in 12. Family studies have shown that, for a woman who has a first-degree relative with breast cancer, the risk that she will also develop breast cancer is between 1.5 and 3 times the risk for the general population. The risk varies according to the age of onset in the affected family member: the earlier the age at diagnosis, the greater the risk to close relatives (p. 217).

Similar studies in gastric cancer have shown that first-degree relatives of persons with cancer of the stomach have a two- to threefold increased risk compared to the general population of developing gastric cancer. The increased risk of developing gastric cancer in close relatives is, however, relatively small, suggesting that environmental factors are likely to be more important.

## TWIN STUDIES

Concordance rates for breast cancer in twins are low for both types of twins, being only slightly greater in monozygotic female twins, at 17%, than 13% in dizygotic female twins, suggesting that, overall, environmental factors are likely to be more important than genetic factors. Twin studies in gastric cancer have not shown an increased concordance rate in monozygotic compared to dizygotic twins.

## DISEASE ASSOCIATIONS

Blood groups are genetically determined, and therefore association of a particular blood group with a disease suggests a possible genetic contribution to the etiology. A large number of studies from a variety of countries have shown an association between blood group A and gastric cancer. It is estimated that persons with blood group A have a 20% increased risk over the general population for developing gastric cancer. Blood group A is associated with an increased risk of developing pernicious anemia, which is also closely associated with chronic gastritis. It appears, however, that pernicious anemia has a separate association with gastric cancer. Persons with pernicious anemia have a three- to sixfold increased risk of developing gastric cancer.

## BIOCHEMICAL FACTORS

Biochemical factors can determine the susceptibility to environmental carcinogens. Examples include the association between slow-acetylator status and debrisoquine metabolizer status (p. 184) and a predisposition to bladder cancer (p. 187), as well as glutathione *S*-transferase activity (p. 187), which influences the risk of developing lung cancer in smokers.

## ANIMAL STUDIES

Certain inbred strains of mice have been developed that have a high chance of developing a particular type of tumor. The A (albino) Bittner strain is especially prone to develop tumors of the lung and breast; the C3H strain is particularly prone to develop breast tumors as well as tumors of the liver; the C58 strain is prone to develop leukemia. Breeding experiments with mice have shown that the tendency to develop cancer is influenced by environmental factors. In strains with a high incidence of breast tumors, the frequency of these tumors is reduced by dietary restrictions and increased by high temperature.

## VIRAL FACTORS

Animal studies undertaken by Peyton Rous early in the twentieth century, among others, showed that transmission of a tumor was possible in the absence of body cells. Bittner later showed that susceptibility to breast tumors in certain strains of mice depended on a combination of genetic factors as well as a transmissible factor present in the milk, known as the 'milk agent'. In high-incidence strains both genetic susceptibility and the milk agent are involved, but in low-incidence strains there is no milk agent. By using foster mothers from cancer-free strains to suckle newborn mice from strains with a high cancer susceptibility it was possible to reduce the incidence of breast cancer from 100% to less than 50%. Conversely, an increased incidence was observed in cancer-free strains by suckling the newborn mice with

**Table 14.1 Human DNA viruses implicated in carcinogenesis**

| Virus family | Type | Tumor |
|---|---|---|
| Papova | Papilloma (HPV) | Warts (plantar and genital), urogenital cancers (cervical, vulval and penile), skin cancer |
| Herpes | Epstein–Barr (EBV) | Burkitt lymphoma*, nasopharyngeal carcinoma, lymphomas in immunocompromised hosts |
| Hepadna | Hepatitis B (HBV) | Hepatocellular carcinoma* |

*For full oncogenicity, 'co-carcinogens' are necessary, e.g. aflatoxin $B_1$ in hepatitis B-associated hepatocellular carcinoma

foster mothers from high cancer-prone strains. The milk agent was shown to be a virus that was usually transmitted by the mother's milk, but could also be transmitted by the father's sperm.

Subsequent studies have shown that certain viruses are tumor forming or *oncogenic* in humans. A limited number of DNA viruses are associated with certain types of human tumors (Table 14.1), while a variety of RNA viruses, or *retroviruses,* cause neoplasia in animals. The study of the genetics and replicative processes of oncogenic retroviruses has revealed some of the cellular biological processes involved in carcinogenesis.

### Retroviruses

Retroviruses have their genetic information encoded in RNA and replicate through DNA by coding for an enzyme known as reverse transcriptase (p. 61), which makes a double-stranded DNA copy of the viral RNA. This DNA intermediate integrates into the host cell genome, allowing the appropriate proteins to be manufactured, resulting in repackaging of new progeny virions.

Naturally occurring retroviruses have only the three genes necessary to ensure replication: *gag*, encoding the structural proteins for the core antigens, *pol*, coding for reverse transcriptase, and *env*, the gene for the glycoprotein envelope proteins (Fig. 14.1). Study of the virus responsible for the transmissible tumor in chickens, the so-called Rous sarcoma virus, identified a fourth gene that results in *transformation* of cells in culture, a model for malignancy in vivo. This viral gene, which *transforms* the host cell, is known as an *oncogene*.

## ONCOGENES

Oncogenes are the altered forms of normal genes – *proto-oncogenes* – that have key roles in cell growth and differentiation pathways. In normal mammalian cells there are sequences of DNA that are homologous to viral oncogenes, and it is these that are named *proto-oncogenes* or *cellular oncogenes*. Although the terms proto-oncogene and cellular oncogene are often used interchangeably, strictly speaking proto-oncogene is reserved for the normal gene and cellular oncogene, or c-*onc*, refers to a mutated proto-oncogene, which has oncogenic properties like the viral oncogenes, or v-*onc*. Some 30 oncogenes have been identified.

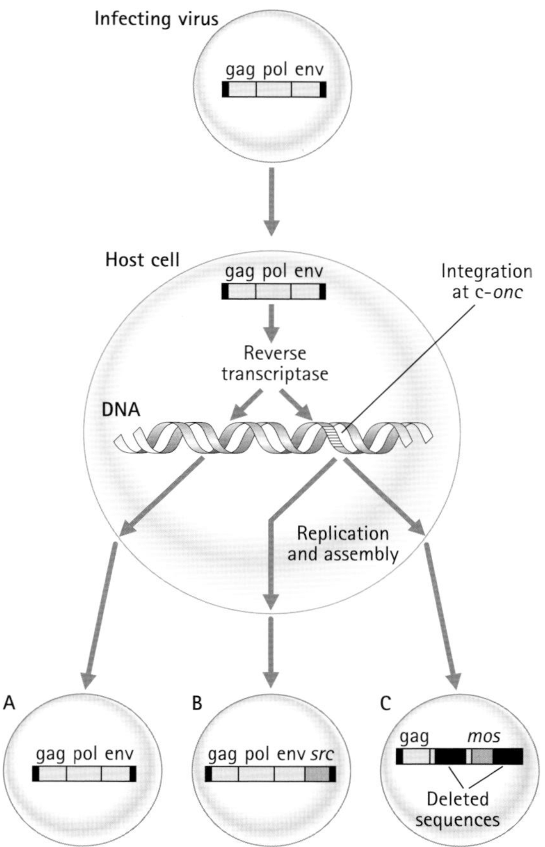


Fig. 14.1
Model for acquisition of transforming ability in retroviruses. (A) Normal retroviral replication. (B) The Rous sarcoma virus has integrated near a cellular oncogene. The transforming ability of this virus is due to the acquired homolog of the cellular oncogene, v-src. (C) A defective transforming virus carries an oncogene similar to src but is defective in the structural genes, e.g. Moloney murine sarcoma virus, which carries *mos.*

## RELATIONSHIP BETWEEN C-*ONC* AND V-*ONC*

Cellular oncogenes are highly conserved in evolution, suggesting that they have important roles as regulators of cell growth, maintaining the ordered progression through the cell cycle, cell division and differentiation. Retroviral oncogenes are thought to acquire their dominant transforming activity during viral transduction through errors in the replication of the retrovirus genome following their random integration into the host DNA. The end result is a viral gene that is structurally similar to its cellular counterpart but is persistently different in its function.

## IDENTIFICATION OF ONCOGENES

Oncogenes have been identified by two types of cytogenetic finding in association with certain types of leukemia and tumor in humans. These include the location of oncogenes at chromosomal translocation break-points, or their amplification in double-minute chromosomes or homogeneously staining regions of chromosomes (p. 207). In addition, a number of oncogenes have also been identified by the ability of tumor DNA to induce tumors in vitro by DNA transfection.

### Identification of oncogenes at chromosomal translocation break-points

Chromosome aberrations are common in malignant cells, which often show marked variation in chromosome number and structure. Certain chromosomes seemed to be more commonly involved and it was initially thought that these changes were secondary to the transformed state rather than causal. This attitude changed when evidence suggested that chromosomal structural changes, often translocations (p. 49), resulted in rearrangements within or adjacent to proto-oncogenes. It has been found that chromosomal translocations can lead to novel chimeric genes with altered biochemical function or level of proto-oncogene activity. There are numerous examples of both types, of which chronic myeloid leukemia is an example of the former and Burkitt lymphoma an example of the latter.

#### *Chronic myeloid leukemia*

In 1960, investigators in Philadelphia were the first to describe an abnormal chromosome in white blood cells from patients with chronic myeloid leukemia. The abnormal chromosome, referred to as the Philadelphia, or $Ph^1$ chromosome, is an acquired abnormality found in blood or bone marrow cells but not in other tissues from these patients. The $Ph^1$ is a tiny chromosome that is now known to be a chromosome 22 from which material from the long arm has been reciprocally translocated to and from the long arm of chromosome 9 (Fig. 14.2), i.e. t(9;22)(q34;q11). This chromosomal rearrangement is seen in 90% of persons with this form of leukemia. This translocation has been found to transfer the cellular *ABL* (*Abelson*) oncogene from chromosome 9 into a region of chromosome 22 known as the *break-point cluster*, or *BCR*, region, resulting in a chimeric transcript derived from both the *c-ABL* (70%) and the *BCR* genes. This results in a chimeric gene expressing a fusion protein consisting of the BCR protein at the amino end and ABL protein at the carboxy end, which is associated with transforming activity.

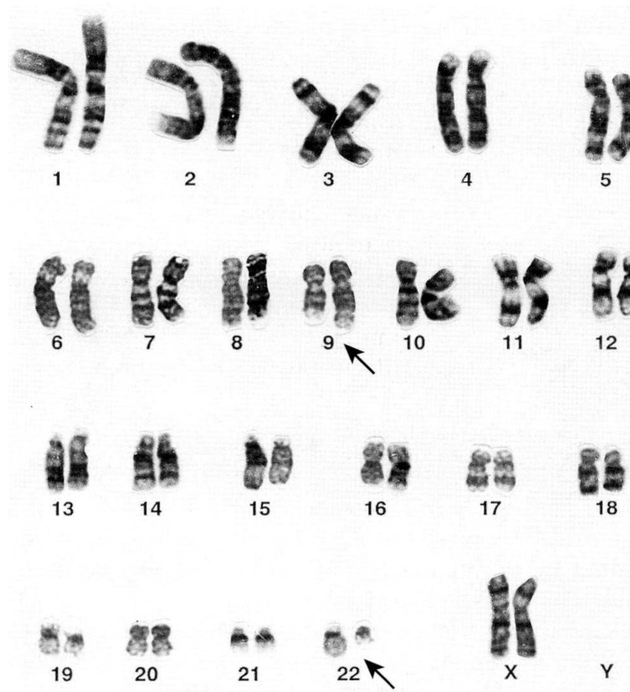


**Fig. 14.2**
Karyotype from a patient with chronic myeloid leukemia, showing the chromosome 22 (arrowed) or Philadelphia chromosome that has material translocated to the long arm of one of the number 9 chromosomes (arrowed).

#### *Burkitt lymphoma*

An unusual form of neoplasia seen in children in Africa is a lymphoma that involves the jaw, known as Burkitt lymphoma, so named after Dennis Burkitt, a medical missionary who first described the condition in the late 1950s. Chromosomal analysis has revealed the majority (90%) of affected children to have a translocation of the *c-MYC* oncogene from the long arm of chromosome 8 on to heavy (H) chain immunoglobulin locus on chromosome 14. Less commonly the *c-MYC* oncogene is translocated to regions of chromosome 2 or 22, which encode genes for the kappa (κ) and lambda (λ) light chains, respectively (p. 191). As a consequence of these translocations *MYC* comes under the influence of the regulatory sequences of the respective immunoglobulin gene and is overexpressed tenfold or more.

## Oncogene amplification

Proto-oncogenes can also be activated by the production of multiple copies of the gene or what is known as *gene amplification*, a mechanism known to have survival value when cells encounter environmental stress. For example, when leukemic cells are exposed to the chemotherapeutic agent methotrexate, the cells acquire resistance to the drug by making multiple copies of the gene for dihydrofolate reductase, the target enzyme for methotrexate.

Gene amplification can increase the number of copies of the oncogene per cell several-fold to several hundred times, leading to greater amounts of the corresponding oncoprotein. In mammals the amplified sequence of DNA in tumor cells can be recognized by the presence of small extra chromosomes known as *double-minute chromosomes* or *homogeneously staining regions* of the chromosomes. These changes are seen in approximately 10% of tumors and are often present more commonly in the later rather than the early stages of the malignant process.

Amplification of specific proto-oncogenes appears to be a feature of certain tumors and is frequently seen with the *MYC* family of genes. For example, N-*MYC* is amplified in approximately 30% of neuroblastomas, but in advanced cases this figure rises to 50%, where gene amplification can be up to 1000-fold. Human small cell carcinomas of the lung also show amplification of c-*MYC*, N-*MYC*, and L-*MYC*.

Amplification of c-*ERB-B2*, c-*MYC* and cyclin D1 is a feature in 20% of breast carcinomas, where it has been suggested that it correlates with a number of well established prognostic factors such as lymph node status, estrogen and progestogen receptor status, tumor size and histological grade.

## Detection of oncogenes by DNA transfection studies

The ability of DNA from a human bladder carcinoma cell line to transform a well established mouse fibroblast cell line called NIH3T3, as demonstrated by the loss of contact inhibition of the cells in culture, or what is known as DNA *transfection*, led to the discovery of the human sequence homologous to the *ras* gene of the Harvey murine sarcoma virus. The human *RAS* gene family consists of three closely related members, c-H-*RAS*, c-K-*RAS* and N-*RAS*. The RAS proteins are closely homologous to their viral counterparts and only differ from one another near the carboxy termini. Oncogenicity of the *RAS* proto-oncogenes has been shown to arise by acquisition of point mutations in the nucleotide sequence. IIn approximately 50% of colorectal cancers and 95% of pancreatic cancers, as well as in a proportion of thyroid and lung cancers, a mutation in a *RAS* gene can be demonstrated.

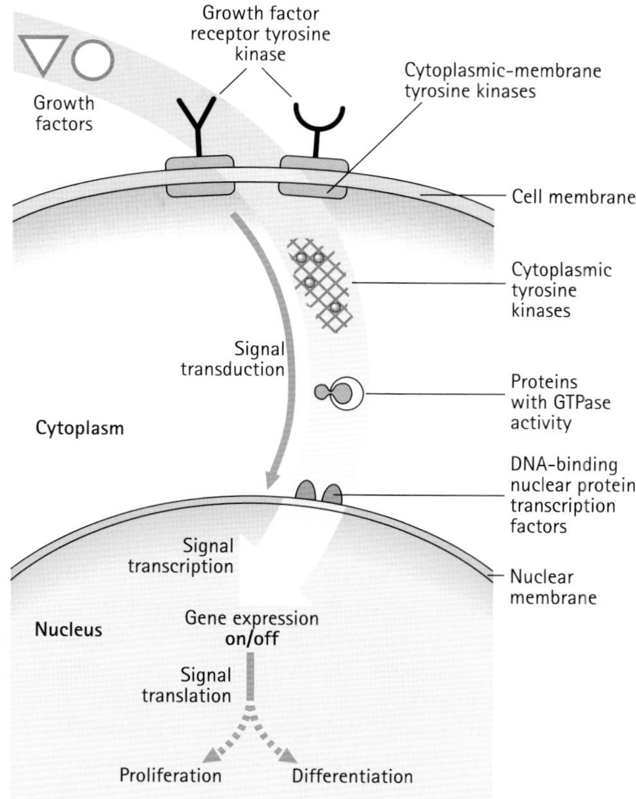


**Fig. 14.3**
Simplified schema of the steps in signal transduction and transcription from cell surface to nucleus. The intracellular pathway amplifies the signal by a cascade which involves one or more of the steps.

DNA transfection studies have also led to identification of other oncogenes that have not been demonstrated through retroviral studies. These include *MET* (hereditary papillary renal cell carcinoma), *TRK*, *MAS* and *RET* (multiple endocrine neoplasia type 2).

# FUNCTION OF ONCOGENES

Cancers have characteristics that indicate, at the cellular level, loss of the normal function of oncogene products consistent with a role in the control of cellular proliferation and differentiation in the process known as *signal transduction*. Signal transduction is a complex multistep pathway from the cell membrane, through the cytoplasm to the nucleus, involving a variety of types of proto-oncogene product involved in positive and negative feedback loops necessary for accurate cell proliferation and differentiation (Fig. 14.3).

Proto-oncogenes have been highly conserved during evolution, being present in a wide variety of different species, indicating that the protein products they encode are likely to have essential biological functions. Proto-oncogenes act in three main ways in the process of signal transduction. The first is through phosphorylation of serine, threonine and tyrosine residues of proteins by the transfer of phosphate groups from ATP. This leads to alteration of the configuration activating the kinase activity of proteins and generating docking sites for target proteins, resulting in signal transduction. The *RAS* family of proto-oncogenes are examples of the second type, which are GTPases and which function as molecular switches through the GDP/GTP cycle as intermediates relaying the transduction signal from membrane-associated tyrosine kinases to serine threonine kinases. The third type involves proteins located in the nucleus that control progress through the cell cycle, DNA replication and the expression of genes.

## TYPES OF ONCOGENE

### Growth factors

The transition of a cell from $G_0$ to the start of the cell cycle (p. 43) is governed by substances called growth factors. Growth factors stimulate cells to grow by binding to growth factor receptors. The best-known oncogene that acts as a growth factor is the v-*SIS* oncogene, which encodes part of the biologically active platelet-derived growth factor (PDG) B subunit. When v-SIS oncoprotein is added to the NIH 3T3 cultures, the cells are transformed, behaving like neoplastic cells, i.e. their growth rate increases and they lose contact inhibition. In vivo they form tumors when injected into nude mice. Oncogene products showing homology to fibroblast growth factors (FGFs) include *HST* and *INT*-2, which are amplified in stomach cancers and in malignant melanomas, respectively.

### Growth factor receptors

Many oncogenes encode proteins that form growth factor receptors, with tyrosine kinase activity possessing tyrosine kinase domains that allow cells to bypass the normal control mechanisms. More than 40 different tyrosine kinases have been identified and can be divided into two main types, those that span the cell membrane (growth factor receptor tyrosine kinases) and those that are located in the cytoplasm (non-receptor tyrosine kinases). Examples of tyrosine kinases include c-*ERB*-B, which encodes the epidermal growth factor (EGFR) receptor and the related c-*ERB*-B2 oncogene. Mutations in, rearrangements of, or amplification of the c-*ERB*-B2 oncogene, result in ligand-independent activation, which has been associated with cancer of the stomach, pancreas and ovary. Mutations in *KIT* occur in the hereditary gastrointestinal stromal tumor syndrome. These oncogenes are not activated by translocation (as in Burkitt lymphoma) but rather by point mutations. When germ line, or inherited, the mutations are not lethal, nor are they sufficient by themselves to cause carcinogenesis. In the case of *MET* (located on chromosome 7), the papillary renal cell carcinoma tumors are trisomic for chromosome 7 and two of the three copies of *MET* are mutant. A ratio of one mutant to one wild-type copy of *MET* is not sufficient for carcinogenesis but a 2:1 ratio is.

### Intracellular signaling transduction factors

Two different types of intracellular signaling transduction factor have been identified, proteins with GTPase activity and cytoplasmic serine threonine kinases.

#### *Proteins with GTPase activity*

Proteins with GTPase activity are intracellular membrane proteins that bind GTP to become active and through their intrinsic GTPase activity generate GDP, which inactivates the protein. Mutations in the *ras* genes result in increased or sustained GTPase activity, leading to unrestrained growth.

#### *Cytoplasmic serine threonine kinases*

A number of soluble cytoplasmic gene products are recognized to be part of the signal transduction pathway. The *RAF* oncogene product modulates the normal signaling transduction cascade. Mutations in the gene can result in sustained or increased transmission of a growth-promoting signal to the nucleus.

### DNA-binding nuclear proteins

The *FOS*, *JUN* and *ERB*-A oncogenes encode proteins which are specific transcription factors that regulate gene expression by activating or suppressing nearby DNA sequences. The function of c-*MYC* and related genes remains uncertain but appears to be related to alterations in control of the cell cycle. The c-*MYC* and *c-MYB* oncoproteins stimulate cells to progress from the $G_1$ into the S phase of the cell cycle (p. 43). Their overproduction prevents cells from entering a prolonged resting phase, resulting in persistent cellular proliferation.

### Cell cycle factors

Cancer cells can increase in number by increased growth and division, or accumulate through decreased cell death. Most cells in vivo are in a non-dividing state. Progress through the cell cycle (p. 43) is regulated at two points, one in $G_1$ when a cell becomes committed to DNA synthesis in the S phase, and another in $G_2$ for cell division in the M (mitosis) phase, through factors known as cyclin-dependent kinases. Abnormalities in regulation of the cell cycle through growth factors, growth factor receptors, GTPases or nuclear proteins or loss of inhibitory factors leads to activation of the cyclin-dependent kinases, such as cyclin D1, resulting in cellular transformation with uncontrolled cell division. Alternatively, loss of the factors that lead to normal programmed cell death, a process known as *apoptosis* (p. 85), can result in the accumulation of cells through prolonged cell survival as a mechanism of development of some tumors. Activation of the *bcl*-2 oncogene through chromosomal rearrangements is associated with inhibition of apoptosis, leading to certain types of lymphoma.

### Signal transduction and phakomatoses

*Phakomatosis* derives from the Greek, *phakos* – mother spot – and originally referred to three diseases that included scattered benign lesions: neurofibromatosis, tuberous sclerosis and von Hippel–Lindau disease. To this list has now been added nevoid basal cell carcinoma (Gorlin) syndrome, Cowden disease, familial adenomatous polyposis, Peutz–Jegher syndrome and juvenile polyposis. The genes for all these conditions are now known and are normally active within intracellular signal transduction and their protein products are tumor suppressors.

## TUMOR SUPPRESSOR GENES

While the study of oncogenes has revealed much about the cellular biology of the somatic genetic events in the malignant process, the study of hereditary cancer in humans has revealed the existence of what are known as *tumor suppressor genes*, which constitute the largest group of cloned hereditary cancer genes.

Studies carried out by Harris and colleagues in the late 1960s, which involved fusion of malignant cells with non-malignant cells in culture, resulted in the suppression of the malignant phenotype in the hybrid cells. The recurrence of the malignant phenotype with loss of certain chromosomes from the hybrid cells suggested that normal cells contain a gene(s) with tumor suppressor activity that, if lost or inactive, can lead to malignancy and that was acting like a recessive trait. Such genes were initially referred to as *antioncogenes*. This term was considered inappropriate since they do not oppose the action of the oncogenes and are more correctly known as tumor suppressor genes. The paradigm for our understanding of the biology of tumor suppressor genes is the eye tumor retinoblastoma. It is important to appreciate, however, that a germline mutation in a tumor suppressor gene (as with an oncogene) does not by itself provoke carcinogenesis: further somatic mutation at one or more loci is necessary and environmental factors, such as ionizing radiation, may be significant in the process. Some 20 tumor suppressor genes have been identified.

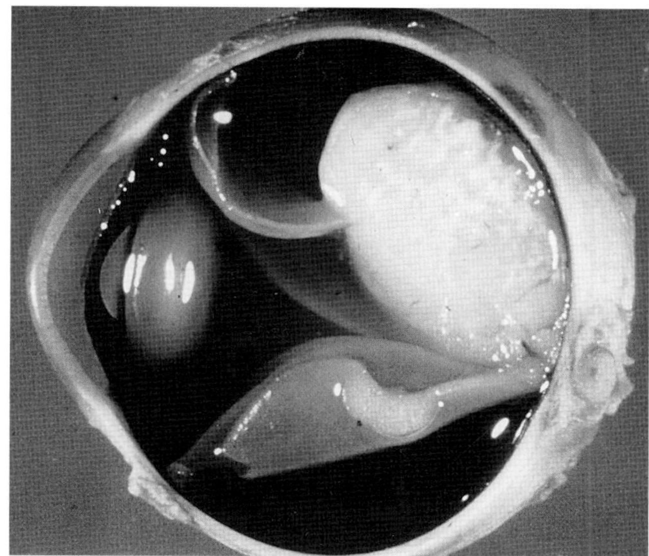

**Fig. 14.4**
Section of an eye showing a retinoblastoma in situ.

## RETINOBLASTOMA

Retinoblastoma (Rb) is a relatively rare, highly malignant childhood cancer of the developing retinal cells of the eye that usually occurs before the age of 5 years (Fig. 14.4). If diagnosed and treated at an early stage, it is associated with a good long-term outcome.

Retinoblastoma can occur either sporadically, the so-called 'non-hereditary' form, or be familial, the so-called 'hereditary' form, which is inherited in an autosomal dominant manner. Non-hereditary cases usually involve only one eye, whereas hereditary cases can be unilateral but are more commonly bilateral or occur in more than one site in one eye, i.e. are multifocal. The familial form also tends to present at an earlier age than the non-hereditary or sporadic form.

### 'Two-hit' hypothesis

In 1971, Knudson carried out an epidemiological study of a large number of cases of both types of retinoblastoma and advanced a 'two-hit' hypothesis to explain the occurrence of this rare tumor in patients with and without a positive family history. He proposed that affected individuals with a positive family history had inherited one non-functional gene that was present in all the cells of the individual, or what is known as a *germline mutation*, with the second gene at the same locus becoming inactivated somatically in a developing retinal cell (Fig. 14.5). The occurrence of a second mutation was likely given the

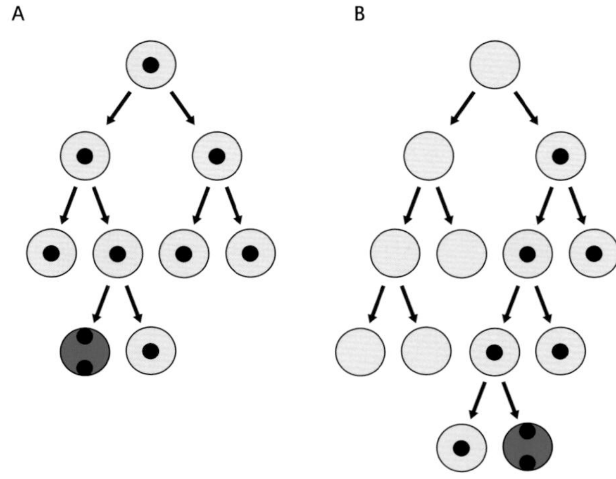


**Fig. 14.5**
Retinoblastoma and Knudson's two-hit hypothesis. All cells in the hereditary form (A) have one mutated copy of the gene, RB1, i.e. the mutation is in the *germline*. In the non-hereditary form (B) a mutation in RB1 arises as a post-zygotic (*somatic*) event sometime early in development. The retinoblastoma tumor will only occur when both RB1 genes are mutated, i.e. after a(nother) *somatic* event, which is more likely to be earlier in life in the hereditary form compared to the non-hereditary form; it is also more likely to give rise to bilateral and multifocal tumors.

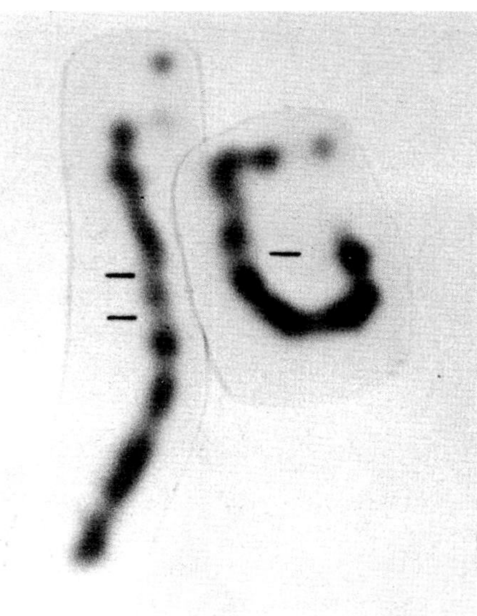

**Fig. 14.6**
Two homologs of chromosome 13 from a patient with retinoblastoma showing an interstitial deletion of 13q14 in the right-hand homolog, as indicated.

large number of retinal cells, explaining the autosomal dominant pattern of inheritance. This would also explain the observation that in hereditary retinoblastoma the tumors were often bilateral and multifocal. In contrast, in the non-heritable or sporadic form, *two* inactivating *somatic mutations* would need to occur independently in the same retinoblast (Fig. 14.5), which was much less likely to occur, explaining the fact that tumors in these patients were often unilateral and unifocal and usually occurred at a later age than in the hereditary form. Hence, although the hereditary form of retinoblastoma follows an autosomal dominant pattern of inheritance, at the molecular level it is *recessive* because a tumor only occurs with loss of both alleles,

It was also recognized, however, that approximately 5% of children presenting with retinoblastoma had other physical abnormalities along with developmental concerns. Detailed cytogenetic analysis of blood samples from these children revealed some of them to have an interstitial deletion involving the long arm of one of their number 13 chromosome pair. Comparison of the regions deleted revealed a common 'smallest region of overlap' involving the sub-band 13q14 (Fig. 14.6). The detection of a specific chromosomal region involved in the etiology of these cases of retinoblastoma (p. 276) suggested that it could also be the locus involved in the autosomal dominant familial form of retinoblastoma. Family studies using a polymorphic enzyme, esterase D, which had previously been mapped to that region, rapidly confirmed linkage of the hereditary form of retinoblastoma to that locus.

## Loss of heterozygosity

Analyses of the DNA sequences in this region of chromosome 13 in the peripheral blood and in retinoblastoma tumor material of children who had inherited the gene for retinoblastoma showed them to have loss of an allele at the retinoblastoma locus in the tumor material, or what is known as *loss of heterozygosity* (LOH), or sometimes loss of *constitutional* heterozygosity. An example of this is shown in Figure 14.7A, in which the mother transmits the retinoblastoma gene along with allele 2 at a closely linked marker locus. The father is homozygous for allele 1 at this same locus, with the result that the child is constitutionally an obligate heterozygote at this locus. Analysis of the tumor tissue reveals apparent homozygosity for allele 2. In fact, there has been loss of the paternally derived allele 1, i.e. LOH in the tumor material. This LOH is consistent with the 'two-hit' hypothesis leading to development of the malignancy as proposed by Knudson.

LOH can occur through several mechanisms, which include loss of a chromosome through mitotic nondisjunction (p. 276), a deletion on the chromosome carrying the corresponding allele, or a cross-over between the two homologous genes leading to homozygosity for the mutant allele (Fig. 14.7B). Observation of consistent cytogenetic rearrangements in other malignancies has led to demonstration of LOH in a number of other cancers

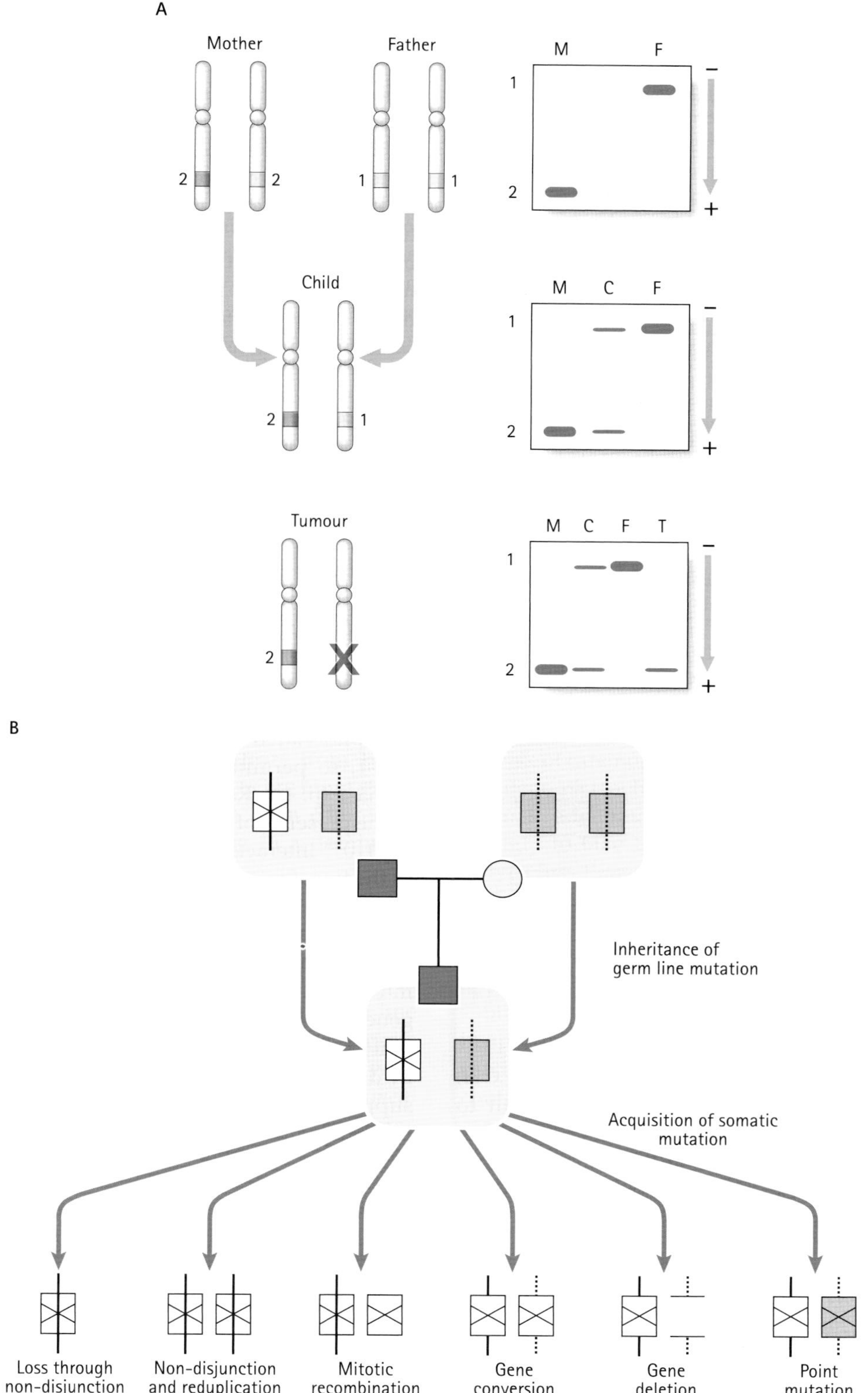


**Fig. 14.7**
(A) Diagrammatic representation of the loss of heterozygosity (LOH) in the development of a tumor. The mother (M) and father (F) are both homozygous for different alleles at the same locus, 2-2 and 1-1, respectively. The child (C) will therefore be constitutionally heterozygous,1-2. If an analysis of DNA from a tumor at that locus reveals only a single allele, 2, this is consistent with LOH. (B) Diagrammatic representations of the mechanisms leading to the 'second hit' leading to the development of retinoblastoma.

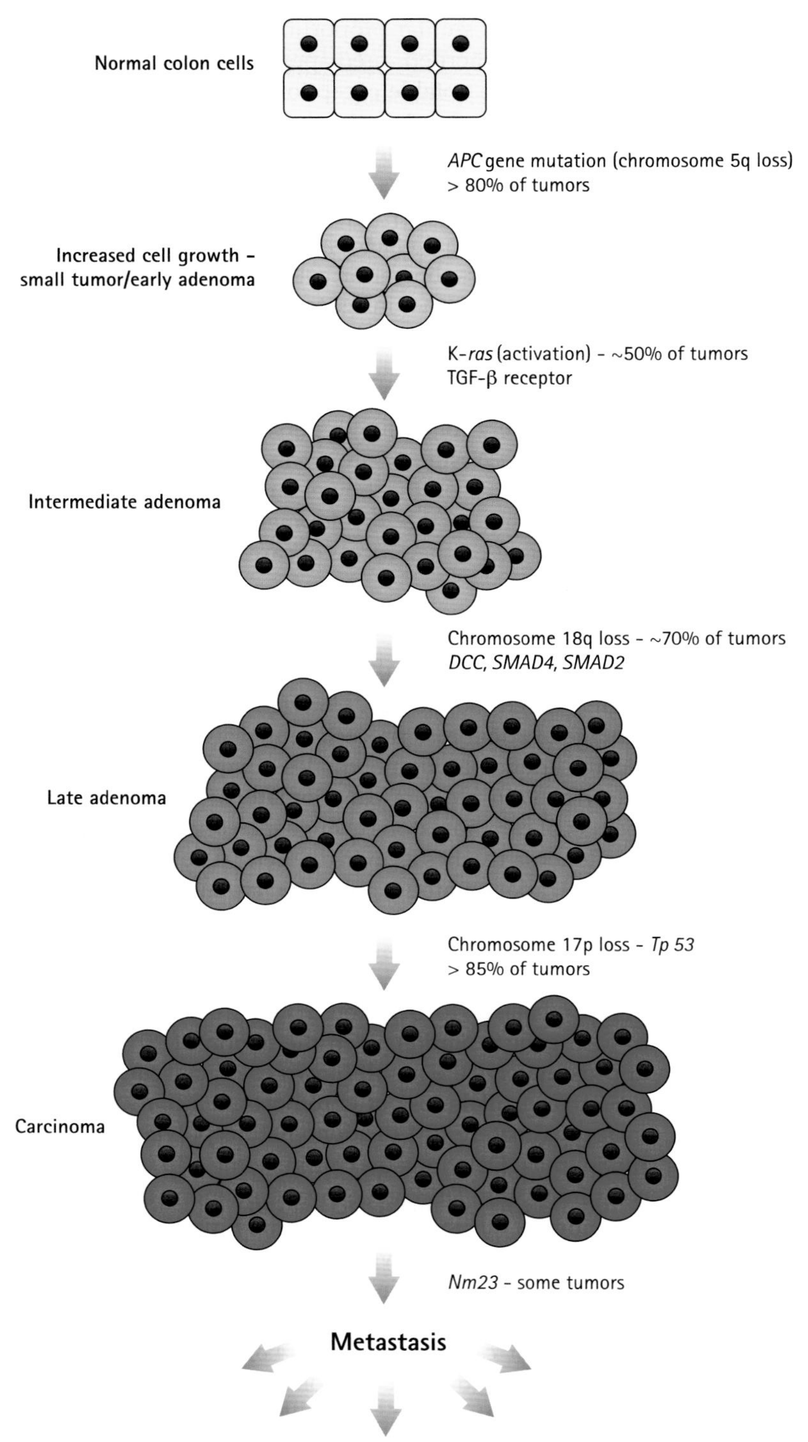


**Fig. 14.8**
The development of colorectal cancer is a multistage process of accumulating genetic errors in cells.

alterations are seen with increasing frequency when adenomas progress in size and show histological features of malignancy. Over 90% of carcinomas show two or more such alterations and approximately 40% show three.

The multistage process of the development of cancer is likely, of course, to be an oversimplification. The distinction between oncogenes and tumor suppressor genes (Table 14.3) has not always been clear-cut, e.g. the *RET* oncogene and MEN2 (p. 92). In addition, the same mutation in some of the inherited cancer syndromes (p. 219) can result in cancers at various sites in different individuals, which could be a consequence of the effect of interactions

**Table 14.3 Some familial cancers or cancer syndromes due to tumor suppressor mutations**

| Disorder | Gene | Locus |
|---|---|---|
| Retinoblastoma | *RB1* | 13q14 |
| Familial adenomatous polyposis | *APC* | 5q31 |
| Li–Fraumeni syndrome | *Tp53* | 17p13 |
| von Hippel–Lindau syndrome | *VHL* | 3p25–26 |
| Multiple endocrine neoplasia type II | *RET* | 10q11.2 |
| Breast–ovarian cancer | *BRCA1* | 17q21 |
| Breast cancer | *BRCA2* | 13q12–13 |
| Gastric cancer | *CDH1* | 16q22.1 |
| Wilms tumor | *WT1* | 11p13 |
| Neurofibromatosis I | *NF1* | 17q12–22 |

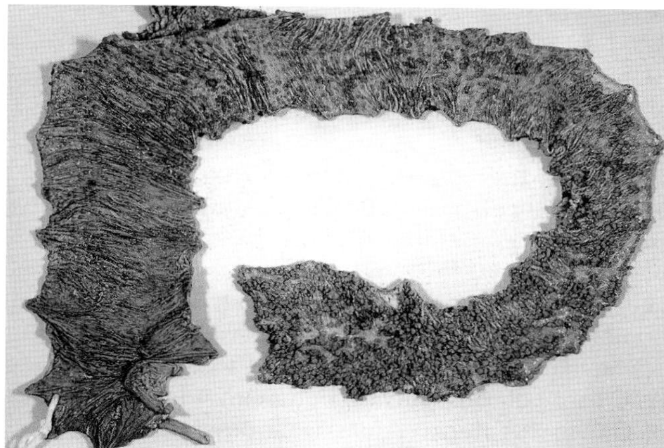

Fig. 14.9
Large bowel from a person with polyposis coli opened up to show multiple polyps throughout the colon. (Courtesy of Mr P. Finan, Department of Surgery, General Infirmary, Leeds.)

with inherited polymorphic variation in a number of other genes or a variety of environmental agents.

Further insight into the processes involved in the development of colorectal cancer came from a rare cause of familial colon cancer known as familial adenomatous polyposis.

## Familial adenomatous polyposis

Approximately 1% of persons who develop colorectal cancer do so through inheritance of an autosomal dominant disorder known as familial adenomatous polyposis (FAP). Affected persons develop numerous polyps of the large bowel, which can involve its entirety (Fig. 14.9). There is a high risk of carcinomatous change taking place in these polyps, with more than 90% of persons with FAP eventually developing bowel cancer.

The identification of an individual with FAP and an interstitial deletion of a particular region of the long arm of chromosome 5 (5q21) led to the demonstration of linkage of FAP to DNA markers in that region (p. 78). Subsequent studies led to the isolation of the adenomatous polyposis coli (*APC*) gene. Analyses of the markers linked to the *APC* gene in cancers from persons who have inherited the gene for this disorder have shown LOH, suggesting a similar mechanism of gene action in the development of this type of bowel cancer.

Studies in the common form of bowel cancer which is not inherited have shown similar LOH at 5q in the tumor material, with the FAP gene being deleted in 40% and 70% of sporadically occurring adenomas and carcinomas of the colon. LOH has also been reported at a number of different sites in colon cancer tumors that include the regions 18q21-qter and 17p12-13, the latter region including the *Tp53* gene, as well as another gene at 5q21 known as the 'mutated in colorectal cancer' (*MCC*) gene, consistent with the development of the common form of colon cancer being a multistage process.

## 'Deleted in colorectal cancer'

Allele loss on chromosome 18q is seen in over 70% of colorectal carcinomas. The original candidate gene for this region, called *deleted in colorectal carcinoma* (*DCC*), has been identified and cloned and has a high degree of homology with the family of genes encoding cell adhesion molecules. The *DCC* gene is expressed in normal colonic mucosa but is either reduced or absent in colorectal carcinomas. As with *Tp53*, somatic mutations in the *DCC* gene of the remaining allele occur in some cancers where gene expression is absent. The known homology suggests that loss of *DCC* plays a role in cell–cell and cell–basement-membrane interactions, features that are lost in overt malignancy. Mutations in the *DCC* gene have only been found, however, in a small proportion of colon cancers. Other genes deleted in this region in colorectal tumors include *DPC4* (renamed *SMAD4*) and *JV18* (renamed *SMAD2*).

## Hereditary non-polyposis colorectal cancer

A proportion of individuals with familial colon cancer may have a small number of polyps and the cancers occur more frequently in the proximal, or right side, of the colon, which is sometimes called 'site-specific' colon cancer. The average age of onset for colon cancer in this condition is the mid-forties. This familial cancer-predisposing syndrome is inherited as an autosomal dominant disorder and is known as hereditary non-polyposis colorectal cancer (HNPCC) – even though polyps may be present

**Table 14.4 Mismatch repair genes associated with hereditary non-polyposis colorectal cancer**

| Human gene | Chromosomal locus | *E. coli* homolog | HNPCC (%) |
|---|---|---|---|
| *hMSH2* | 2p15–16 | MutS | 31 |
| *hMSH6* | 2p15-16 | MutS | Rare |
| *hMLH1* | 3p21 | MutL | 33 |
| *hPMS1* | 2q31 | MutL | Rare |
| *hPMS2* | 7p22 | MutL | 4 |
| Undetermined loci | | | ~32 |

(the name helps to distinguish the condition from FAP). There is also a risk of small intestinal cancers, including stomach, endometrial cancer, and a variety of other cancers (see Table 14.6).

### *DNA mismatch repair genes*

Comparison of polymorphic microsatellite markers in tumor tissue and constitutional cells in persons with HNPCC, looking for LOH, somewhat surprisingly revealed the presence of new rather than fewer alleles in the DNA from tumor tissue. In contrast to the site-specific chromosome rearrangements seen with certain malignancies (p. 206), this phenomenon, known as *microsatellite instability* (MSI) or *replication error* (RER), is generalized, occurring with all microsatellite markers analyzed, irrespective of their chromosomal location.

This phenomenon was recognized to be similar to that seen in association with mutations in genes known as mutator genes, such as the *MutHLS* genes in yeast and *E. coli*. In addition, the human homolog of the mutator genes were located in regions of the human chromosomes to which HNPCC had previously been mapped, rapidly leading to the cloning of the genes responsible for HNPCC in humans (Table 14.4). The mutator genes code for a system of 'proof-reading' enzymes and are usually known as *mismatch repair genes*, which detect mismatched base pairs arising through errors in DNA replication or acquired causes, e.g. mutagens.

Individuals who inherit a mutation in one of the mismatch repair genes responsible for HNPCC are constitutionally heterozygous for a loss-of-function mutation (p. 23). Loss-of-function of the second copy through any of the mechanisms discussed in relation to LOH (p. 210) results in defective mismatch repair leading to an increased mutation rate associated with an increased risk of developing malignancy. Certain germline mutations, however, seem to have dominant-negative effects. Although HNPCC accounts for a small proportion of colon cancers, estimated to be between 2 and 4% overall, approximately 15% of *all* colorectal cancers exhibit MSI, the proportion being greater in tumors from persons who develop colorectal cancer at a younger age. Some of these individuals will have inherited constitutional mutations in one of the mismatch repair genes in the absence of a family history of colon cancer. In addition, for women with a constitutional mismatch repair gene mutation, the lifetime risk of endometrial cancer is up to 50%.

## OTHER POLYPOSIS SYNDROMES

Whilst isolated intestinal polyps are common, even occurring in about 1% of children, there are familial forms of multiple polyposis that are distinct from FAP but showing heterogeneity.

### MYH polyposis

In a recent large study nearly 20% of familial polyposis cases showed neither dominant inheritance nor evidence of an *APC* gene mutation. Of these families more than 20% were found to have mutations in the *MYH* gene, and affected individuals were compound heterozygotes. In contrast to the other polyposis conditions described below, MYH polyposis is, therefore, an autosomal recessive trait, thus significantly affecting genetic counseling as well as the need for screening in the wider family. The gene, located on chromosome band 1p33, is the human homolog of *mutY* in *E. coli*. This bacterial mismatch repair operates in conjunction with *mutM* to correct A/G and A/C base-pair mismatches. In tumors studied, an excess of G:C to T:A transversions were observed in the *APC* gene. Mutations that effectively knock out the *MYH* gene, therefore, lead to defects in the base excision repair pathway, and this is a form of DNA mismatch repair but, unusually, follows autosomal recessive inheritance.

### Juvenile polyposis syndrome

Autosomal dominant transmission is well described for a rare form of juvenile polyposis that may present in variety of ways, including bleeding with anemia, pain, intussusception and failure to thrive. The polyps carry an approximate 13-fold increased cancer risk and, once diagnosed, regular surveillance and polypectomy should be undertaken. The average age at diagnosis of cancer is in the third decade, so that colectomy in adult life may be advisable. Two genes have been identified as causative – *SMAD4* (18q), previously known as *DPC4*, and *BMPR1A* (10q22). Both are components of the TGF-β signaling pathway and *SMAD4* mutations, which account for about 60% of cases, appear to carry a higher malignancy potential and the possibility of large numbers of gastric polyps.

### Cowden disease

Also known as *multiple hamartoma syndrome*, Cowden disease is autosomal dominant but very variable. Gastrointestinal polyps are found in about half of the cases and are generally benign hamartomas or adenomas. Multiple lipomas occur with similar frequency and the oral mucosa may have a 'cobblestone' appearance. Macrocephaly is common in this condition. Importantly, however, there is a high incidence (50%) of breast cancer in females, usually occurring at a young age, and papillary thyroid carcinoma affects about 7% of cases. Mutations in the tumor suppressor *PTEN* gene on chromosome 10q23, encoding a tyrosine phosphatase, cause Cowden disease. A related phenotype with many overlapping features, which glories in the eponymous name Bannayan–Riley–Ruvalcaba syndrome, has also been shown to be due to mutations in *PTEN* in a large proportion of cases.

### Peutz–Jegher syndrome

Also autosomal dominant, this condition is characterized by the presence of dark melanin spots on the lips, around the mouth, on the palms and plantar areas, and other extremities. These are usually present in childhood and can fade in adult life. Patients often present with colicky abdominal pain from childhood due to the development of multiple polyps that occur throughout the gastrointestinal tract, though they are most common in the small intestine. These are hamartomas but there is a significant risk of malignant transformation. There is an increased risk of cancers at other sites, particularly breast, uterus, ovary and testis, and these tend to occur in early adult life. Regular screening for these cancers throughout life, from early adulthood, is warranted. Mutations in a novel serine threonine kinase gene, *STK11*, located on chromosome 19p, cause PJS.

## BREAST CANCER

Approximately 1 in 12 women in Western societies will develop breast cancer, this being the most common cancer in women between 40 and 55 years of age, with approximately 1 in 3 affected women going on to develop metastatic disease. Fifteen to 20% of women who develop breast cancer have a family history of the disorder. Family studies have shown that the risk of a woman developing breast cancer is greater when one or more of the following factors is present in the family history: (1) a clustering of cases in close female relatives; (2) early age (<50 years) of presentation; (3) the occurrence of bilateral disease; (4) the additional occurrence of ovarian cancer.

Molecular studies of breast cancer tumors have revealed a variety of different findings that included amplification of *erb*-B1, *erb*-B2, *myc* and *int*-2 oncogenes as well as LOH at a number of chromosomal sites, including (in descending order of frequency) 7q, 16q, 13q, 17p, 8p, 21q, 3p, 18q, 2q, and 19p, as well as several other regions with known candidate genes or fragile sites. In many breast tumors showing LOH, allele loss occurs at between two and four of the sites, again suggesting that the accumulation of alterations, rather than their order, is important in the evolution of breast cancer. One potentially key element in the development of sporadic breast cancer, and sporadic ovarian cancer, is a newly discovered gene named *EMSY*. This was found to be amplified in 13% of breast cancers and 17% of ovarian cancers, and was ascertained through looking for DNA sequences that interact with *BRCA2*. The normal function of *EMSY* may be to switch off *BRCA2*, which may point to an important pathway of control of cell growth in these tissues.

### *BRCA1* and *BRCA2* genes

Family studies of early-onset or premenopausal breast cancer showed that it behaved like a dominant trait in many families. Linkage analysis in these families showed that the tendency to develop breast cancer mapped to the long arm of chromosome 17, eventually leading to identification of the *BRCA1* gene. A proportion of families with early-onset breast cancer that did not show linkage to this region showed linkage to the long arm of chromosome 13 resulting in the identification of the *BRCA2* gene.

Approximately 40–50% of families with early-onset autosomal dominant breast cancer have a mutation in the *BRCA1* gene and have been shown to have a 60–85% lifetime risk of developing breast cancer. Individuals with a mutation in the *BRCA1* gene also have an increased risk of developing bowel cancer, females an increased risk of developing ovarian cancer, and males an increased risk of developing prostate cancer. Mutations in the *BRCA2* gene account for 30–40% of families with early-onset autosomal dominant breast cancer and the lifetime risk of developing breast cancer is similar. Although initially mutations in the *BRCA2* gene were not thought to be associated with an increased risk of other cancers, women heterozygous for a mutation have a slightly increased risk of developing ovarian cancer. In some of the original families with familial breast cancer collected for linkage studies, a number had males who developed breast cancer. Although breast cancer in males is very rare, males with mutations in the *BRCA2* gene have been shown to have a 6% lifetime risk of developing breast cancer, approximately a 100-fold increase in the population risk of breast cancer in males.

## OVARIAN CANCER

Approximately one in 70 women develops ovarian cancer, the incidence increasing with age. The majority arise as a result of genetic alterations within the ovarian surface epithelium and are therefore referred to as *epithelial* ovarian cancer. In general it is a poorly understood disease, though recent studies have shown a high frequency of LOH at 11q25 in tumor tissue. A possible tumor suppressor gene at this locus is *OPCML*, which encodes a cell adhesion molecule that includes an immunoglobulin domain. Approximately 5% of women with ovarian cancer have a family history of the disorder and it is estimated that 1% of all ovarian cancer follows dominant inheritance because it is strongly predisposed by single gene mutations. In families with multiple women affected with ovarian cancer, the age of presentation is 10–15 years earlier than with non-hereditary ovarian cancer in the general population. Mutations in *BRCA1*, *BRCA2*, and less commonly the genes responsible for HNPCC, will be responsible for a proportion of these families, but a susceptibility gene locus for site-specific ovarian cancer has yet to be identified.

## PROSTATE CANCER

Prostate cancer is the most common cancer affecting men, being the most common cancer after breast, with men having a lifetime risk of 10% of developing prostate cancer and a 3% chance of dying from it. Enquiries into the family history of males presenting with prostate cancer have revealed a significant proportion – in the region of 15% – to have a first-degree male relative with prostate cancer. Family studies have shown that first-degree male relatives of a man presenting with prostate cancer have between two and five times the population risk of developing prostate cancer. Analysis of prostate cancer tumor material has revealed LOH at several chromosomal locations. Segregation analysis of family studies of prostate cancer suggested that a single dominant susceptibility locus could be responsible, accounting for 9% of all prostate cancers and up to 40% of early-onset prostate cancers (diagnosed under age 55 years). Linkage analysis studies identified two major susceptibility loci, hereditary prostate cancer-1 and 2 (HPC1 and HPC2), and a number of other more minor susceptibility loci have been reported. Recently mutations in the ribonuclease L gene (*RNASEL*) were identified in two families showing linkage to the HPC1 locus at 1q25. Mutations have been found in the *ELAC2* gene at 17p11, the HPC2 locus, and, rarely, mutations in three genes – *PTEN*, *MXI1* and *KAI1* – have been identified in a minority of families with familial prostate cancer. A small proportion of familial prostate cancer is associated with *BRCA1* or *BRCA2*. Men who carry mutations in either *BRCA1* or *BRCA2* have an increased risk and in one study, conducted in Ashkenazi Jews, men with such mutations had a 16% risk of prostate cancer by age 70 years, compared with 3.8% for the general population.

**Table 14.5 Features suggestive of an inherited cancer susceptibility syndrome in a family**

| |
|---|
| Several close (first- or second-degree) relatives with a common cancer |
| Several close relatives with related cancers, e.g. breast and ovary or bowel and endometrial |
| Two family members with the same rare cancer |
| An unusually early age of onset |
| Bilateral tumors in paired organs |
| Synchronous or successive tumors |
| Tumors in two different organ systems in one individual |

Although the majority of prostate cancers occur in men after the age of 65 years, individuals with a family history of prostate cancer consistent with the possibility of a dominant gene being responsible have a significantly increased risk of developing prostate cancer at a relatively younger age (less than 55 years). Screening by measuring prostate-specific antigen (PSA) levels has been suggested, but problems with specificity and sensitivity mean that this has limited value.

## GENETIC COUNSELING IN FAMILIAL CANCER

Recognition of individuals with an inherited susceptibility to cancer usually relies on taking a careful family history to document the presence or absence of other family members with similar or related cancers. The malignancies which develop in susceptible individuals are often the same as those that occur in the population in general. There are a number of other features that can suggest an inherited cancer susceptibility syndrome in a family (Table 14.5).

### INHERITED CANCER-PREDISPOSING SYNDROMES

While most cancers due to an inherited cancer syndrome occur at a specific site, families have been described in which cancers occur at more than one site in an individual or at different sites in various members of the family more commonly than would be expected. These families are referred to as having a familial cancer-predisposing syndrome. The majority of the rare inherited familial cancer-predisposing syndromes currently recognized are dominantly inherited, with offspring of affected individuals having a 50% chance of inheriting the gene and therefore of being at increased risk of developing cancer (Table 14.6). There are also a number of syndromes usually inherited as autosomal recessive disorders with an increased risk of developing cancer associated with an increased number of abnormalities in the chromosomes

**Table 14.6 Inherited family cancer syndromes, mode of inheritance, gene responsible and chromosomal site**

| Syndrome | Mode of inheritance* | Gene | Chromosomal site | Main cancer(s) |
|---|---|---|---|---|
| Breast/ovary families | AD | *BRCA1* | 17q21 | Breast, ovary, colon, prostate |
| Breast families | AD | *BRCA2* | 13q12 | Breast, ovary |
| Familial adenomatous polyposis | AD | *APC* | 5q21 | Colorectal, duodenal, thyroid |
| Turcot's | AD | *APC*<br>*hMLH1*<br>*hMSH2* | 5q21<br>3p21<br>2p15–16 | Colorectal, brain |
| Hereditary non-polyposis colorectal cancer (HNPCC) | | | | |
| • Lynch I | AD | *hMSH2*<br>*hMSH6*<br>*hMLH1*<br>*hPMS1*<br>*hPMS2* | 2p15–16<br>2p15-16<br>3p21<br>2q31<br>7p22 | Colorectal |
| • Lynch II | AD | *hMSH2*<br>*hMLH1*<br>*hPMS1*<br>*hPMS2* | 2p15–16<br>3p21<br>2q31<br>7p22 | Colorectal, endometrial, urinary tract, ovarian, gastric, small bowel, hepatobiliary |
| MYH polyposis | AR | *MYH* 1p33 | | |
| Muir–Torre | AD | *hMSH2* | 2p15–16 | As Lynch II plus sebaceous tumors, laryngeal |
| Juvenile polyposis | AD | *SMAD4/DPC4*<br>*BMPR1A* | 18q21.1<br>10q22 | Colorectal |
| Peutz–Jeghers | AD | *STK11* | 19p13.3 | Gastrointestinal, breast, uterus, ovary, testis |
| Cowden disease | AD | *PTEN* | 10q23 | |
| Familial retinoblastoma | AD | *RB1* | 13q14 | Retinoblastoma |
| Li–Fraumeni | AD | *Tp53* | 17p13 | Sarcoma, breast, brain, leukemia, adrenal cortex |
| Multiple endocrine neoplasia (MEN) Type 1 (MEN1) | AD | *MEN1* | 11q13 | Parathyroid, thyroid, anterior pituitary, pancreatic islet cells, adrenal |
| Type II (MEN2) | AD | *RET* | 10q11.2 | Thyroid (medullary), pheochromocytoma |
| von Hippel–Lindau | AD | *VHL* | 3p25–26 | CNS hemangioblastoma, renal, pancreatic, pheochromocytoma |
| Gorlin (nevoid basal cell carcinoma) syndrome | AD | *PTCH* | 9q22 | Basal cell carcinomas, medulloblastoma, ovarian fibromas, (odontogenic keratocysts) |
| Dysplastic nevus syndrome | AD | *CMM1* | 1p | Melanoma (familial atypical mole melanoma, FAMM) |

*AD: autosomal dominant

when they are cultured, or what are known as the chromosomal breakage syndromes. These are discussed in detail in Chapter 18 (p. 287).

Persons with an inherited familial cancer-predisposing syndrome are at risk of developing a second tumor (multifocal or bilateral in the case of breast cancer), have an increased risk of developing a cancer at a relatively younger age than persons with the sporadic form, and can develop tumors at different sites in the body, although one type of cancer is usually predominant.

A number of different familial cancer-predisposing syndromes have been described, depending on the patterns of cancer occurring in a family. For example, persons with the Li–Fraumeni syndrome (p. 213) are at risk of developing adrenocortical tumors, soft-tissue sarcomas, breast cancer, brain tumors and leukemia – sometimes at a strikingly young age. The cancer-predisposing syndrome HNPCC used to be clinically separated into Lynch type I, in which family members appear to only be at risk for cancer of the colon, and Lynch type II (sometimes, confusingly, known as the *cancer family syndrome*), in which family members are also at risk for a number of other cancers, including stomach, endometrial, breast and renal transitional cell carcinomas. However, progress at the molecular level has highlighted the difficulty of the Lynch classification as individuals from families with both type I and II characteristics have been found to have mutations in any one of the mismatch repair genes (Table 14.4). Furthermore, Turcot syndrome is due to mutations in the *APC* gene and two of the mismatch repair genes, whilst Muir–Torre syndrome results from mutations in the *hMSH2* mismatch repair gene. Individuals at risk in such families should, however, be screened for the appropriate cancers (p. 222).

**Table 14.7 Lifetime risk of colorectal cancer for an individual according to the family history of colorectal cancer**

| | |
|---|---|
| Population risk | 1 in 50 |
| One first-degree relative affected | 1 in 17 |
| One first-degree relative and one second-degree relative affected | 1 in 12 |
| One relative aged under 45 affected | 1 in 10 |
| Two first-degree relatives affected | 1 in 6 |
| Three or more first-degree relatives affected | 1 in 2 |

From Houlston R S, Murday V, Harocopos C, Williams C B, Slack J 1990 Screening and genetic counselling for relatives of patients with colorectal cancer in a family screening clinic. Br Med J 301: 366–368

**Table 14.8 Lifetime risk of breast cancer in females according to the family history of breast cancer**

| | |
|---|---|
| Population risk | 1 in 12 |
| Sister diagnosed 65–70 years of age | 1 in 8 |
| Sister diagnosed under 40 years of age | 1 in 4 |
| Two first-degree relatives affected under 40 years of age | 1 in 3 |

## INHERITED SUSCEPTIBILITY FOR THE COMMON CANCERS

The majority of persons at an increased risk of developing cancer because of their family history do not have one of the cancer-predisposing syndromes. The level of risk for persons with a family history of one of the common cancers such as bowel or breast cancer depends on a number of factors. These include the number of persons with cancer in the family, how closely related the person at risk is to the affected individuals, and the age at which the affected family member(s) developed cancer. A few families with a large number of members affected with one of the common cancers are consistent with a dominantly inherited cancer susceptibility gene. In most instances there are only a few individuals with cancer in a family, and there is doubt about whether a cancer susceptibility gene is responsible or not. In such an instance one relies on empirical data gained from epidemiological studies to provide risk estimates (Tables 14.7 and 14.8).

## SCREENING FOR FAMILIAL CANCER

Prevention or early detection of cancer is the ultimate goal of screening individuals at risk of familial cancer. The means of prevention for certain cancers can include a change in lifestyle or diet, drug therapy, prophylactic surgery or screening.

Screening of persons at risk for familial cancer is usually directed at detecting the phenotypic expression of the genotype, i.e. surveillance for a particular cancer or its precursor. Screening can also include diagnostic tests that indirectly reveal the genotype, looking for other clinical features that are evidence of the presence or absence of the gene. For example, individuals at risk for familial adenomatous polyposis can be screened for evidence of the *APC* gene by retinal examination looking for areas of *c*ongenital *h*ypertrophy of the *r*etinal *p*igment *e*pithelium, or what is known as *CHRPEs*. The finding of CHRPEs increases the likelihood of an individual at risk being heterozygous for the *APC* gene and therefore developing polyposis and malignancy. We now know that CHRPEs are seen in persons with FAP when mutations occur in the first part of the *APC* gene, an example of a genotype–phenotype correlation (p. 27).

More recently, identification of the gene responsible for a number of the cancer-predisposing syndromes, and determination of the genotypic status, i.e. presymptomatic testing (p. 318), of an individual at risk allows more efficient delivery of surveillance screening for the phenotypic expression, e.g. renal cancer, CNS tumors and pheochromocytomas in VHL disease (Table 14.9). For those who test negative for the family mutation, expensive and time-consuming screening is unnecessary. As more genes for cancer susceptibility are discovered there will be an increasing number of conditions for which DNA testing will enable presymptomatic determination of genotypic status.

While the potential for prevention of cancer through screening persons at high risk is considerable, it is important to remember that the impact on the overall rate of cancer in the population in general will be small as only a minority of all common cancers are due to gene mutations following straightforward Mendelian inheritance.

## Familial cancer-predisposing syndromes

Many familial cancer-predisposing syndromes are inherited as autosomal dominant traits that are fully penetrant, with the consequent risk for heterozygotes of developing cancer approaching 100%. This level of risk means that more invasive means of screening with more frequent and earlier initiation of screening protocols are justified than would be acceptable for the population in general (Table 14.9).

## Inherited susceptibility for the common cancers

Screening for the common cancers arising from inherited susceptibility has only relatively recently been established and by its very nature involves a long-term undertaking for the individual at risk as well as his/her physician or surgeon. It is important to emphasize that the natural enthusiasm for screening needs to be balanced with the paucity of hard data in many instances on the relative benefits and risks. Recommended screening protocols at present are often based on current opinion rather than on formal evidence-based medicine (Table 14.10).

## Who should be screened?

In the case of the rare dominantly inherited single-gene familial cancer-predisposing syndromes such as FAP, VHL and MEN, those who should be screened can be identified on a simple Mendelian basis. However, for retinoblastoma, for example, the situation is more complex. If no *RB1* mutation has been identified presymptomatic genetic testing cannot be offered. Some individuals with the non-hereditary form have bilateral tumors whilst some with the hereditary form have no tumor (i.e. the condition is non-penetrant) or a unilateral tumor. It may be impossible to distinguish which form is present, and screening of second-degree, as well as first-degree, relatives may be appropriate given that early detection can successfully prevent blindness. For persons with a family history of the common cancers, such as bowel or breast cancer, the risk levels at which screening is recommended and below which screening is not likely to be of benefit will vary. At each extreme of risk the decision is usually straightforward, but with intermediate-level risks there can be doubt as to relative benefits and risks of screening.

## What age and how often?

Cancer in persons with a familial cancer-predisposing syndrome tends to occur at a relatively earlier age than in the general population and screening programs must reflect this. With the exception of familial adenomatous polyposis, in which it is recommended that sigmoidoscopy to detect rectal polyps should start in the teenage years, most cancer screening programs do not start until 25 years of age or later. The highest-risk age band for most inherited susceptibilities is 35–50 years, but because cancer can still develop in those at risk at a later age, screening is usually continued thereafter. In some families the age of onset of cancer can be especially early and it is recommended that screening of at-risk individuals in these families commences 5 years before the age of onset in the earliest affected member of the family. Again, retinoblastoma is an exception to the usual rule because, as it is a cancer of early childhood, screening starts in the postnatal period with frequent ophthalmic examination.

The recommended interval between repeated screening procedures should be determined from the natural history of the particular cancer. The development of colorectal cancer from an adenoma is believed to take place over a number of years and as a result it is thought that 5-yearly screening intervals will suffice. If, however, a polyp is found, then the interval between screening procedures is usually brought down to 3 years. Breast cancer is not detectable in a premalignant stage and early diagnosis is critical if there is to be a good prognosis. Annual mammography for females at high risk is therefore recommended from the age of 35 years.

## What sites should be screened?

Having decided who is at risk within a family, one has to judge which types of cancer are most likely to occur and which systems of the body should be screened.

### *Familial cancer-predisposing syndromes*

This can be a very difficult problem with some of the family cancer syndromes, such as the old Lynch type II form of HNPCC, in which a person at risk can develop cancer at a number of different sites. Screening for every possible cancer that can occur would mean frequent investigation by a variety of different specialists and/or investigations. This would result in an unwieldy and unpleasant protocol. Persons at risk for HNPCC should have regular colonoscopy, and females may be offered pelvic screening for gynecological malignancies, although the efficacy is very debatable. Some of the other cancers that can occur in persons at risk for Lynch type II, such as stomach cancer, are not seen in every family,

**Table 14.9 Suggested guidelines for screening persons at risk for the familial cancer-predisposing syndromes or for one of the common cancers**

| Condition/cancer | Screening test | Frequency | Starting age |
|---|---|---|---|
| **Familial susceptibility for the common cancers** | | | |
| **Breast cancer** | | | |
| Breast | Mammography | Annual | 35 (2 yearly from 50) |
| **Breast/ovary** | | | |
| Breast | Mammography | Annual | 35 (2 yearly from 50) |
| Ovary | US/Doppler, CA125 | Annual | 25 |
| **Familial cancer-predisposing syndromes** | | | |
| Familial adenomatous polyposis | Retinal examination (CHRPE)* | | Childhood |
| Colorectal | Sigmoid/colonoscopy*+ | Annual | 12 |
| Duodenal | Gastroscopy | 3 yearly | 20 |
| Thyroid (women) | None/US? | Annual | 20 |
| **HNPCC–Lynch I** | | | |
| Colorectal | Colonoscopy | 3–5 yearly | 35 |
| **HNPCC–Lynch II** | | | |
| Colorectal | Colonoscopy | 3–5 yearly | 35 |
| Endometrial | US | Annual | 35 |
| Ovary | US | Annual | 25 |
| Renal tract | US | Annual | 35 |
| Gastric | Gastroscopy | 1–2 yearly | 35 |
| Small bowel | None | | |
| Hepatobiliary | None | | |
| Breast | Mammography | Annual | 35 (2 yearly from 50) |
| **Li–Fraumeni** | | | |
| Breast | Mammography | Annual | 35? (2 yearly from 50) |
| Sarcoma | None | | |
| Brain | None | | |
| Leukemia | None | | |
| Adrenal cortex | None | | |
| **Retinoblastoma** | Retinal examination | Frequently | From birth |
| **Multiple endocrine neoplasia** | | | |
| Type 1 | $Ca^{2+}$, PTH, pituitary hormones, | Annual | 8 years, up to 50 |
| **Pancreatic hormones** | | | |
| Type 2 | Calcitonin provocation test* | | 10 years |
| Medullary thyroid | US | ? | 10 |
| Pheochromocytoma | Urinary VMA | Annual | 10 |
| Parathyroid adenoma | $Ca^{2+}$, $PO_4$, PTH | Annual | 10 |
| **von Hippel–Lindau** | | | |
| Retinal angioma | Retinal examination* | Annual | 5 |
| Hemangioblastoma | CNS CT/MRI | 3 yearly | 15 (5 yearly from 40 years) |
| Pheochromocytoma | Urinary VMA | Annual | 10 |
| Renal | Abdominal CT | 3 yearly | 20 |
| Abdominal US | Annual | 20 | |
| **Gorlin (nevoid basal cell carcinoma) syndrome** | | | |
| BCCs | Clinical surveillance | Annual | 10 |
| Medulloblastoma | Clinical surveillance | Annual | Infancy |
| Odontogenic keratocysts | Orthpantomogram | 6-monthly | 10 |

*Test to detect heterozygous state

+ In individuals found to be affected, annual colonoscopy prior to colectomy and lifelong 4–6-monthly surveillance of the rectal stump, after subtotal colectomy

US: ultrasound; CHRPE: congenital hypertrophy of the retinal pigment epithelium; CT: computed tomography; MRI: magnetic resonance imaging; PTH: parathyroid hormone; VMA: vanillyl mandelic acid

**Table 14.10 Requirements of a screening test for persons at risk for a familial cancer-predisposing syndrome or at increased risk for the common cancers**

| |
|---|
| The test should detect a malignant or premalignant condition at a stage prior to its producing symptoms, with high sensitivity and specificity |
| The treatment of persons detected by screening should improve the prognosis |
| The benefit of early detection should outweigh potential harm from the screening test |
| The test should preferably be non-invasive since most at-risk individuals require long-term surveillance |
| Adequate provision for prescreening counseling and follow-up should be available |

and so screening is usually restricted to persons from those families to those cancers that have affected at least one family member. In persons at risk for the Li–Fraumeni syndrome, a wide spectrum of cancers can occur. However, apart from regular mammography, no satisfactory screening is available for the other malignancies (Table 14.9).

## *Inherited susceptibility for the common cancers*

### Colorectal cancer

Colorectal carcinoma holds the greatest promise for prevention by screening. Endoscopy provides a sensitive and specific means of examination of the colorectal mucosa and polypectomy can be carried out with relative ease so that screening, diagnosis and treatment can take place concurrently. While colonoscopy is the preferred screening method, it requires a skilled operator and, as it is an invasive procedure, it has a small but consequent morbidity. Because of this, and in order to target screening to those most likely to benefit, most genetic centers have adopted the so-called *Amsterdam criteria* to select the high-risk individual. These minimal criteria suggest a familial form of colon cancer:

1. At least three affected relatives (related to each other by first-degree relationships), one a first-degree relative of the other two; FAP excluded.
2. At least two successive generations affected.
3. Cancer diagnosed before age 50 in at least one relative.

Failure to visualize the right side of the colon with colonoscopy necessitates a barium enema to view this region, particularly in persons at risk for HNPCC, in which proximal right-sided involvement commonly occurs. For persons with a moderately increased risk of developing colorectal cancer, the majority of cancers occur in the distal (left-sided) colon and at a relatively later age. Flexible sigmoidoscopy, which is much less invasive than colonoscopy, provides an adequate screening tool for persons in this risk group and can be employed from the age of 50 years.

### Breast cancer

In the UK screening of women aged 50 years and over for breast cancer by regular mammography has become established as a national program as a result of studies demonstrating improved survival of women detected as having early breast cancer. For women with an increased risk of developing breast cancer because of their family history, there is conflicting evidence of the relative benefit of screening with respect to the frequency of mammography and the chance of developing breast cancer in the interval between the screening procedures, or what is termed interval cancer. One reason is that cancer detection rates are lower in premenopausal than in postmenopausal breast tissue.

It is also argued that the radiation exposure associated with annual mammography could be detrimental if started at an early age, leading to an increased risk of breast cancer through the screening when carried out over a long period of time. This is of particular concern in families with the Li–Fraumeni syndrome because mutations in the *Tp53* gene have been shown experimentally in vitro to impair the repair of DNA damaged by X-irradiation. However, most experts currently believe that there is a greater relative benefit than risk in identifying and treating breast cancer in women from this high-risk group, although formal evaluation of such screening programs continues.

Mammography is usually only offered to women at increased risk of breast cancer after the age of 35 years, since interpretation of mammograms is difficult before this age because of the density of the breasts. As a consequence, women at increased risk of developing breast cancer should be taught breast self-examination and undergo regular clinical examination.

### Ovarian cancer

Ovarian cancer in the early stages is frequently asymptomatic and often incurable by the time a woman presents with symptoms. Early diagnosis of ovarian cancer in individuals at high risk is vital, with prophylactic oophorectomy being the only logical, if radical, alternative. The position of the ovaries within the pelvis makes screening difficult. Ultrasound imaging provides the most sensitive means of screening. Transvaginal scanning is more sensitive than conventional transabdominal scanning, and the use of color Doppler blood flow imaging further enhances screening of women at increased risk. If a suspicious feature is seen on scanning and confirmed on further investigation, then laparoscopy or a laparotomy is usually required to confirm the diagnosis. Screening should be carried out annually as

CHAPTER

# 15 Genetic factors in common diseases

Medical genetics usually concentrates on the study of rare unifactorial chromosomal and single-gene disorders. Diseases such as diabetes, cancer, cardiovascular and coronary artery disease, mental health and neuro-degenerative disorders are responsible, however, for the majority of the morbidity and mortality in developed countries. These so-called *common* diseases are likely to be of even greater importance in the future, with the elderly accounting for an increasing proportion of the population.

The common diseases do not usually show a simple pattern of inheritance. Instead the contributing genetic factors are often multiple, interacting with each other and environmental factors in a complex manner. In fact, it is uncommon for either genetic or environmental factors to be entirely responsible for a particular common disorder or disease in a single individual. In most instances both genetic and environmental factors are contributory, although sometimes one can appear more important than the other (Fig. 15.1).

At one extreme are diseases such as Duchenne muscular dystrophy; these are exclusively genetic in origin and the environment plays little or no direct part in the etiology. At the other extreme are infectious diseases that are almost entirely the result of environmental factors. Between these two extremes are the common diseases and disorders such as diabetes mellitus, hypertension, cerebrovascular and coronary artery disease, schizophrenia, the common cancers and the congenital abnormalities, in which both genetic and environmental factors are involved.

## GENETIC SUSCEPTIBILTY TO COMMON DISEASE

For many of the common diseases a small but significant proportion of cases have single-gene causes, but the major proportion of the genetic basis of common diseases can be considered to be the result of an inherited predisposition or genetic susceptibility. Common diseases result from a complex interaction of the effects of multiple different genes, or what is known as *polygenic inheritance*, with environmental factors and influences, due to what is known as *multifactorial inheritance* (p. 139).

If the underlying genetic factors were understood, it would be possible to offer genetic testing to identify those persons genetically susceptible to a particular disorder.

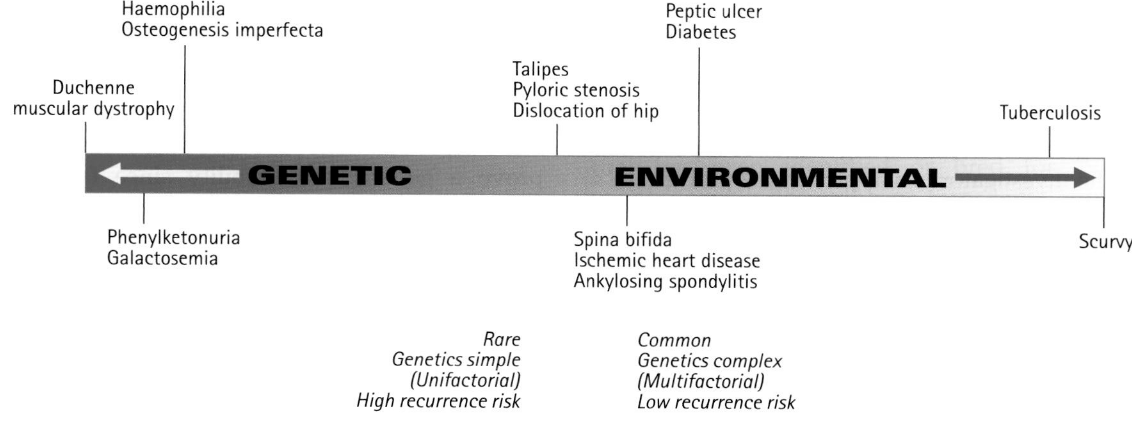


**Fig. 15.1**
Human disease represented as being on a spectrum ranging from those that are largely environmental in causation to those that are entirely genetic.

mellitus (T1DM) accounts for 5–10% of diabetes. T1DM has a peak age of onset in adolescence and can only be controlled by regular injection of insulin. The second more common form is known as type 2 or non-insulin-dependent diabetes mellitus (T2DM). T2DM usually affects older persons and may respond to simple dietary restriction of carbohydrate intake, although many persons with T2DM require oral hypoglycemic medication, and some require insulin.

An additional 1–2% of persons with diabetes have a *monogenic* (single-gene) form of diabetes called maturity-onset diabetes of the young (MODY).

Lastly, 1–3% of women develop glucose intolerance during pregnancy. This is known as *gestational diabetes*. Their abnormal glucose tolerance usually reverts to normal after the pregnancy, although approximately one-half to three-quarters of these women go on to develop diabetes later in life.

Diabetes can also occur secondary to a variety of other rare genetic syndromes and non-genetic disorders. Examples include Prader–Willi syndrome (p. 118), Bardet–Biedl syndrome, Wolfram syndrome and Friedreich ataxia (p. 25) Diabetes mellitus is therefore etiologically heterogeneous.

**Table 15.2 Population and recurrence risks for T2DM and T1DM**

| Group | % |
|---|---|
| **T2DM** | |
| **Population** | **4–5 (ages 20–74)** |
| First-degree relatives | 10–15 |
| **T1DM** | |
| **Population** | **0.2** |
| 1 high-risk allele (DR3 or DR4) | 0.25 |
| HLA DR3/3 or HLA DR4/4 | 0.75 |
| HLA DR3/4 | 2.5 |
| **Relatives** | |
| **Siblings** | **7** |
| No antigens shared | 1 |
| 1 antigen shared | 5 |
| 2 antigens shared | 16 |
| 2 antigens shared — DR3/4 | 20–25 |
| **Offspring** | **4** |
| Offspring of affected female | 2–2.5 |
| Offspring of affected male | 5 |

From Rotter J I, Vadhein C M, Rimoin D L Diabetes mellitus, Chapter 21 in King, Rotter and Motulsky 1992

## EVIDENCE FOR GENETIC FACTORS

Diabetes can affect up to 10% of the population in developed countries with the prevalence varying between different population and ethnic groups. For example, T1DM is 20 times more common in North America than in China. While migration studies are consistent with a significant environmental contribution, particularly in T2DM, the evidence from family and twin studies suggests that there is a significant genetic contribution to the etiology of diabetes mellitus.

### Family studies

Between 25% and 50% of diabetics have a family history of diabetes as opposed to less than 15% in the general population. A variety of formal family studies have shown a prevalence of diabetes in relatives that ranges from 10% to 30% compared to between 1% and 6% in relatives of non-diabetics (Table 15.2). The criteria for the diagnosis of diabetes used in the different studies have not, however, always been the same, ranging from frank clinical diabetes through formal glucose tolerance tests to random blood sugars. In addition, while some studies looked at risks in relatives dependent on the type or age of onset of the diabetes in the proband, many of the studies considered all ages of onset and different types of diabetes together. These factors can account, to some extent, for the differences seen in the percentage of affected relatives in the various studies.

### Twin studies

A number of surveys have shown that between 45% and 96% of identical twins are concordant for diabetes whereas between only 3% and 37% of non-identical twins are. More recent twin studies in which the concordance rates for insulin-dependent and non-insulin-dependent diabetes have been looked at separately have shown concordance rates in identical twins for the former to be in the region of 30–50% while for the latter they have been in excess of 90%. These data indicate that genetic factors are important in both forms of diabetes. The fact that a significant proportion of the identical twins were discordant for IDDM suggests that environmental factors have a significant influence in that form of diabetes. The very high concordance rate of MZ twins for T2DM suggests that the primary determining factor is genetic, although a diabetogenic diet is necessary for the susceptibility to be expressed.

## SINGLE-GENE DISORDERS

Rare forms of diabetes which show high penetrance within families are usually due to mutations in single genes. Maturity-onset diabetes of the young (MODY) is an example of a monogenic form of diabetes (see Table 15.3).

### Maturity-onset diabetes of the young

MODY is an autosomal dominant form of diabetes characterized by β-cell dysfunction. It shows clinical heterogeneity that can now be explained by genetic heterogeneity. Mutations in the glucokinase gene cause

**Table 15.3 Subtypes of diabetes**

| | Type 1 diabetes | Type 2 diabetes | MODY |
|---|---|---|---|
| Prevalence | <1% | <10% | <0.01% |
| Age of onset | Childhood/ adolescence | Middle/ old age | Adolescence/ early adulthood |
| Inheritance | Polygenic | Polygenic | Monogenic |
| Number of genes | >20 loci | Numerous | At least 7 genes |
| Pathophysiology | Autoimmune | Insulin secretion/ resistance | β Cell dysfunction |

mild hyperglycemia (usually between 5.5 and 8 mmol/l), which is stable throughout life and often treated by diet alone. Glucokinase is described as the pancreatic glucose sensor because it catalyses the rate-limiting step of glucose metabolism in the pancreatic β cell. It was therefore an obvious candidate gene. Many patients with glucokinase mutations are asymptomatic and their hyperglycemia is detected during routine screening, for example during pregnancy or employment medicals. The mild phenotype means that finding a glucokinase mutation is 'good news'.

Mutations in five additional genes that encode transcription factors required for development of the β cell have been reported. The hepatocyte nuclear factor 1 α (*HNF-1α*) and hepatocyte nuclear factor 4 α (*HNF-4α*) genes were identified through positional cloning efforts and are associated with a more severe, progressive form of diabetes usually diagnosed during the teens or early adulthood. These patients are sensitive to treatment with sulfonylurea tablets; this is an example of pharmacogenetics. Good glycemic control is important as patients have a long duration of diabetes and may suffer from diabetic complications. Mutations in the *HNF-1α* gene are the most common cause of MODY in most populations (65% of UK MODY), but *HNF-4α* mutations are less frequent.

Hepatocyte nuclear factor 1 β (HNF-1β) plays a key role in development of the kidney. Mutations cause renal cysts and diabetes (RCAD) and some female patients also have genital tract malformations. Insulin promoter factor 1 (*IPF-1*) and *NEURO D1* mutations are rare causes of MODY but highlight the possibility that further genes encoding β-cell transcription factors may be mutated in MODY (so called MODYX genes).

## ASSOCIATED RISK FACTORS

Monogenic forms of diabetes account for only 1–2% of diabetes. The remainder is multifactorial in origin and a number of loci have been shown to be associated with an increased risk of developing diabetes.

### T1DM

Persons with T1DM are recognized to have an increased risk of developing autoimmune disorders such as autoimmune thyroiditis, pernicious anemia and Addison disease. A significant proportion of persons with T1DM also develop pancreatic islet cell antibodies. Not surprisingly, perhaps, T1DM has been found to be associated with specific HLA antigens, with 95% of persons with T1DM having the HLA DR3 and/or DR4 antigens. The reported peak of onset of T1DM in the autumn and winter seasons, along with the autoimmune observations have suggested the possibility that viral infections, such as mumps, Coxsackie B or cytomegalovirus infection, act as a trigger in genetically susceptible individuals.

Siblings with T1DM have HLA haplotypes (p. 144) in common more frequently than would be expected by chance. An individual with either the DR3 or DR4 HLA antigens has a slightly increased risk of developing T1DM compared to the general population (Table 15.2). The presence of either of these two antigens in siblings of an individual with T1DM significantly increases their chance of developing diabetes, and if a sibling has both high-risk antigens the risk is greatly increased. Linkage studies have shown that the HLA susceptibility locus (*IDDM1*) has the major role in T1DM, accounting for between 30 and 40% of the genetic predisposition. A large number of other loci have been identified as candidate susceptibility genes for T1DM, the only significant one being a VNTR (p. 146) 5′ to the insulin gene on the short arm of chromosome 11, which accounts for around 10% of the genetic susceptibility.

### T2DM

T2DM is not a single disease but rather a genetically heterogeneous group of metabolic disorders sharing glucose intolerance. It remains a diagnosis of exclusion. Genome scanning linkage studies have identified numerous putative loci but the strongest evidence currently supports susceptibility loci on chromosomes 2q, 12q, 20q, and 1q. The gene on 2q has been identified as calpain 10, and an intronic SNP accounts for the linkage observed in the Mexican-American population in which it was mapped (p. 146). Missense variants in the *PPARG* (P12A), *KCNJ11* (E23K), *IPF-1* (D76N) and *HNF-1α* (G319S) genes are associated with a modest increased risk of T2DM (p. 147), but the relative importance of these loci varies between populations.

## ANIMAL MODELS FOR DIABETES

A number of spontaneously occurring animal models for diabetes have been identified which include the non-obese diabetic (nod) mouse for T1DM and the obese diabetic (ob) mouse and GK rat for T2DM. Studies of the genetics of the tendency to diabetes in these animal models are consistent with a minimum of two and up to six or more genes being involved, suggesting that orthologous regions for genes for which linkage is shown would be candidate regions for genes leading to diabetes susceptibility in humans.

## HYPERTENSION

Various studies have shown that between 10% and 25% of the population is hypertensive but the prevalence is age dependent, with up to 40% of 75–79-year-olds being hypertensive. Hypertension leads to an increased morbidity and mortality through a greater risk of stroke, coronary artery and renal disease. Blood pressure may contribute up to 50% of the global cardiovascular epidemic. There is substantial evidence that treatment of hypertension prevents the development of these complications.

Persons with hypertension fall into two groups. In one the onset is usually in early adult life and is a consequence of another disorder, such as kidney disease or abnormalities of certain endocrine glands. This is referred to as *secondary hypertension*. In the second, more common group hypertension usually begins in middle age and there is no recognized cause. This is known as *essential hypertension*. The following discussion is concerned with only essential hypertension.

### ENVIRONMENTAL FACTORS IN HYPERTENSION

Environmental factors, such as high sodium levels in the diet, obesity, alcohol intake and reduced exercise, are recognized as being associated with an increased risk of hypertension. Hypertension is also more prevalent in persons from poorer socioeconomic groups. Studies of adopted children have shown lower correlation of their blood pressure with their biological parents than with children remaining with their biological parents. In addition, migration studies involving persons moving from a population with a low prevalence to one with a high prevalence of hypertension have shown that the immigrant group acquires the frequency of hypertension of their new population group during the course of one to two generations. This suggests that environmental factors are of major importance in the etiology of hypertension.

### GENETIC FACTORS IN HYPERTENSION

Family and twin studies have shown that hypertension is familial (Table 15.4) and that blood pressure correlates with the degree of relationship (Table 15.4). These findings suggest the importance of genetic factors in the etiology of hypertension. In addition, there are differences in the prevalence of hypertension between populations, hypertension being more common in persons of Afro-Caribbean origin and less common in Eskimos, Australian Aborigines and Central and South American Indians.

**Table 15.4 Recurrence risks for hypertension**

| Group | % |
|---|---|
| Population | 5 |
| 2 Normotensive parents | 4 |
| 1 Hypertensive parent | 8–28 |
| 2 Hypertensive parents | 25–45 |

From Burke W, Motulsky A G Hypertension. Chapter 10 in King, Rotter and Motulsky 1992

### POSSIBLE SINGLE-GENE MODELS OF INHERITANCE

If blood pressure measurements are made on a large enough number of persons, the results are normally distributed and show no evidence of any bimodality. Hypertension could therefore be considered to represent one extreme of the normal distribution curve and to be due to the action of many genes that interact with environmental factors, consistent with a multifactorial or polygenic basis.

Another school of thought considers that essential hypertension could be due to a common dominant gene. It is argued that if essential hypertension is a disorder of middle age resulting from the action of a dominant gene, it would be expected that the siblings of hypertensive patients would segregate into two groups: those who inherit the gene for hypertension and those who do not. Analysis of blood pressure readings from siblings of persons known to have hypertension, excluding as far as possible cases of secondary hypertension by choosing all cases from the age group 45–60 years, showed that the blood pressure values of the siblings were not normally distributed but had a bimodal distribution, with two peaks corresponding to systolic blood pressures of 130 and 160 mmHg (Fig. 15.2). This suggested that those with systolic blood pressure values around 130 mmHg had inherited the normal gene, whereas those with systolic blood pressure values around 160 mmHg had inherited the gene for hypertension.

Much of the controversy between these two schools of thought concerning the hereditary nature of hypertension revolves around the definition of bimodality. Critics of the single-gene theory claim that what others have interpreted as bimodality are merely irregularities in the distribution curve that are of no significance. It is argued that with small sample sizes the distribution curve of any variable can show small dips and irregularities, and that if a large

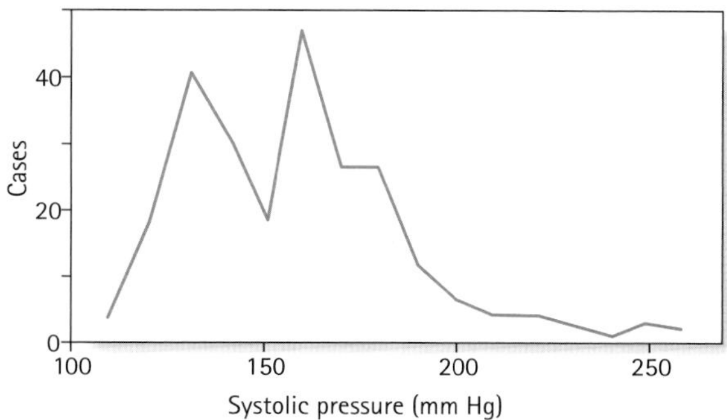


Fig. 15.2
Distribution of systolic blood pressures in 252 siblings of persons aged 45–60 with hypertension. (After Platt R 1959 Lancet ii: 57, with permission.)

enough sample is taken then the resultant distribution curve would be less likely to show any evidence of bimodality.

## BIOCHEMICAL STUDIES

Biochemical studies supported the possibility of a common autosomal dominant gene being responsible for hypertension. Dietary salt has long been recognized as a contributory factor in hypertension and a salt-free diet has been used in its treatment. In some persons with hypertension there appeared to be defective extrusion of sodium from red cells because of an abnormality in the sodium–potassium cotransport in the red cell membrane, resulting in an increased intracellular sodium. This defect was proposed as a major biochemical determinant of hypertension on the basis that this could reflect a generalized membrane abnormality in vessel walls. Family studies showed that this abnormality appeared to be inherited in an autosomal dominant manner.

In communities that use little salt the incidence of hypertension is less than, for example, among the Japanese, who eat large amounts of salty foods. It was proposed that individuals with a defect in sodium–potassium cotransport can eat little salt and develop hypertension. Conversely, persons with normal cotransport can eat large amounts of salt yet remain normotensive.

A second assay of red cell ion transport was developed, known as the sodium–lithium countertransport system. This involved loading red blood cells with lithium and measuring the rate of efflux of lithium from the red cells in high and low sodium concentrations. Increased sodium–lithium countertransport correlated positively with hypertension. Studies of the correlation of sodium–lithium countertransport in different types of biological relatives of hypertensives were compatible with a genetic rather than an environmental basis. Segregation analysis testing different models of inheritance suggested that sodium–lithium countertransport was compatible with a recessive gene of major effect on a polygenic background.

Studies in North American individuals of Afro-Caribbean origin suggested that differences in sodium–lithium countertransport were not as important a factor in that population as in other population groups, even though they were twice as likely to develop hypertension as North Americans of Caucasian origin. This emphasized the importance of possible differences between various population groups in genetic susceptibility.

A third assay, known as the ouabain-sensitive sodium–potassium ATPase system, was investigated as a possible indicator of genetic susceptibility. Attempts to correlate the findings from these various assay systems have not been straightforward, and it is fair to say that these findings have not provided clear evidence for the role of a single gene of major importance in determining predisposition to essential hypertension.

## ASSOCIATED RISK FACTORS

The renin–angiotensin system is integrally involved in the biological control of blood pressure and would seem to provide an obvious series of candidate susceptibility genes for hypertension.

### The renin–angiotensin system

Renin catalyses the cleavage of angiotensinogen to angiotensin I, which is converted to angiotensin II by the angiotensin I converting enzyme (ACE).

### Renin gene

The renin–angiotensin system is rate limiting in angiotensin II production. Although one study has shown that approximately one-third of persons with essential hypertension have elevated renin levels compared to normotensive controls, no association between renin gene polymorphisms or renin levels and hypertension has been demonstrated in a number of different studies.

### Angiotensinogen gene

Angiotensinogen is the substrate for renin. Correlation between angiotensinogen levels and blood pressure suggested that it could have a role in hypertension. Two studies of a microsatellite dinucleotide polymorphism in the 3′ end of the angiotensinogen gene in hypertensive sibling pairs in the USA and France showed a significant frequency of allele sharing in hypertensive sibling pairs. A polymorphic sequence variant has been identified in the angiotensinogen gene that leads to methionine or threonine being present at position 235 in the angiotensinogen protein. The threonine variant has been found to be associated with increased angiotensinogen levels and hypertension in a number of different studies.

### Angiotensin I gene

There is evidence that the angiotensin I gene contributes to the normal control of blood pressure, as well as polymorphic variants in the gene being associated with hypertension in studies of some populations.

### Angiotensin I converting enzyme

Angiotensin I converting enzyme (ACE) converts angiotensin I into angiotensin II and inactivates bradykinin. ACE levels can vary as much as fivefold between different individuals. The variation in ACE levels is, in part, associated with the presence or absence of a polymorphic DNA deletion (D)/insertion (I) in the ACE gene (p. 236), with individuals homozygous for the D allele having ACE levels twice as high as those homozygous for the I allele. A number of different association studies of the ACE polymorphisms with hypertension have not shown consistent results, suggesting they do not play a major role in determining blood pressure.

### Angiotensin II type 1 receptor

The angiotensin II type 1 receptor mediates the biological and physiological effects of the renin–angiotensin system and is, therefore, an obvious candidate gene for genetic susceptibility to hypertension. Increased activity of the receptor could lead to hypertension. Preliminary studies have shown a possible association between hypertension and polymorphic variants in the angiotensin II type 1 receptor.

## PREGNANCY-INDUCED HYPERTENSION

Women who develop pre-eclampsia in pregnancy were thought to have an increased risk of hypertension after the pregnancy. A familial tendency to pre-eclampsia is well recognized. Hormonal influences, such as the elevated estrogen levels of pregnancy, are associated with stimulation of angiotensinogen expression. Preliminary evidence of inherited variation in the angiotensinogen gene has been demonstrated in familial pre-eclampsia.

## ANIMAL MODELS

Animal models of hypertension, such as the SA locus and the α-adducin gene, identified from strains of genetically hypertensive rats, have led to the suggestion that the orthologous regions could contain susceptibility loci for hypertension in humans.

## SUSCEPTIBILITY GENES

To date, there is some evidence for three loci contributing to the predisposition to hypertension, one on the long arm of chromosome 17 (*HYT1*), another on chromosome 16 that is homologous to the SA locus in rats (*HYT3*), and one-third on the long arm of chromosome 15 (*HYT2*). A recent genome-wide scan in 2010 affected sibling pairs (p. 144) failed to confirm these loci but found a major locus on 6q and minor loci on 2q, 5q and 9q.

# CORONARY ARTERY DISEASE

Coronary artery disease is a major cause of morbidity and mortality, accounting for up to 50% of deaths in many of the developed countries. It results from atherosclerosis, a process taking place over many years which involves deposition of lipid in the subendothelial space (intima) of arteries with a consequent narrowing of their lumina. The first stage involves the deposition of lipid in the arterial wall that is determined by hemodynamic factors. Monocytes adhere to areas of the endothelial surface of arterial walls with lipid deposits and enter the vessel wall, proliferate and differentiate into macrophages. The macrophages scavenge the lipids, producing the classic fatty streaks, and through the action of cytokines, growth factors and adhesion molecules induce smooth muscle proliferation and the formation of extracellular matrix that results in the development of the fibrous atherosclerotic plaques. The narrowing of the coronary arteries compromises the metabolic needs of the heart muscle, leading to myocardial ischemia which, if severe, results in myocardial infarction.

## LIPID METABOLISM

The metabolic pathways by which the body absorbs, synthesizes, transports and catabolizes dietary and endogenous lipids are complex. Lipids are packaged in intestinal cells as a complex with various proteins known as *apolipoproteins* to form triglyceride-rich chylomicrons. These are secreted into the lymph and transported to the liver, where, in association with endogenous synthesis of triglyceride and cholesterol, they are packaged and secreted into the circulation as triglyceride-rich very low-density lipoproteins (VLDLs). VLDL is degraded to intermediate-density lipoprotein (IDL), which is further broken down into cholesterol-rich low-density lipoprotein (LDL). High-density lipoproteins (HDLs) are formed from lipoproteins secreted by the liver, chylomicrons and VLDL remnants.

High levels of LDLs are associated with an increased risk of coronary artery disease. Conversely, high levels of

**Table 15.5 Coefficient of correlation for blood pressure in various relatives**

| Group | Correlation coefficient |
|---|---|
| Siblings | 0.12–0.34 |
| Parent/child | 0.12–0.37 |
| Dizygotic twins | 0.25–0.27 |
| Monozygotic twins | 0.55–0.72 |

From Burke W, Motulsky A G Hypertension. Chapter 10 in King, Rotter and Motulsky 1992

**Table 15.6 Recurrence risks for premature coronary artery disease**

| Proband | Relative risk |
|---|---|
| **Male (< 55 years)** | |
| Brother | 5 |
| Sister | 2.5 |
| **Female (< 65 years)** | |
| Siblings | 7 |

Data from Slack J, Evans K A 1966 The increased risk of death from ischaemic heart disease in first degree relatives of 121 men and 96 women with ischaemic heart disease. J Med Genet 3: 239–257

HDLs are inversely correlated with a risk of coronary artery disease. Consequently, the LDL:HDL ratio has been used as a risk predictor for coronary artery disease and as an indicator for therapeutic intervention.

## EPIDEMIOLOGY OF CORONARY ARTERY DISEASE

The incidence of coronary artery disease varies greatly between different population groups, being one-sixth as common in Japan as in many Western countries. These differences can, in part, be attributed to well-known environmental risk factors. Support for this comes from the results of migration studies which show that persons moving from populations with a low risk of coronary artery disease to areas with a high risk acquire the higher risk of their new population group within 10–20 years.

Coronary artery disease can occur secondary to other diseases, such as diabetes mellitus and hypertension. It is also more common in males than in females. After the menopause, the risk for females increases and approaches that of males within 10–15 years as a result of the associated hormonal changes.

Although there are well-recognized environmental factors associated with an increased risk of developing coronary artery disease, it is clear that genetic factors are also important in its etiology.

## FAMILY AND TWIN STUDIES

The familial nature of coronary artery disease has been recognized since the early part of the twentieth century. The risk to a first-degree relative of a person with premature coronary artery disease, defined as occurring before age 55 in males and age 65 in females, varies between two and seven times that for the general population (Table 15.6). Twin studies of concordance for coronary artery disease vary from 15% to 25% for dizygotic twins and from 39% to 48% for monozygotic twins. Although these figures support the involvement of genetic factors, the low concordance rate for monozygotic twins clearly supports the importance of environmental factors.

## SINGLE-GENE DISORDERS OF LIPID METABOLISM LEADING TO CORONARY ARTERY DISEASE

Although there are a number of individually rare inherited disorders of specific lipoproteins, levels of the various lipoproteins and the hyperlipidemias are determined by a complex interaction of genetic and environmental factors. Family studies of some of the hyperlipidemias are, however, consistent with a single gene being a major factor determining genetic susceptibility.

### Familial combined hyperlipidemia

The most common disorder of lipid metabolism associated with an increased risk of early coronary artery disease is familial combined hyperlipidemia (FCH). FCH affects 1 in 200 of the population, is inherited as an autosomal dominant disorder, is associated with elevated triglyceride and cholesterol levels and accounts for approximately 10% of premature coronary artery disease. It has been shown to be genetically heterogeneous, with at least four loci being involved.

### Familial hypercholesterolemia

The best known disorder of lipid metabolism is familial hypercholesterolemia (FH) (p. 170). FH is associated with a significantly increased risk of early coronary artery disease and is inherited as an autosomal dominant disorder. It has been estimated that about 1 person in 500 in the general population, and about 1 in 20 persons presenting with early coronary artery disease, are heterozygous for a mutation in the gene for FH. Molecular studies in FH have revealed that it is due to a variety of defects in the number, function or processing of the LDL receptors on the cell surface (p. 170).

## ASSOCIATED RISK FACTORS

For the majority of persons their risk of coronary artery disease is multifactorial or polygenic in origin. A variety refers to the schizophrenia-like traits often seen in relatives of schizophrenics. The problem arises because clinical criteria to distinguish schizoid from normal personality are lacking. For the sake of simplicity we can regard the term schizoid as referring to a person with the fundamental symptoms of schizophrenia but in a milder form. It has been estimated that roughly 4% of the general population have schizophrenia or a schizoid personality disorder.

### Family and twin studies

The results of several studies of the prevalence of schizophrenia and schizoid disorder among the relatives of schizophrenics are summarized in Table 15.8. If only schizophrenia is considered, the concordance rate for identical twins is only 46%, suggesting the importance of environmental factors. If, however, schizophrenia and schizoid personality disorder are considered together, then almost 90% of identical co-twins are concordant.

### Adoption studies

Other evidence that provides compelling support for genetic factors in the causation of schizophrenia is provided by the results of adoption studies. The nature of schizophrenia can result in disruption of the family, with children being placed with adoptive parents. Any differences in the frequency of schizophrenia between individuals adopted away from their biological parents and their siblings can help to differentiate genetic and environmental influences.

**Table 15.8 Proportions (%) of first-degree relatives of individuals with schizophrenia who are similarly affected or have a schizoid disorder**

| | Proportion (%) of relatives | | |
|---|---|---|---|
| **Relatives** | **Schizophrenia*** | **Schizoid** | **Total schizophrenia + schizoid** |
| Identical twins | 46 | 41 | 87 |
| Offspring (of 1 schizophrenic) | 16 | 33 | 49 |
| Siblings | 14 | 32 | 46 |
| Parents | 9 | 35 | 44 |
| Offspring (of 2 schizophrenics) | 34 | 32 | 66 |
| General population | 1 | 3 | 4 |

*Age corrected
From Heston L L 1970 The genetics of schizophrenia and schizoid disease. Science 167: 249–256

In one study of 47 offspring of schizophrenic mothers separated shortly after birth, five of the offspring developed schizophrenia compared to none of 50 offspring of age- and sex-matched control mothers. Another study looked at the prevalence of schizophrenia in the relatives of adoptees who were schizophrenic compared to matched-control adoptees who were not schizophrenic. This showed a fivefold increase in the prevalence of schizophrenia in the biological relatives of the schizophrenic adoptees compared to biological relatives of the control adoptees, the prevalence in the latter group being the same as that seen in the adoptive relatives in both groups. Another study showed similar concordance rates of schizophrenia in identical twin offspring born to a schizophrenic parent, whether reared together or separated at birth. These findings provide compelling evidence that genetic factors are important in the causation of schizophrenia.

## POSSIBLE SINGLE-GENE MODELS OF INHERITANCE

What interpretation can be put on these results? The simplest would be that schizophrenia and schizoid disorders are both inherited as an autosomal dominant trait with almost complete penetrance. The idea that schizophrenia and schizoid disorders represent a single genetic disease is supported by their clinical similarity and the fact that both occur with almost equal frequency in identical co-twins of schizophrenics. If the two conditions are considered together, then the proportion of affected first-degree relatives fits well with the hypothesis of autosomal dominant inheritance, with 50% of first-degree relatives of an affected individual and 75% of the offspring of two affected individuals being affected. However, the proportion of more distant relatives being affected does not fit this mode of inheritance so well.

Schizophrenia has been associated with a number of complex traits, such as body build and intelligence. It is clear from twin studies and other findings that environmental factors also play an important part in the etiology of schizophrenia. The prevalence of schizophrenia among close relatives could partly be the result of sharing a common environment, but most investigators consider that schizophrenia is, in fact, determined in a multifactorial manner, the genetic contribution being on a polygenic basis.

## LINKAGE AND ASSOCIATION STUDIES

The observation of differences in concentrations of neurotransmitter substances, such as dopamine or 5-hydroxytryptamine (serotonin), in various parts of the brains of schizophrenics at autopsy, and the pharmacological action of antipsychotic drugs, has suggested that genes for CNS neurotransmitter substances and their receptors could be possible candidate genes for linkage studies. No confirmed linkage has been found, but some studies have shown evidence of possible associations with particular allelic variants, e.g. the 5-hydroxytryptamine type 2a receptor.

The report of a proband and his maternal uncle with schizophrenia, both of whom had an unbalanced translocation leading to partial trisomy for part of the long arm of chromosome 5, led molecular geneticists to look for linkage to that region of the genome in schizophrenia. There were, however, conflicting results. In several Icelandic and two English families with schizophrenia there was evidence supporting linkage of schizophrenia to DNA markers on the long arm of chromosome 5, but studies in Swedish, Scottish and North American families did not show linkage to this locus (SCZD1). It is a similar story for a 30–50 cM region on chromosome 6p, which includes the HLA locus. In some populations, in particular an Irish family with many affected members, linkage was promising but not subsequently borne out by studies in other families, including further Irish kindreds. Overall, a dozen or so loci show some significance through linkage studies but it is thought likely that different susceptibility loci are present in different populations. A number of other cytogenetic abnormalities have been reported with familial schizophrenia, most of which appear to have been coincidental rather than causal, although a locus on the long arm of chromosome 11 (SCZD2) has been reported to be associated with a predisposition to schizophrenia in a number of studies.

The highest risk factor for schizophrenia is for the monozygotic twin of an affected co-twin, followed by being the child of two schizophrenic parents. A similar risk also applies to individuals with deletion 22q11 (DiGeorge/Sedlácková/velocardiofacial) syndrome. This chromosome region has therefore been of great interest and systematic approaches have focused on the genes encoding PRODH (proline dehydrogenase) and COMT (catechol-*O*-methyl transferase). Once again, however, promising results from some studies have not been replicated in others, and if one thing is clear, it is that there are no simple solutions to the cause(s) of schizophrenia.

### ANTICIPATION

More recently, observations in several studies of an earlier age of onset and an increase in severity in affected individuals in subsequent generations with familial schizophrenia have suggested the possibility of anticipation (p. 116). Although care has to be taken with regard to possible ascertainment bias, these observations introduce unstable mutations (p. 24) as a possible mutational mechanism.

## AFFECTIVE DISORDERS

Affective disorders include purely depressive, or *unipolar* illness, and manic–depressive or *bipolar* illness. Both are episodic disorders characterized by a persistent lowering of feeling, emotion and desire, resulting in difficulty in performing routine tasks at the usual rate and expected quality. The manic phase of bipolar illness is characterized by elevation of affect, euphoric emotions, pathological desire and rapid speech. In the absence of a laboratory test a diagnosis is made on clinical grounds using symptomology rating defined by the Diagnostic and Statisticial Manual (DSM) devised by the American Psychiatric Association. This is currently in its fourth revision (DSM IV). Manic–depressive illness is associated with a significant risk of suicide. Bipolar and unipolar illness show differences in the length and number of episodes and age of onset.

### EPIDEMIOLOGY

Affective disorders are universal, occurring in all societies. The lifetime risk of developing bipolar depressive illness is between 0.5% and 1%, while unipolar depressive illness ranges from 2% to 25%, the latter variation probably being due to different cultural and environmental influences.

### FAMILY STUDIES

Familial occurrence of affective disorders has been reported in a number of studies. Relatives of persons with unipolar and bipolar affective disorders have an increased risk of similar problems compared to the general population. Although there is a tendency for recurrence of the same type of affective disorder in affected relatives, unipolar depressive illness is the most common disorder in first-degree relatives of persons with both unipolar and bipolar affective disorder.

### TWIN STUDIES

Concordance rates in monozygotic and dizygotic twins are 67% and 20%, respectively, being slightly higher for bipolar illness and lower for unipolar illness. Although concordance for the polarity of the affective disorder occurs in the majority of the familial recurrences, approximately one-quarter are for unipolar affective disorder when the proband has bipolar affective disorder, and vice versa.

### ADOPTION STUDIES

The results of adoption studies, which have shown a high prevalence of affective disorder in the biological parents and other relatives of adoptees with bipolar affective possible role in the acceleration of the neurodegenerative process in AD.

In addition, there is an association with polymorphisms in the $\alpha_2$-macroglobulin gene and the LDL-related protein, both of which interact with components involved in the clearance and degradation of amyloid protein.

Although it is clear that the APOE ε4 allele is the most significant risk factor for late-onset AD, accounting for up to 40% of cases, it is neither necessary nor sufficient for the development of AD, emphasizing the importance of other genetic and environmental etiological factors. This underlies the recommendation of the US National Institute on Aging and the Alzheimer Association Working Group that APOE testing is *not* used to predict whether an asymptomatic person is likely to develop AD.

### ANIMAL MODELS

Transgenic mice with mutations in the presenilin-1 and -2 genes resulting in their overexpression showed an increase in the rate of deposition of amyloid in the brain, suggesting that mutations in the presenilin genes could cause AD through a gain of function. Generation of a transgenic mouse expressing the APP gene will allow a better understanding of the pathogenesis of AD and the assessment of possible therapeutic interventions.

## HEMOCHROMATOSIS

Hemochromatosis is a common disorder of iron metabolism that results in accumulation of iron. The liver is the most commonly damaged tissue, with iron deposition leading to cirrhosis and liver failure. Patients are at increased risk of hepatocellular carcinoma. Other organs that may be affected include the pancreas, heart, pituitary gland, skin and joints. The iron overload is easily treated by venesection and this is very effective at reducing morbidity and mortality. The ratio of affected males:females is 5:1 and the disease is underdiagnosed in the general population but overdiagnosed in patients with secondary iron overload.

### LINKAGE AND GENE IDENTIFICATION

In 1996 the *HFE* gene was discovered close to the HLA region on 6p21. Two variants were described, *C282Y* and *H63D*. Between 85 and 100% (depending on population) of affected individuals were found to be homozygous for *C282Y*, and the carrier frequency in Northern Europe is approximately 1 in 10. *H63D* is more common in the general population, and homozygosity for this variant is associated with only a modest increased (about fourfold) risk of hemochromatosis. Compound heterozygosity for *C282Y* and *H63D* is associated with reduced penetrance; only 1% are thought likely to develop symptoms. Homozygosity for *C282Y* was thought to confer a high risk of hemochromatosis and it was suggested that population screening would be useful since the iron overload is easily treated. However, recent population-based studies have suggested that the penetrance of hereditary hemochromatosis due to homozygosity for *C282Y* may be as low as 1%.

### GENETIC TESTING

Genetic testing is now commonplace in families where an index case is found to be homozygous for *C282Y* or compoundly heterozygous for *C282Y* and *H63D*. Current strategy involves first testing the spouse for carrier status, as there is a 1 in 10 chance they will be heterozygous for *C282Y*. If the offspring have inherited a predisposing genotype, annual monitoring of serum ferritin is recommended in order to detect iron overload at an early stage and initiate prompt treatment.

### GENETIC HETEROGENEITY

Hemochromatosis is a genetically heterogeneous disorder (Table 15.10) with mutations also reported in the transferrin receptor 2 gene and the *SLC11A3* gene, which encodes ferroportin. In addition to the common recessive adult-onset form, there is a rare juvenile form with iron overload and organ failure before the age of 30 years, which is lethal if untreated. Neonatal hemochromatosis is a severe form of unknown etiology.

## VENOUS THROMBOSIS

Venous thrombosis represents a major health problem worldwide, with increasing incidence from 1 in 100 000

**Table 15.10 Genetic heterogeneity in hemochromatosis**

| Type | Inheritance | Gene | Chromosome location | Age of onset |
|---|---|---|---|---|
| HFE | Autosomal recessive | *HFE* | 6p21.3 | 40–60 years |
| HFE2A | Autosomal recessive | Not known | 1q21 | <30 years (Juvenile) |
| HFE2B | Autosomal recessive | *HAMP* | 19q13 | <30 years (Juvenile) |
| HFE3 | Autosomal recessive | *TFR2* | 7q22 | 40–60 years |
| HFE4 | Autosomal dominant | *SLC11A3* | 2q32 | up to 60/70* years |

*Up to 60 years in males and 70 years in females.

**Table 15.11 Inherited and acquired causes of venous thrombosis**

**Inherited**
***Common***
Factor V Leiden (R506Q)
Prothrombin variant G20210A
Homozygous C677T mutation in the methylenetetrahydrofolate reductase gene (*MTHFR*)
***Rare***
Antithrombin deficiency
Protein C deficiency
Protein S deficiency

**Acquired**
Surgery and trauma
Prolonged immobilization
Previous thrombosis
Pregnancy
Oral contraceptives or hormone replacement therapy
Older age

during childhood to 1 in 100 in old age. Venous thromboembolism, including deep-vein thrombosis and pulmonary embolism, is a complex disease that results from multiple interactions between inherited and acquired risk factors (Table 15.11). Inherited thrombophilias also increase the risk of fetal loss, both stillbirths and early miscarriages.

## IDENTIFICATION OF GENES

In the last decade the identification of two mutations prevalent in European Caucasians has paved the way for a number of large cohort studies that have increased our understanding of venous thrombosis. The factor V Leiden mutation (R506Q) renders the factor V protein resistant to cleavage by activated protein C, thus increasing generation of thrombin. The prothrombin variant G20210A is located in the 3′ UTR and is associated with increased prothrombin levels. These variants confer a four- to fivefold increased risk of thrombosis in the heterozygous state (Table 15.12), but individuals homozygous for one or heterozygous for both are at significantly elevated risk (up to 80-fold).

**Table 15.12 Frequency of factor V Leiden and prothrombin 20210A variant in the UK population and corresponding risk of venous thrombosis**

| Risk factor | Status | Population frequency | Approximate increased risk* |
|---|---|---|---|
| Factor V Leiden | Heterozygous | 4% (1 in 25) | 4.9 |
| | Homozygous | 0.15% (1 in 625) | 10–80 |
| Prothrombin | Heterozygous | 2% (1 in 50) | 3.8 |
| | Homozygous | 0.04% (1 in 2500) | Not known |
| FVL and prothrombin | Heterozygous for both | 0.08% (1 in 1250) | 20 |

* These figures will be increased in the presence of antithrombin, protein C or protein S deficiency

## GENETIC TESTING

More than 50% of venous thromboembolism cases can be explained by factor V Leiden and the prothrombin variant. Testing is now commonplace, but there is no evidence that the detection of a heritable thrombophilic defect alters management of the index case. However, if an inherited predisposition is identified, testing can be offered to first-degree relatives. Those who test positive may be able to reduce their risk of developing thrombosis by, for example, short-term thromboprophylaxis in periods of increased thrombotic risk, e.g. surgery. Knowledge of a genetic predisposition to thrombosis will also influence the choice of oral contraceptives.

## FURTHER READING

Adams PC 2002 Hemochromatosis: clinical implications. Medscape Gastroenterology eJournal 4
*A summary of clinical aspects of hemochromatosis and the role of genetic testing.*

Heston L L 1966 Psychiatric disorders in foster home reared children of schizophrenic mothers. Br J Psychiatry 112: 819–825
*A classic paper demonstrating genetic factors in the etiology of schizophrenia.*

Jameson J L (ed) 1998 Principles of molecular medicine. Humana Press, Totowa, New Jersey
*A large multiauthor text covering in detail the molecular basis of the common diseases as well as many of the more common single-gene and chromosome disorders.*

King R A, Rotter J I, Motulsky A G (eds) 1992 The genetic basis of common diseases. Oxford University Press, Oxford
*An excellent multiauthor text covering the principles of analysis with an extensive review of the genetic basis of the common diseases plus an exhaustive reference list.*

Plomin R, De Fries J C, McClearn G E, Rutter M 1997 Behavioral genetics. W H Freeman, New York
*A multiauthor text covering the approaches to studying behavioral genetics.*

Seligsohn MD, Lubetsky A 2001 Genetic susceptibility to venous thrombosis. N Engl J Med 344: 1222–1231
*A comprehensive review of hereditary thrombophilia.*

CHAPTER 16

# Congenital abnormalities and dysmorphic syndromes

*"They certainly give very strange names to diseases."*

Plato

The formation of a human being, a process sometimes known as *morphogenesis*, involves an extremely complicated and as yet very poorly understood interaction of genetic and environmental factors. Given the extraordinary complexity of this process it is not surprising that on occasion it can go wrong. Nor is it surprising that in many congenital abnormalities genetic factors can clearly be implicated. Approximately 2400 dysmorphic syndromes are described that are believed to be due to molecular pathology in single genes, and for about 500 the genes have been identified and a further 200 or so mapped. A further 500 or so sporadically occurring syndromes are recognized, for which the precise cause remains elusive. In this chapter we shall consider the overall impact of abnormalities in morphogenesis by reviewing:

1. The incidence of abnormalities at various stages from conception onwards.
2. Their nature and the ways in which they can be classified.
3. Their causes, when known, with particular emphasis on the role of genetics.

## INCIDENCE

### SPONTANEOUS FIRST-TRIMESTER PREGNANCY LOSS

It has been estimated that around 50% of all human conceptions are lost either before implantation at 5–6 days post conception or shortly afterwards before the mother realizes that she is pregnant. Among recognized pregnancies at least 15% end in spontaneous miscarriage before 12 weeks' gestation. Even if material from the abortus can be obtained it is often very difficult to establish why a pregnancy loss has occurred. However, careful study of large numbers of spontaneously aborted embryos has shown that gross structural abnormalities are present in between 80% and 85%. These abnormalities vary from complete absence of an embryo in the developing pregnancy sac – a *blighted ovum* – to a very distorted body shape, or a specific abnormality in a single body system.

Chromosome abnormalities such as trisomy, monosomy or triploidy are found in about 50% of all spontaneous abortions. This incidence rises to 60% when a gross structural abnormality is present and it is very likely that submicroscopic or de novo single-gene abnormalities account for a proportion of the remainder.

### CONGENITAL ABNORMALITIES AND PERINATAL MORTALITY

Perinatal mortality figures include all infants who are stillborn after 28 weeks' gestation plus all babies who die during the first week of life. Studies undertaken in several centres in Europe and North America have shown that between 25% and 30% of all perinatal deaths occur as a result of a serious structural abnormality. In 80% of these cases genetic factors can be implicated, with a recurrence risk to future pregnancies equal to 1% or greater. The relative contribution of structural abnormalities to perinatal mortality is lower in developing countries, where environmental factors play a much greater role.

### NEWBORN INFANTS

Surveys reviewing the incidence of both major and minor anomalies in newborn infants have been undertaken in many parts of the world. A major anomaly is defined as one which has an adverse outcome on either the function or the social acceptability of the individual (Table 16.1). In contrast, minor abnormalities are of neither medical nor cosmetic importance (Table 16.2). However, the division between major and minor abnormalities is not always straightforward: an inguinal hernia occasionally leads to strangulation of bowel and always requires surgical correction, so there is a small risk of serious sequelae.

These surveys have consistently shown that between 2% and 3% of all newborns have at least one major abnormality apparent at birth. The true incidence, taking into account abnormalities that present later in life, such

**Table 16.1 Examples of major congenital structural abnormalities**

| System and abnormality | Incidence per 1000 births |
|---|---|
| Cardiovascular | 10 |
| Ventricular septal defect | 2.5 |
| Atrial septal defect | 1 |
| Patent ductus arteriosus | 1 |
| Fallot tetralogy | 1 |
| Central nervous system | 10 |
| Anencephaly | 1 |
| Hydrocephaly | 1 |
| Microcephaly | 1 |
| Lumbo-sacral spina bifida | 2 |
| Gastro-intestinal | 4 |
| Cleft lip/palate | 1.5 |
| Diaphragmatic hernia | 0.5 |
| Esophageal atresia | 0.3 |
| Imperforate anus | 0.2 |
| Limb | 2 |
| Transverse amputation | 0.2 |
| Urogenital | 4 |
| Bilateral renal agenesis | 2 |
| Polycystic kidneys (infantile) | 0.02 |
| Bladder exstrophy | 0.03 |

**Table 16.2 Examples of minor congenital structural abnormalities**

Preauricular pit or tag
Epicanthic folds
Lacrimal duct stenosis
Brushfield spots in the iris
Lip pits
Single palmar crease
Fifth finger clinodactyly
Syndactyly between second and third toes
Supernumerary nipple
Umbilical hernia
Hydrocele
Sacral pit or dimple

as brain malformations, is probably close to 5%. Minor abnormalities are found in approximately 10% of all newborn babies. If two or more minor abnormalities are present in a newborn infant there is a 10–20% risk that the baby will also have a major malformation.

The long-term outlook for a baby with a major abnormality obviously depends on the nature of the specific birth defect and whether it can be treated successfully. Taken together, the overall prognosis for this group of newborns is relatively poor, with 25% dying in early infancy, 25% having subsequent mental or physical disability, and the remaining 50% having a fair to good outlook after treatment.

**Table 16.3 The incidence of structural abnormalities**

| Incidence | (%) |
|---|---|
| **Spontaneous miscarriages** | |
| First trimester | 80–85 |
| Second trimester | 25 |
| **All babies** | |
| Major abnormality apparent at birth | 2–3 |
| Major abnormality apparent later | 2 |
| Minor abnormality | 10 |
| Deaths in perinatal period | 25 |
| Deaths in first year of life | 25 |
| Deaths from 1 to 9 years | 20 |
| Deaths from 10 to 14 years | 7.5 |

## CHILDHOOD MORTALITY

Congenital abnormalities make a significant contribution to mortality throughout childhood. During the first year of life approximately 25% of all deaths are the result of major structural abnormalities. This figure falls to 20% between the ages of 1 and 10 years and to around 7.5% for children aged between 10 and 15 years.

Taking into account the incidence of major and minor abnormalities noted in newborn surveys and the high incidence of defects observed in early spontaneous miscarriages, it is evident that at least 15% of all recognized human conceptions are structurally abnormal (Table 16.3). It is probable that genetic factors are involved in the causation of at least 50% of all structural abnormalities.

## DEFINITION AND CLASSIFICATION OF BIRTH DEFECTS

So far in this chapter the terms *congenital abnormality* and *birth defect* have been used in a general sense to describe all types of structural abnormality that can occur in an embryo, fetus or newborn infant. While these terms are perfectly acceptable for the purpose of lumping together all these abnormalities when studying their overall incidence, they do not provide any insight into possible underlying mechanisms. More specific definitions have been devised that have the added advantage of providing a combined clinical and etiological classification.

## SINGLE ABNORMALITIES

Single abnormalities may have a genetic or non-genetic basis. The system of terms used help us to understand the different mechanisms that might be implicated, and these can be illustrated in schematic form (Fig. 16.1).

### Malformation

A *malformation* is a primary structural defect of an organ, or part of an organ, which results from an inherent abnormality in development. This used to be known as a primary or intrinsic malformation. The presence of a malformation implies that the early development of a particular tissue or organ has been arrested or misdirected. Common examples of malformations include congenital heart abnormalities such as ventricular or atrial septal defects, cleft lip and/or palate (p. 142), and neural tube defects such as anencephaly or lumbo-sacral myelomeningocele (Fig. 16.2). Most malformations involving only a single organ show multifactorial inheritance, implying an interaction of many genes with other factors (p. 141). Multiple malformations are more likely to be due to chromosomal abnormalities.

### Disruption

The term *disruption* refers to an abnormal structure of an organ or tissue as a result of external factors disturbing the normal developmental process. This used to be known as a secondary or extrinsic malformation. Extrinsic factors that can disrupt normal development include ischemia, infection and trauma. An example of a disruption is the effect seen on limb development when a strand or band of amnion becomes entwined around a baby's forearm or digits (Fig. 16.3). By definition a disruption is not genetic, although occasionally genetic factors can predispose to

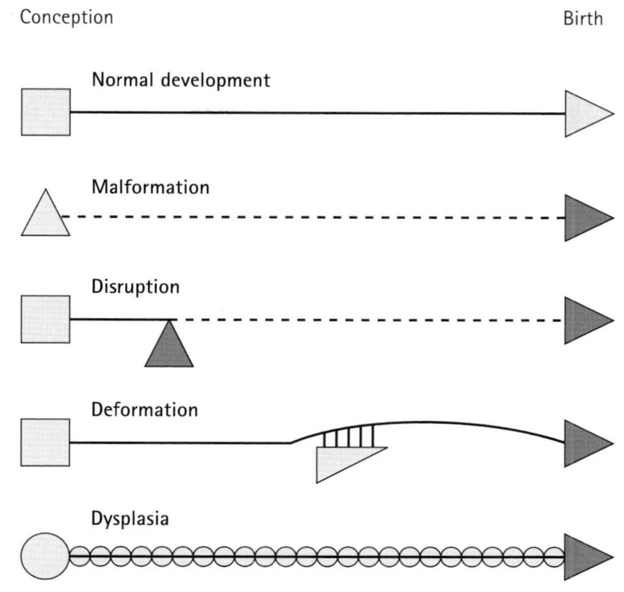


**Fig. 16.1**
Schematic representation of the different mechanisms in morphogenesis. For malformation, disruption and dysplasia, the broken line symbolizes developmental potential rather than timing of the manifestation of the defect, which might be late in embryogenesis. (Adapted from Springer et al 1982 Errors of morphogenesis: concepts and terms. J Pediatr 100: 160–165)

disruptive events. For example, a small proportion of amniotic bands are caused by an underlying genetically determined defect in collagen, which weakens the amnion making it more liable to tear or rupture spontaneously.

### Deformation

A *deformation* is a defect which results from an abnormal mechanical force which distorts an otherwise normal

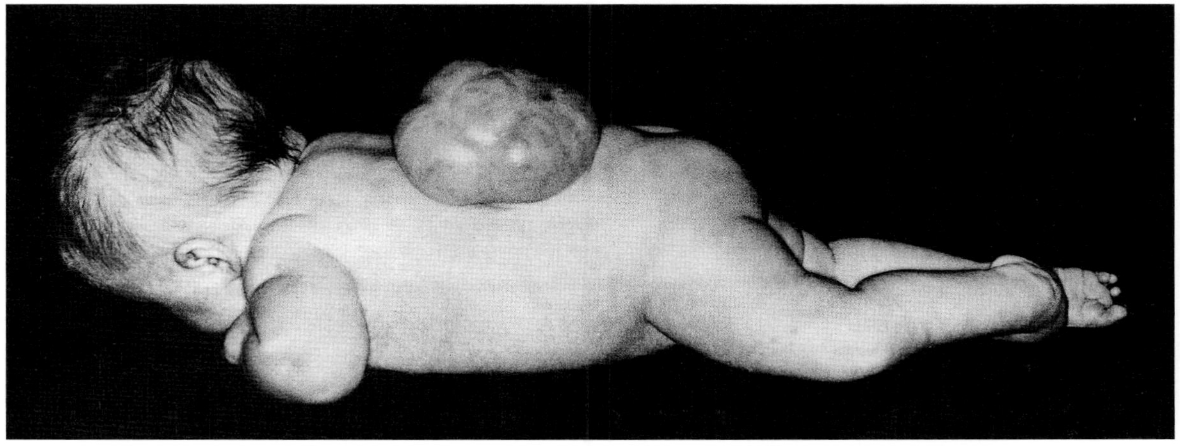

**Fig. 16.2**
Child with a large thoraco-lumbar myelomeningocele consisting of protruding spinal cord covered by meninges.

A

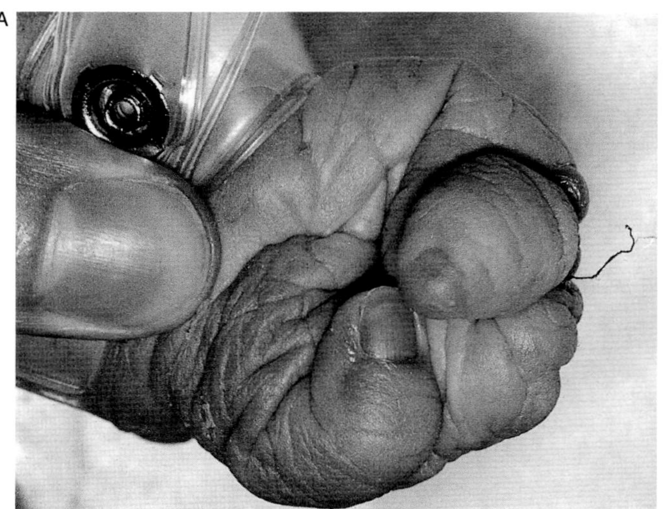

B

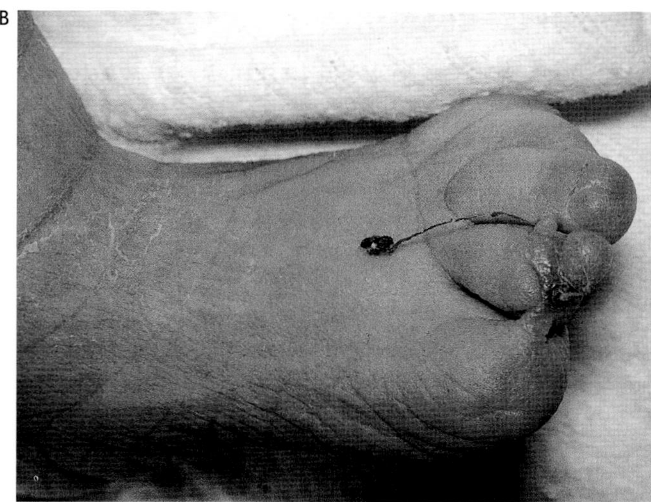

**Fig. 16.3**
(A) Hand and (B) foot of a baby with digital amputations due to amniotic bands showing residual strands of amnion. (Courtesy of Dr Una MacFadyen, Leicester Royal Infirmary.)

structure. Well-recognized examples include dislocation of the hip and mild 'positional' talipes ('club foot') (Fig. 16.4), both of which can be caused by lack of amniotic fluid (oligohydramnios) or intra-uterine crowding due to twinning or a structurally abnormal uterus. Deformations usually occur late in pregnancy and convey a good prognosis with appropriate treatment, e.g. gentle splinting for talipes, since the underlying organ is fundamentally normal in structure.

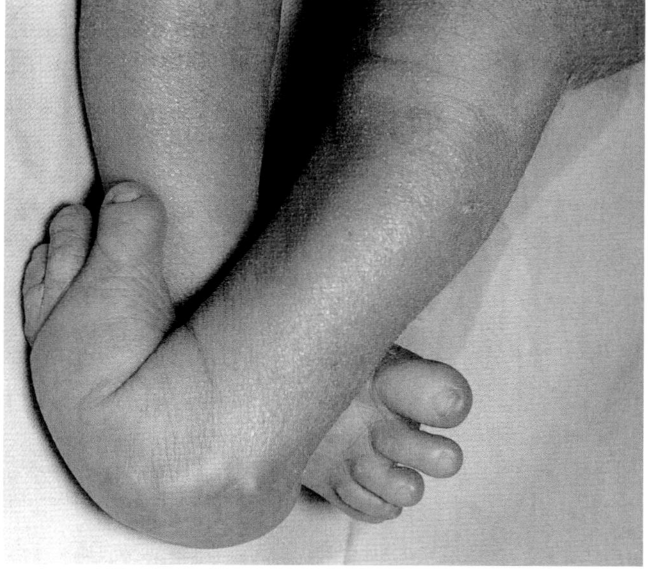

**Fig. 16.4**
The lower limbs of a baby with talipes equinovarus.

### Dysplasia

A *dysplasia* is an abnormal organization of cells into tissue. Usually the effects are seen in all parts of the body in which that particular tissue is present. For example, in a skeletal dysplasia such as thanatophoric dysplasia, which is caused by mutations in *FGFR3* (p. 92), almost all parts of the skeleton are affected (Fig. 16.5). Similarly, in an ectodermal dysplasia, widely dispersed tissues of ectodermal origin, such as hair, teeth, skin and nails, are involved (Fig. 16.6). Most dysplasias are caused by single-gene defects and are associated with high recurrence risks for siblings and/or offspring.

## MULTIPLE ABNORMALITIES

### Sequence

The most logical and easily understood pattern of multiple abnormalities is the concept of a *sequence*. This describes the findings that occur as a consequence of a cascade of events initiated by a single primary factor. This can often be a single organ malformation. In the 'Potter' sequence, chronic leakage of amniotic fluid or defective urinary output results in oligohydramnios (Fig. 16.7). This, in turn, leads to fetal compression, resulting in squashed facial features, dislocation of the hips, talipes and pulmonary hypoplasia (Fig. 16.8) which usually results in early neonatal death from respiratory failure.

### Syndrome

In practice the term *syndrome* is used very loosely (e.g. the amniotic band 'syndrome'), but in theory it should be

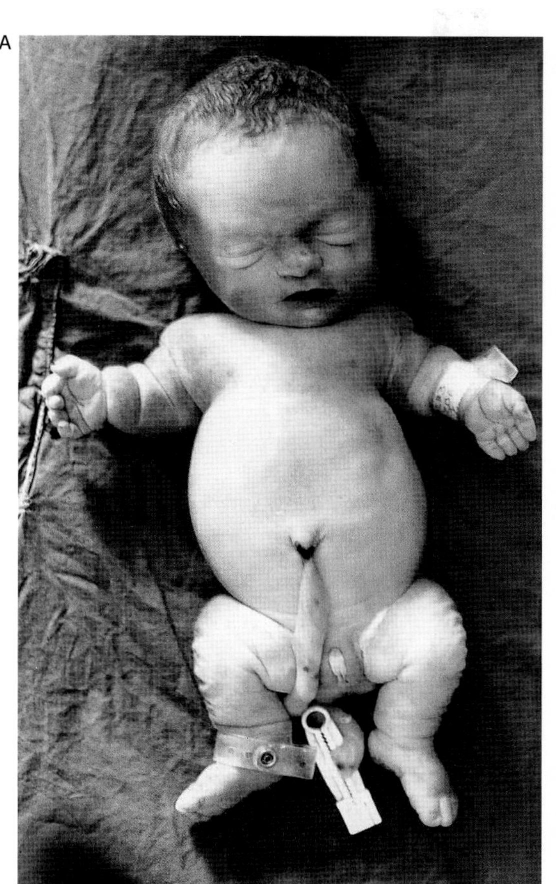
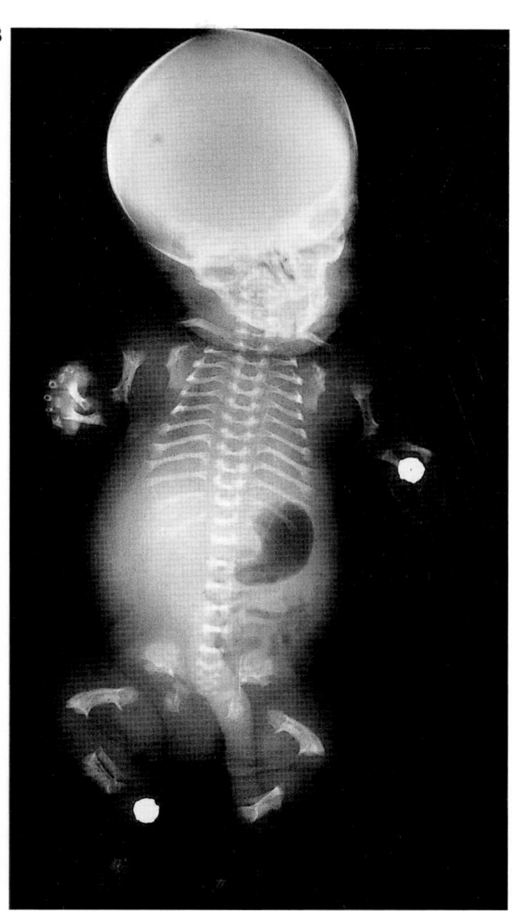

Fig. 16.5
(A) Infant with thanatophoric dysplasia; (B) X-ray of the infant showing short ribs, flat vertebral bodies and curved femora.

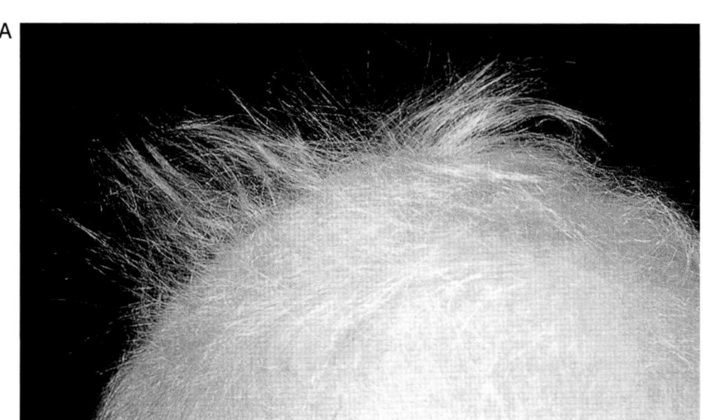
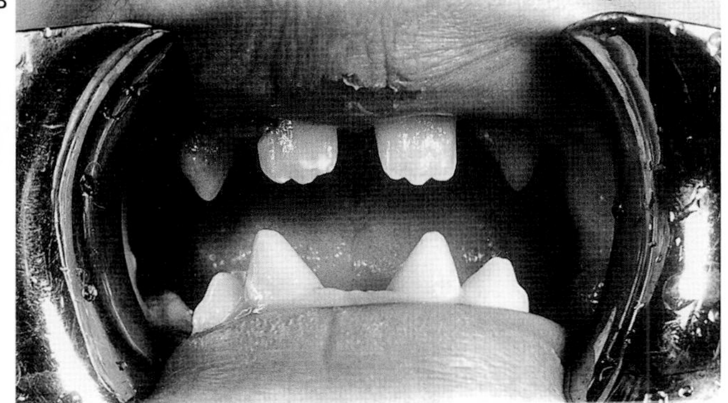

Fig. 16.6
(A) Hair and (B) teeth of a male with ectodermal dysplasia.

reserved for consistent and recognizable patterns of abnormalities for which there will often be a known underlying cause. These underlying causes can include chromosome abnormalities, as in Down syndrome, or single-gene defects, as in the Van der Woude syndrome, in which cleft lip and/or palate occurs in association with pits in the lower lip (Fig. 16.9).

Several thousand multiple malformation syndromes are now recognized. This field of study is known as dysmorphology. The diagnosis of individual syndromes

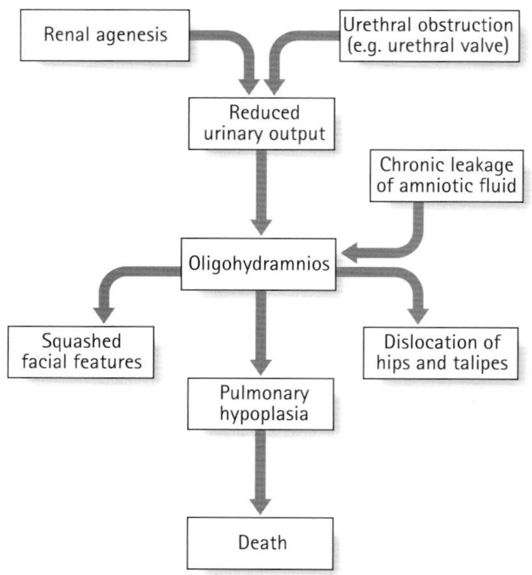


**Fig. 16.7**
The 'Potter' sequence showing the cascade of events leading to and resulting from oligohydramnios (reduced volume of amniotic fluid).

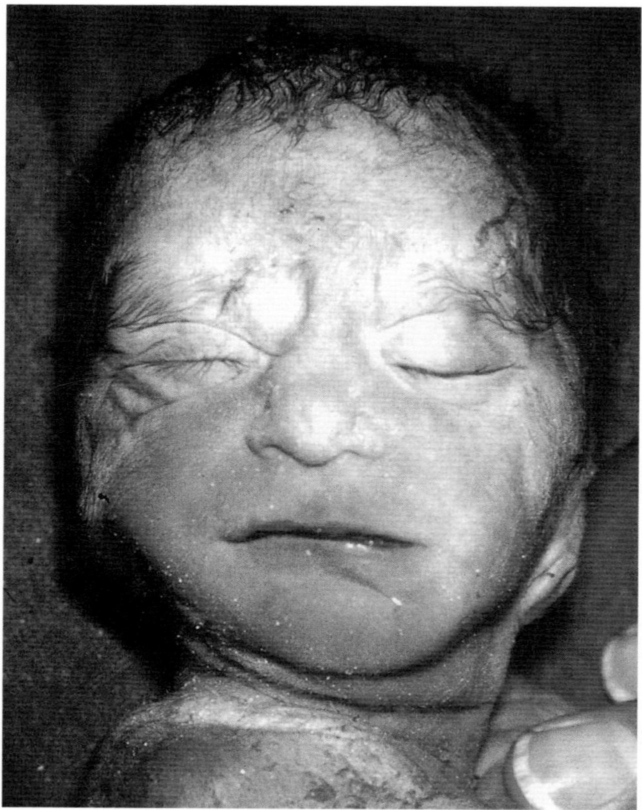

**Fig. 16.8**
Facial appearance of a baby with Potter sequence due to oligohydramnios as a consequence of bilateral renal agenesis. Note the squashed appearance caused by in utero compression.

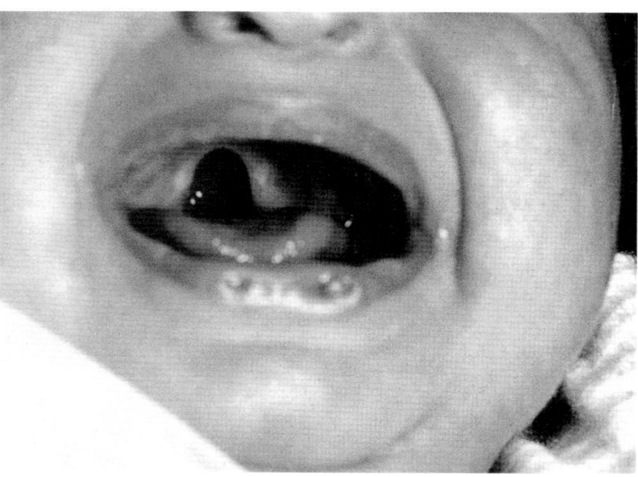

**Fig. 16.9**
A posterior cleft palate and lower lip pits in a child with Van der Woude syndrome.

has been greatly helped by the development of computerized databases (see Appendix). It is possible to obtain a list of differential diagnoses by providing the search facility of the database with details of key abnormal clinical features. Even with the help of this extremely valuable diagnostic tool, there are, unfortunately, many dysmorphic children for whom no diagnosis can be reached, so that it can be very difficult to provide accurate information about the likely prognosis and recurrence risk (p. 341).

## Association

The term *association* has been introduced in recognition of the fact that certain malformations tend to occur together more often than would be expected by chance, yet this non-random occurrence of abnormalities cannot be explained on the basis of a sequence or a syndrome. The main differences from a syndrome are the lack of consistency of abnormalities from one affected individual to another and the absence of a satisfactory underlying explanation. The names of associations are often acronyms devised by juggling the first letters of the organs or systems most commonly involved: for example, the VATER association features *V*ertebral, *A*nal, *T*racheo-*E*sophageal and *R*enal abnormalities. Associations convey a low risk of recurrence and are generally thought not to be genetic in origin even though the underlying cause is usually unknown.

It is recognized that this classification of birth defects is not perfect. It will be readily apparent that it is far from being either fully comprehensive or mutually exclusive. For example, bladder outflow obstruction caused by a primary malformation such as a urethral valve will result in the oligohydramnios or Potter sequence, leading to secondary deformations such as dislocation of the hip and talipes. To complicate matters further, the absence of both kidneys, which will result in the same sequence of events, is usually erroneously referred to as Potter's syndrome. Despite this semantic confusion, adherence to this classification is important since it serves as an aid to understanding and recurrence risks (Ch. 17).

## GENETIC CAUSES OF MALFORMATIONS

There are many recognized causes of congenital abnormalities, although it is notable that in up to 50% of all cases no clear explanation can be established (Table 16.4).

### CHROMOSOME ABNORMALITIES

These account for approximately 6% of all recognized congenital abnormalities. As a general rule any perceptible degree of autosomal imbalance, such as duplication, deletion, trisomy or monosomy, will result in severe structural and developmental abnormality. If very severe this can lead to early spontaneous miscarriage. Common chromosome syndromes are described in detail in Chapter 18. It is not known whether malformations caused by a significant chromosome abnormality, such as a trisomy, are the result of dosage effects of the individual genes involved ('additive' model) or general developmental instability caused by a large number of abnormal developmental gene products ('interactive' model).

### SINGLE-GENE DEFECTS

These account for approximately 7.5% of all congenital abnormalities. Some of these are isolated, i.e. they involve only one organ or system (Table 16.5). Other single-gene defects result in multiple congenital abnormality syndromes involving many organs or systems that do not have any obvious underlying embryological relationship. For example, ectrodactyly (Fig. 16.10) in isolation can be inherited as an autosomal dominant trait, occasionally autosomal recessive, and rarely X-linked. It can also occur as one manifestation of the EEC syndrome (*E*ctodermal dysplasia, *E*ctrodactyly and *C*left lip/palate), which also shows autosomal dominant inheritance. There is abundant evidence from the study of dysmorphology that several different mutations, allelic or non-allelic, can cause similar if not identical malformations.

**Table 16.4 Causes of congenital abnormalities**

| Cause | % |
|---|---|
| **Genetic** | |
| Chromosomal | 6 |
| Single gene | 7.5 |
| Multifactorial | 20–30 |
| Subtotal | 30–40 |
| **Environmental** | |
| Drugs and chemicals | 2 |
| Infections | 2 |
| Maternal illness | 2 |
| Physical agents | 1 |
| **Subtotal** | **5–10** |
| Unknown | 50 |
| **Total** | **100** |

**Table 16.5 Congenital abnormalities that can be caused by single-gene defects**

| | Inheritance | Abnormalities |
|---|---|---|
| **Isolated** | | |
| **Central nervous system** | | |
| Hydrocephalus | XR | |
| Megalencephaly | AD | |
| Microcephaly | AD/AR | |
| **Ocular** | | |
| Aniridia | AD | |
| Cataracts | AD/AR | |
| Microphthalmia | AD/AR | |
| **Limb** | | |
| Brachydactyly | AD | |
| Ectrodactyly | AD/AR/XR | |
| Polydactyly | AD | |
| **Other** | | |
| Infantile polycystic kidneys | AR | |
| **Syndromes** | | |
| Apert | AD | Craniosynostosis, syndactyly |
| EEC | AD | Ectodermal dysplasia, ectrodactyly, cleft lip/palate |
| Meckel | AR | Encephalocele, polydactyly, polycystic kidneys |
| Roberts | AR | Cleft lip/palate, phocomelia |
| Van der Woude | AD | Cleft lip/palate, lip pits |

AD: autosomal dominant; AR: autosomal recessive; XR: sex-linked recessive

The importance of identifying birth defects that show single-gene inheritance is twofold. From the family's point of view it is essential that correct counseling is available so that close relatives can be alerted to possible risks. From the academic point of view, the identification of a molecular defect causing an isolated single-gene abnormality in a particular organ can provide a clue as to the locus of a susceptibility gene for similar malformations affecting the same organ, which appear to show multifactorial inheritance.

Many examples of progress in identifying the genes that cause congenital abnormalities could be given. However,

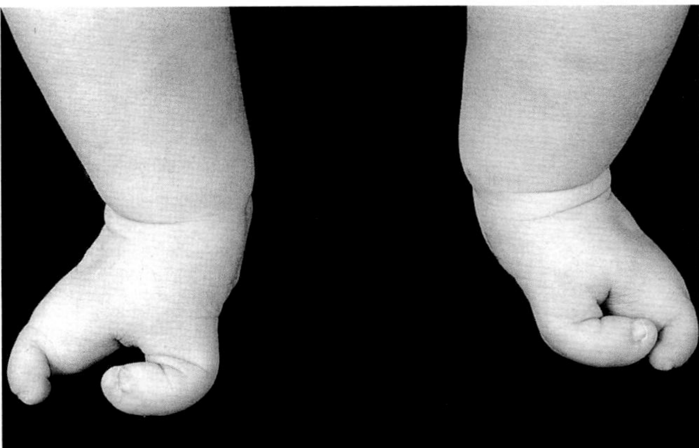

Fig. 16.10
Appearance of the feet in a child with ectrodactyly.

progress has been particularly impressive in relation to well-defined syndromes, and two recent examples from the field of pediatric genetics are highlighted. In both cases the function of the gene in relation to widespread expression in many tissues has yet to be determined.

## Noonan syndrome

First described by Noonan and Ehmke in 1963, this condition is well known to pediatricians. The incidence may be as high as 1 in 2000 births, affecting males and females equally. The clinical features bear a resemblance to those of Turner syndrome in females – short stature, neck webbing, increased carrying angle at the elbow, and congenital heart disease. Pulmonary stenosis (PS) is the most common lesion but ASD, VSD and occasionally hypertrophic cardiomyopathy occur. A characteristic pectus deformity may be seen, as well as the face, which includes hypertelorism, down-slanting palpebral fissures and low-set ears (Fig. 16.11). Some patients have a mild bleeding diathesis and learning difficulties are present in about one-quarter.

In a three-generation Dutch family NS was mapped to 12q22 in 1994 but it was not until 2001 that mutations were identified in the protein-tyrosine phosphatase, non-receptor-type, 11 (*PTPN11*) gene. Attention has turned rapidly to phenotype–genotype correlation. *PTPN11* does not account for all cases of NS, but mutation-positive cases have a much higher frequency of PS than mutation-negative cases, and very few mutations have been found in cases with cardiomyopathy. Facial features are similar, whether or not a mutation is found.

## Sotos syndrome

First described in 1964, this is one of the 'overgrowth' syndromes, previously known as cerebral gigantism. Birth weight is usually increased and macrocephaly noted. Early feeding difficulties and hypotonia may prompt many investigations and there is often motor delay and ataxia. Height progresses along the top of, or above, the normal centile lines but final adult height is not necessarily increased. Advanced bone age may be present, large hands and feet, and the cerebral ventricles

A
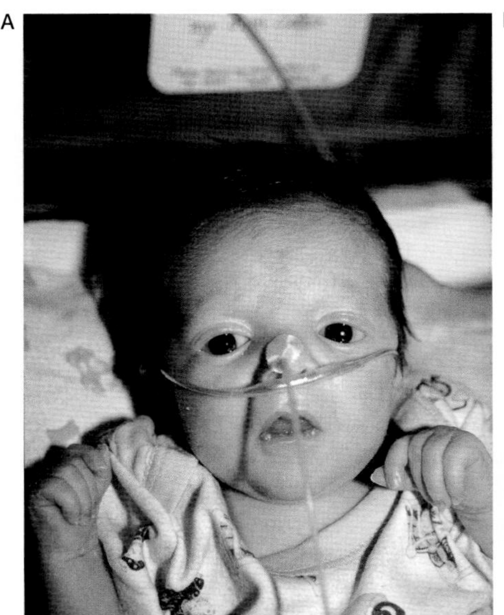
B
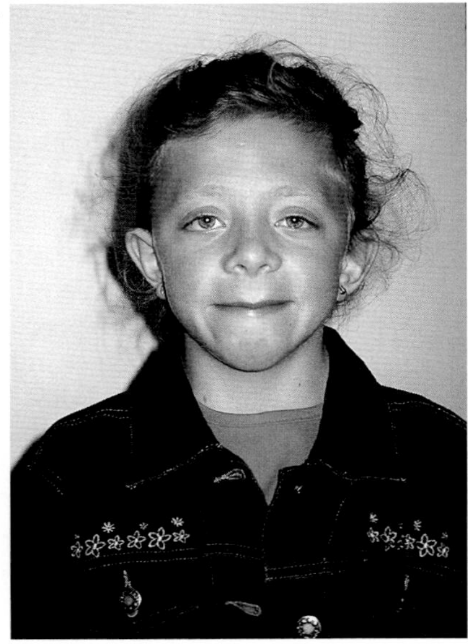
C
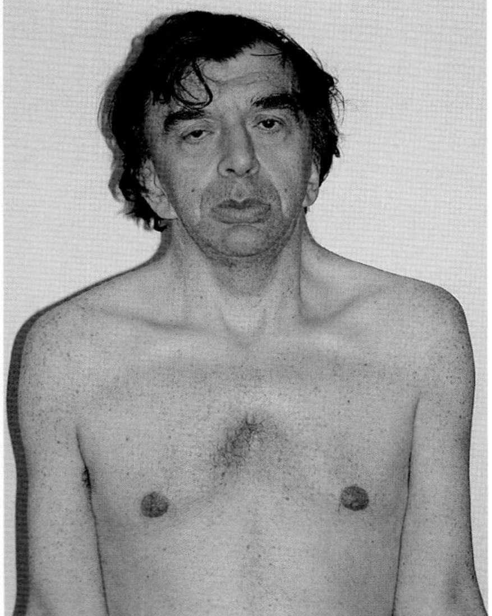

Fig. 16.11
Noonan syndrome. (A) In a baby presenting with cardiomyopathy at birth (which later resolved). (B) In a child. (C) In a 57-year-old man.

A
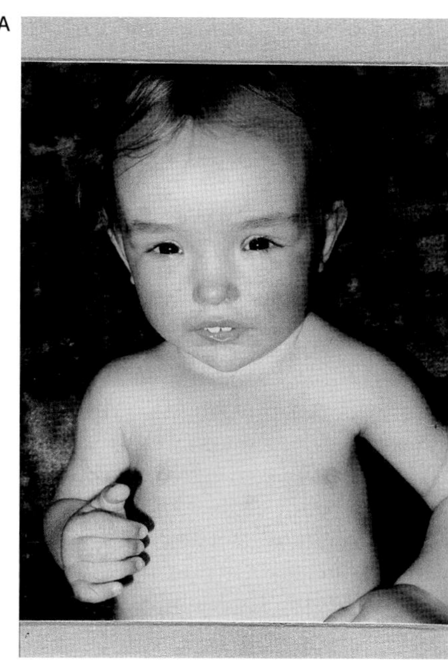

B
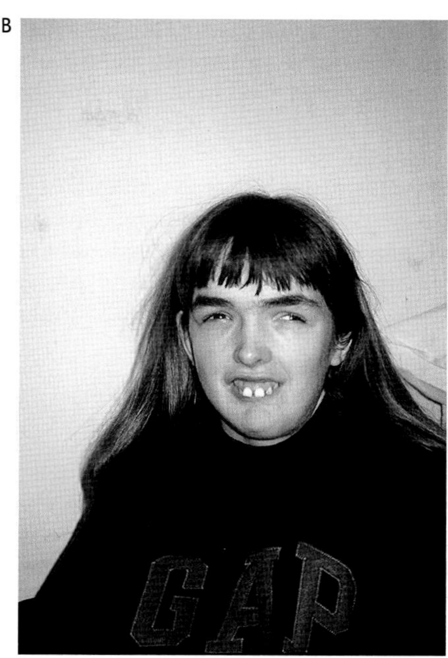


**Fig. 16.12**
Sotos syndrome. (A) In a young child – she has the typical high forehead, large head, characteristic tip to the nose. (B) The same individual aged 18 years, with learning difficulties and a spinal curvature (scoliosis).

may be mildly dilated on MRI or CT scan. The face is characteristic (Fig. 16.12) with a high prominent forehead, hypertelorism with down slanting palpebral fissures, a characteristic nose in early childhood, and a long pointed chin. Scoliosis develops in some cases during adolescence. Parent–child transmission is rare, probably because most patients have learning difficulties.

Among SS patients reported to have balanced chromosome translocations were two with break-points at 5q35. From these crucial patients a Japanese group in 2002 went on to identify a 2.2 Mb deletion in a series of SSb cases. The deletion takes out a gene called *NSD1*, an androgen receptor-associated coregulator with 23 exons. The Japanese found a small number of frameshift mutations in their patients but, interestingly, a study of European cases found that mutations were far more common than deletions. For the large majority of cases the mutations and deletions occur de novo.

## MULTIFACTORIAL INHERITANCE

This accounts for the majority of congenital abnormalities in which genetic factors can clearly be implicated. These include most isolated ('non-syndromal') malformations involving the heart, central nervous system and kidneys (Table 16.6). For many of these conditions empirical risks have been derived (p. 348) based on large epidemiological family studies, so that it is usually possible to provide the parents of an affected child with a clear indication of the likelihood that a future child will be similarly affected. Risks to the offspring of patients who were themselves treated successfully in childhood are becoming available. These are usually similar to the risk figures, which apply to siblings as would be predicted by the multifactorial model (p. 141).

## GENETIC HETEROGENEITY

It has long been recognized that specific congenital malformations can have many different causes (p. 109), hence the importance of trying to distinguish between

**Table 16.6 Isolated (non-syndromal) malformations that show multifactorial inheritance**

**Cardiac**
Atrial septal defect
Fallot tetralogy
Patent ductus arteriosus
Ventricular septal defect

**Central nervous system**
Anencephaly
Encephalocele
Spina bifida

**Genitourinary**
Hypospadias
Renal agenesis
Renal dysgenesis

**Other**
Cleft lip/palate
Congenital dislocation of hips
Talipes

syndromal and isolated cases. This causal diversity has become increasingly apparent as developments in molecular biology have led to the identification of highly conserved families of genes which play crucial roles in early embryogenesis.

This subject is discussed at length in Chapter 6. In this chapter two specific malformations, holoprosencephaly and neural tube defects, will be considered to demonstrate the rate of progress in this field and the extent of the challenge that lies ahead before full understanding is achieved.

## Holoprosencephaly

This severe and often lethal malformation is caused by a failure of cleavage of the embryonic forebrain or prosencephalon. Normally this divides transversely into the telencephalon and the diencephalon. The telencephalon divides in the sagittal plane to form the cerebral hemispheres and the olfactory tracts and bulbs. The diencephalon develops to form the thalamic nuclei, the pineal gland, the optic chiasm and the optic nerves. In holoprosencephaly there is incomplete or partial failure of these developmental processes, and in the severe alobar form this results in an abnormal facial appearance (Fig. 6.1) and profound neurodevelopmental impairment.

Etiologically, holoprosencephaly can be classified as chromosomal, syndromal or isolated. Chromosomal causes account for around 30–40% of all cases, with the most common abnormality being trisomy 13 (p. 274). Other chromosomal causes include deletions of 18p, 2p21, 7q36, and 21q22.3, duplication of 3p24-pter, duplication or deletion of 13q, and triploidy (p. 280). Syndromal causes of holoprosencephaly are numerous and include relatively well known conditions such as the DiGeorge/ velocardiofacial syndrome (pp. 197, 277) and a host of much rarer multiple malformation syndromes, some of which show autosomal recessive inheritance. One of these, the Smith–Lemli–Opitz syndrome (SLOS) (p. 287), is associated with low levels of cholesterol, which is relevant in that it is known that cholesterol is necessary for normal functioning of the hedgehog development gene family (p. 86).

This leads conveniently to the third group consisting of isolated holoprosencephaly, which until recently was largely unexplained. However, over the last few years three genes have been identified. Heterozygous mutations in these genes can cause very variable degrees of holoprosencephaly, ranging from mild 'microforms' with minimal features such as anosmia to the full-blown lethal alobar form. They are sonic hedgehog (*SHH*) on chromosome 7q36, *ZIC2* on chromosome 13q32 and *SIX3* on chromosome 2p21. Of these *SHH* is thought to make the greatest contribution, accounting for up to 20% of all familial cases and between 1 and 10% of isolated cases. Some sibling recurrences of holoprosencephaly, not due to SLOS, have been shown to be due to germline mutations in these genes

The fact that so many familial cases remain unexplained indicates that more holoprosencephaly genes await identification. The extent of causal heterogeneity shown by this condition is further illustrated by its association with poorly controlled maternal insulin-dependent diabetes mellitus (p. 249).

## Neural tube defects

Neural tube defects, such as spina bifida and anencephaly, illustrate many of the underlying principles of multifactorial inheritance and emphasize the importance of trying to identify possible adverse environmental factors. These conditions result from defective closure of the developing neural tube during the first month of embryonic life. A defect occurring at the upper end of the developing neural tube results in either anencephaly or an encephalocele (Fig. 16.13). A defect occurring at the lower end of the developing neural tube leads to a spinal

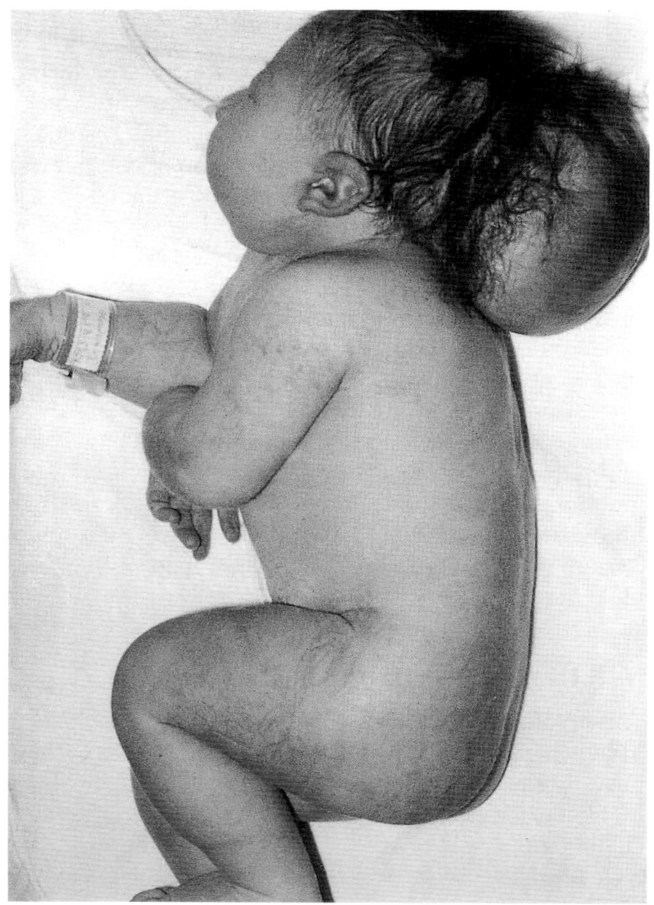

Fig. 16.13
A baby with a large occipital encephalocele.

lesion such as a lumbo-sacral myelocele or meningomyelocele (Fig. 16.2). Most NTDs have serious consequences. Anencephaly is not compatible with survival for more than a few hours after birth. Large lumbo-sacral lesions usually cause partial or complete paralysis of the lower limbs with impaired bladder and bowel continence.

As with many malformations neural tube defects can be classified etiologically under the headings of chromosomal, syndromal and isolated. Chromosomal causes include trisomy 13 and trisomy 18 in both of which NTDs show an incidence of around 5–10%. Syndromal causes include the relatively rare autosomal recessive disorder Meckel syndrome in which an encephalocele occurs in association with polycystic kidneys and polydactyly. However, most NTDs represent isolated malformations in otherwise normal infants and most isolated NTDs are believed to show multifactorial inheritance.

The empiric recurrence risks to first-degree relatives (siblings and offspring) vary according to the local population incidence and are as high as 4–5% in areas where NTDs are common. The incidence in the UK is highest in people of Celtic origin. If such individuals move from their country of origin to another part of the world, the incidence of NTDs in their offspring declines but remains higher than amongst the indigenous population. These observations suggest that there is a relatively high incidence of adverse susceptibility genes in the Celtic populations.

No single NTD susceptibility genes have been identified in humans, although there is some evidence that the common 677C>T polymorphism in the methylenetetrahydrofolate reductase (*MTHFR*) gene can be a susceptibility factor in some populations. Reduction in MTHFR activity results in decreased plasma folate levels, which are known to be causally associated with NTDs (see below). Research efforts have also focused on developmental genes, such as the *PAX* family (p. 90), which are expressed in the embryonic neural tube and vertebral column. To date, understanding of the processes involved in humans is very limited. In contrast, studies in mice have revealed that an interaction between mutations of *PAX1* and the platelet-derived growth factor α gene (*Pdgfra*) results in severe NTDs in 100% of double mutant embryos. This rare example of digenic inheritance serves as a useful illustration of the difficulties posed by a search for susceptibility genes in a multifactorial disorder.

Environmental factors involved in the etiology of NTDs that have been identified include poor socioeconomic status, multiparity and valproic acid embryopathy. Firm evidence has also emerged that periconceptional multivitamin supplementation reduces the risk of recurrence by a factor of 70–75% when a woman has had one affected child. Several studies have shown that folic acid is likely to be the effective constituent in multivitamin preparations. In both the UK and the USA it is recommended that all women who have had a previous child with an NTD should take 4–5 mg of folic acid daily both before and during the early stages of all subsequent pregnancies. Similarly in the UK it has been recommended that all women who are trying to conceive should take 0.4 mg folic acid daily. In the USA, where bread is fortified with folic acid, this recommendation applies to all women of reproductive age throughout their reproductive years. In the UK this recommendation has not as yet resulted in a noticeable decline in the incidence of NTDs, although a longer period may be necessary to show any such effect.

## ENVIRONMENTAL AGENTS (TERATOGENS)

An agent that can cause a birth defect by interfering with normal embryonic or fetal development is known as a teratogen. Many teratogens have been identified and exhaustive tests are now undertaken before any new drug is approved for use by pregnant women. The potential effects of any particular teratogen will usually depend on the dosage and timing when it is administered during the pregnancy, along with the susceptibility of both the mother and her unborn baby.

An agent that conveys a high risk of teratogenesis, such as the rubella virus or thalidomide, will usually be identified relatively quickly. Unfortunately, it is much more difficult to detect a low-grade teratogen that causes an abnormality in only a small proportion of cases. This is because of the relatively high background incidence of congenital abnormalities, and also because many pregnant women take medication at some time in pregnancy, often for an ill-defined 'flu-like' illness. Despite extensive study, controversy still **surrounds** the use of a number of drugs in pregnancy. The antinausea drug Debendox has been the subject of successful litigation in the USA despite the absence of firm evidence to support a definite teratogenic effect.

### DRUGS AND CHEMICALS

Drugs and chemicals which have a proven teratogenic effect in humans are listed in Table 16.7. Overall, these account for approximately 2% of all congenital abnormalities.

Many other drugs have been proposed as possible teratogens but the relatively small numbers of reported cases make it difficult to confirm that they are definitely teratogenic. This applies to many anticancer drugs, such as methotrexate and chlorambucil, and to anticonvulsants, such as sodium valproate, carbamazepine and primadone. Exposure to environmental chemicals is also an area of widespread concern. Organic mercurials ingested in

**Table 16.7 Drugs with a proven teratogenic effect in humans**

| Drug | Effects |
|---|---|
| ACE inhibitors | Renal dysplasia |
| Alcohol | Cardiac defects, microcephaly, characteristic facies |
| Chloroquine | Chorioretinitis, deafness |
| Diethylstilbestrol | Uterine malformations, vaginal adenocarcinoma |
| Lithium | Cardiac defects (Ebstein's anomaly) |
| Phenytoin | Cardiac defects, cleft palate, digital hypoplasia |
| Retinoids | Ear and eye defects, hydrocephalus |
| Streptomycin | Deafness |
| Tetracycline | Dental enamel hypoplasia |
| Thalidomide | Phocomelia, cardiac and ear abnormalities |
| Valproic acid | Neural tube defects, characteristic facies |
| Warfarin | Nasal hypoplasia, stippled epiphyses |

contaminated fish in Minamata, Japan, as a result of industrial pollution caused a 'cerebral palsy-like' syndrome in babies who had been exposed in utero. Controversy surrounds the use of agents used in warfare such as dioxin (Agent Orange) in Vietnam and various nerve gases in the Gulf War.

## The thalidomide tragedy

Thalidomide was used widely in Europe during the years 1958 to 1962 as a sedative. In 1961 an association with severe limb anomalies in babies whose mothers had taken the drug during the first trimester was recognized and the drug was subsequently withdrawn from use. It has been estimated that during this short period over 10 000 babies were damaged by this drug. Review of these babies' records indicated that the critical period for fetal damage was between 20 and 35 days from conception, i.e. 34–50 days after the beginning of the last menstrual period.

The most characteristic abnormality caused by thalidomide was phocomelia (Fig. 16.14). This is the name given to a limb that is malformed due to absence of some or all of the long bones, with retention of digits giving a 'flipper' or 'seal-like' appearance. Other external abnormalities included ear defects, microphthalmia and cleft lip/palate. In addition, approximately 40% of 'thalidomide babies' died in early infancy as a result of severe internal abnormalities affecting the heart, kidneys or gastrointestinal tract. Some 'thalidomide babies' have grown up and had children of their own, and in some cases these offspring have also had similar defects. It is therefore most likely, not surprisingly, that thalidomide was wrongly blamed in a proportion of cases that were in fact due to single-gene defects following autosomal dominant inheritance.

The thalidomide tragedy focused attention on the importance of avoiding all drugs in pregnancy as far as is possible, unless absolute safety has been established. Drug manufacturers undertake extensive research trials before releasing a drug for general use, and invariably urge caution about the use of any new drug in pregnancy. Monitoring systems, in the form of congenital abnormality registers, have been set up in most Western countries so that it is unlikely that an 'epidemic' on the scale of the thalidomide tragedy could ever happen again.

## The fetal alcohol syndrome

Children born to mothers who have consistently consumed large quantities of alcohol during pregnancy tend to show a distinctive facial appearance, with short palpebral fissures (eye apertures) and a long smooth philtrum (upper lip).

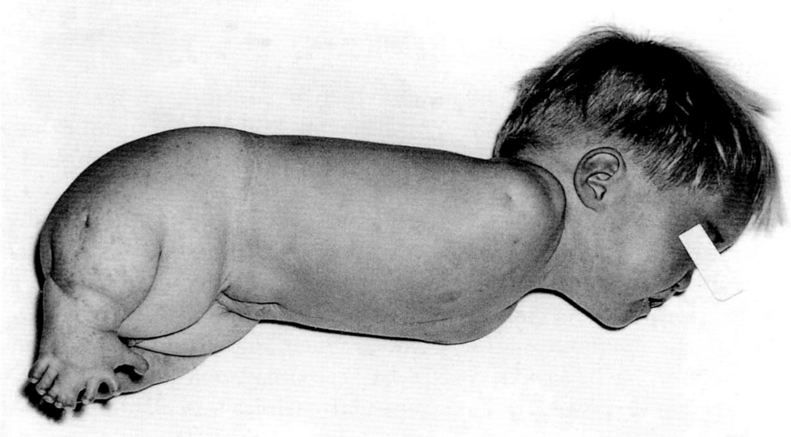

**Fig. 16.14**
A child with thalidomide embryopathy. There is absence of the upper limbs (amelia). The lower limbs show phocomelia and polydactyly. (Courtesy of Emeritus Professor R W Smithells, University of Leeds.)

They also show mild developmental delay and are often hyperactive and clumsy in later childhood. This condition is referred to as the fetal alcohol syndrome. There is uncertainty about the level of alcohol consumption that is 'safe' in pregnancy and there is evidence that even mild-to-moderate ingestion can be harmful. Generally, it is advised that all women should try to abstain from alcohol intake completely throughout pregnancy.

## MATERNAL INFECTIONS

Several infectious agents can interfere with embryogenesis and fetal development (Table 16.8). The developing brain, eyes and ears are particularly susceptible to damage by infection.

### Rubella

The rubella virus, which damages between 15% and 25% of all babies infected during the first trimester, also causes cardiovascular malformations such as patent ductus arteriosus and peripheral pulmonary artery stenosis. Congenital rubella infection can be prevented by the widespread use of immunization programs based on administration of either the measles, mumps, rubella (MMR) vaccine in early childhood or the rubella vaccine alone to young adult women.

### Cytomegalovirus

At present no immunization is available against the cytomegalovirus (CMV) and naturally occurring infection does not always produce long-term immunity. The risk of abnormality is greatest if infection occurs during the first trimester. Overall this virus causes damage in only 5% of infected pregnancies.

### Toxoplasmosis

Maternal infection with the parasite causing toxoplasmosis conveys a risk of 20% that the fetus will be infected during the first trimester, rising to 75% in the second and third trimesters. Vaccines against toxoplasmosis are not available.

If a woman is exposed to any of these infectious agents during pregnancy then an attempt can be made to establish whether the fetus has been infected by sampling fetal blood to look for specific IgM antibodies. Fetal blood analysis can also reveal generalized evidence of infection, such as abnormal liver function and thrombocytopenia.

There is some evidence to suggest that maternal infection with *listeria* can cause a miscarriage, and a definite association has been established between maternal infection with this agent and neonatal meningitis. Maternal infection with parvovirus can cause severe anemia in the fetus, resulting in hydrops fetalis and pregnancy loss.

**Table 16.8 Infectious teratogenic agents**

| Infection | Effects |
|---|---|
| **Viruses** | |
| Cytomegalovirus | Chororetinitis, deafness, microcephaly |
| Herpes simplex | Microcephaly, microphthalmia |
| Rubella | Microcephaly, cataracts, retinitis, cardiac defects |
| Varicella zoster | Microcephaly, chorioretinitis, skin defects |
| **Bacteria** | |
| Syphilis | Hydrocephalus, osteitis, rhinitis |
| **Parasites** | |
| Toxoplasmosis | Hydrocephalus, microcephaly, cataracts, chorioretinitis, deafness |

## PHYSICAL AGENTS

Women who have had babies with congenital abnormalities are often understandably anxious that exposure to agents such as radiowaves, ultrasound or magnetic fields could have caused their babies' problems. Unfortunately, it is difficult to prove or disprove any of these possibilities as exposure to these physical agents is almost universal.

However, there is evidence that two specific physical agents, ionizing radiation and prolonged hyperthermia, can have teratogenic effects.

### Ionizing radiation

Heavy doses of ionizing radiation, far in excess of those used in routine diagnostic radiography, can cause microcephaly and ocular defects in the developing fetus. The most sensitive time of exposure is from 2 to 5 weeks after conception. Ionizing radiation can also have mutagenic (p. 27) and carcinogenic effects, and although the risks associated with low-dose diagnostic procedures are minimal, radiography should always be avoided during pregnancy if at all possible.

### Prolonged hyperthermia

There is evidence that prolonged hyperthermia in early pregnancy can cause microcephaly and microphthalmia as well as neuronal migration defects. Consequently it is recommended that care should be taken to avoid excessive use of hot baths and saunas during the first trimester.

## MATERNAL ILLNESS

A number of maternal illnesses are associated with an increased risk of an untoward pregnancy outcome.

### Diabetes mellitus

Maternal insulin-dependent diabetes mellitus is associated with a two- to threefold increase in the incidence of congenital abnormalities in offspring. Malformations which occur most commonly in such infants include congenital heart disease, neural tube defects, sacral agenesis, femoral hypoplasia, holoprosencephaly and sirenomelia ('mermaidism'). The likelihood of an abnormality is inversely related to the quality of the control of the mother's blood glucose levels during early pregnancy. This can be assessed by regular monitoring of blood glucose and glycosylated hemoglobin levels. Non-insulin-dependent diabetes and gestational diabetes do not convey an increased risk for congenital malformations in offspring.

### Phenylketonuria

The other main maternal metabolic condition that conveys a risk to offspring is untreated phenylketonuria (p. 161). A high serum level of phenylalanine in a pregnant woman with phenylketonuria who is not on a special diet will almost invariably result in serious damage to the fetus, with the incidence of mental retardation in the offspring close to 100%. Structural abnormalities can include microcephaly and congenital heart defects. All women with phenylketonuria should be strongly advised to adhere to a strict and closely monitored low phenylalanine diet both before and during pregnancy.

### Maternal epilepsy

There is a large body of literature devoted to the question of maternal epilepsy, the link with congenital abnormalities, and the teratogenic effects of antiepileptic drugs (AEDs). The largest and best-controlled studies suggest that maternal epilepsy itself is not associated with an increased risk of congenital abnormalities. However, all studies have shown an increased incidence of birth defects in babies exposed to AEDs. The risks are in the region of 5–10%, which is 2–4 times the background population risk. These figures apply mainly to single drug therapy but can be doubled if the fetus is exposed to more than one AED. Some drugs are more teratogenic than others, and data suggest that, of the AEDs currently most commonly prescribed, the highest risks apply to sodium valproate. The range of abnormalities occurring in the 'fetal anticonvulsant syndromes' (FACS) are wide, including neural tube defect (~2%), oral clefting, genitourinary abnormalities such as hypospadias, congenital heart disease and limb defects. The abnormalities themselves are not specific to FACS; making a diagnosis in an individual case can therefore be difficult. Sometimes characteristic facial features are seen, particularly in fetal valproate syndrome (Fig. 16.15).

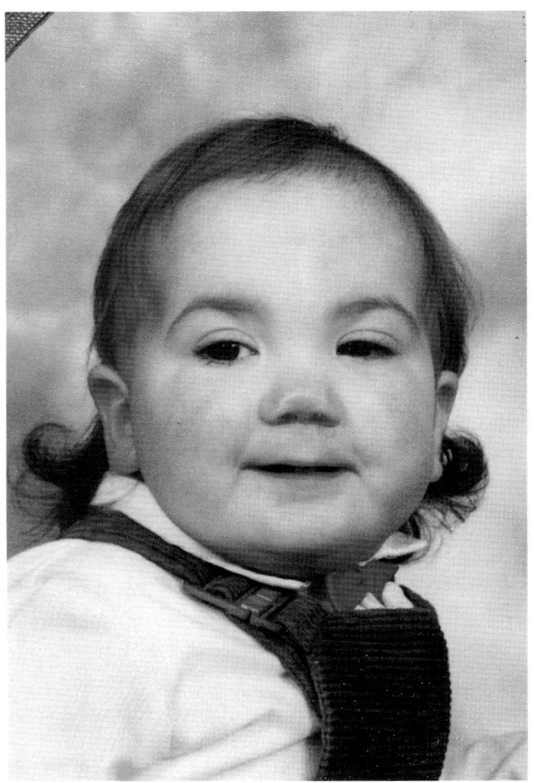

Fig. 16.15
A child with fetal valproate syndrome. She has a broad nasal root, blunt nasal tip and a thin upper lip.

The most controversial aspect of AEDs and FACS is the risk of learning difficulties and behavioral problems. Controlled studies in this area are difficult to set up but many reports, and much clinical experience, strongly suggest that the incidence of these problems is significantly higher than in the general population. For practical purposes, potential risks to the fetus have to be weighed against the dangers of stopping AED treatment and risking seizures during pregnancy. If the patient has been seizure free for at least 2 years she can be offered withdrawal of anticonvulsant treatment before proceeding with a pregnancy. If therapy is essential, then single-drug treatment is much preferred and sodium valproate should be avoided if possible.

## MALFORMATIONS OF UNKNOWN CAUSE

In up to 50% of all congenital abnormalities no clear cause can be established. This applies to many relatively common conditions such as isolated diaphragmatic hernia, tracheo-esophageal fistula, anal atresia and single limb reduction defects. For an isolated limb defect, such as absence of a hand, it is reasonable to postulate that loss of vascular supply at a critical time during the development of the limb bud leads to developmental arrest, with the formation of only vestigial digits. It is much more difficult to envisage how vascular occlusion could result in an abnormality such as esophageal atresia with an associated tracheo-esophageal fistula.

## SYMMETRY AND ASYMMETRY

In trying to assess whether a birth defect is genetic or non-genetic it can be very helpful to consider aspects of symmetry. As a broad generalization, symmetrical and midline abnormalities frequently have a genetic basis. Asymmetrical defects are less likely to have a genetic basis. In the examples shown in Figure 16.16 the child with cleidocranial dysplasia (Fig. 16.16A) has symmetrical defects (absent or hypoplastic clavicles) and other features indicating a generalized tissue disorder that is overwhelmingly likely to have a genetic basis. The striking asymmetry of the limb deformities in Figure 16.16B is very likely to have a non-genetic basis.

## COUNSELING

In cases where the precise diagnosis is uncertain an assessment of symmetry and midline involvement may be helpful for genetic counseling. While it is obviously frustrating for the parents of a child with one of these abnormalities that no factual explanation can be given, in many cases they can at least be reassured that the empiric risk of recurrence for siblings is very low. It is worth noting that this does not necessarily mean that genetic factors are irrelevant. Some 'unexplained' malformations and syndromes could well be due to new dominant mutations (p. 108), submicroscopic microdeletions or uniparental disomy (p. 117).

All of these would convey negligible recurrence risks to future siblings, although those cases due to new mutations or microdeletions would be associated with a significant risk to offspring of affected individuals. There is optimism that molecular techniques will provide at least some of the answers to these many unresolved issues.

A

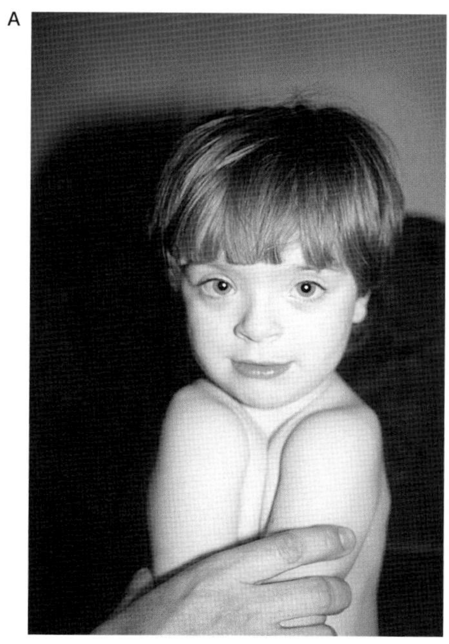

B

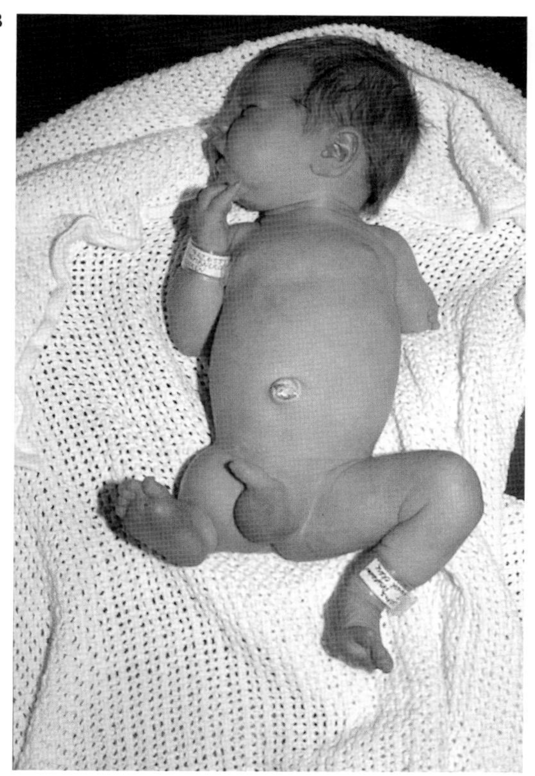

**Fig. 16.6**
(A) A boy with cleidocranial dysplasia in whom the clavicles have failed to develop, hence the remarkable mobility of his shoulders. He also has a relatively large head with widely spaced eyes (hypertelorism). He presented with ear problems – conductive deafness is a recognized feature. Skeletal dysplasias usually manifest in one main tissue and are symmetrical, thus suggesting a genetic basis. (B) A child with congenital limb deformities due to amniotic bands. The complete lack of symmetry suggests a non-genetic cause.

## FURTHER READING

Aase J 1990 Diagnostic dysmorphology. Plenum, London
*A detailed text of the art and science of dysmorphology.*

Hanson J W 1997 Human teratology. In: Rimoin D L, Connor J M, Pyeritz R E (eds) Principles and practice of medical genetics, 3rd edn. Churchill Livingstone, New York, pp. 697–724
*A comprehensive balanced overview of known and suspected human teratogens.*

Jones K L 1996 Smith's recognizable patterns of human malformation, 5th edn. Saunders, Philadelphia
*The standard pediatric textbook guide to syndromes.*

Smithells R W, Newman C G H 1992 Recognition of thalidomide defects. J Med Genet 29: 716–723
*A comprehensive account of the spectrum of abnormalities caused by thalidomide.*

Spranger J, Benirschke K, Hall J G et al 1982 Errors of morphogenesis: concepts and terms. Recommendations of an international working group. J Pediatr 100: 160–165
*A short paper providing a classification and clarification of the terms used in describing birth defects.*

Stevenson R E, Hall J G, Goodman R M 1993 Human malformations and related anomalies. Oxford University Press, New York
*The definitive guide, in two volumes, to human malformations.*

## ELEMENTS

1. Congenital abnormalities are apparent at birth in 1 in 40 of all newborn infants. They account for 20–25% of all deaths occurring in the perinatal period and in childhood up to the age of 10 years.

2. A single abnormality can be classified as a malformation, a deformation, a dysplasia or a disruption. Multiple abnormalties can be classified as a sequence, a syndrome or an association.

3. Congenital abnormalities can be caused by chromosome imbalance, single-gene defects, multifactorial inheritance or non-genetic factors. Most isolated malformations, including isolated congenital heart defects and neural tube defects, show multifactorial inheritance, whereas most dysplasias have a single-gene etiology.

4. Many congenital malformations, including cleft lip/palate, congenital heart defects and neural tube defects, show etiological heterogeneity, so that when counseling it is important to establish whether these malformations are isolated or are associated with other abnormalities.

5. Many environmental agents have been shown to have a teratogenic effect and, if at all possible, great care should be taken to avoid exposure to these agents during pregnancy.

CHAPTER 17

# Genetic counseling

*Q. "What's the difference between ... a doctor ... and God?"*
*A. "God doesn't think He's a doctor."*

Anon

Any couple who have had a child with a serious abnormality must inevitably reflect on why this has happened and whether any child(ren) they choose to have in future could be similarly affected. Similarly, individuals with a family history of a serious disorder are likely to be concerned that they could either develop the disorder or transmit it to future generations. They are also very concerned about the risk that their normal children might transmit the condition to their offspring. For all those affected by a genetic condition that is serious to them, great sensitivity is needed in communication. Just a few words spoken with genuine caring concern can put patients at ease and allow a meaningful session to proceed; just a few careless words that make light of a serious situation can damage communication irrevocably. The importance of confidence and trust in the relationship between patient and health professional can never be underestimated.

Realization of the needs of such individuals and couples, together with awareness of the importance of providing them with accurate and appropriate information, has led to the widespread introduction of genetic counseling clinics in parallel with the establishment of clinical genetics as a recognized medical specialty.

## DEFINITION

Since the first introduction of genetic counseling services approximately 40 years ago many attempts have been made to devise a satisfactory and all-embracing definition. A theme common to all is the concept of genetic counseling being a process of communication and education which addresses concerns relating to the development and/or transmission of a hereditary disorder.

An individual who seeks genetic counseling is known as a *consultand*. During the genetic counseling process it is widely agreed that the counselor should try to ensure that the consultand is provided with information that enables him or her to understand:

1. The medical diagnosis and its implications in terms of prognosis and possible treatment.
2. The mode of inheritance of the disorder and the risk of developing and/or transmitting it.
3. The choices or options available for dealing with the risks.

It is also agreed that genetic counseling should include a strong communicative and supportive element, so that those who seek information are able to reach their own fully informed decisions without undue pressure or stress (Table 17.1).

**Table 17.1 Steps in genetic counseling**

| |
|---|
| Diagnosis — based on accurate family history, medical history, examination and investigations |
| Risk assessment |
| Communication |
| Discussion of options |
| Long-term contact and support |

## ESTABLISHING THE DIAGNOSIS

The most crucial step in any genetic consultation is that of establishing the diagnosis. If this is incorrect, then inappropriate and totally misleading information could be given, with potentially tragic consequences.

Reaching a diagnosis in clinical genetics usually involves the three fundamental steps of any medical consultation, i.e. taking a history, carrying out an examination and undertaking appropriate investigations. Often, detailed information about the consultand's family history will have been obtained by a skilled genetic nurse counselor as part of a preclinic home visit. A full and accurate family history is a cornerstone in the whole genetic assessment and counseling process. Further information about the family and personal medical history often emerges at the clinic visit, when a full examination can be undertaken and appropriate investigations initiated. These can include chromosome and molecular studies as well as referral on to specialists in other fields, such as neurology and ophthalmology.

It cannot be overemphasized that the quality of genetic counseling is dependent upon the availability of facilities that ensure an accurate diagnosis can be made.

Even when a firm diagnosis has been made, problems can arise if the disorder in question shows etiological heterogeneity. Common examples include hearing loss and non-specific mental retardation, both of which can be caused by either environmental or genetic factors. In these situations empiric risks can be used (p. 348), although these are not as satisfactory as risks based on a precise and specific diagnosis.

A disorder is said to show genetic *heterogeneity* if it can be caused by more than one genetic mechanism (p. 109). Many such disorders are recognized, and counseling can be extremely difficult if the heterogeneity extends to different modes of inheritance. Commonly encountered examples include the various forms of Ehlers–Danlos syndrome (Fig. 17.1), Charcot–Marie–Tooth disease (p. 297) and retinitis pigmentosa, all of which can show autosomal dominant, autosomal recessive and X-linked recessive inheritance (Table 17.2). Fortunately, progress in molecular genetics is providing solutions to some of these problems. For example, mutations in the gene that codes for rhodopsin, a retinal pigment protein, are found in approximately 30% of families showing autosomal dominant inheritance of retinitis pigmentosa (Fig. 17.2) and the molecular basis of the most common forms of Charcot–Marie–Tooth disease (type 1), also known as hereditary motor and sensory neuropathy (HMSN), is now understood (p. 297).

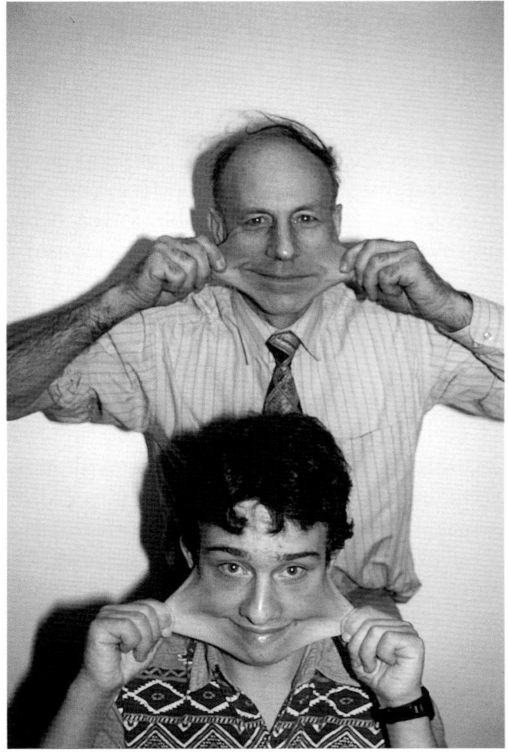

**Fig. 17.1**
Ehlers–Danlos syndrome. The inheritance pattern in this case is autosomal dominant because father and son are affected.

**Table 17.2 Hereditary disorders that can show different patterns of inheritance**

| Disorder | Inheritance patterns |
|---|---|
| Cerebellar ataxia | AD, AR |
| Charcot–Marie–Tooth disease (HMSN) | AD, AR, XR |
| Congenital cataract | AD, AR, XR |
| Ehlers–Danlos syndrome | AD, AR, XR |
| Ichthyosis | AD, AR, XR |
| Microcephaly | AD, AR |
| Polycystic kidney disease | AD, AR |
| Retinitis pigmentosa | AD, AR, XR, M |
| Sensorineural hearing loss | AD, AR, XR, M |

AD: autosomal dominant; AR: autosomal recessive; XR: X-linked recessive; M: mitochondrial

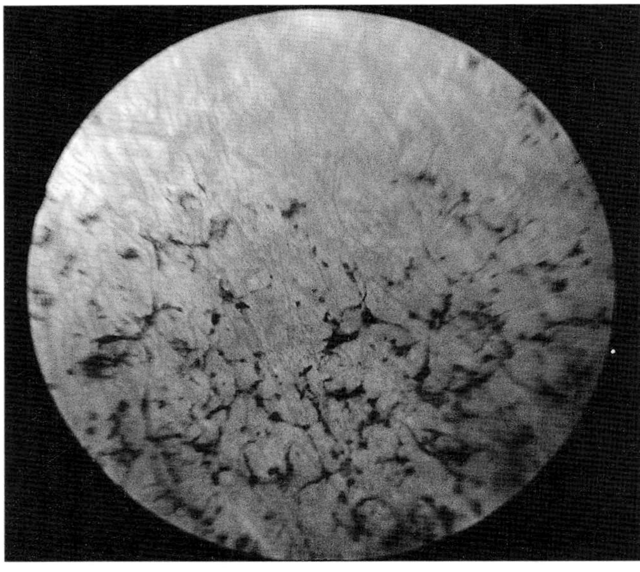

**Fig. 17.2**
Fundus showing typical pigmentary changes of retinitis pigmentosa.

## CALCULATING AND PRESENTING THE RISK

In some counseling situations, calculation of the recurrence risk is relatively straightforward and requires little more than a reasonable knowledge of Mendelian inheritance. However, many factors, such as delayed age of onset, reduced penetrance and the use of linked DNA markers, can result in the calculation becoming much more complex. The theoretical aspects of risk calculation are considered in more detail in Chapter 22.

The provision of a recurrence risk does not simply involve conveying a stark risk figure in isolation. It is very important that information that is provided is understood and that parents are given as much background information as possible to help them reach their own decision. As a working rule of thumb, recurrence risks should be quantified, qualified and placed in context.

## QUANTIFICATION – THE NUMERICAL VALUE OF A RISK

Most prospective parents will be familiar to some degree with the concept of risks, but not everyone is comfortable with probability theory and the alternative ways of expressing risk, such as in the form of odds or as a percentage. Thus, for example, a risk of 1 in 4 can be presented as an odds ratio of 3 to 1 against, or numerically as 25%. Consistency and clarity are important if confusion is to be avoided. It is also essential to emphasize that a risk applies to *each* pregnancy and that chance does not have a memory. For example, the fact that parents have just had a child with an autosomal recessive disorder (recurrence risk equals 1 in 4) does not mean that their next three children will be unaffected. A useful analogy is that of the tossed coin that cannot be expected to remember whether it landed heads or tails at the last throw and cannot therefore be expected to know what it should do at the next throw.

It is also important that genetic counselors should not be seen exclusively as prophets of doom. Continuing the penny analogy, the good side of the coin should also be emphasized, particularly if the odds strongly favor a successful outcome. For example, a couple faced with a probability of 1 in 25 that their next baby will have a neural tube defect should be reminded that there are 24 chances out of 25 that their next baby will not be affected.

## QUALIFICATION – THE NATURE OF A RISK

Several studies have indicated that the factor which most influences parents when deciding whether or not to have another child is the nature of the long-term burden, or severity, associated with a risk rather than its precise numerical value. Therefore a 'high' risk of 1 in 2 for a trivial problem such as an extra digit (polydactyly) will deter very few parents. In contrast a 'low' risk of 1 in 25 for a disabling condition such as a neural tube defect can have a very significant deterrent effect. A woman who grew up watching her brother develop Duchenne muscular dystrophy and subsequently die from the condition aged 21 years, may not risk having children even if there is only a 1% chance that she is a carrier. Other factors, such as whether a condition can be successfully treated, whether it is associated with pain and suffering, and whether prenatal diagnosis is available, will all be relevant to the decision-making process.

## PLACING RISKS IN CONTEXT

Prospective parents seen at a genetic counseling clinic should be provided with information that enables them to put their risks in context so as to be able to decide for themselves whether a risk is 'high' or 'low'. For example, it can be helpful (but also alarming) to point out that approximately 1 in 40 of all babies has a congenital malformation or handicapping disorder. Therefore an additional quoted risk of 1 in 50, while initially alarming, might on reflection be perceived as relatively low. As an arbitrary guide, risks of 1 in 10 or greater tend to be regarded as high, 1 in 20 or less as low, and intermediate values as moderate.

# DISCUSSING THE OPTIONS

Having established the diagnosis and discussed the risk of occurrence/recurrence, the counselor is then obliged to ensure that the consultands are provided with all of the information necessary for them to make their own informed decisions. This should include details of all the choices open to them. For example, if relevant, the availability of prenatal diagnosis should be discussed, together with details of the techniques, limitations and risks associated with the various methods employed (Ch. 21). Mention will sometimes be made of other reproductive options. These can include alternative approaches to conception, such as artificial insemination using donor sperm (AID), the use of donor ova and preimplantation genetic diagnosis (p. 336). These techniques can be used when one partner is infertile, as in the case of Klinefelter syndrome and Turner syndrome (Ch. 18), or simply to bypass the possibility that one or other partner will transmit his or her disadvantageous gene(s) to the baby.

These are issues that should be broached with great care and sensitivity. For some couples the prospect of prenatal diagnosis followed by selective termination of pregnancy is unacceptable, whereas others view this as their only means of ensuring that any children they do have will be healthy. Whatever the personal views of the counselor, the consultands are entitled to knowledge of those prenatal diagnostic procedures that are both technically feasible and legally permissible.

## COMMUNICATION AND SUPPORT

The ability to communicate is essential in genetic counseling. Communication is a two-way process. Not only does the counselor provide information, he or she also has to be receptive to the fears and aspirations, expressed or unexpressed, of the consultand. A readiness to listen is a key attribute for anyone involved in genetic counseling, as is an ability to present information in a clear, sympathetic and appropriate manner.

Often an individual or couple will be extremely upset when first made aware of a genetic diagnosis, and it is very common for guilt feelings to set in. The individual or couple may look back and scrutinize every event and happening, for example during a pregnancy. The delivery of potentially distressing information cannot be carried out in isolation. Genetic counselors need to take into account the complex psychological and emotional factors that can influence the counseling dialog. The setting should be agreeable, private and quiet, with ample time for discussion and questions. When possible, technical terms should be avoided or, if used, fully explained. Questions should be answered openly and honestly, and if information is lacking it is certainly not a fault or sign of weakness to admit that this is so. Most couples respect and recognize the truth, and some parents of children whose condition cannot be diagnosed derive a curious pleasure from knowing that their child appears to be unique and has bamboozled the medical profession (unfortunately, this is not particularly difficult!).

Despite all these measures, a counseling session can be so intense and intimidating that the amount and accuracy of information retained on follow-up at a later date can be very limited. For this reason a letter summarizing the topics discussed at a counseling session is usually sent to the family afterwards. In addition, they are often contacted at a later date by a member of the counseling team, either by telephone or by a home visit, thereby providing an opportunity for clarification of any confusing issues and for further questions to be answered.

It would be wrong to simply convey information of a distressing nature without offering an opportunity for further discussion and long-term support. Most genetic counseling centres maintain informal contact with relevant families through a network of genetic nurse counselors who are familiar with the family and their particular circumstances. This is especially valuable for prospective parents who subsequently request specific prenatal diagnostic investigations and for presymptomatic adults who are shown to be at high risk of developing late-onset autosomal dominant disorders such as Alzheimer disease and Huntington disease (p. 293). Genetic registers (p. 324) provide a very useful means of ensuring that effective contact can be maintained with all such relevant family members.

### PATIENT SUPPORT GROUPS

Finally, mention should be made of the widespread network of support groups that now exists. These organizations have usually been established by highly motivated and well-informed parents or affected families who can provide enormous support and companionship for others affected by a particular genetic condition or syndrome. When confronted by a new diagnosis of a rare disorder many families feel very isolated, and if at all possible they should be given contact information so that they have the option of communicating with other affected families who have had similar experiences. Referral to an appropriate support group would now be viewed as an essential integral component of the genetic counseling process. As well as providing support and information for affected families these groups have often been very successful in fostering research.

## GENETIC COUNSELING – DIRECTIVE OR NON-DIRECTIVE?

It has already been emphasized that genetic counseling should be viewed as a communication process that provides information. The ultimate goal is to ensure that an individual or couple can reach their own decisions based on full information about risks and options. There is universal agreement that genetic counseling should be non-directive, with no attempt being made to steer the consultand along a particular course of action. In the same spirit the genetic counselor should also strive to be non-judgmental, even if a decision is reached that seems ill-advised or is contrary to the counselor's own beliefs. Thus the role of the genetic counselor is to facilitate and enhance individual autonomy rather than give advice or recommend a particular course of action.

Genetic counselors are sometimes asked what they themselves would do if placed in the consultand's position. Generally it is preferable to avoid being drawn into expressing an opinion, opting instead to suggest that the consultand try to imagine how he or she might feel in the future having pursued each of the available options. This approach, sometimes referred to as 'scenario-based decision counseling', provides individuals with an opportunity for careful reflection. This is particularly important if one of the options under consideration involves a potentially irreversible reproductive decision such as sterilization. There is a well-established maxim that it is the consultands and not the counselors who have to live with the consequences of their decisions and, indeed, consultands should be encouraged to make the decision that they can best live with – the one that they are least likely to regret.

## OUTCOMES IN GENETIC COUNSELING

The issue of defining outcomes in genetic counseling is difficult and contentious, but also topical in today's climate of health economy where everything has to be justified. The difficulty arises because of the rather nebulous nature of genetic counseling, which in contrast to most medical activities does not have any easily quantified end points, such as rate of infection or survival after surgery. The issue is topical because of the increasing pressure being applied by funding authorities, with emphasis on demonstrable quality and effectiveness. Finally, the issue is contentious because it raises serious questions about the purpose of genetic counseling and whether this should be viewed as simply the provision of information or whether there should be identified benefits for society in terms of a reduction in the incidence of genetic disease.

In practice the three main outcome measures that have been assessed are recall, impact on subsequent reproductive behavior, and patient satisfaction. Most studies have shown that the majority of individuals who have attended a genetic counseling clinic have a reasonable recall of the information given, particularly if this was reinforced by a personal letter or follow-up visit. Nevertheless, confusion can arise, and as many as 30% of counselees have difficulty in remembering a precise risk figure. Studies that have focused on the subsequent reproductive behavior of couples who have attended a genetic counseling clinic have shown that approximately 50% have been influenced to some extent. Those factors that have been shown to be influential are the severity of the disorder, the desire of the parents to have children, and whether prenatal diagnosis and/or treatment are available. Finally, studies that have attempted to assess patient satisfaction have struggled to address the problem of how this should best be defined. For example, an individual could be very satisfied with the way in which they were counseled but remain very dissatisfied by lack of a precise diagnosis or the availability of subsequent prenatal diagnostic tests.

In an increasingly cost-conscious society it is not surprising that the purchasers of health care, whether privately or state funded, are keen to identify quantifiable targets with which they can assess the 'effectiveness' of genetics services, and genetic counseling in particular. Outcomes such as the number of abnormal pregnancies terminated or individuals screened can seem attractive to administrators and politicians who are preoccupied with balancing budgets and cost–benefit analyses. In contrast, clinical geneticists and non-medical counselor colleagues universally reject the use of these outcome criteria on the grounds that they hint at a eugenics philosophy that is totally unacceptable in a society in which patient autonomy is a guiding ethical principle. Instead they emphasize the benefits of an educated informed community with enhanced individual autonomy. The goals of satisfaction as expressed by the users of genetic services and their ability to make informed decisions are seen as much more acceptable than a reduction in the financial and personal burdens caused by genetic disease.

In the future it is possible that an outcome measure such as 'perceived personal control' will be developed. This will almost certainly incorporate both information and satisfaction criteria, together with an assessment of whether individuals have been able to understand the information and come to terms with their situation, thereby enabling them to make appropriate life decisions with which they are comfortable. The idea is also consistent with general government policy to encourage individuals to take more personal control of their own health agenda.

## SPECIAL PROBLEMS IN GENETIC COUNSELING

There are a number of special problems that can arise in genetic counseling.

### CONSANGUINITY

A consanguineous relationship is one between blood relatives who have at least one common ancestor no more remote than a great-great grandparent. Consanguineous marriage is widespread in many parts of the world (Table 17.3). In Arab populations the most common type of consanguineous marriage occurs between first cousins who are the children of two brothers, whereas in the Indian subcontinent uncle–niece marriages are the most commonly encountered form of consanguineous relationship. While there is in these communities some recognition of the potential disadvantageous genetic effects of consanguinity, there is also a strongly held view that these are greatly outweighed by social advantages such as greater family and marital stability.

**Table 17.3 Worldwide incidence of consanguineous marriage**

| Country | Incidence (%) |
|---|---|
| Kuwait | 54 |
| Saudi Arabia | 54 |
| Jordan | 50 |
| Pakistan | 40–50 |
| India | 5–60 |
| Syria | 33 |
| Egypt | 28 |
| Lebanon | 25 |
| Algeria | 23 |
| Japan | 2–4 |
| France, UK, USA | 2 |

Data adapted from various sources including Jaber L, Halpern G J, Shohat M 1998 The impact of consanguinity worldwide. Community Genet 1: 12–17

Many studies have shown that among the offspring of consanguineous marriages there is an increased incidence of both congenital malformations and other conditions that will present later, such as hearing loss and mental retardation. For the offspring of first cousins the incidence of congenital malformations is increased to approximately twice that seen in the offspring of unrelated parents. Almost all of this increase in morbidity and mortality is attributed to homozygosity for autosomal recessive disorders, a finding consistent with Garrod's original observation that 'the mating of first cousins gives exactly the conditions most likely to enable a rare, and usually recessive, character to show itself' (p. 109).

On the basis of studies of children born to consanguineous parents it has been estimated that the average human carries between one and two genes for a harmful autosomal recessive disorder, together with several mutations for conditions that result in lethality before birth. Most prospective consanguineous parents are concerned primarily with the risk that they will have a handicapped child, and fortunately the overall risks are usually relatively small. When estimating a risk for a particular consanguineous relationship it is generally assumed that each common ancestor carried one deleterious recessive mutation.

Therefore, for first cousins, the probability that their first child will be homozygous for their common grandfather's deleterious gene will be 1 in 64 (Fig. 17.3). Similarly, the risk that this child will be homozygous for the common grandmother's recessive gene will also be 1 in 64. This gives a total probability that the child will be homozygous for one of the grandparent's deleterious genes of 1 in 32. This risk should be added to the general population risk of 1 in 40 that any baby will have a major congenital abnormality (p. 247), to give an overall risk of approximately 1 in 20 that a child born to first-cousin parents will be either malformed or handicapped in some way. Risks arising from consanguinity for more distant relatives are much lower.

For consanguineous marriages there is also a slightly increased risk that a child will have a multifactorial disorder. In practice this risk is usually very small. In contrast, a close family history of an autosomal recessive disorder can convey a relatively high risk that a consanguineous couple will have an affected child. For example, if the sibling of someone with an autosomal recessive disorder marries a first cousin, the risk that their first baby will be affected equals 1 in 24 (p. 344).

## INCEST

Incestuous relationships are those which occur between first-degree relatives (in other words, brother/sister or parent/child – see Table 17.4). Marriage between first-degree relatives is forbidden, both on religious grounds and by legislation in almost every culture. Incestuous relationships are associated with a very high risk of abnormality in offspring, with less than half the children of such unions being entirely healthy (Table 17.5).

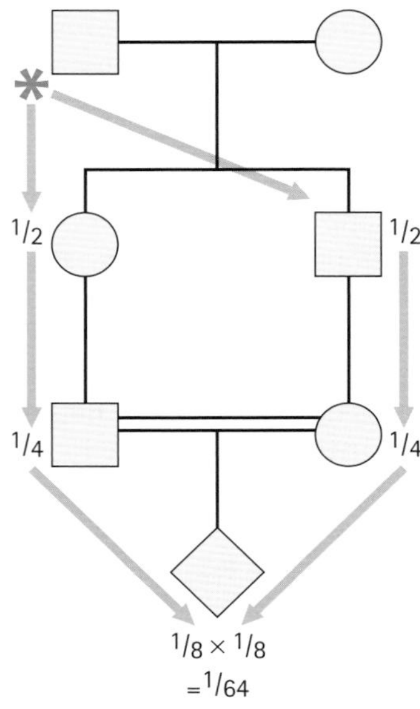


**Fig. 17.3**
Shows the probability that the first child of first cousins will be homozygous for the deleterious allele* carried by the common great-grandfather. A similar risk of 1 in 64 will apply to the deleterious allele belonging to the common great-grandmother, giving a total risk of 1 in 32.

**Table 17.4 Genetic relationship between relatives and risk of abnormality in their offspring**

| Genetic relationship | Proportion of shared genes | Risk of abnormality in offspring (%) |
|---|---|---|
| **First degree**<br>Parent/child<br>Brother/sister | 1/2 | 50 |
| **Second degree**<br>Uncle/niece<br>Aunt/nephew<br>Double first cousins | 1/4 | 5–10 |
| **Third degree**<br>First cousins | 1/8 | 3–5 |

**Table 17.5 Frequencies of the three main types of abnormality in the children of incestuous relationships**

| Abnormality | Frequency (%) |
|---|---|
| **Mental retardation** | |
| Severe | 25 |
| Mild | 35 |
| **Autosomal recessive disorder** | **10–15** |
| **Congenital malformation** | **10** |

## ADOPTION AND GENETIC DISORDERS

The issue of adoption can arise in several situations relating to genetics. Firstly, parents at high risk of having a child with a serious abnormality often express interest in adopting rather than running the risk of having an affected baby. In genetic terms this is a perfectly reasonable option, although in practice the number of couples wishing to adopt usually far exceeds the number of babies and children available for adoption.

The physician with a knowledge of genetics can also be called upon to try to determine whether a child who is being placed for adoption will develop a genetic disorder. For the offspring of consanguineous or incestuous matings, risks can be given as outlined previously (Tables 17.4 and 17.5). Adoption societies sometimes also wish to place a child with a family history of a particular hereditary disorder. This raises the difficult ethical dilemma of predictive testing in childhood for conditions showing onset in adult life (p. 371). Increasingly it is felt that such testing should not be undertaken unless this will be of direct medical benefit to the child. In practice, even when a child is actually affected by a genetic disorder, suitable adoptive parents can usually be found.

Concern about the possible misuse of genetic testing in neonates and young children who are up for adoption has prompted the American Society of Human Genetics and the American College of Medical Genetics to issue joint recommendations. These are based on the best interests of the child. They can be summarized as supporting genetic testing in such children only when the testing would be appropriate for all children of that age and when the tests are undertaken for disorders that manifest during childhood and for which preventive measures can be undertaken during childhood. The joint statement does not support testing for untreatable disorders of adult onset or for detecting predispositions to 'physical, mental or behavioral traits within the normal range'.

## DISPUTED PATERNITY

This presents a difficult problem for which the help of a clinical geneticist is sometimes sought. Until recently paternity could never be proved with absolute certainty, although it could be disproved or excluded in two ways. If a child was found to possess a blood group or other polymorphism not present in either the mother or the putative father, then paternity could be confidently excluded. For example, if the mother and putative father both lacked blood group B, but this was present in the child, then the putative father could be excluded. Similarly, if a child lacked a marker that the putative father would have had to transmit to all of his children, then once again paternity could be excluded. As an example, a putative father with blood group AB could not have a child with blood group O.

Until recently attempts to establish paternity were based on analysis of several different polymorphic systems, such as blood groups, isoenzymes and HLA haplotypes. The results of these studies can be consistent with paternity but cannot give absolute proof of it. Depending on the number of polymorphic systems analyzed and their frequencies in the general population, it is possible to calculate the relative probability that a particular male is the father compared with any male taken at random from the general population.

The limitations of these approaches have been overcome by the development of genetic fingerprinting using minisatellite repeat sequence probes (pp. 18, 72). The

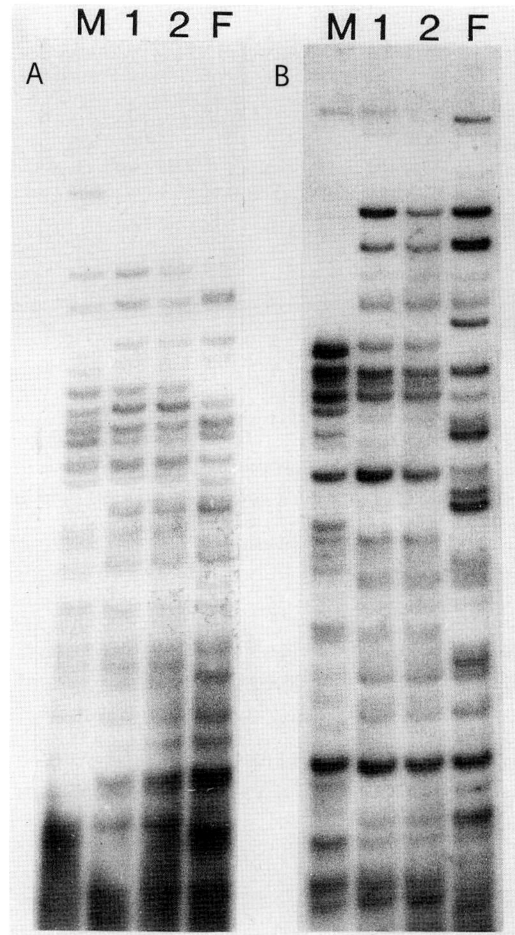


**Fig. 17.4**
Genetic fingerprint obtained using two minisatellite probes with DNA from a mother (M), father (F) and their twins (1 and 2). The twins have an identical set of bands and each band in the twins originates from one of the parents. Reproduced with permission from the American Journal of Medical Genetics. (Courtesy of Dr Raymond Dalgleish and Professor Sir Alec Jeffreys, University of Leicester, reproduced from Young I D, Dalgleish R, Mackay E H, MacFadyen U M 1988 Discordant expression of the G syndrome in monozygotic twins. Am J Med Genet 29: 863–869.)

pattern of DNA fragments generated by these probes is so highly polymorphic that the restriction map obtained is unique to each individual, with the exception of identical twins (Fig. 17.4). If DNA from the child and the mother is analyzed then the bands inherited from the biological father can be analyzed and compared with those present in DNA from the putative father(s). If these match, this gives an extremely high mathematical probability that the putative and biological fathers are the same individual.

## FURTHER READING


ASHG/ACMG. Statement 2000. Genetic testing in adoption. Am J Hum Genet 66: 761–767

*The joint recommendations of the American Society of Human Genetics and the American College of Medical Genetics on genetic testing in young children who are being placed for adoption.*

Clarke A (ed) 1994 Genetic counselling. Practice and principles. Routledge, London

*A thoughtful and provocative multi-author text that addresses difficult issues such as predictive testing, screening, prenatal diagnosis and confidentiality.*

Clarke A, Parsons E, Williams A 1996 Outcomes and process in genetic counseling. Clin Genet 50: 462–469

*A critical review of previous studies of the outcomes of genetic counseling.*

Frets P G, Niermeijer M F 1990. Reproductive planning after genetic counselling: a perspective from the last decade. Clin Genet 38: 295–306

*A review of studies undertaken between 1980 and 1989 to determine that factors are most important in influencing reproductive decisions.*

Harper P S 1998 Practical genetic counselling, 5th edn. Butterworth-Heinemann, Oxford

*An extremely useful practical guide to all aspects of genetic counseling.*

Jaber L, Halpern G J, Shohat M 1998 The impact of consanguinity worldwide. Community Genet 1: 12–17

*A review of the incidence and consequences of consanguinity in various parts of the world.*

Jeffreys A J, Brookfield J F Y, Semeonoff R 1985 Positive identification of an immigration test-case using human DNA fingerprints. Nature 317: 818–819

*A clever demonstration of the value of genetic fingerprinting in analyzing alleged family relationships.*

Turnpenny P (ed) 1995 Secrets in the genes: adoption, inheritance and genetic disease. British Agencies for Adoption and Fostering, London

*A multi-author basic text covering aspects of genetics relevant to the adoption process.*


## ELEMENTS

1. Genetic counseling may be defined as a communication process that deals with the risk of developing or transmitting a genetic disorder.

2. The most important steps in genetic counseling are the establishment of a diagnosis, estimation of a recurrence risk, communication of relevant information and the provision of long-term support.

3. Genetic counseling should be non-directive and the genetic counselor should be non-judgmental. The goal of genetic counseling is to provide accurate information that enables counselees to make their own fully informed decisions.

4. Marriage between blood relatives conveys an increased risk for an autosomal recessive disorder in future offspring. The probability that first cousins will have a child with an autosomal recessive condition is approximately 3%, although this risk can be greater if there is a family history of a specific genetic disorder.

5. The most sensitive technique for paternity testing is genetic fingerprinting. Other polymorphic systems can disprove paternity but cannot establish with such a high statistical probability that a particular male is the biological father.

CHAPTER

# 18 Chromosome disorders

The development of a reliable technique for chromosome analysis in 1956 soon led to the discovery that several previously described conditions were due to an abnormality in chromosome number. Within 3 years the causes of Down syndrome (47,XX/XY, +21), Klinefelter syndrome (47,XXY) and Turner syndrome (45,X) had been established. Shortly afterwards other autosomal trisomy syndromes were recognized, and gradually over the ensuing years many other multiple malformation syndromes were described in which there was loss or gain of chromosome material.

To date, around 20 000 chromosomal abnormalities have been registered on laboratory databases. While on an individual basis most of these are very rare, together they make a major contribution to human morbidity and mortality. Chromosome abnormalities account for a large proportion of spontaneous pregnancy loss and childhood disability, and also contribute to the genesis of a significant proportion of malignancy in both childhood and adult life as a consequence of acquired somatic chromosome aberrations.

In Chapter 3 the basic principles of chromosome structure and function were described. Details of chromosome behavior during cell division were also provided, along with a theoretical account of the nature of chromosome abnormalities and how these can both arise and be transmitted in families. In this chapter the medical aspects of chromosome abnormalities are considered and specific chromosome abnormality syndromes described.

## INCIDENCE OF CHROMOSOME ABNORMALITIES

Chromosome abnormalities are present in at least 10% of all spermatozoa and 25% of mature oocytes. Between 15% and 20% of all recognized pregnancies end in spontaneous miscarriage, and many more zygotes and embryos are so abnormal that survival beyond the first few days or weeks after fertilization is not possible. Approximately 50% of all spontaneous miscarriages have a chromosome abnormality (Table 18.1) and the incidence of chromosomal abnormalities in morphologically normal embryos is around 20%. These observations indicate that chromosome abnormalities account for the loss of a very high proportion of all human conceptions.

From conception onwards the incidence of chromosome abnormalities falls rapidly. By birth it has declined to a level of 0.5–1%, although the total is much higher (5%) in stillborn infants. Table 18.2 lists the incidence figures for chromosome abnormalities based on newborn surveys. It is notable that among the commonly recognized aneuploidy syndromes there is also a high proportion of spontaneous pregnancy loss (Table 18.3). This is illustrated by comparison of the incidence of conditions such as Down syndrome at the time of chorionic villus sampling (11–12 weeks), amniocentesis (16 weeks) and term (Fig. 18.1).

## DOWN SYNDROME (TRISOMY 21)

This condition derives its name from Dr Langdon Down, who first described it in the Clinical Lecture Reports of the London Hospital in 1866. The chromosomal basis of

**Table 18.1 Chromosome abnormalities in spontaneous abortions (percentage figures relate to total of chromosomally abnormal abortuses)**

| Abnormality | Incidence (%) |
|---|---|
| Trisomy 13 | 2 |
| Trisomy 16 | 15 |
| Trisomy 18 | 3 |
| Trisomy 21 | 5 |
| Trisomy other | 25 |
| Monosomy X | 20 |
| Triploidy | 15 |
| Tetraploidy | 5 |
| Other | 10 |

**Table 18.2 Incidence of chromosome abnormalities in the newborn**

| Abnormality | Incidence per 10 000 births |
|---|---|
| **Autosomal** | |
| Trisomy 13 | 2 |
| Trisomy 18 | 3 |
| Trisomy 21 | 15 |
| **Sex chromosomes** | |
| **Female births** | |
| 45,X | 1–2 |
| 47,XXX | 10 |
| **Male births** | |
| 47,XXY | 10 |
| 47,XYY | 10 |
| **Other unbalanced rearrangements** | 10 |
| **Balanced rearrangements** | 30 |
| **Total** | 90 |

**Table 18.3 Spontaneous pregnancy loss in commonly recognized aneuploidy syndromes**

| Disorder | Proportion undergoing spontaneous pregnancy loss (%) |
|---|---|
| Trisomy 13 | 95 |
| Trisomy 18 | 95 |
| Trisomy 21 | 80 |
| Monosomy X | 98 |

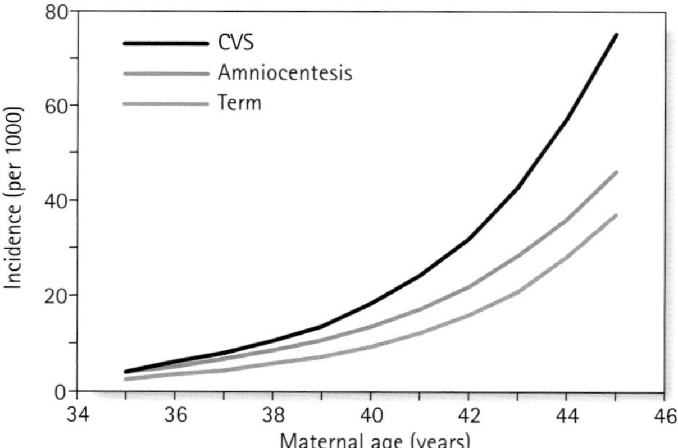


Fig. 18.1
Approximate incidence of trisomy 21 at the time of chorionic villus sampling (CVS) (11–12 weeks), amniocentesis (16 weeks) and delivery. (Data from Hook E B, Cross P K, Jackson L, Pergament E, Brambati B 1988 Maternal age-specific rates of 47, +21 and other cytogenetic abnormalities diagnosed in the first trimester of pregnancy in chorionic villus biopsy specimens. Am J Hum Genet 42: 797–807; and Cuckle H S, Wald N J, Thompson S G 1987 Estimating a woman's risk of having a pregnancy associated with Down syndrome using her age and serum alpha-fetoprotein level. Br J Obstet Gynaecol 94: 387–402.)

Down syndrome was not established until 1959 by Lejeune and his colleagues in Paris.

## Incidence

The overall incidence, when adjusted for the impact of antenatal screening, is approximately 1 in 650 to 1 in 700. In the UK approximately 50% of Down syndrome cases are detected prenatally. There is a strong association between the incidence of Down syndrome and advancing maternal age (Table 18.4).

## Clinical features

These are summarized in Table 18.5. The most common finding in the newborn period is severe hypotonia. Usually the facial characteristics of upward sloping palpebral fissures, small ears and protruding tongue (Figs 18.2 and 18.3) prompt rapid suspicion of the diagnosis, although this can be delayed in very small or premature babies. Single palmar creases are found in 50% of Down syndrome children (Fig. 18.4) in contrast to 2–3% of the general population. Congenital cardiac abnormalities are present in 40–45% of babies with Down syndrome, with the three most common lesions being atrioventricular canal defects, ventricular septal defects and patent ductus arteriosus.

**Table 18.4 Incidence of Down syndrome in relation to maternal age**

| Maternal age at delivery (years) | Incidence of Down syndrome |
|---|---|
| 20 | 1 in 1500 |
| 25 | 1 in 1350 |
| 30 | 1 in 900 |
| 35 | 1 in 400 |
| 36 | 1 in 300 |
| 37 | 1 in 250 |
| 38 | 1 in 200 |
| 39 | 1 in 150 |
| 40 | 1 in 100 |
| 41 | 1 in 85 |
| 42 | 1 in 65 |
| 43 | 1 in 50 |
| 44 | 1 in 40 |
| 45 | 1 in 30 |

Adapted from Cuckle H S, Wald N J, Thompson S G 1987 Estimating a woman's risk of having a pregnancy associated with Down syndrome using her age and serum alpha-fetoprotein level. Br J Obstet Gynaecol 94: 387–402

**Table 18.5 Common findings in Down syndrome**

**Newborn period**
Hypotonia, sleepy, excess nuchal skin

**Craniofacial**
Brachycephaly, epicanthic folds, protruding tongue, small ears, upward sloping palpebral fissures

**Limbs**
Single palmar crease, small middle phalanx of fifth finger, wide gap between first and second toes

**Cardiac**
Atrial and ventricular septal defect, common atrioventricular canal, patent ductus arteriosus

**Other**
Anal atresia, duodenal atresia, Hirschsprung disease, short stature, strabismus

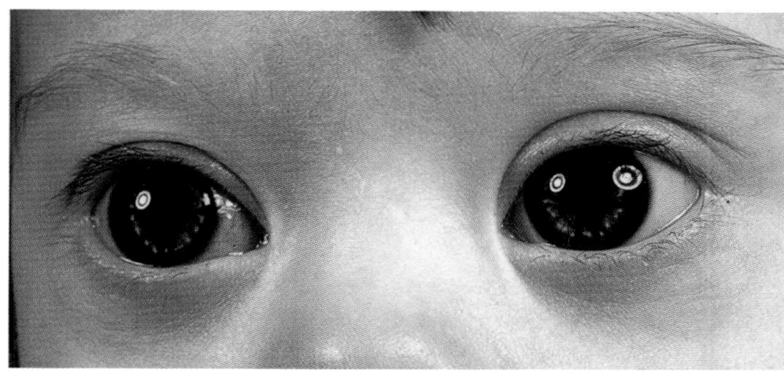

Fig. 18.3
Close-up view of the eyes and nasal bridge of a child with Down syndrome showing upward sloping palpebral fissures, Brushfield spots and bilateral epicanthic folds.

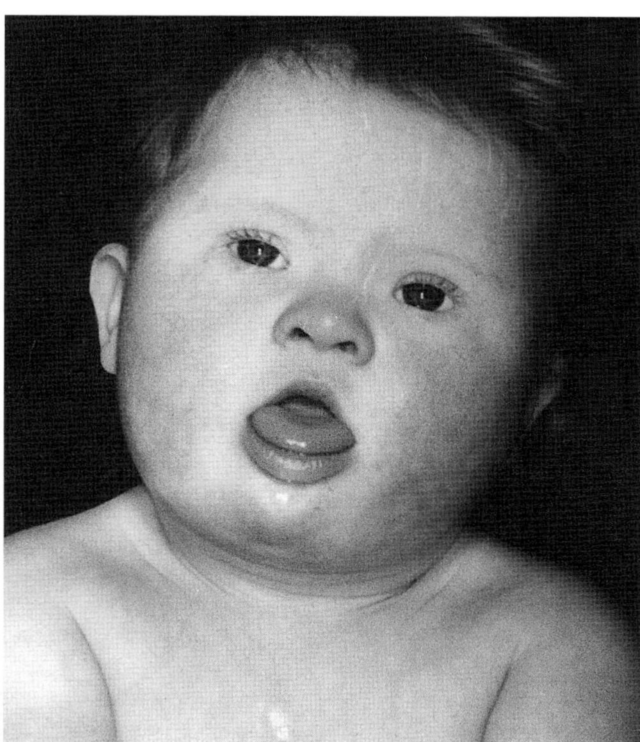

Fig. 18.2
A child with Down syndrome.

## Natural history

Affected children show a broad range of intellectual ability with IQ scores ranging from 25 to 75. The average IQ of young adults with Down syndrome is around 40 to 45. Social skills are relatively well advanced and most children with Down syndrome are happy and very affectionate. Adult height is usually around 150 cm. In the absence of a severe cardiac anomaly, which leads to early death in 15–20% of cases, average life expectancy is 50–60 years. Most affected adults develop Alzheimer disease in later life, possibly because of a gene dosage

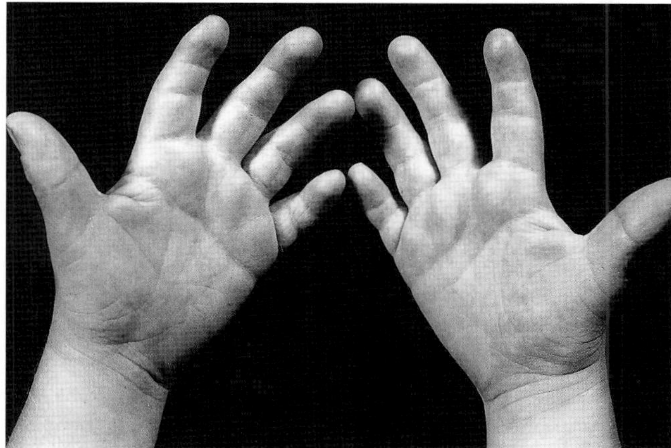

Fig. 18.4
The hands of an adult with Down syndrome. Note the single palmar crease in the left hand plus bilateral short curved fifth fingers (clinodactyly).

effect as the locus for the amyloid precursor protein gene is on chromosome 21. This gene has been implicated in some familial cases of Alzheimer disease (p. 241)

## Chromosome findings

These are listed in Table 18.6. In cases resulting from trisomy 21, the additional chromosome is maternal in origin in over 90% of cases, and DNA studies have shown

**Table 18.6 Chromosome abnormalities in Down syndrome**

| Abnormality | Frequency (%) |
|---|---|
| Trisomy | 95 |
| Translocation | 4 |
| Mosaicism | 1 |

that this arises most commonly as a result of non-disjunction in maternal meiosis I (p. 47). Robertsonian translocations (p. 51) account for approximately 4% of all cases, in roughly one-third of which one of the parents is found to be a carrier of the translocation. Children with mosaicism are often less severely affected than in the full syndrome.

Efforts have been made to correlate the various clinical features in Down syndrome with trisomy for specific regions of chromosome 21, by studying children with partial trisomy for different regions. There is some support for a Down syndrome 'critical region' at the distal end of the long arm (21q22) as children with trisomy for this region usually have typical Down syndrome facial features. Chromosome 21 is a 'gene-poor' chromosome with a high ratio of AT to GC sequences (p. 39). At present the only reasonably well-established genotype–phenotype correlation in trisomy 21 is the high incidence of Alzheimer disease, which is attributed to an amyloid precursor protein gene dosage effect.

### Recurrence risk

For straightforward trisomy 21 the recurrence risk is related to maternal age and is usually of the order of 1/200 to 1/100. In translocation cases similar figures apply if neither parent is a carrier. In familial translocation cases, the recurrence risks vary from around 1–3% for male carriers up to 10–15% for female carriers, with the exception of very rare carriers of a 21q21q translocation, for whom the recurrence risk is 100% (p. 52).

Prenatal diagnosis can be offered based on analysis of chorionic villi or cultured amniotic cells. Prenatal screening programs have been introduced based on the so-called 'triple' or 'quadruple' tests of maternal serum at 16 weeks' gestation (p. 330).

## PATAU SYNDROME (TRISOMY 13) AND EDWARDS SYNDROME (TRISOMY 18)

These very severe conditions were first described in 1960 and share many features in common (Figs 18.5 and 18.6). They both show incidence figures of approximately 1 in 5000 and convey a very poor prognosis, with most affected infants dying during the first days or weeks of life. In the unusual event of long-term survival there are severe learning difficulties. Cardiac abnormalities occur in at least 90% of all cases.

Usually chromosome analysis reveals straightforward trisomy. Both of these disorders show an association between increasing incidence and advanced maternal age, and in both the additional chromosome is usually of maternal origin (Table 3.4, p. 48). Approximately 10% of cases are caused by mosaicism or unbalanced rearrangements, particularly Robertsonian translocations in cases of Patau syndrome.

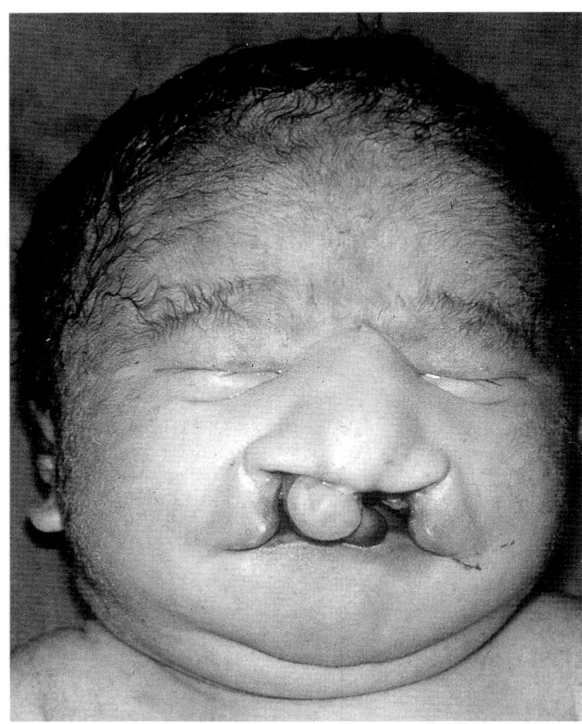

Fig. 18.5
Facial view of a child with trisomy 13 showing severe bilateral cleft lip and palate.

## CHROMOSOME DELETION AND MICRODELETION SYNDROMES

Microscopically visible deletions of the terminal portions of chromosomes 4 and 5 cause the Wolf–Hirschhorn (4p-) (Fig. 18.7) and Cri du chat (5p-) (Fig. 18.8) syndromes respectively. In both conditions there are usually severe learning difficulties, often in association with failure to thrive. However, there is considerable variability, particularly in Wolf–Hirschhorn syndrome, and there is a poor correlation of the phenotype with the precise loss of chromosomal material as determined by molecular analysis. The Cri du chat syndrome derives its name from the characteristic cat-like cry of affected neonates that results from underdevelopment of the larynx. Both conditions are rare, with estimated incidences of approximately 1 in 50 000 births. In some children with clinical features of one of these syndromes but apparently normal chromosomes, the presence of a very subtle deletion can be demonstrated by FISH (p. 35) using locus-specific probes for 4p or 5p (Fig. 18.9).

### Microdeletions

Through a combination of high-resolution prometaphase banding (p. 34) and FISH (p. 35), several previously unexplained syndromes have been shown to be due to

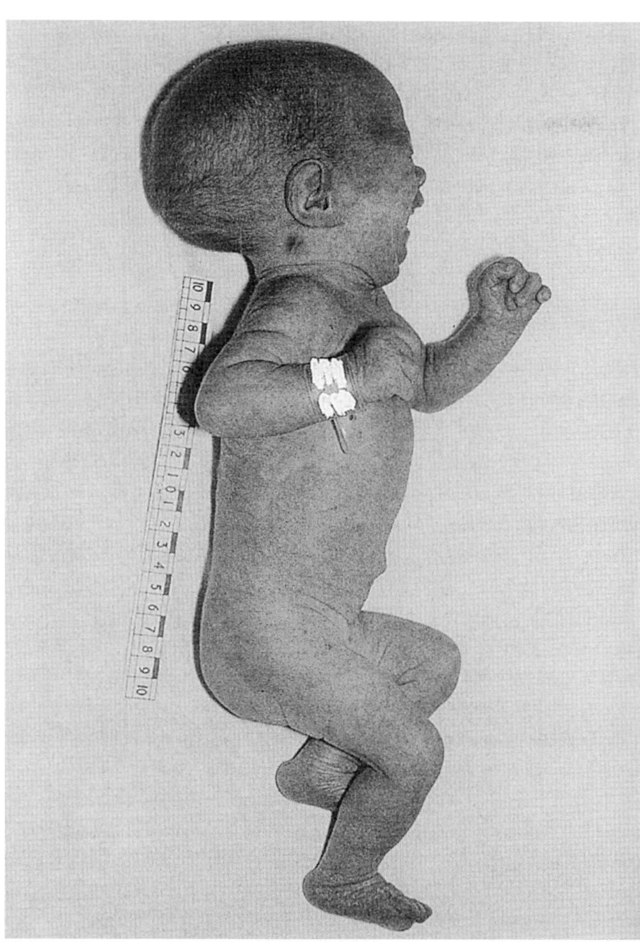

Fig. 18.6
A baby with trisomy 18. Note the prominent occiput and tightly clenched hands.

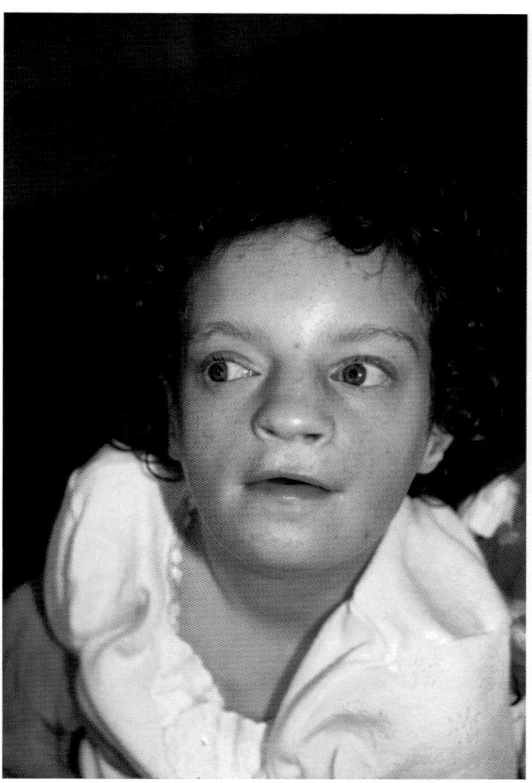

Fig. 18.7
A child with deletion 4p syndrome – Wolf-Hirschhorn syndrome.

submicroscopic or 'micro-'deletions. Some of these *microdeletions* involve loss of only a few genes at closely adjacent loci, resulting in what are known as *contiguous gene syndromes*. For example, several boys with Duchenne muscular dystrophy (DMD) have been described who also have other X-linked disorders, such as retinitis pigmentosa and glycerol kinase deficiency (p. 78). The loci for these disorders are known to be very close to the DMD locus on Xp21.

In several other microdeletion syndromes it is likely that more than a few loci are involved. Examples are given in Table 18.7. Even when considered together these conditions are rare, but improvements in molecular technology will probably reveal that microdeletion syndromes, and possibly microduplication syndromes also, are more common than is realized. Many malformations and syndromes have been described for which there is as yet no recognized cause (p. 253), but some of these will turn out to be due to microdeletions.

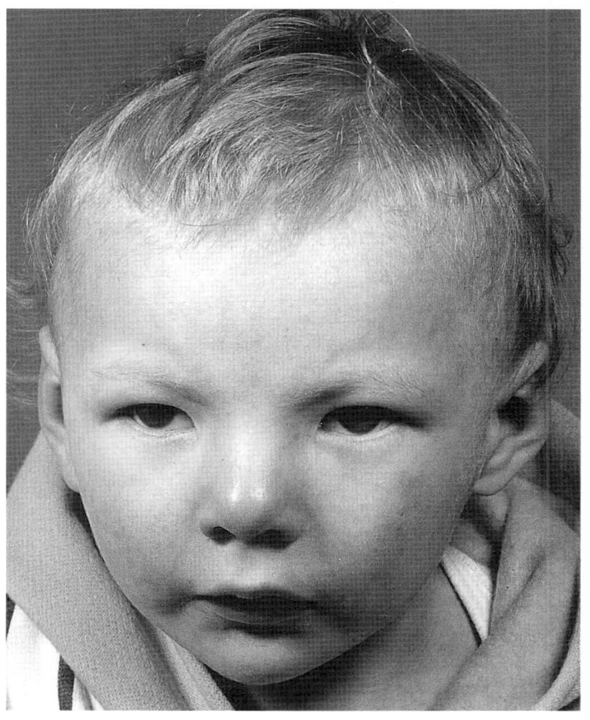

Fig. 18.8
Facial view of a 2-year-old boy with the Cri du chat syndrome.

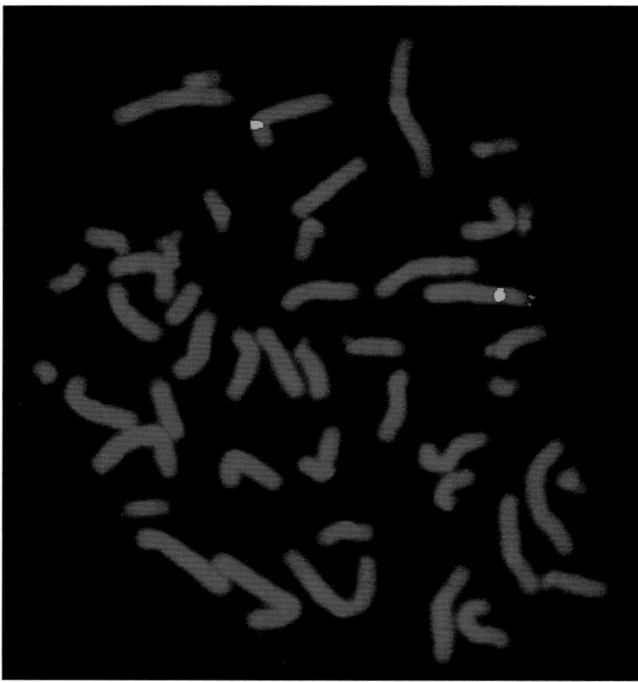

Fig. 18.9
FISH showing failure of a chromosome 4p locus-specific probe (red) to hybridize to one number 4 chromosome in a child with the Wolf–Hirschhorn syndrome. The yellow probe acts as a marker for the centromere of each number 4 chromosome. (Courtesy of Nigel Smith, City Hospital, Nottingham.)

**Table 18.7 Microdeletion syndromes**

| Syndrome | Chromosome |
|---|---|
| Deletion 1p36 | 1 |
| Williams | 7 |
| Langer–Giedion | 8 |
| WAGR* | 11 |
| Angelman | 15 |
| Prader–Willi | 15 |
| Rubinstein–Taybi | 16 |
| Miller–Dieker | 17 |
| Smith–Magenis | 17 |
| DiGeorge/Sedlácková/VCFS | 22 |

*WAGR: *W*ilms tumor, *A*niridia, *G*enitourinary malformations and *R*etardation of growth and development.

## Lessons from microdeletion syndromes

### *Retinoblastoma*

The first clue to the location of the gene for retinoblastoma was provided by the discovery that approximately 5% of children presenting with the condition had other abnormalities, including learning difficulties. In several of these children a constitutional interstitial deletion of a region of the long arm of chromosome 13 was identified. The smallest region of overlap was 13q14, which was subsequently shown to be the position of the locus for the autosomal dominant form of retinoblastoma. This in turn led to the cloning of the gene and identification of the gene product (pp. 210, 212).

### *Wilms' tumor*

A proportion of children who develop the rare renal embryonal neoplasm known as *W*ilms' tumor (or hypernephroma) also have *A*niridia (= absent iris, see Fig. 18.11), *G*enitourinary abnormalities and *R*etardation of growth and development. This combination of findings is referred to as the WAGR syndrome. Chromosome analysis in these children reveals an interstitial deletion of chromosome 11p13 (Fig. 18.10). Molecular studies have identified several genes within this deletion. Loss of one of these, *PAX6*, is responsible for the aniridia (Fig. 18.11) and can be established by FISH probe analysis. Loss of another, known as *WT1*, causes the development of Wilms' tumor. This knowledge can now be used to predict whether a newly diagnosed child with an 11p13 deletion is at high risk of developing a Wilms' tumor, and this can also be achieved by a separate FISH analysis using *WT1* as a locus, specific probe. Failure of *WT1* to hybridize to the deletion site indicates that the risk for developing Wilms' tumor is high.

It is important to note that in contrast to retinoblastoma the genetic aspects of Wilms' tumor have proved to be extremely complicated, with several different autosomal loci involved. Nevertheless, these discoveries based on the study of microdeletion syndromes have proved to be extremely valuable in leading to the isolation of genes that cause these two embryonal tumors.

### *Angelman and Prader–Willi syndromes*

Recent developments in these disorders have generated particular interest. Children with Angelman syndrome (Fig. 7.22, p. 119) show inappropriate laughter, with convulsions, poor coordination (ataxia) and learning difficulties. Children with the Prader–Willi syndrome (Fig. 7.21, p. 119) are extremely floppy (hypotonic) in early infancy and develop quite marked obesity and mild-to-moderate learning difficulties in later years. A large proportion of children with these disorders have a microdeletion involving the proximal part of the long arm of chromosome 15q (15q11-12).

It is now known that if the deletion occurs de novo on the paternally inherited number 15 chromosome the child will have the Prader–Willi syndrome. In contrast, a deletion occurring at the same region on the maternally

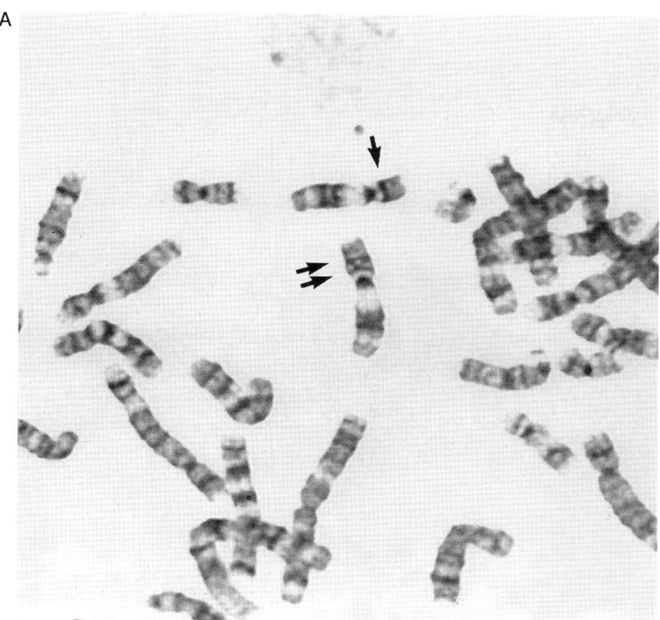


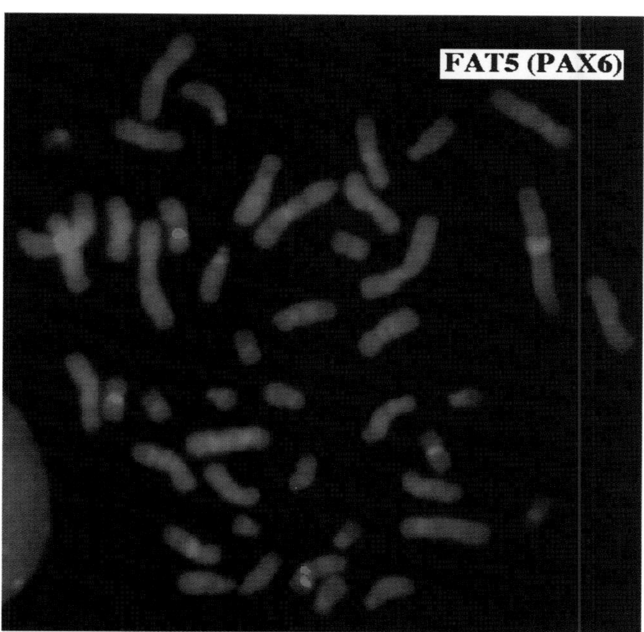


**Fig. 18.10**
(A) Metaphase spread showing the number 11 chromosomes (arrowed). The chromosome indicated by the single arrow has an interstitial deletion in the short arm. See Figures 18.11 and 18.12. (Courtesy of Meg Heath, City Hospital, Nottingham.) (B) FISH showing failure of a *PAX6* locus specific probe (red) to hybridize to the deleted number 11 chromosome shown in Figure 18.10(A) from a child with WAGR syndrome. The green probe acts as a marker for the centromere of each number 11 chromosome. (Courtesy of Dr John Crolla, Salisbury and Dr Veronica van Heyningen, Edinburgh.)

inherited number 15 chromosome causes Angelman syndrome. Non-deletion cases also exist and are often due to uniparental disomy (p. 117), with both number 15 chromosomes being paternal in origin in Angelman syndrome and maternal in origin in the Prader–Willi syndrome. Thus loss of a critical region from a paternal number 15 chromosome causes the Prader–Willi syndrome. Loss of an identical or similar region from a maternally inherited number 15 chromosome causes Angelman syndrome. These observations are fundamental to the concept of imprinting (p. 118) and illustrate how new technological developments coupled with clinical observation have helped identify new underlying genetic mechanisms.

**Fig. 18.11**
A baby with deletion 11p13 presenting with aniridia on routine neonatal examination.

## *DiGeorge/Sedlácková/Velocardiofacial syndrome*

DiGeorge syndrome is a disorder affecting approximately 1 in 4000 births, usually occurring sporadically, characterized by a high incidence of heart malformations, particularly those involving the cardiac outflow tract, along with thymic and parathyroid hypoplasia (p. 197). Molecular and FISH studies have shown that most if not all cases are due to a microdeletion involving the proximal long arm of chromosome 22 (22q11.2). Dr Eva Sedlácková from Prague reported a large series of children with a congenitally short palate in 1955, 10 years earlier than DiGeorge, and these patients clearly had the same condition. A similar phenotype was described by Shprintzen, with cardiac malformations, cleft palate and a recognizable facial appearance – now usually referred to as velocardiofacial syndrome (VCFS). Figure 18.12 shows individuals with deletion 22q11 at different ages. Because it is the most

often cytogenetically visible on a good quality karyotype. As with DiGeorge syndrome the mechanism of deletion in many cases involves homologous recombination between flanking repeat gene clusters. The physical characteristics are not convincingly distinctive (Fig. 18.14) but congenital heart disease occurs in a third, scoliosis develops in late childhood in more than a half, and hearing impairment in about two-thirds. The syndrome is most likely to be recognized by the behavioral characteristics, for as children these patients exhibit self-harming (head-banging, pulling out nails and inserting objects into orifices), a persistently disturbed sleep pattern, and characteristic 'self-hugging'. Some degree of learning difficulty is the norm. The sleep pattern can often be managed by judicious use of melatonin.

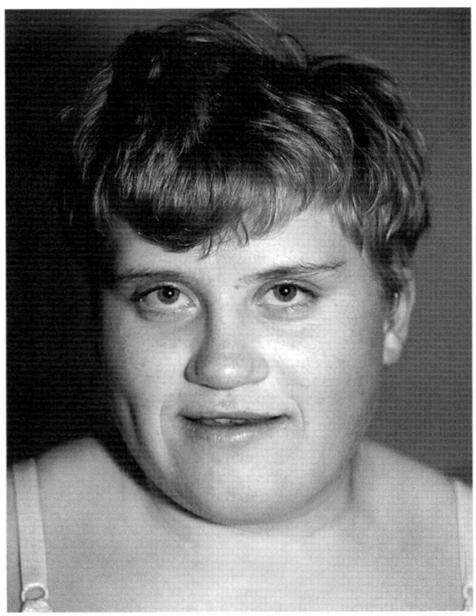

**Fig. 18.14**
A young person with Smith–Magenis syndrome; the facial features are not highly distinctive, but the philtrum is usually short. As babies chromosome studies are often requested because the possibility of Down syndrome is raised.

### *Deletion 1p36 syndrome*

Improvements in cytogenetic techniques and the use of FISH is leading to the identification and characterization of additional rare microdeletion syndromes. One of these to emerge during the 1990s is deletion 1p36 syndrome. The features are hypotonia, microcephaly, growth delay, severe learning difficulties, epilepsy (including infantile spasms), and characteristically straight eyebrows with slightly deep-set eyes, and midface hypoplasia (Fig. 18.15).

## MULTITELOMERIC PROBES AND LEARNING DIFFICULTIES

A key development in the use of FISH technology has been a set of subtelomeric probes for all chromosomes. Their use has begun to be routine in the investigation of non-specific learning difficulties with or without dysmorphic features, especially when there is a family history of similar problems that follows a pattern that could be explained by the segregation of balanced and unbalanced forms of a reciprocal translocation (p. 49). The rationale is based on the observation that the most viable unbalanced translocations are those that are small and therefore involve very terminal (telomeric) chromosome segments. A review of the use of the system has shown that abnormalities are found in about 5% of cases analyzed, though the figure is slightly higher for cases of severe learning difficulties. About half the positive cases are de novo whilst the remainder are familial. Positive findings are especially important for familial cases in order to identify balanced carriers.

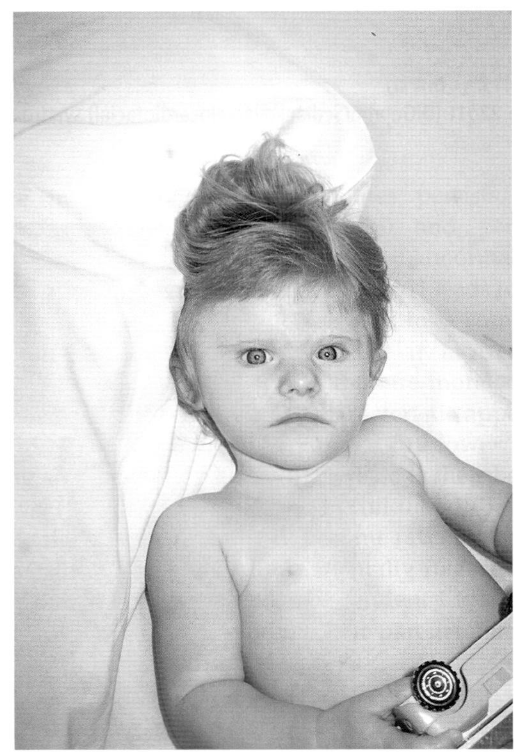

**Fig. 18.15**
A child with deletion 1p36 syndrome – very straight eyebrows, epilepsy and learning difficulties.

## TRIPLOIDY

Triploidy (69,XXX, 69,XXY, 69,XYY) is a relatively common finding in material cultured from spontaneous abortions, but is seen only rarely in a liveborn infant. Such a child will almost always show severe intra-uterine growth retardation with relative preservation of head growth at the expense of a small thin trunk. Syndactyly involving the third and fourth fingers and/or the second and third toes is a common finding. Cases of triploidy due to a double paternal contribution usually miscarry in early to mid-pregnancy and are associated with partial hydatidiform changes in the placenta (p. 96). Cases with a double maternal contribution survive for longer but rarely beyond the early neonatal period.

### Hypomelanosis of Ito

Several children with mosaicism for diploidy/triploidy have been identified. These can demonstrate the clinical picture seen in full triploidy but in a milder form. An alternative presentation occurs as the condition known as hypomelanosis of Ito. In this curious disorder the skin shows alternating patterns of normally pigmented and depigmented streaks that correspond to the embryological developmental lines of the skin known as Blaschko's lines (Fig. 7.17, 18.16). Most children with hypomelanosis of Ito have moderate learning difficulties and have convulsions that can be particularly difficult to treat. There is increasing evidence that this clinical picture represents a non-specific embryological response to cell or tissue mosaicism. A similar pattern of skin pigmentation is sometimes seen in women with one of the rare X-linked dominant disorders (p. 113) with skin involvement, such as incontinentia pigmenti (Fig. 7.17). Such women can be considered as being mosaic, as some cells will be expressing the normal gene whereas others will be expressing only the mutant gene.

# DISORDERS OF THE SEX CHROMOSOMES

## KLINEFELTER SYNDROME (47,XXY)

First described in 1942, this relatively common condition with an incidence of 1 in 1000 male live births was in 1959 shown to be due to the presence of an additional X chromosome.

### Clinical features

In childhood the diagnosis can be suspected in a male presenting with clumsiness or mild learning difficulties, particularly in relation to verbal skills. The overall verbal IQ is reduced by 10–20 points below that of unaffected siblings and controls, and they can be rather self-obsessed in their behavior. Adults with Klinefelter syndrome tend to be slightly taller than average with long lower limbs. Approximately 30% of adult males with Klinefelter syndrome show moderately severe gynecomastia (enlargement of the breasts) and all are infertile, with small soft testes. There is an increased incidence of leg ulcers, osteoporosis and carcinoma of the breast in adult life. Treatment with testosterone from puberty onwards is beneficial for the development of secondary sexual characteristics and the long-term prevention of osteoporosis. Males with Klinefelter syndrome are usually infertile due to the absence of sperm in their semen (*azoospermia*), although fertility has been achieved for a small number of affected males using the techniques of testicular sperm aspiration and ICSI (*intra-cytoplasmic sperm injection*).

### Chromosome findings

Usually the karyotype shows an additional X chromosome. Molecular studies have shown that there is a roughly equal chance that this will have been inherited from the mother or from the father. The maternally derived cases are associated with advancing maternal age. A small proportion of cases show mosaicism, i.e. 46,XY/47,XXY. Rarely, a male with more than two X chromosomes can be encountered, e.g. 48,XXXY or 49,XXXXY. These individuals are usually quite severely retarded and also share physical characteristics with Klinefelter men, often to a more marked degree.

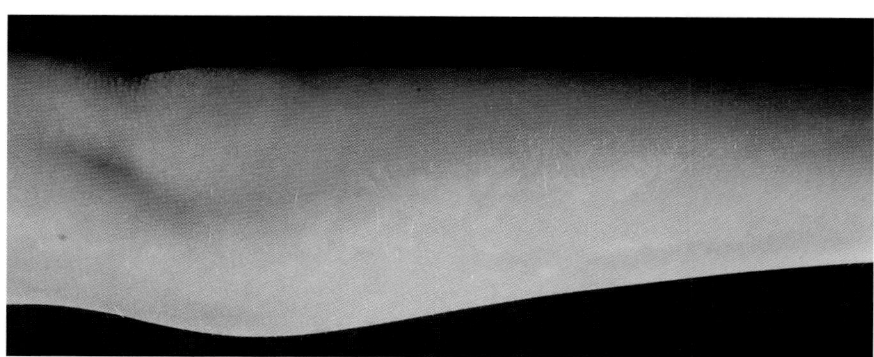

**Fig. 18.16**
Mosaic pattern of skin pigmentation on the arm of a child with hypomelanosis of Ito. (Reproduced with permission from Jenkins D, Martin K, Young I D 1993 Hypomelanosis of Ito associated with mosaicism for trisomy 7 and apparent 'pseudomosaicism' at amniocentesis. J Med Genet 30: 783–784.)

## TURNER SYNDROME (45,X)

This condition was first described in 1938. The absence of a Barr body, consistent with the presence of only one X chromosome, was noted in 1954 and cytogenetic confirmation was forthcoming in 1959. While common at conception and in spontaneous abortions (Table 18.1), the incidence in liveborn female infants is low, with estimates ranging from 1 in 5000 to 1 in 10 000.

### Clinical features

Presentation can be at any time from pregnancy to adult life. Increasingly, Turner syndrome is being detected during the second trimester as a result of routine detailed ultrasound scanning, which can reveal either generalized edema (hydrops) or swelling localized to the neck (nuchal cyst or thickened nuchal pad) (Fig. 18.17). At birth many babies with Turner syndrome look entirely normal. Others show the residue of intra-uterine edema with puffy extremities (Fig. 18.18) and neck webbing. Other findings can include a low posterior hair-line, increased carrying angles at the elbows, short fourth metacarpals, widely spaced nipples and coarctation of the aorta, which is present in 15% of cases.

Intelligence in Turner syndrome is normal. However, studies have shown some differences in social cognition and higher-order executive function skills according to whether their X chromosome was paternal or maternal in origin (Ch. 6, p. 101). The two main medical problems are short stature and ovarian failure. The short stature becomes apparent by mid-childhood, and without growth hormone treatment the average adult height is 145 cm. This short stature is due, at least in part, to haploinsufficiency for the *SHOX* gene, which is located in the pseudoautosomal region (p. 114). Ovarian failure commences during the second half of intra-uterine life and almost invariably leads to primary amenorrhea and infertility. Estrogen replacement therapy should be initiated at adolescence for the development of secondary sexual characteristics and long-term prevention of osteoporosis. In vitro fertilization using donor eggs offers the prospect of pregnancy for women with Turner syndrome.

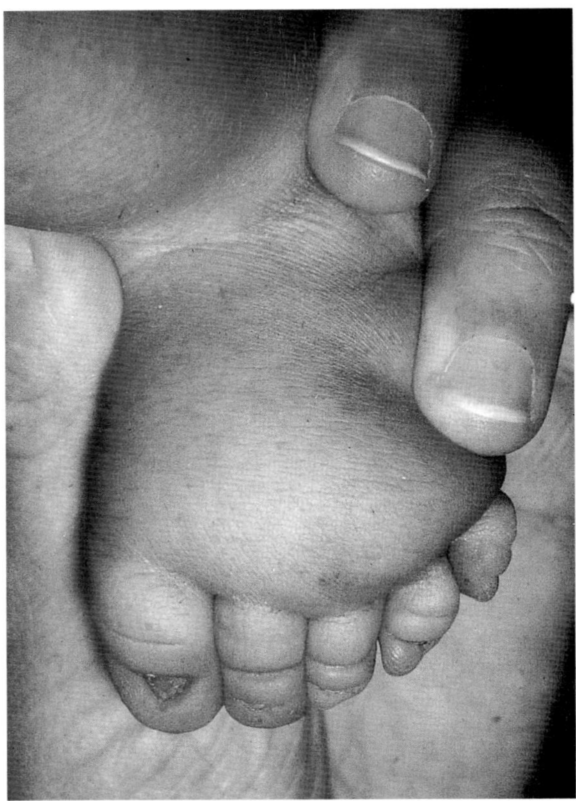

**Fig. 18.18**
The foot of an infant with Turner syndrome showing edema and small nails.

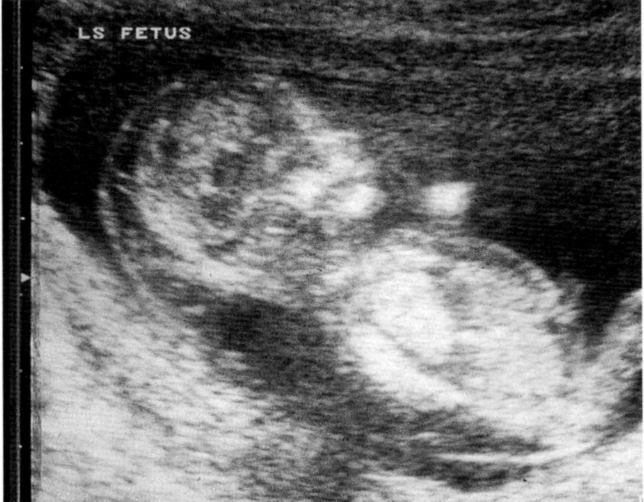


**Fig. 18.17**
Ultrasound scan at 18 weeks' gestation showing hydrops fetalis. Note the halo of fluid surrounding the fetus. (Courtesy of Dr D Rose, City Hospital, Nottingham.)

### Chromosome findings

These are summarized in Table 18.8. The most common finding is 45,X, sometimes erroneously referred to as 45,XO. It has been shown that Turner syndrome arises in 80% of instances through a sex chromosome (X or Y) being lost in paternal meiosis. In a significant proportion of cases there is chromosome mosaicism and those with a normal cell line (46,XX) have a chance of being fertile. Those with some Y chromosome material in their second cell line must be investigated for possible gonadal dysgenesis; intracellular male gonads can occasionally become malignant and need to be surgically removed.

**Table 18.8 Chromosome findings in Turner syndrome**

| Karyotype | Frequency (%) |
|---|---|
| Monosomy X — 45,X | 50 |
| Mosaicism — e.g. 45,X/46,XX | 20 |
| Isochromosome — 46,X,i(Xq) | 15 |
| Ring — 46,X,r(X) | 5 |
| Deletion — 46,X,del(Xp) | 5 |
| Other | 5 |

## XXX FEMALES

Birth surveys have shown that approximately 0.1% of all females have a 47,XXX karyotype. These women usually have no physical abnormalities but can show a mild reduction of between 10 and 20 points in intellectual skills and sometimes quite oppositional behavior. This is rarely of sufficient severity to require special education. Studies have shown that the additional X chromosome is of maternal origin in 95% of cases and usually arises from an error in meiosis I. Women with a 47,XXX karyotype usually show normal fertility and have children with normal karyotypes.

As with males who have more than two X chromosomes, women with more than three X chromosomes show a high incidence of learning difficulties, the severity of which is directly related to the number of X chromosomes present.

## XYY MALES

This condition shows an incidence of 1 in 1000 in males in newborn surveys but is found in 2–3% of males who are in institutions because of learning difficulties or antisocial criminal behavior. However, it is important to stress that most 47,XYY men have neither learning difficulty nor a criminal record, although they can show emotional immaturity and impulsive behavior. Fertility is normal.

Physical appearance is normal and stature is usually above average. Intelligence is mildly impaired, with an overall IQ score of 10–20 points below a control sample. The additional Y chromosome must arise as a result of non-disjunction in paternal meiosis II or as a post-zygotic event.

## FRAGILE X SYNDROME

This condition, which could equally well be classified as a single-gene disorder rather than a chromosome abnormality, has the unique distinction of being both the most common inherited cause of learning difficulties and the first disorder in which a dynamic mutation was identified (p. 25). Martin and Bell described the condition in the 1940s before the chromosome era, and it has also been known as Martin–Bell syndrome. The chromosomal abnormality was first described in 1969 but the significance not fully realized until 1977. In 1991 the underlying molecular defect was discovered.

### Incidence

Fragile X syndrome affects approximately 1 in 5000 males and accounts for 4–8% of all males with learning difficulties.

### Clinical features

Older boys and adult males usually have a recognizable facial appearance with high forehead, large ears, long face and prominent jaw (Fig. 18.19). After puberty most affected males have large testes (macro-orchidism). There can also be evidence of connective tissue weakness, with hyperextensible joints, stretch marks on the skin (striae) and mitral valve prolapse. The learning difficulties are moderate to severe and many affected boys show autistic features and/or hyperactive behavior. Speech tends to be halting and repetitive. Female carriers can show some of the facial features, and approximately 50% of women with the full mutation show mild-to-moderate learning difficulties.

### The Fragile X chromosome

The Fragile X syndrome takes its name from the appearance of the X chromosome, which shows a *fragile site* close

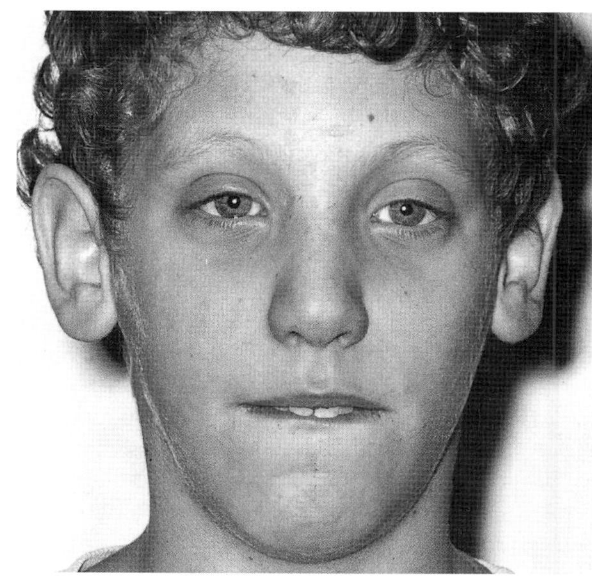

**Fig. 18.19**
Facial view of a boy with the Fragile X syndrome.

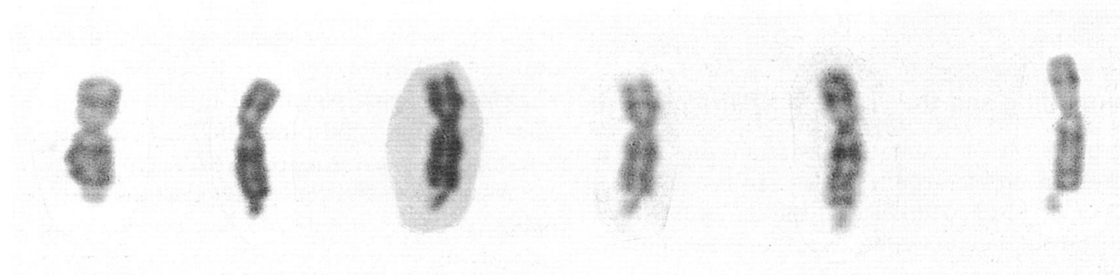

**Fig. 18.20**
X chromosome from several males with Fragile X syndrome. (Courtesy of Ashley Wilkinson, City Hospital, Nottingham.)

to the telomere at the end of the long arm at Xq27.3 (Fig. 18.20). A fragile site is a non-staining gap usually involving both chromatids at a point at which the chromosome is liable to break. In this condition, detection of the fragile site involves the use of special culture techniques such as folate or thymidine depletion, which can result in the fragile site being detectable in up to 50% of cells from affected males. Demonstration of the fragile site in female carriers is much more difficult and cytogenetic studies alone are not a reliable means of carrier detection, in that although a positive result confirms carrier status, the absence of the fragile site does not exclude a woman from being a carrier.

### The molecular defect

In gene mapping the Fragile X locus is known as *FRAXA*. The FRAXA mutation consists of an increase in the size of a region in the 5′-untranslated region of the Fragile X learning difficulties (*FMR-1*) gene. This region contains a long CGG trinucleotide repeat sequence. In the DNA of a normal person there are between 10 and 50 copies of this triplet repeat and these are inherited in a stable fashion. However, a small increase to between 50 and 200 renders this repeat sequence unstable, a condition in which it is referred to as a *premutation*.

A man who carries a premutation is known as a 'normal transmitting male', although it has recently been recognized that these premutation carriers are at increased risk of a late-onset neurological condition named 'Fragile X tremor/ataxia syndrome'. All of his daughters will inherit the premutation and will be of normal intelligence, but when these daughters come to have sons there is a high risk that the premutation will undergo a further increase in size during meiosis. If this reaches a critical size of greater than 200 CGG triplets it becomes a full mutation. This process is sometimes referred to as expansion of the triplet repeat sequence.

The full mutation is unstable not only during female meiosis but also in somatic mitotic divisions. Consequently, in an affected male gel electrophoresis shows a 'smear' of DNA consisting of many different sized alleles rather than a single band (Fig. 18.21). Note that a normal allele and premutation can be identified by PCR, whereas Southern blotting is necessary to detect full mutations as the long GCC expansion is often refractory to PCR amplification. At the molecular level a full mutation suppresses transcription of the *FMR-1* gene by hypermethylation, and this in turn is thought to be responsible for the clinical

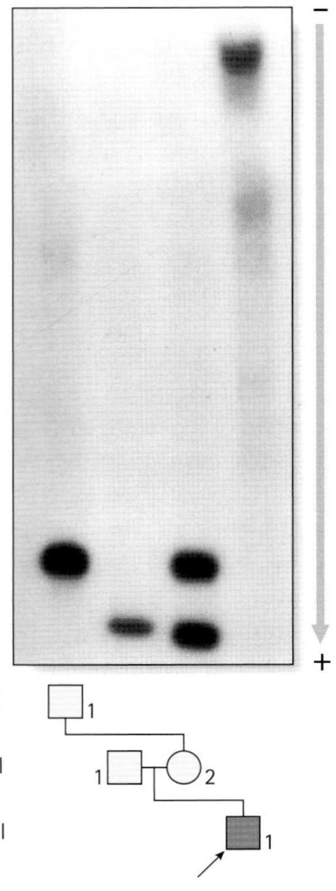


**Fig. 18.21**
Southern blot of DNA from a family showing expansion of the CGG triplet repeat being passed from a normal transmitting male through his obligate carrier daughter to her son with Fragile X learning difficulties. (Courtesy of Dr G Taylor, St James's Hospital, Leeds.)

**Table 18.9 The Fragile X syndrome — genotype–phenotype correlations**

| Number of triplet repeats (normal range = 10–50) | Fragile site | Intelligence detectable |
|---|---|---|
| **Males** | | |
| 50–200 (premutation) | No | Normal (normal transmitting male) |
| 200–2000 (full mutation) | Yes (in up to 50% of cells) | Moderate-to-severe learning difficulties |
| **Females** | | |
| 50–200 (premutation) | No | Normal |
| 200–2000 (full mutation) | Yes (usually <10% of cells) | 50% normal, 50% mild learning difficulties |

features seen in males, and in some females with a large expansion (Table 18.9). The *FMR-1* gene contains 17 exons that encode a cytoplasmic protein that plays a crucial role in the development and function of cerebral neurons. The FMR-1 protein can be detected in blood using specific monoclonal antibodies.

Another fragile site closely adjacent to FRAXA has been identified at Xq28. This is known as *FRAXE*. The expansion mutations at FRAXE also involve CGG triplet repeats and occur at approximately one-quarter the frequency of FRAXA mutations, or less. Some males with these mutations have mild learning difficulties, whereas others are just as severely affected as men with FRAXA. These men are usually ascertained through the discovery of a fragile site on chromosome analysis with a normal result on FRAXA mutation analysis. A third fragile site, FRAXF, has recently been identified close to FRAXA and FRAXE. This does not seem to cause any clinical abnormality.

### Genetic counseling and the Fragile X syndrome

This common cause of learning difficulties presents a major counseling problem. Inheritance can be regarded as modified or atypical X-linked. All the daughters of a normal transmitting male will carry the premutation. Their male offspring are at risk of inheriting either the premutation or a full mutation. This risk is dependent on the size of the premutation in the mother, with mutations greater than 100 CGG repeats almost invariably increasing in size to become full mutations.

For a woman who carries a full mutation there is a 50% risk that each of her sons will be affected with the full syndrome and that each of her daughters will inherit the full mutation. Since approximately 50% of females with the full mutation have mild learning difficulties, the risk that a female carrier of a full mutation will have a daughter with learning difficulties equals $\frac{1}{2} \times \frac{1}{2}$, i.e. $\frac{1}{4}$.

Prenatal diagnosis can be offered based on analysis of DNA from chorionic villi, but in the event of a female fetus with a full mutation accurate prediction of phenotype cannot be made.

The Fragile X syndrome is a condition for which population screening could be offered, either among selected high-risk groups such as males with learning difficulties, or on a widespread general population basis. Such programs will have to surmount major ethical, financial and logistical concerns if they are to achieve widespread acceptance (p. 375).

## CHROMOSOME DISORDERS AND BEHAVIORAL PHENOTYPES

The distinctive behavior of children with Williams syndrome – their outgoing 'cocktail party manner' – has been recognized as part of the condition for a long time. As the microdeletion conditions have emerged it has been increasingly clear that patterns of behavior can reliably be attributed to certain disorders. This is very striking in Smith–Magenis syndrome but also apparent to a lesser extent in deletion 22q11, Cri-du-chat, Angelman and Prader–Willi syndromes. It is also apparent in the aneuploidies – Down syndrome, Klinefelter syndrome – as well as 47,XXX and 47,XYY and Fragile-X syndrome. Behavioral phenotypes have therefore become an area of considerable interest to clinical scientists and the observations lend support to the belief that behavior, to some extent at least, is genetically determined. In studying chromosome disorders we are of course looking at genetically abnormal situations, and from this we cannot necessarily extrapolate directly to 'normal' situations. For the latter, twin studies have provided substantial and valuable information. This field of study remains complex and understandably controversial. However, most now accept that behavior is a complex interaction of genetic background, physical influences during early development (e.g. fetal well-being), nurturing experiences, family size, culture and belief systems.

## DISORDERS OF SEXUAL DIFFERENTIATION

The process of sexual differentiation has been described in Chapter 6 (p. 97). Given the complexity of the sequential cascade of events that takes place between 6 and 14 weeks of embryonic life it is not surprising that errors can occur. Many of these errors can lead to sexual ambiguity or to discordance between the chromosomal sex and the appearance of the external genitalia. These disorders are also sometimes referred to as various forms of intersex (Table 18.10).

**Table 18.10 Disorders of sexual differentiation and development**

**Seminiferous tubule dysgenesis (Klinefelter syndrome)**
47,XXY, 48,XXXY, 48,XXYY, 49,XXXXY

**Ovarian dysgenesis (Turner syndrome)**
45,X, 46,X,i(Xq), 46,X,del(Xp), 46,X,r(X)

**True hermaphroditism**
46,XX with Y-derived sequences
46,XX/46,XY chimerism

**Male pseudohermaphroditism**
***Androgen insensitivity***
Complete — testicular feminization
Incomplete — Reifenstein syndrome

***Inborn errors of testosterone biosynthesis***
e.g. 5α-reductase deficiency
45,X/46,XY mosaicism

**Female pseudohermaphroditism**
Congenital adrenal hyperplasia
Maternal androgen ingestion or androgen-secreting tumor

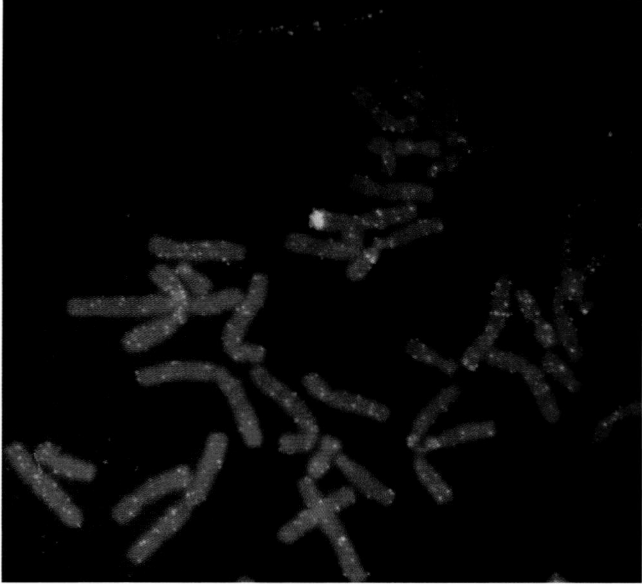

**Fig. 18.22**
FISH showing hybridization of a Y chromosome paint to the short arm of an X chromosome in a 46,XX male. (Courtesy of Nigel Smith, City Hospital, Nottingham.)

## TRUE HERMAPHRODITISM

In this extremely rare condition an individual has both testicular and ovarian tissue, often in association with ambiguous genitalia. When an exploratory operation is carried out in these patients an ovary can be found on one side and a testis on the other. Alternatively, there can be a mixture of ovarian and testicular tissue in the gonad, which is known as an ovotestis. Most patients with true hermaphroditism have a 46,XX karyotype, and in many of these individuals the paternally derived X chromosome carries Y chromosome-specific DNA sequences as a result of illegitimate crossing over between the X and Y chromosomes during meiosis I in spermatogenesis (Fig. 18.22).

A small proportion of patients with true hermaphroditism are found to be chimeras with both 46,XX and 46,XY cell lines, a situation analogous to freemartins in cattle (p. 56).

## MALE PSEUDOHERMAPHRODITISM

In pseudohermaphroditism there is gonadal tissue of only one sex. The external genitalia can be ambiguous or of the sex opposite to that of the chromosomes. Thus in male pseudohermaphroditism there is a 46,XY karyotype with ambiguous or female genitalia.

The most widely recognized cause of male pseudohermaphroditism is androgen insensitivity (p. 169). In this condition, which is also known as *testicular feminization syndrome*, the karyotype is normal male and the external phenotype is essentially that of a normal female. Internally the vagina ends blindly and the uterus and fallopian tubes are absent. Testes are located in the abdomen or in the inguinal canal, where they can be mistaken for inguinal herniae. This condition is caused by the absence of androgen receptors in the target organs, so that, although testosterone is formed normally, its peripheral masculinizing effects are blocked. These androgen receptors are coded for by a gene on the X chromosome in which both deletions and point mutations have been identified. Curiously, expansion of a CAG repeat in the first exon of this androgen receptor gene causes a neurological disorder known as Kennedy disease, or spinobulbar muscular atrophy (SBMA). This is a rare example of the phenomenon referred to as a 'gene within a gene' (p. 17).

Other causes of male pseudohermaphroditism include:

1. An incomplete form of androgen insensitivity known as Reifenstein syndrome in which affected males have hypospadias, small testes and gynecomastia.
2. Enzyme defects in testosterone synthesis such as 5α-reductase deficiency, in which the external genitalia are ambiguous at birth but undergo masculinization (virilization) at puberty.
3. Chromosome mosaicism (45,X/46,XY), in which most individuals are normal males but a small proportion have ambiguous or female external genitalia.
4. Campomelic dysplasia, which is caused by mutations in the *SOX9* gene on chromosome 17. *SOX9* is believed to be an important gene in the regulatory pathway by which *SRY* causes masculinization of the undifferentiated fetal gonads (p. 90).

5. The Smith–Lemli–Opitz syndrome, which is caused by deficiency of 7-dehydrocholesterol reductase, an enzyme involved in cholesterol biosynthesis. Some severely affected male infants have female external genitalia.

### FEMALE PSEUDOHERMAPHRODITISM

In female pseudohermaphroditism, the karyotype is female and the external genitalia are virilized so that they either resemble those of a normal male or are ambiguous.

Congenital adrenal hyperplasia (CAH) is by far the most important cause of female pseudohermaphroditism (p. 168). This can be caused by several different enzyme defects in the adrenal cortex, all of which show autosomal recessive inheritance. Reduced cortisol production leads to an increase in ACTH secretion, which in turn causes hyperplasia of the adrenal glands. In the most common form of CAH, due to 21-hydroxylase deficiency, hormone synthesis switches from the manufacture of cortisol and aldosterone to the androgen pathway (Fig. 11.5, p. 169), leading to striking virilization of a female fetus (Fig. 11.6, p. 170). The lack of cortisol and aldosterone usually leads to rapid collapse shortly after birth, which can prove fatal unless appropriate hormone and electrolyte supplementation is initiated (p. 170).

Rarer causes of female pseudohermaphroditism include an androgen-secreting tumor and maternal androgen ingestion during pregnancy.

## CHROMOSOMAL BREAKAGE SYNDROMES

Constitutional and acquired chromosome abnormalities which predispose to malignancy are considered in Chapter 14. In addition to these conditions, it is recognized that a small number of hereditary disorders are characterized by an excess of chromosome breaks and gaps as well as an increased susceptibility to neoplasia.

### ATAXIA TELANGIECTASIA

This is an autosomal recessive disorder that presents in early childhood with ataxia, oculocutaneous telangiectasia (Fig. 18.23), radiation sensitivity and susceptibility to sinus and pulmonary infection (p. 197). There is a 10–20% risk of leukemia or lymphoma. Cells from patients show an increase in spontaneous chromosome abnormalities, such as chromatid gaps and breaks, which are enhanced by radiation. The gene for ataxia telangiectasia is called *ATM* (M = mutation) and maps to chromosome 11q23. The protein product is thought to act as a 'check-point' protein kinase which interacts with the *Tp53* and *BRCA1* gene products to arrest cell division and thereby allow repair of radiation-induced chromosome breaks before the S phase in the cell cycle.

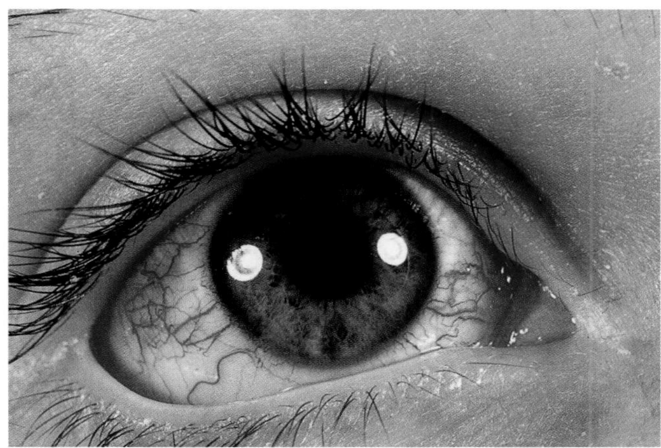

Fig. 18.23
Ocular telangiectasia in a child with ataxia telangiectasia.

### BLOOM SYNDROME

Children with this autosomal recessive disorder are small with a light-sensitive facial rash and reduced immunoglobulin levels (IgA and IgM). The risk of lymphoreticular malignancy is approximately 20%. Cultured cells show an increased frequency of chromosome breaks, particularly if they are exposed in vitro to ultraviolet light. The gene for Bloom syndrome maps to chromosome 15q26, where it encodes one member of a group of enzymes called the DNA helicases (p. 15). These are responsible for unwinding double-stranded DNA prior to replication, repair and recombination. Normally the Bloom syndrome gene plays a major role in maintaining genome stability. When defective in the homozygous state, DNA repair is impaired and the rate of recombination between sister chromatids is increased dramatically. This can be demonstrated by looking for sister chromatid exchanges – see below.

### FANCONI ANEMIA

This autosomal recessive disorder is associated with upper limb abnormalities involving the radius and thumb (Fig. 18.24), increased pigmentation and bone marrow failure leading to deficiency of all types of blood cells, i.e. pancytopenia. There is also an increased risk of neoplasia, particularly leukemia, lymphoma and hepatic carcinoma. Multiple chromosomal breaks are observed in cultured cells (Fig. 18.25) and the basic defect lies in the repair of DNA strand cross-links. There are five known subtypes of Fanconi anemia, each caused by recessive

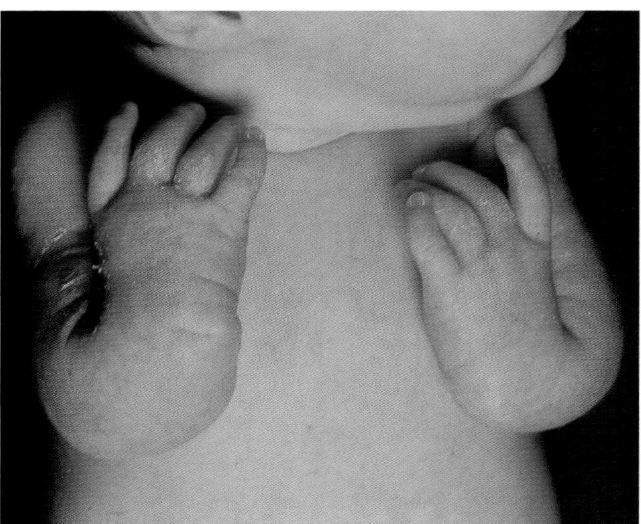

Fig. 18.24
Bilateral radial aplasia with absent thumbs in an infant with Fanconi anaemia.

mutations at different autosomal loci. The commonest, type A, maps to chromosome 16q24. It is not known how any of the Fanconi anemia genes are involved in maintaining the integrity of DNA cross-links.

## XERODERMA PIGMENTOSA

This exists in at least seven different forms, all of which show autosomal recessive inheritance. Patients present with a light-sensitive pigmented rash and usually die of skin malignancy in sun-exposed areas before the age of 20 years. Cells cultured from these patients only show chromosome abnormalities after exposure to ultraviolet light. These disorders are due to defects in the nucleotide excision repair pathway. This involves endonuclease cleavage 5′ and 3′ to each damaged nucleotide, excision of the damaged nucleotide(s), and finally restoration of the damaged strand using the intact opposite strand as a template.

## CHROMOSOME BREAKAGE AND SISTER CHROMATID EXCHANGE

Strong evidence of increased *chromosome instability* is provided by the demonstration of an increased number of *sister chromatid exchanges* (SCEs) in cultured cells. An SCE is an exchange (crossing-over) of genetic material between the two chromatids of a chromosome in mitosis, in contrast to recombination in meiosis I that is between homologous chromatids. SCEs can be demonstrated by differences in the uptake of certain stains by the two

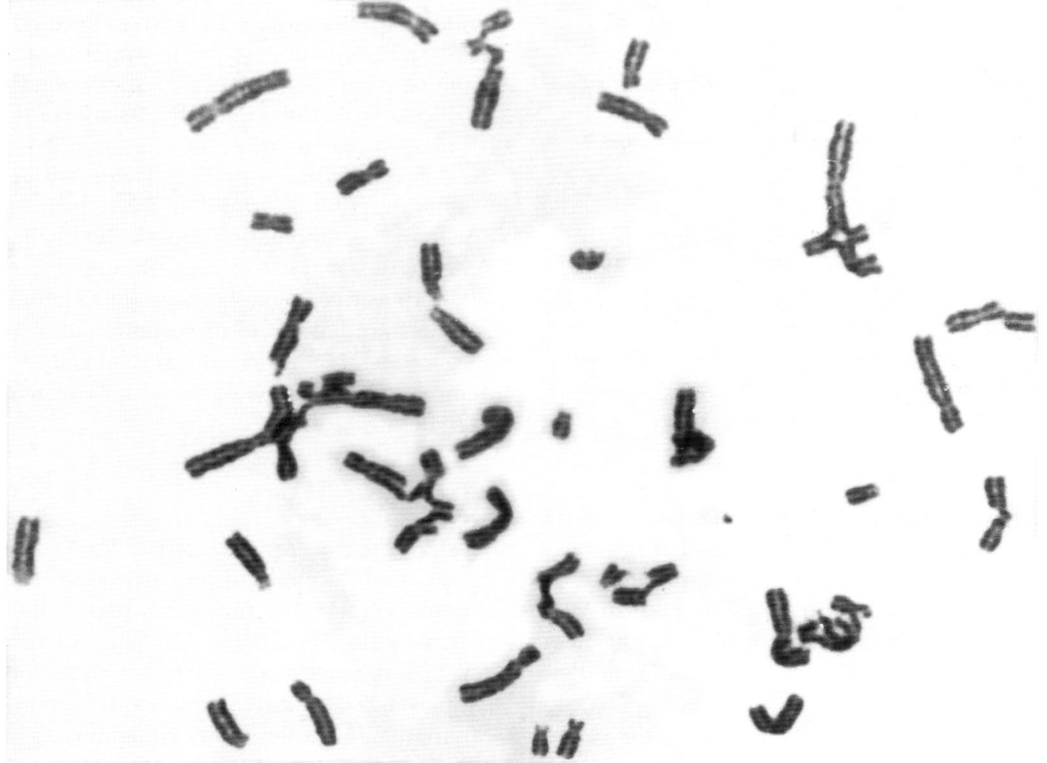

Fig. 18.25
Multiple chromosome breaks and gaps in a metaphase spread prepared from a child with Fanconi anemia.

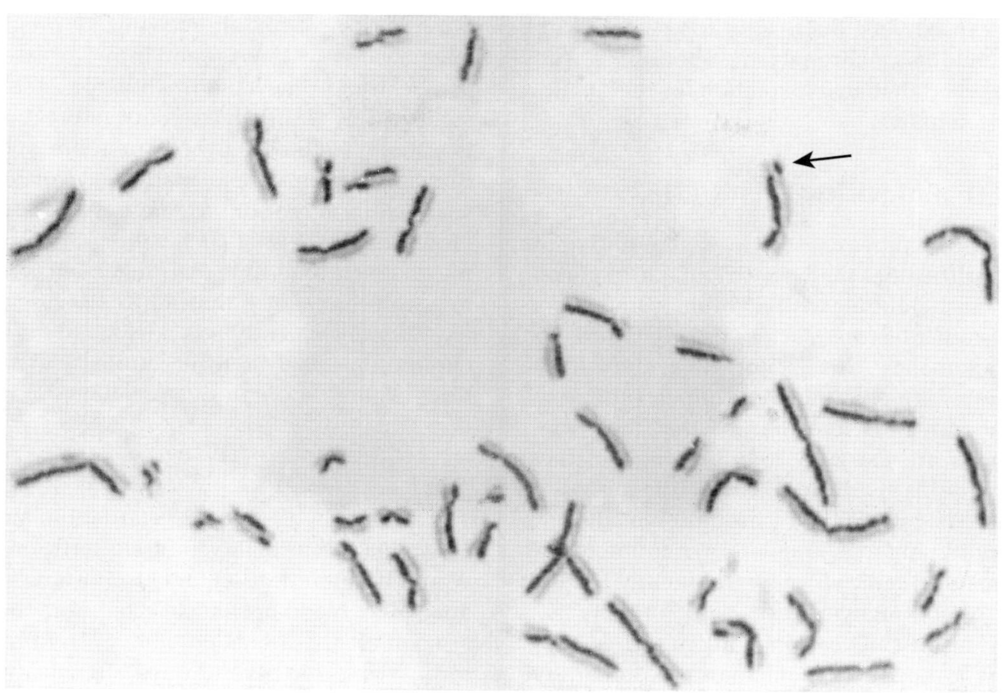

Fig. 18.26
Chromosome preparation showing sister chromatid exchanges (arrowed).

chromatids of each metaphase chromosome after two rounds of cell division in the presence of the thymidine analogue 5-bromodeoxyuridine (BudR), which becomes incorporated in the newly synthesized DNA (Fig. 18.26). There are normally about 10 SCEs per cell but the number is greatly increased in cells from patients with Bloom syndrome and xeroderma pigmentosa. In the latter condition this is only apparent after the cells have been exposed to ultraviolet light.

At present it is not clear how SCEs relate to the increase in chromosome breakage observed in these two disorders, but it is thought that the explanation could involve one of the steps in DNA replication. It is also of interest that the number of SCEs in normal cells is increased on exposure to certain carcinogens and chemical mutagens. For this reason the frequency of SCEs in cells in culture has been suggested as a useful in vitro test of the carcinogenicity and mutagenicity of chemical compounds (p. 29).

## INDICATIONS FOR CHROMOSOMAL ANALYSIS

It should be apparent from the contents of this chapter that chromosome abnormalities can present in many different ways. Consequently it is appropriate to consider the indications for chromosome analysis under a number of different headings (Table 18.11).

### MULTIPLE CONGENITAL ABNORMALITIES

Every child with multiple congenital abnormalities should have chromosome studies undertaken. This is important for several reasons:

1. Establishing a chromosomal diagnosis will prevent further potentially unpleasant investigations being undertaken.
2. Information about the prognosis can be provided, along with details of the relevant support group and an offer of contact with other families.
3. A chromosomal diagnosis should facilitate the provision of accurate information about the recurrence risk for future siblings.

**Table 18.11 Indications for chromosome analysis**

| |
|---|
| **Multiple congenital abnormalities** |
| Unexplained mental retardation |
| Sexual ambiguity or abnormality in sexual development |
| Infertility |
| Recurrent miscarriage |
| Unexplained stillbirth |
| Malignancy and chromosome breakage syndromes |

Although it can be very distressing for parents to be told that their child has a chromosome abnormality they will often be relieved that an explanation for their child's problems has been found.

## UNEXPLAINED LEARNING DIFFICULTIES

Chromosome abnormalities cause at least one-third of the 50% of learning difficulties that are attributable to genetic factors. While most children with a chromosome abnormality will have other features such as growth retardation and physical anomalies, this is not always so. If the Fragile X syndrome is a possibility it is important that the cytogenetics laboratory is informed so that the correct culture conditions are used (p. 284), although in most centres the Fragile X syndrome is now diagnosed by molecular methods rather than chromosome analysis. If standard karyotyping and Fragile X syndrome testing is negative, many geneticists now frequently request multitelomeric probe analysis, especially if there is a positive family history of learning difficulties (p. 280). In the future it is hoped that microarray comparative genomic hybridization (p. 40) will resolve many diagnostic problems in individuals and families with learning difficulties.

## SEXUAL AMBIGUITY

The birth of a child with ambiguous genitalia should be regarded as a medical emergency, not only because of the inevitable parental anxiety, but also because of the importance of ruling out the potentially life-threatening diagnosis of salt-losing congenital adrenal hyperplasia (p. 169). A chromosome analysis should be among the first investigations undertaken.

Disorders of sexual development presenting in later life with problems such as delayed puberty, primary amenorrhea or male gynecomastia are also strong indications for chromosome analysis as a first-line investigation. This can provide a diagnosis such as Turner syndrome (45,X) or Klinefelter syndrome (47,XXY). Alternatively a normal karyotype will stimulate a search for other possible explanations, such as an endocrine abnormality.

## INFERTILITY AND RECURRENT MISCARRIAGE

Unexplained involuntary infertility should prompt a request for chromosome studies, particularly if investigations reveal evidence of azoospermia in the male partner. At least 5% of such men are found to have Klinefelter syndrome. More rarely a complex chromosome rearrangement such as a translocation can cause such severe mechanical disruption in meiosis that complete failure of gametogenesis ensues.

At least 15% of all recognized pregnancies end in spontaneous miscarriage and in 50% of cases this is because of a chromosome abnormality (p. 247). Unfortunately, some couples experience recurrent pregnancy loss, which is usually defined as three or more spontaneous miscarriages. Often no explanation is ever found and many such couples go on to have successful pregnancies. However, in 3–6% of such couples, one partner is found to carry a chromosome rearrangement which predisposes to severe imbalance through malsegregation at meiosis (p. 49). Consequently it is now standard practice to offer chromosome analysis to all couples who have experienced three or more spontaneous pregnancy losses.

## UNEXPLAINED STILLBIRTH/NEONATAL DEATH

The presence of growth retardation and at least one congenital abnormality in a stillbirth or neonatal death would be an indication for chromosome studies based on analysis of blood or skin collected from the baby before or as soon after death as possible. Skin fibroblasts continue to be viable for several days after death. Chromosome abnormalities account for 5% of all stillbirths and neonatal deaths, and not all of these babies have multiple abnormalities that would immediately suggest a chromosomal cause.

## MALIGNANCY AND CHROMOSOME BREAKAGE SYNDROMES

Certain types of leukemia (p. 206) and many solid tumors, such as retinoblastoma (p. 209) and Wilms' tumor (p. 276), are associated with specific chromosomal abnormalities that can be of both diagnostic and prognostic value. Clinical features suggestive of a chromosome breakage syndrome (p. 287), such as a combination of photosensitivity and short stature, should also lead to appropriate chromosome fragility studies, such as analysis of sister chromatid exchanges.

## FURTHER READING

De Grouchy J, Turleau C 1984 Clinical atlas of human chromosomes, 2nd edn. John Wiley, Chichester

*A lavishly illustrated atlas of known chromosomal syndromes.*

Donnai D, Karmiloff-Smith A 2000 Williams syndrome: from genotype through to the cognitive phenotype. Am J Med Genet (Semin Med Genet) 97: 164–171

*A review dealing with one microdeletion syndrome in detail and the efforts to understand how the phenotype can be explained by the molecular findings.*

Gardner R J M, Sutherland G R 1996 Chromosome abnormalities and genetic counselling, 2nd edn. Oxford University Press, Oxford

*A useful updated guide to genetic counseling in families with a chromosome disorder.*

Hagerman R J, Silverman A C (eds) 1991 Fragile X syndrome. Diagnosis, treatment and research. Johns Hopkins University Press, Baltimore

*A detailed account of the clinical and genetic aspects of the Fragile X syndrome.*

Jacobs P A, Browne C, Gregson N, Joyce C, White H 1992 Estimates of the frequency of chromosome abnormalities detectable in unselected newborns using moderate levels of banding. J Med Genet 29: 103–108

*A review of the results of over 14 000 prenatal diagnoses with estimates of the incidence of chromosome abnormalities in term infants.*

Ratcliffe S 1999 Long term outcome of children of sex chromosome abnormalities. Arch Dis Child 80: 192–195

*A very useful and clear description of the cognitive and social outcomes of long term follow-up studies of sex chromosome aneuploidies.*

Schinzel A 1994 Human cytogenetics database. Oxford University Press, Oxford

*A regularly updated computerized database of all known chromosome abnormalities. This is an invaluable aid to diagnosis and counseling.*

## ELEMENTS

1. Chromosome abnormalities account for 50% of all spontaneous miscarriages and are present in 0.5–1.0% of all newborn infants.

2. Down syndrome is the most common autosomal chromosomal syndrome and shows a strong association between increasing incidence and advancing maternal age. Ninety-five per cent of all cases are caused by trisomy 21. Chromosome studies are necessary in all cases so that the rare but important cases due to unbalanced familial Robertsonian translocations can be identified.

3. An increasing number of chromosome microdeletion syndromes are being recognized. These have helped in gene mapping and in enhancing understanding of underlying genetic mechanisms such as imprinting. Microdeletions of chromosome 15 are found in both Angelman and the Prader–Willi syndrome and are maternally and paternally derived, respectively.

4. Triploidy is a common finding in spontaneously aborted products of conception but rare in a live-born infant. Some children with diploidy/triploidy mosaicism present with learning difficulties and areas of depigmentation, a condition known as hypomelanosis of Ito.

5. Sex chromosome abnormalities include Klinefelter syndrome (47,XXY), Turner syndrome (45,X), the XYY syndrome (47,XYY) and the triple X syndrome (47,XXX). In all of these conditions intelligence is either normal or only mildly impaired. Infertility is the rule in Klinefelter and Turner syndromes. Fertility is normal in the XYY and the triple X syndrome.

6. The Fragile X syndrome is the most common inherited cause of learning difficulties. It is associated with a fragile site on the long arm of the X chromosome and shows modified X-linked inheritance. Affected males have moderate-to-severe learning difficulties; carrier females can show mild learning difficulties. At the molecular level there is expansion of a CGG triplet repeat which can exist as a premutation or a full mutation.

7. Disorders of sexual differentiation include true and pseudohermaphroditism. True hermaphroditism is extremely rare. Male pseudohermaphroditism is caused most commonly by androgen insensitivity, an X-linked disorder involving the formation of androgen receptors. The most common cause of female pseudohermaphroditism is congenital adrenal hyperplasia, in which virilized infants can collapse with adrenal failure during the first week of life.

8. The chromosome breakage syndromes are rare autosomal recessive disorders characterized by increased chromosome breakage in cultured cells and an increased tendency to neoplasia, such as leukemia and lymphoma. They are caused by underlying defects in DNA repair.

CHAPTER 19

# Single-gene disorders

To date, over 10 000 single-gene traits and disorders have been identified. Most of these are individually rare, but together they affect between 1% and 2% of the general population at any one time. The management of these disorders in affected individuals and in their extended families presents a major challenge for clinical genetics and allied relevant specialties.

A wide variety of single-gene disorders have been mentioned throughout this book. In this chapter some of the more common and important single-gene disorders will be described, besides a small number that hold particular interest to clinicians, with particular emphasis on their basic molecular defects. Each of these disorders illustrates important genetic principles, and for many the identification of the mutational basis and isolation of the associated protein product represent some of the most notable scientific achievements of the last decade.

## HUNTINGTON DISEASE

Huntington disease (HD), also known as Huntington chorea, derives its eponymous title from Dr George Huntington, who described multiple affected individuals in a large North American kindred in 1872. George Huntington's paper, which was published in the Philadelphia journal *The Medical and Surgical Reporter*, gave a graphic description of the progressive neurological disability that has endowed HD with the unenviable reputation of being one of the most feared and unpleasant hereditary disorders encountered in humans. The natural history is characterized by slowly progressive selective cell death in the central nervous system, for which there is no effective treatment or cure. The prevalence in most parts of the world is approximately 1 in 10 000, although in some areas, such as Tasmania and the Lake Maracaibo region of Venezuela, much higher figures have been noted.

Generally, HD is a disorder of middle to late adult life. However, HD can start at virtually any age, including a rare juvenile form that presents much younger and with different clinical features. This is one of several enigmatic aspects of HD that have been explained, at least in part, by the discovery of the underlying molecular defect.

### CLINICAL FEATURES

In the common adult-onset form of HD the disease course is characterized by a slowly progressive movement disorder and an insidious impairment of intellectual function with psychiatric disturbance and eventual dementia. The average age of onset is around 40 years and the mean duration of the illness is approximately 15 years. Chorea is the most common movement abnormality. This takes the form of subtle involuntary movements such as facial grimacing, twitching of the face and limbs, folding of the arms and crossing of the legs. As the disease progresses the gait becomes very unsteady and speech becomes unclear.

Intellectual changes in the early stages of HD include memory impairment and poor concentration span. Anxiety, aggressive behavior, paranoia, irrationality, increased libido and alcohol abuse can also occur. There is a gradual deterioration in intellectual function, leading eventually to total incapacitation and dementia.

#### Juvenile Huntington disease

In recent studies (since 1970) up to 5% of HD cases have presented before the age of 20 years; in some earlier studies the figure was up to 10%. Instead of chorea there is rigidity, with slowing of voluntary movement and clumsiness. A decline in school performance heralds the onset of a severe progressive dementia, often in association with epileptic seizures. The average duration of the illness is around 10–15 years.

### GENETICS

Traditionally HD has been said to show autosomal dominant inheritance with a variable age of onset, close to complete penetrance, and a very low mutation rate. In addition, it has been noted that the disorder often shows

**Table 19.1 Comparison of genetic aspects of Huntington disease and myotonic dystrophy**

| | Huntington disease | Myotonic dystrophy |
|---|---|---|
| Inheritance | Autosomal dominant | Autosomal dominant |
| Chromosome locus | 4p16.3 | 19q13.3 |
| Trinucleotide repeat | CAG in 5′ translated region | CTG in 3′ untranslated region |
| Repeat sizes | Normal ≤26<br>Mutable 27–35<br>Reduced penetrance 36–39<br>Fully penetrant ≥40 | Normal < 37<br><br>Full mutation 50–2000+ |
| Protein product | Huntingtin | MD protein kinase (DMPK) |
| Early-onset form | Juvenile<br>Usually paternally transmitted | Congenital<br>Usually maternally transmitted |

anticipation, whereby the onset is at a younger age in succeeding generations, particularly when transmitted by a male. The recent discovery of the HD gene has provided an explanation for some of these observations.

## Mapping and isolation of the Huntington disease gene

HD was one of the first disorders to be mapped by linkage analysis using polymorphic DNA markers when, in 1983, the disorder was found to show close linkage with a probe known as G8 on the short arm of chromosome 4. This initial search for the HD locus was helped enormously by the collection of blood samples from a huge pedigree containing over 100 affected subjects living on the shores of Lake Maracaibo in Venezuela. As well as providing the first means of predictive testing for HD, this work also revealed that HD homozygotes are no more severely affected than heterozygotes. This is in contrast to most other autosomal dominant disorders (p. 108). Ten years later, in 1993, the gene itself was isolated and found to contain a highly polymorphic CAG (polyglutamine) repeat sequence located in the 5′ region. The messenger RNA codes for a protein of approximately 350 kDa, known as *huntingtin* (also IT15). Huntingtin is expressed in many different cells throughout the central nervous system, as well as other tissues, although its function remains unclear. One proposed role, as yet unproven, is that it is involved in apoptosis, i.e. cell death.

## The mutation in Huntington disease

Almost all individuals with HD possess an expansion of a CAG polyglutamine repeat sequence located in the 5′ region of the HD gene. HD is thus an example of a disorder caused by expansion of a triplet repeat (p. 24), a mutational mechanism that was first identified in humans in contrast to almost all other types of mutation that were first reported in other species such as *Drosophila* and mice. A recent joint working party of the American College of Medical Genetics and the American Society of Human Genetics recommended that HD genes should be categorized under four headings on the basis of CAG repeat length (Table 19.1).

### *Normal alleles*

Alleles containing 26 or fewer CAG repeats are not associated with disease manifestations and are stable in meiosis.

### *Mutable alleles*

Allele sizes of 27 to 35 CAG repeats do not cause disease but show meiotic instability with a potential to increase or decrease in size. These 'mutable' alleles thus constitute a reservoir for new mutations. When an affected individual presents with what appears to be a new mutation, it usually emerges that the father carries a mutable allele. Furthermore, there is evidence that mutable alleles that expand are associated with a particular haplotype as identified by intragenic and flanking DNA markers. This implies that certain haplotypes are more mutable than others.

### *Reduced penetrance alleles*

This third category consists of alleles containing 36 to 39 CAG repeats. These are associated with either late-onset disease or complete absence of disease expression, i.e. non-penetrance.

### *Disease alleles*

The final group of HD genes contains 40 or more CAG repeats. These are invariably associated with disease, although sometimes this may not develop until the seventh or eighth decade. There is a direct relationship between length of repeat and disease expression, with the average age of onset for repeat sizes of 40, 45 and 50 being 57, 37 and 26 years, respectively. Most affected adults have repeat sizes of between 36 and 50, whereas juvenile cases often have an expansion greater than 55 repeats.

### Parent of origin effect in disease transmission

Autosomal dominant inheritance is well established, with an offspring risk of 1 in 2 regardless of whether the affected parent is male or female. However, for reasons that are not understood, meiotic instability appears to be much greater in spermatogenesis than in oogenesis. This is reflected in anticipation, occurring mainly when the mutant allele is transmitted by a male. Juveniles with the rigid form of HD have almost always inherited the mutant allele from their more mildly affected father.

Several possible explanations have been suggested for this preferential transmission of expanded alleles by the male. One possibility is that expansion caused by *slippage* (p. 24) of DNA polymerase simply reflects the number of mitoses undergone during gametogenesis. In Chapter 3 it was pointed out that spermatogenesis involves a much larger number of mitotic divisions than oogenesis (p. 45). An alternative possibility is based on the observation that huntingtin is expressed in oocytes, so that there could be selection against oocytes with large expansions as a consequence of preferential apoptosis.

## CLINICAL APPLICATIONS AND FUTURE PROSPECTS

The discovery of the HD gene has meant that accurate predictive testing is possible, although there is universal agreement that this should only be offered as part of a well-planned and carefully monitored counseling package. Experience to date indicates that more women than men take up the offer of predictive testing, with the degree of psychological disturbance in those given positive results being less than was expected. Sixty per cent of candidates test negative, i.e. they receive good news, and the reasons for this departure from the expected 50% are not clear.

Prenatal diagnosis is also possible for those couples for whom this is acceptable, though only 20–25 such tests are performed in the UK annually. Obviously there are considerable emotional and ethical issues associated with termination of pregnancy, on the grounds that a child could go on to develop a neurodegenerative disease in middle age. This will be particularly pertinent when effective therapeutic strategies have been devised. One appealing approach is based on the observation that large CAG repeats result in intracellular accumulation of huntingtin 'aggregates', which are cleaved by a protease known as caspase to form a toxic product that causes cell death (apoptosis). Caspase inhibitors have been shown to have a beneficial effect in an HD mouse model. Another therapeutic approache undergoing trial is fetal neuronal cell transfer into regions of the brain, such as the caudate nucleus and putamen, which become atrophic in the early stages of the disease. This approach carries ethical considerations that will be difficult for some couples.

## MYOTONIC DYSTROPHY

Myotonic dystrophy (MD) is the most common form of muscular dystrophy seen in adults, with an overall incidence of approximately 1 in 8000. MD shares many features in common with HD (Table 19.1). In particular both disorders show autosomal dominant inheritance with anticipation and an early-onset form with rather different clinical features. However, in MD the early-onset form is transmitted almost exclusively by the mother and presents at birth, in contrast to juvenile HD, which is generally paternally transmitted with an age of onset in the teens.

## CLINICAL FEATURES

In contrast to most forms of muscular dystrophy, these are not limited exclusively to the neuromuscular system. Most commonly persons with MD present in adult life with slowly progressive weakness and myotonia. This latter term refers to tonic muscle spasm with prolonged relaxation, which can manifest as a delay in releasing the grip on shaking hands. Other clinical abnormalities can include cataracts (Fig. 19.1), cardiac conduction defects, disturbed gastrointestinal peristalsis (dysphagia, consti-

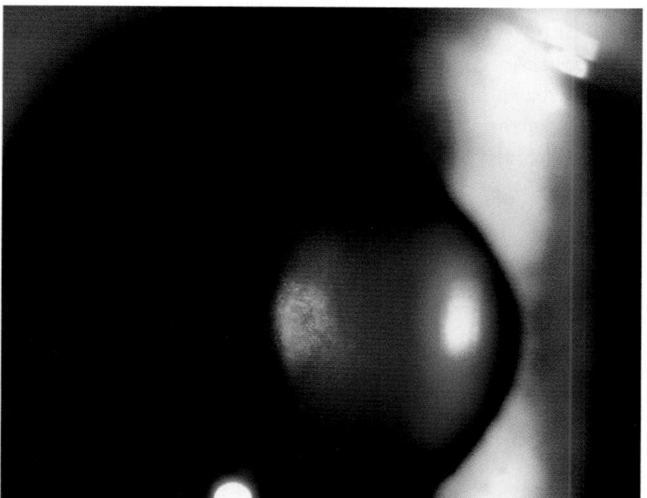

**Fig. 19.1**
Refractile lens opacities in an asymptomatic person with myotonic dystrophy. (Courtesy of Mr R Doran and Mr M Geall, Department of Ophthalmology, General Infirmary, Leeds.)

pation, diarrhea), weak sphincters, increased risk of diabetes mellitus and gallstones, somnolence, frontal balding and testicular atrophy. The age of onset is very variable and in its mildest form usually runs a relatively benign course. However, as the age of onset becomes earlier, so the clinical symptoms increase in severity and more body systems are involved. In the 'congenital' form affected babies present at birth with hypotonia, talipes and respiratory distress that can prove life threatening (Fig. 7.18). Children who survive tend to show a lack of facial expression ('myopathic facies') with delayed motor development and learning difficulties.

The diagnosis of MD used to be based on the finding of myotonic discharges seen on electromyography. This unpleasant investigation has now been superseded by mutation analysis.

## GENETICS

It has long been recognized that MD shows autosomal dominant inheritance, with increasing severity in succeeding generations. At one time it was thought that this phenomenon of *anticipation* (p. 116) was a reflection of ascertainment bias, caused by the greater likelihood of detecting a mildly affected parent having a severely affected child, rather than the other way round. However, studies in the 1980s confirmed that anticipation is a real phenomenon in MD.

### Mapping and isolating the myotonic dystrophy gene

Genetic linkage of MD to the secretor and Lutheran blood group loci was established in 1971, and the MD locus was mapped to chromosome 19 in 1982. As with HD, 10 years elapsed before the gene itself was isolated. This was achieved by an international collaborative effort whereby most of the relevant region of chromosome 19 was cloned. The mutational basis of MD was shown in 1992 to be instability in a CTG repeat sequence which is present in the 3′ untranslated region of a protein kinase gene – dystrophia myotonica protein kinase (*DMPK*).

### Genotype–phenotype correlation in myotonic dystrophy

In unaffected persons the CTG sequence lying 3′ to the *DMPK* gene consists of up to 37 repeats (Table 19.1). Affected individuals have an expansion of at least 50 copies of the CTG sequence. There is a close correlation between disease severity and the size of the expansion, which can exceed 2000 repeats. The severe congenital cases show the largest repeat copy number, with almost invariable inheritance from the mother. Thus meiotic or germ line instability is greater in the female for alleles containing a large number of sequences. Curiously, expansion of a relatively small number of repeats appears to occur more commonly in the male, and most MD mutations are thought to have occurred originally during meiosis in the male. One possible explanation for these observations is that mature spermatozoa can only carry small expansions whereas ova can accommodate much larger expansions; hence congenital onset cases are almost exclusively maternally transmitted.

Yet another puzzling feature of MD is the reported tendency for healthy individuals who are heterozygous for MD alleles in the normal size range to preferentially transmit alleles that are greater than 19 CTG repeats in size. This possible example of meiotic drive (p. 130) could explain the relatively high frequency of MD with constant replenishment of a reservoir of potential MD mutations.

### The myotonic dystrophy protein kinase

At present it is not known precisely how, or indeed if, the MD protein kinase causes muscular weakness or the other clinical problems. Rather surprisingly, it has been shown that mice with both overexpression and underexpression of DMPK do not show myotonia and other typical clinical features of MD. It is now believed that abnormal protein kinase activity is not the main cause of MD, but that instead the RNA produced by the expanded *DMPK* allele somehow interferes with the cellular processing of RNA produced by a variety of other genes. It has been shown that expanded *DMPK* transcripts accumulate in the nuclei of cells, and this is believed to have a gain-of-function effect through its binding with a CUG RNA-binding protein (CUG-BP) that has been identified. Excess CUG-BP has been shown to interfere with a number of genes relevant to MD, which is not surprising because CUG repeats are known to exist in various alternately spliced muscle-specific enzymes. An additional possibility is that expansion of the CTG sequence in the 3′ region of the *DMPK* gene influences expression not only of the protein kinase but also of other closely adjacent genes, such as the recently identified homeobox-containing gene known as *DMAHP* (= DM locus-associated homeodomain protein).

## CLINICAL APPLICATIONS AND FUTURE PROSPECTS

The development of a reliable molecular diagnostic test for MD has meant that both presymptomatic testing and prenatal diagnosis can be offered to those families for whom it is appropriate and acceptable. This is particularly relevant for couples who have had a child with the severe congenital form, for whom it is known that the risk of recurrence is relatively high. As in HD, presymptomatic testing should not be undertaken without an offer of long-term support and medical care, and in both HD and MD the possibility of difficulty in obtaining both life and health insurance should be discussed before predictive testing is undertaken (p. 373).

Important components of the management of MD include regular surveillance for cardiac conduction defects and the provision of information about risks associated with general anesthesia. Logical approaches to gene therapy will almost certainly have to await a better understanding of the mechanism whereby expansion of the repeat sequence in the 3′ untranslated region of the *DMPK* gene causes such diverse and variable clinical abnormalities.

### Type 2 myotonic dystrophy

Some families with a variable presentation of similar features to MD, but without the $(CTG)_n$ expansion of *DMPK*, have been shown to link to 3q21. Originally referred to as *proximal myotonic myopathy* (PROMM), these cases are designated type 2 MD to distinguish them from the more common type 1 MD. The molecular defect has been shown to be a $(CCTG)_n$ expansion mutation in intron 1 of a gene called *ZNF9*. Most families are of German descent, and haplotype studies suggest a single founder mutation occurring between 200 and 500 generations ago.

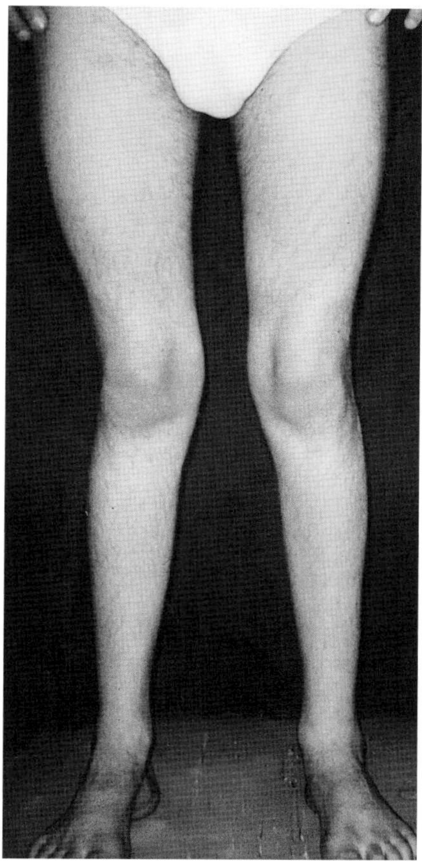

**Fig. 19.2**
Lower limbs of a male with hereditary motor and sensory neuropathy (HMSN) showing severe muscle wasting below the knees.

## HEREDITARY MOTOR AND SENSORY NEUROPATHY

Hereditary motor and sensory neuropathy (HMSN) comprises a group of clinically and genetically heterogeneous disorders characterized by slowly progressive distal muscle weakness and wasting. Other names for these disorders include *Charcot–Marie–Tooth disease* and *peroneal muscular atrophy*. Their overall incidence is approximately 1 in 2500.

HMSN can be classified on the basis of the results of motor nerve conduction velocity (MNCV) studies. In HMSN type I MNCV is reduced, and nerve biopsies from patients show segmental demyelination accompanied by hypertrophic changes with 'onion bulb' formation. In HMSN type II MNCV is normal or only slightly reduced and nerve biopsies show axonal degeneration.

### CLINICAL FEATURES

In autosomal dominant HMSN I, which is the most common form, there is onset of slowly progressive distal muscle weakness and wasting in the lower limbs between the ages of 10 and 30 years. Similar changes occur later in the upper limbs in many patients, often in association with ataxia and tremor. The appearance of the lower limbs has been likened to that of an 'inverted champagne bottle' (Fig. 19.2). With age, locomotion becomes more difficult and the feet tend to show exaggeration of their normal arch, known as 'pes cavus'. Despite these quite striking changes most patients retain reasonable muscle strength and are not too seriously disabled. Other faculties such as vision, hearing and intellect are not impaired. In keeping with the pathological changes of hypertrophy, palpable thickening of peripheral nerves can be detected in around one-third of cases.

The clinical features in other forms of HMSN are relatively similar but differ in the age of onset, rate of progression and presence of other neurological involvement. For example, in HMSN II onset is usually later than in HMSN I and the disease course is milder to the extent that some affected individuals are asymptomatic. By contrast, in HMSN III, which is very rare, onset is in early childhood and there is severe delay in achieving motor milestones.

### GENETICS

HMSN can show autosomal dominant, autosomal recessive or X-linked inheritance, although autosomal

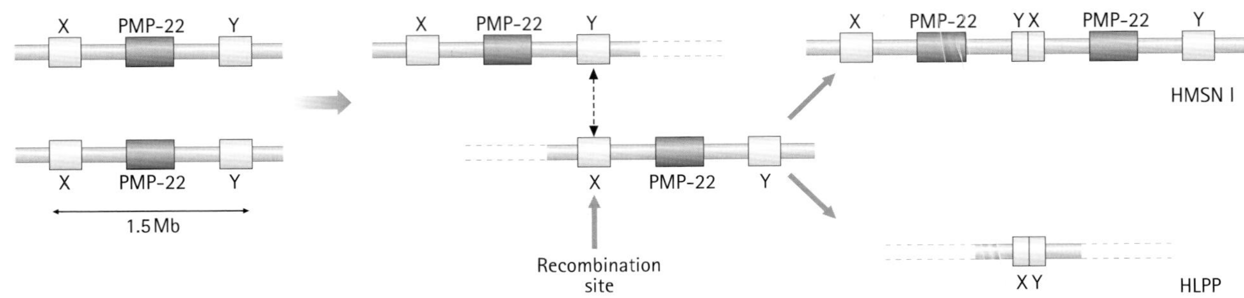


**Fig. 19.3**
Mechanism by which misalignment and recombination with unequal crossing over lead to the formation of the duplication and deletion that cause hereditary motor and sensory neuropathy type I (HMSN I) and hereditary neuropathy with liability to pressure palsies (HNPP). X and Y represent homologous sequences flanking the *PMP-22* gene.

dominant forms are by far the most common. In over 70% of cases of HMSN I the disorder arises as the result of a duplication of 1.5 megabases of genomic DNA on the short arm of chromosome 17. This is seen both in familial cases and in most sporadic cases, implying a common causal mechanism with a high mutation rate. Located within this 1.5 Mb region on 17p is the gene which codes for a 22 kDa glycoprotein known as peripheral myelin protein-22 (*PMP-22*). This is present in the myelin membranes of peripheral nerves, where it plays a major role in arresting Schwann cell division. Changes in this protein cause a peripheral neuropathy in a mutant strain of mice known as 'trembler'. HMSN I in humans is thought to be the result of a *PMP-22* dosage effect. Point mutations have been identified in the *PMP-22* gene in a small number of non-duplication HMSN I patients.

Recent studies have shown that the HMSN I duplication is generated by misalignment and subsequent recombination between homologous sequences which flank the *PMP-22* gene (Fig. 19.3). For reasons which are not understood this recombination event usually occurs in male gametogenesis (rather than in the female, as is the case in Duchenne muscular dystrophy (p. 308)). The reciprocal deletion product of this unequal crossing-over event causes a relatively mild disorder known as *hereditary neuropathy with liability to pressure palsies* (HNPP), in which minor nerve trauma, such as pressure from prolonged sitting on a long-haul flight, causes focal numbness and weakness. The mechanism whereby duplication and deletion products result from misalignment and recombination is identical to that which produces Hb Lepore and anti-Lepore (Fig. 10.3, p. 151), congenital adrenal hyperplasia (p. 169), and deletion 22q11 syndrome (p. 277).

### Other forms of hereditary motor and sensory neuropathy

In a small proportion of families with typical features of HMSN I, linkage analysis indicated that the disease locus was on chromosome 1 rather than on chromosome 17. This led to chromosome 17 cases being referred to as HMSN Ia and chromosome 1 cases as HMSN Ib. It is now known that HMSN Ib is caused by mutations in the gene which codes for another major myelin protein, known as myelin protein zero (*MPZ*). This plays a crucial role as an adhesion molecule in the compaction of myelin in peripheral nerves.

A rare form of HMSN shows X-linked inheritance, with males having typical HMSN I features and females being more mildly affected (sometimes with HMSN II features). This form of HMSN is caused by mutations in the gene that encodes a gap junction protein called *connexin 32*. Previously it was not known that gap junctions existed in peripheral nerves and the role of connexin 32 in causing HMSN is not fully understood at present.

### FUTURE PROSPECTS

The discovery of the chromosome 17 duplication in HMSN Ia has dramatically improved diagnostic precision and has removed the need for nerve conduction studies as a presymptomatic test for family members at risk. Unfortunately successful treatment remains elusive. Efforts at gene therapy in mouse models such as 'trembler' will almost certainly be directed at trying to achieve a reduction in gene dosage by switching off or 'down-regulating' *PMP-22* expression.

## NEUROFIBROMATOSIS

References to the clinical features of neurofibromatosis (NF) first appeared in the eighteenth century medical literature, but historically the disorder is most commonly associated with the name Von Recklinghausen, a German pathologist who coined the term 'neurofibroma' in 1882.

Neurofibromatosis is now known to be one of the most common genetic disorders in humans and gained public notoriety when it was suggested that Joseph Merrick, the 'elephant man' was probably affected. However, subsequent review of Merrick's photographs and skeleton led to the conclusion that he did not have neurofibromatosis but instead had a much rarer disorder known as *Proteus syndrome*.

There are two main types of neurofibromatosis, NF1 and NF2. Both conditions, especially NF2, could be included under familial cancer syndromes (Ch. 14) but are covered in more detail here. NF1 is by far the more common, with an incidence at birth of approximately 1 in 3000. NF2 has an incidence of approximately 1 in 35 000 and a prevalence of around 1 in 200 000.

## CLINICAL FEATURES

The most notable features of NF1 are small pigmented skin lesions, known as *café-au-lait spots*, and small soft fleshy growths known as neurofibromata (Fig. 19.4). Café-au-lait spots first appear in early childhood and continue to increase in both size and number until puberty. A minimum of six café-au-lait spots at least 5 mm in diameter are required to support the diagnosis in childhood, and axillary and/or inguinal freckling should be present. Neurofibromata are benign tumors that arise most commonly in the skin. They usually appear in late childhood and adult life and show an increase in number with age.

Other clinical findings in NF1 include axillary freckling, relative macrocephaly (large head) and Lisch nodules. These are small harmless raised pigmented hamartomata of the iris (Fig. 19.5). The most common complication, occurring in a third of childhood cases, is mild developmental delay characterized by a non-verbal learning disorder. For many significant improvement is seen through the school years. Most individuals with NF1 enjoy a normal healthy life and are not unduly inconvenienced by their condition. However, a small number of patients develop one or more major complications, such as epilepsy, a central nervous system tumor or a scoliosis.

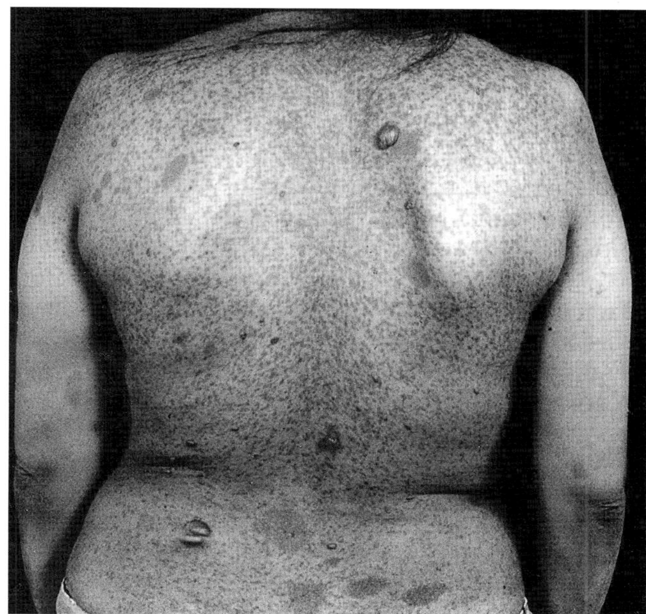

**Fig. 19.4**
A patient with neurofibromatosis type I showing truncal freckling, café-au-lait spots and multiple neurofibromata.

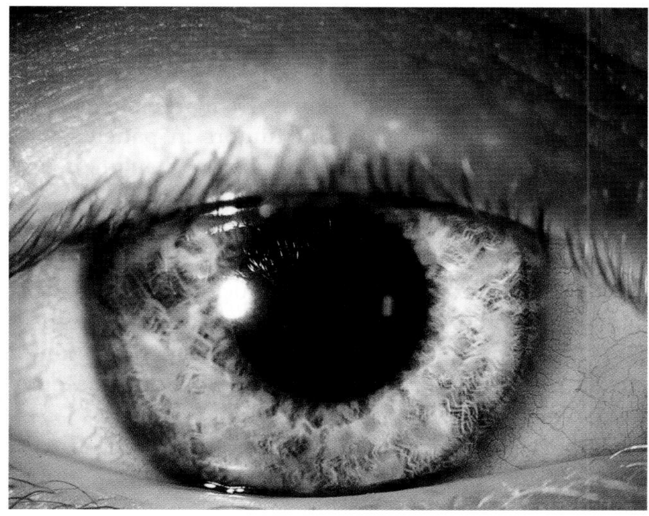

**Fig. 19.5**
Lisch nodules seen in neurofibromatosis type I. (Courtesy of Mr R Doran, Department of Ophthalmology, General Infirmary, Leeds.)

## GENETICS

NF1 shows autosomal dominant inheritance and probably complete penetrance by the age of 5 years. Expression is very variable and affected members of the same family can show quite striking differences in disease severity. The features in affected identical twins are usually very similar so that variable expression in family members, who must have the same mutation, is probably due to the effects of modifying genes at other loci. Approximately 50% of cases of NF1 are due to new mutations, with the estimated mutation rate being approximately 1 per 10 000 gametes. This is around 100 times greater than the average mutation rate per generation per locus in humans.

There are a few reports of multiple affected children born to unaffected healthy parents. These probably represent examples of parental gonadal mosaicism (p. 117). Somatic mosaicism in NF1 can manifest with features limited to a particular part of the body. This is referred to as *segmental* NF.

A

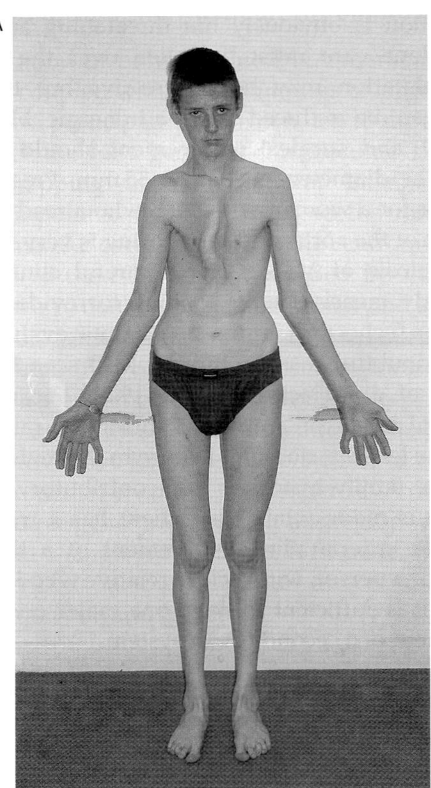

B

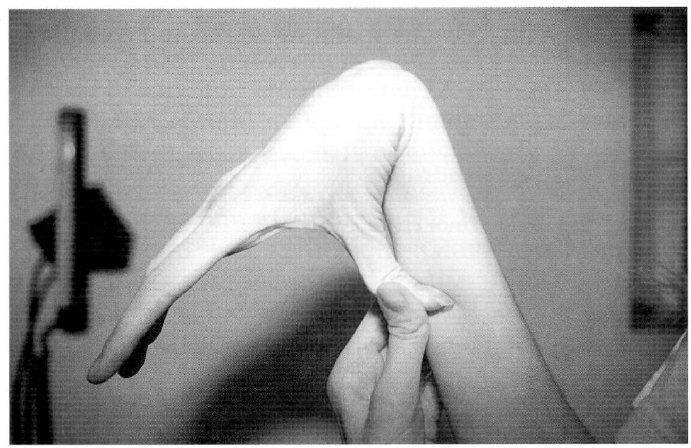

**Fig. 19.6**
(A) An adolescent with Marfan syndrome. He shows disproportionately long limbs (arachnodactyly) and a very extreme example of chest bone deformity; he also has a dilated aortic root. (B) Joint hypermobility at the wrist in a woman with Marfan syndrome, although this appearance might also be seen in other joint laxity conditions, e.g. Ehlers–Danlos syndrome.

five distinct regions, or domains. The largest of these, occupying about 75% of the gene, comprises about 46 epidermal growth factor repeats. Finding the causative mutations in affected patients was initially very difficult but well in excess of 300 are now reported. Most are missense and have a dominant-negative effect, resulting in less than 35% of the expected amount of fibrillin in the extracellular matrix. Mutations have also been found in related phenotypes such as neonatal MFS, familial ectopia lentis, Shrintzen–Goldberg syndrome, and the MASS phenotype. In one study a Marfan family not showing linkage to 15q was found to link to 3p25, suggesting a second locus in a minority of cases.

### Congenital contractural arachnodactyly

Also known as Beal syndrome, this is probably the condition originally described by Marfan in 1896. Many features overlap with MFS, but there is less tendency to aortic dilatation and its catastrophic consequences. Individuals have congenital contractures of their digits, a crumpled ear helix, and sometimes marked scoliosis. It is due to mutated *type 2 fibrillin*, which shares the same organizational structure as fibrillin-1 and maps to 5q23.

## CYSTIC FIBROSIS

Cystic fibrosis (CF) was first recognized as a discrete entity in 1936 and used to be known as 'mucoviscidosis' because of the accumulation of thick mucous secretions that lead to blockage of the airways and secondary infection. Although antibiotics and physiotherapy have been very effective in increasing the average life expectancy of a child with CF from less than 5 years in 1955 to around 30 years at present, CF remains a significant cause of chronic ill health and mortality in childhood and early adult life.

CF is one of the most common autosomal recessive disorders encountered in individuals of Western European origin, in whom the incidence varies from 1 in 2000 to 1 in 3000. The incidence is slightly lower in Eastern and Southern European populations and much lower in African-Americans (1 in 15000) and Asian-Americans (1 in 31 000).

### CLINICAL FEATURES

The organs most commonly affected in CF are the lungs and the pancreas. Chronic lung disease caused by recurrent infection eventually leads to fibrotic changes in the lungs with secondary cardiac failure, a condition known as cor pulmonale. When this complication occurs the only hope for long-term survival rests in a successful heart–lung transplant.

In 85% of persons with CF pancreatic function is impaired, with reduced enzyme secretion due to blockage of the pancreatic ducts by inspissated secretions. This leads to malabsorption with an increase in the fat content of the stools. This complication of CF is readily amenable to treatment with oral supplements of pancreatic enzymes.

Other problems which are commonly encountered in CF include nasal polyps, rectal prolapse, cirrhosis and diabetes mellitus. Around 10% of children with CF present in the newborn period with obstruction of the small bowel due to thickened meconium, a condition known as meconium ileus. Almost all males with CF are sterile because of congenital bilateral absence of the vas deferens (CBAVD). It is now recognized that a small subset of males have a very mild form of CF in which CBAVD is the only significant clinical problem. Other rare presentations of CF include chronic pancreatitis, diffuse bronchiectasis and bronchopulmonary allergic aspergillosis.

## GENETICS

CF shows autosomal recessive inheritance. Other autosomal recessive disorders, such as hemochromatosis, which causes tissue iron overload, show a higher incidence, but CF is by far the most serious autosomal recessive disorder encountered in children of Western European origin. Possible explanations that have been proposed for this high incidence include multiple CF loci, a high mutation rate, meiotic drive and heterozygote advantage. This latter explanation, possibly mediated by increased heterozygote resistance to chloride-secreting bacterially induced diarrhea, is thought to be the most likely, although absolute proof is lacking.

### Mapping and isolation of the cystic fibrosis gene

The CF locus was mapped to chromosome 7q31 in 1985 by the demonstration of linkage to the gene for a polymorphic enzyme known as paraoxanase. Shortly afterwards two polymorphic DNA marker loci, known as MET and D7S8, were shown to be closely linked flanking markers. The region between these markers was scrutinized for the presence of HTF or CpG islands, which are known to be present close to the 5′ end of many genes (p. 77). This led to the identification of several new DNA markers which were shown to be very tightly linked to the CF locus with recombination frequencies of less than 1%. These loci were found to be in linkage disequilibrium (p. 134) with the CF locus, and the CF mutation was found to be associated with one particular haplotype in 84% of cases. This discovery of linkage disequilibrium was consistent with the concept of a single original mutation being responsible for a large proportion of all CF genes. The identification of loci tightly linked to the CF locus narrowed its location down to a region of approximately 500 kb. Genes expressed in tissues involved in CF, such as lung and pancreas, and conserved between species were identified. The CF gene was eventually cloned by two groups of scientists in North America in 1989 by a combination of chromosome jumping, physical mapping, isolation of exon sequences and mutation analysis. It was named the CF transmembrane conductance regulator (*CFTR*) gene and was shown to span a genomic region of approximately 250 kb and to contain 27 exons.

### The cystic fibrosis transmembrane conductance regulator protein

The structure of *CFTR* is consistent with a protein product containing 1480 amino acids with a molecular weight of 168 kDa. It is believed to consist of two transmembrane (TM) domains that anchor it to the cell membrane, two nucleotide binding folds (NBF) which bind ATP, and a regulatory (R) domain, which is phosphorylated by protein kinase-A (Fig. 19.7).

The primary role of the CFTR protein is to act as a chloride channel. Activation by phosphorylation of the regulatory domain, followed by binding of ATP to the NBF domains, opens the outwardly rectifying chloride

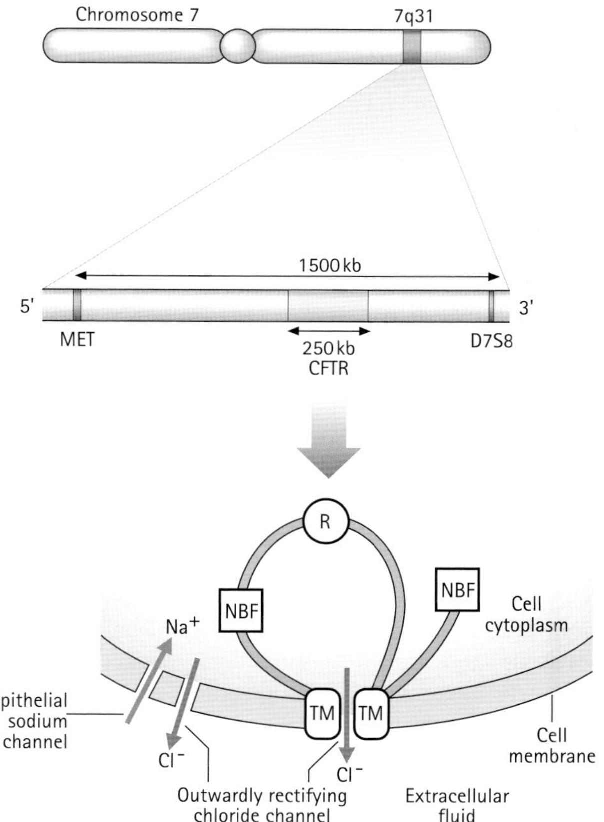


**Fig. 19.7**
The cystic fibrosis locus, gene and protein product that influences closely adjacent epithelial sodium and outwardly rectifying chloride channels. R: regulatory domain; NBF: nucleotide binding fold; TM: transmembrane domain.

**Table 19.3 Contribution of ΔF508 mutation to all CF mutations**

| Country | % |
|---|---|
| Denmark | 88 |
| Netherlands | 79 |
| UK | 78 |
| Ireland | 75 |
| France | 75 |
| USA | 66 |
| Germany | 65 |
| Poland | 55 |
| Italy | 50 |
| Turkey | 30 |

Data from European Working Group on CF Genetics (EWGCFG) Gradient of distribution in Europe of the major CF mutation and of its associated haplotype. Hum Genet 1990 85: 436–441, and Worldwide survey of the ΔF508 mutation – report from the cystic fibrosis genetic analysis consortium. Am J Hum Genet 1990 47: 354–359

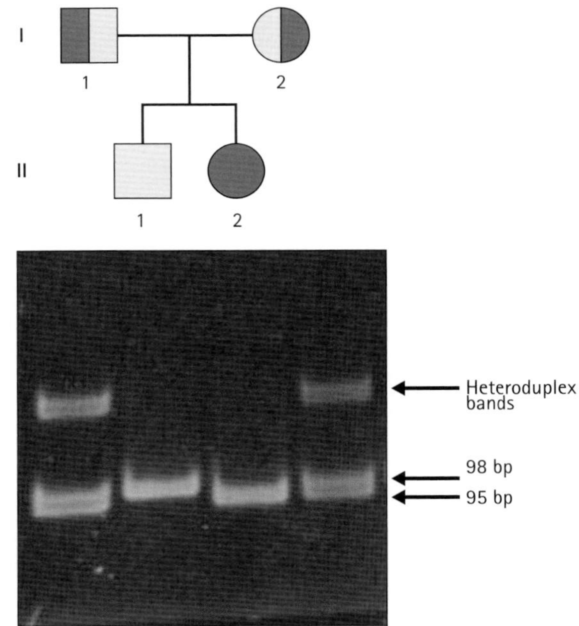


**Fig. 19.8**
PCR amplification of 98 and 95 bp DNA fragments surrounding the ΔF508 mutation site in the *CFTR* gene from a child with cystic fibrosis and her parents. The child, $II_2$, is homozygous for ΔF508. Her parents, $I_1$ and $I_2$, are heterozygous, and her brother, $II_1$, is homozgous for the normal allele. Heterozygotes are readily identified by the presence of heteroduplex bands formed between 95 and 98 bp products and electrophoresed on a non-denaturing gel.

channel and exerts a negative effect on intracellular sodium absorption by closure of the epithelial sodium channel. The net effect is to reduce the level of intracellular sodium chloride, which improves the quality of cellular mucous secretions.

## Mutations in the cystic fibrosis transmembrane conductance regulator gene

The first mutation to be identified in *CFTR* was a deletion of three adjacent base pairs at the 508th codon which results in the loss of a phenylalanine residue. This mutation is known as ΔF508 (Δ for deletion and F for phenylalanine) and it has been shown to account for approximately 70% of all mutations in *CFTR*, with the highest incidence of 88% being in Denmark (Table 19.3). The ΔF508 mutation can be demonstrated relatively simply by PCR (p. 62) using primers which flank the 508th codon (Fig. 19.8).

Over 1300 other mutations in the *CFTR* gene have been identified. These include missense, frameshift, splice-site, nonsense and deletion mutations. Most of these are extremely uncommon, although a few can account for a small but significant proportion of mutations in a particular population. For example, the G542X and G551D mutations account for 12% and 3% of all CF mutations in the Ashkenazi Jewish and North American Caucasian populations, respectively. Commercial multiplex PCR-based kits have been developed that detect approximately 90% of all carriers. Using these it is possible to reduce the carrier risk for a healthy individual from a population risk of 1 in 25 to less than 1 in 200 (p. 345).

## Genotype–phenotype correlation

Mutations in *CFTR* can influence the function of the protein product by:

1. causing a complete or partial reduction in its synthesis, e.g. G542X and IVS8-6(5T)
2. preventing it from reaching the epithelial membrane, e.g. ΔF508
3. causing it to function incorrectly when it reaches its final location, e.g. G551D and R117H.

The net effect of all these mutations is to reduce the normal functional activity of the CFTR protein. The extent to which normal CFTR protein activity is reduced correlates well with the clinical phenotype. Levels of less than 3% are associated with severe 'classic' CF, sometimes referred to as the PI type because of associated pancreatic insufficiency. Levels of activity between 3% and 8% cause a milder 'atypical' form of CF in which there is respiratory disease but relatively normal pancreatic function. This is referred to as the PS (pancreatic sufficient) form. Finally, levels of activity between 8% and 12% cause the mildest CF phenotype, in which the only clinical abnormality is CBAVD in males.

The relationship between genotype and phenotype is complex. Homozygotes for ΔF508 almost always have severe classical CF, as do compound heterozygotes with ΔF508 and G551D or G542X. The outcome for other compound heterozygote combinations can be much more difficult to predict. The complexity of the interaction between *CFTR* alleles is illustrated by the IVS8-6 poly T variant. This contains a polythymidine tract in intron 8 that influences the splicing efficiency of exon 9, resulting in reduced synthesis of normal CFTR protein. Three variants consisting of 5T, 7T and 9T have been identified. The 9T variant is associated with normal activity but the 5T allele leads to a reduction in the number of transcripts containing exon 9. The 5T variant has a population frequency of approximately 5%, but is more often found in patients with CBAVD (40–50%) or disseminated bronchiectasis (30%). Curiously, it has been shown that the number of thymidine residues influences the effect of another mutation, R117H. When R117H is in *cis* with 5T (i.e. in the same allele) it causes the PS form of CF when another CF mutation is present on the other allele. However, in compound heterozygotes (eg. ΔF508/R117H) where R117H is in *cis* with 7T it can result in a milder but variable phenotype, ranging from CBAVD to PS CF. The milder phenotype is likely to result from the expression of higher levels of full-length R117H protein with some residual activity. The increasing number of *CFTR* mutations and variability of the associated phenotypes has led some authors to propose a spectrum of 'CFTR disease', recognizing that a label of CF may be inappropriate for patients with milder symptoms.

## CLINICAL APPLICATIONS AND FUTURE PROSPECTS

Prior to the mapping of the CF locus and the subsequent isolation of *CFTR*, it was not possible to offer either carrier detection or reliable prenatal diagnosis. Now parents of an affected child can almost always be offered prenatal diagnosis, either by direct mutational analysis of DNA from chorionic villi, or by linkage analysis using polymorphic intragenic markers if one or both of the mutations in the affected child cannot be identified. Similarly, knowledge of one or both of the mutations in an affected child now permits the offer of carrier detection to close family relatives. In many parts of the world it is now standard practice to offer what is known as *cascade screening* to all families in which a mutation has been identified. Population screening for carriers of CF (p. 324) and neonatal screening for CF homozygotes (p. 323) have been widely implemented and are discussed elsewhere.

CF is a prime candidate for gene therapy because of the relative accessibility of the crucial target organs, i.e. the lungs. Gene transfer studies carried out using adenoviruses and *CFTR* cDNA liposome complexes have resulted in the restoration of chloride secretion in CF transgenic mice. Several clinical trials have been undertaken in small groups of volunteer CF patients. Although there has been experimental evidence of *CFTR* expression in the treated patients, this has generally been transient. Problems have been encountered with poor vector efficiency and inflammatory reactions, particularly when adenoviruses have been used as the vector. Despite these initial problems there is cautious optimism that effective gene therapy for CF will be developed within the next decade.

# INHERITED CARDIAC ARRHYTHMIAS AND CARDIOMYOPATHIES

In about 4% of sudden cardiac death in the 16–64 age group no explanation is evident, which is enormously traumatic for the family left behind. In England this equates to about 200 such deaths annually. Understandably, there can be great anxiety when this is familial and affects young adults. Over the last few years the term *sudden adult death syndrome* (SADS) has been applied, but as several inherited cardiac arrhythmias have been delineated the term *sudden arrythmic death syndrome* is preferred, thus retaining the same acronym. This group of conditions includes the long QT syndromes (LQTS), Brugada syndrome, and arrhythmogenic right ventricular cardiomyopathy (ARVC). LQTS and Brugada syndrome are *ion channelopathies*. In ARVC there is overlap with the inherited cardiomyopathies, in most of which there is pathological evidence of either a hypertrophic or a dilated myocardium.

## INHERITED ARRHYTHMIAS

### Clinical features

When sudden unexplained death occurs a careful review of the postmortem findings, exploration of the deceased's history, as well as the family history, are all indicated. Most of those who die are young males and death occurs during sleep or while inactive. In a proportion of cases death occurs while swimming, especially in LQT1. Emotional stress can be a trigger, especially in LQT2, and cardiac events are more likely in sleep for LQT2 and LQT3. Careful investigation and questioning may reveal an antecedent history of episodes of syncope, palpitation, chest discomfort and dyspnea, and these symptoms should be explored in the relatives in relation to possible triggers. If the deceased had a 12-lead electrocardiogram (ECG) this may hold some key evidence, but a normal ECG is present in about 30% of proven LQTS and possibly a higher proportion of Brugada syndrome cases.

In LQTS, also known as Romano–Ward syndrome, the ECG findings are dominated by, as the name suggests, a

QT interval outside the normal limits, remaining long when the heart rate increases. They are classified according to the gene involved (Table 19.4). The inheritance is overwhelmingly autosomal dominant but a rare recessive form exists, combined with sensorineural deafness, which is known as *Jervell and Lange-Nielsen syndrome*. The ECG changes may be evident from a young age and a cardiac event occurs by age 10 years in about 50%, and by age 20 in 90%. First cardiac events tend to be later in LQT2 and LQT3. Predictive genetic testing, where possible, is helpful to identify those at risk in affected families, and decisions about prophylactic β-blockade can be made. β-Blockers are particularly useful in LQT1 but less so in LQT2 and LQT3; indeed, it is possible that β-blockers may be harmful in LQT3.

Brugada syndrome also follows autosomal dominant inheritance and was first described in 1992. The cardiac event is characterized by a proneness to idiopathic ventricular techycardia (VT), and there may be abnormal ST wave elevation in the right chest leads with incomplete right bundle branch block. In at-risk family members with a normal ECG the characteristic abnormalities can usually be unmasked by the administration of potent sodium channel blockers such as flecainide. The condition is relatively common in Southeast Asia, there is a male predominance of 8:1, and the average age of arrhythmic events is 40 years. The definitive treatment is an implantable defibrillator and exercise is not a particular risk factor. So far, the only gene implicated is *SCN5A*, which is also implicated in some cases of LQT3 (Table 19.4). Indeed, there are families where both electrocardiographic abnormalities occur.

ARVC, mainly following dominant inheritance, is characterized by localized or diffuse atrophy and fatty infiltration of the right ventricular myocardium. It can lead to VT and sudden cardiac death in young people, especially athletes with apparently normal hearts. The ECG shows right precordial T-wave inversion and prolongation of the QRS complex. ARVC appears to demonstrate substantial genetic heterogeneity (Table 19.4) with three genes identified, one of which, encoding *plakoglobin*, is implicated in the rare recessive form found on the island of Naxos. The *RYR2* gene, for ARVC2, is also mutated in catecholaminergic polymorphic ventricular tachycardia (CPVT), also known as Coumel's VT.

### Genetics

These are genetically heterogeneous conditions. Nearly all follow autosomal dominant inheritance and the genes and their loci are summarized in Table 19.4.

## INHERITED CARDIOMYOPATHIES

Dilated cardiomyopathy is characterized by cardiac dilation and reduced systolic function. Causes include myocarditis, coronary artery disease, systemic and metabolic diseases, and toxins. When these are excluded the prevalence of idiopathic dilated cardiomyopathy is 35–40 per 100 000 and familial cases account for about 25%. Like the inherited cardiac arrhythmias they are genetically heterogeneous but nearly always follow autosomal dominant inheritance. They are also very variable, and even within the same family affected members may show

**Table 19.4 The inherited cardiac arrhythmias**

| Arrhythmia | Onset | Triggers | Gene | Locus |
|---|---|---|---|---|
| LQT1 (Romano-Ward) | 90% by age 20 | Exercise (swimming) | *KCNQ1* | 11p15 |
| LQT2 | Early adult life | Stress/sleep | *KCNH2 (HERG)* | 7q35 |
| LQT3 | Early adult life | Stress/sleep | *SCN5A* | 3p21 |
| LQT4 | Adulthood | | *Ankyrin-B* | 4q25 |
| LQT5 | Childhood | | *KCNE1* | 21q22 |
| LQT6 | Adulthood | | *KCNE2* | 21q22 |
| LQT7 (Andersen syndrome) | Adulthood | | *KCNJ2* | 17q23 |
| Brugada syndrome | Adulthood | | *SCN5A* | 3p21 |
| ARVC1 | Childhood/adolescence | | | 14q23 |
| ARVC2 | Childhood/adolescence | | *RYR2* | 1q42 |
| ARVC3, 4, 5, 6, 7 | Childhood/adolescence | | | 14q12, 2q32, 10p14, 10q22 |
| ARVC8 | Childhood/adolescence | | *Desmoplakin* | 6p24 |
| Naxos disease (autosomal recessive) | Childhood | | *Plakoglobin* | 17q21 |

symptoms in childhood at one end of the spectrum, whilst in other individuals the onset of cardiac symptoms may not occur until late in adult life. At least 10 different loci have been mapped in different family studies. One cause is the result of mutations in the *LMNA* gene (which encodes Lamin A/C), noted for its pleiotropic effects (p. 107), of which dilated cardiomyopathy is one and may occasionally be isolated.

Hypertrophic cardiomyopathy is similarly genetically heterogeneous but the large majority follow autosomal dominant inheritance. The group includes asymmetric septal hypertrophy, hypertrophic subaortic stenosis and ventricular hypertrophy. The most common single gene involved appears to be that which encodes the cardiac β-myosin heavy chain (*MYH7*) on chromosome 14q but, again, there are at least another eight loci mapped for genes encoding different cardiac muscle proteins. Sudden death can occur, especially in young athletes. Notable is cardiomyopathy due to mutations in the gene encoding the 'T' isoform of cardiac troponin (*TNNT2*), located on chromosome 1q32. This isoform is not expressed in skeletal muscle but, when mutated, a mild and sometimes subclinical hypertrophy results. Unfortunately, there is a high incidence of sudden death.

Because of the vast genetic heterogeneity genetic testing is not readily available as a routine service, but once a diagnosis has been made in an index case a detailed family history is indicated and investigation by ECG and echocardiogram should be offered. Screening may need to continue well into adult life.

## SPINAL MUSCULAR ATROPHY

Spinal muscular atrophy (SMA) is the term used to describe a clinically and genetically heterogeneous group of disorders that are among the most common genetic causes of death in childhood. The disease is characterized by degeneration of the anterior horn cells of the spinal cord leading to progressive muscle weakness and ultimately death.

Three common childhood forms of SMA are recognized with a collective incidence of approximately 1 in 10 000 and carrier frequency of 1 in 50. Of these type I SMA is the most common and the most severe.

### CLINICAL FEATURES

#### Type I spinal muscular atrophy (Werdnig–Hoffmann disease)

Children with type I SMA present at birth or in the first 6 months of life with severe hypotonia and lack of spontaneous movement. Sometimes the mother will have noticed that intrauterine fetal movements were reduced in both strength and frequency. These children show normal intellectual activity but their profound muscle weakness, which affects swallowing and respiratory function, leads to death within the first 2 years of life. The diagnosis is confirmed by electromyography and there is no effective means of treating the disorder or even delaying its rate of progression.

#### Type II spinal muscular atrophy

This is less severe than type I, with an age of onset between 6 and 18 months. As in type I SMA, muscle weakness and hypotonia are the main presenting features. These children are able to sit unaided but are never able to achieve independent locomotion. The rate of progression is slow and most affected children survive into early adult life.

#### Type III spinal muscular atrophy (Kugelberg–Welander disease)

In this relatively mild form of childhood or juvenile-onset SMA the age of onset is after 18 months and all patients are able to walk without support. Slowly progressive muscle weakness results in many affected individuals having to use a wheelchair by early adult life. Long-term survival can be jeopardized by recurrent respiratory infection and the development of a scoliosis caused by weakness of the spinal muscles.

### GENETICS

All three types of childhood-onset SMA show autosomal recessive inheritance. Several other much rarer forms of SMA have been described, and among these all forms of Mendelian inheritance have been noted. Type I SMA generally shows a high degree of intrafamilial concordance, with affected siblings showing an almost identical clinical course. In types II and III SMA, intrafamilial variation can be quite marked.

#### Mapping the spinal muscular atrophy locus

Using linkage analysis all three childhood forms of SMA were mapped to the long arm of chromosome 5 in 1990. Subsequently linkage analysis and physical mapping narrowed the disease locus down to a region of approximately 1000 kb, which has been shown to consist of a 500 kb inverted duplication (Fig. 19.9). This region of chromosome 5q is notable for its high rate of instability, with several DNA duplications and a relatively large number of pseudogenes (p. 17).

#### Isolating the spinal muscular atrophy gene(s)

The search for the childhood SMA gene(s) within this 500 kb inverted duplication region has yielded confusing

practice deletions are usually detected by a multiplex-PCR technique in which multiple exons within the 5′ and 3′ deletion 'hot spots' are amplified simultaneously. Mutations identified in the remaining one-third of affected boys include stop codons, frameshift mutations, altered splicing signals and promoter mutations. Most point mutations in DMD lead to premature translational termination, resulting in the production of little if any protein product. In contrast to deletions, point mutations in the DMD gene usually arise in paternal meiosis, most probably due to a copy error in DNA replication.

### The gene product dystrophin

The DMD gene encodes a 427 kDa protein known as *dystrophin*. This is located close to the muscle membrane, where it links intracellular actin with extracellular laminin. Absence of dystrophin, as occurs in males with DMD, results in gradual muscle cell degeneration. The presence of dystrophin in a muscle biopsy sample can be assessed by immunofluorescence. Levels of less than 3% are diagnostic of DMD. In muscle biopsies from males with BMD the dystrophin shows qualitative rather than gross quantitative abnormalities.

Dystrophin binds to a glycoprotein complex in the muscle membrane through its C-terminal domain (Fig. 19.11). This glycoprotein complex consists of several subunits, abnormalities of which cause other rare genetic muscle disorders, including several different types of autosomal recessive and congenital MD.

### Carrier detection

Until molecular methods were available carrier detection was based on pedigree analysis combined with creatine kinase assay in serum (p. 316). Creatine kinase is grossly elevated in the serum of boys with DMD and is marginally increased in approximately two-thirds of all carriers (Fig. 20.1, p. 316). Creatine kinase assay is still used occasionally as an adjunct in carrier detection and family studies, but its lack of sensitivity has led to it being superseded by DNA analysis.

Accurate carrier detection can now be achieved for most female relatives of affected DMD/BMD males by direct mutation/deletion analysis or indirectly by linkage studies using polymorphic intragenic markers. If a microsatellite maps to the site of a deletion, then study of the segregation of the microsatellite marker in a family will often provide conclusive evidence of carrier status in relevant female relatives (Fig. 20.2, p. 317). Care has to be taken when using linkage for carrier detection because there is a high recombination rate of 12% across the DMD gene.

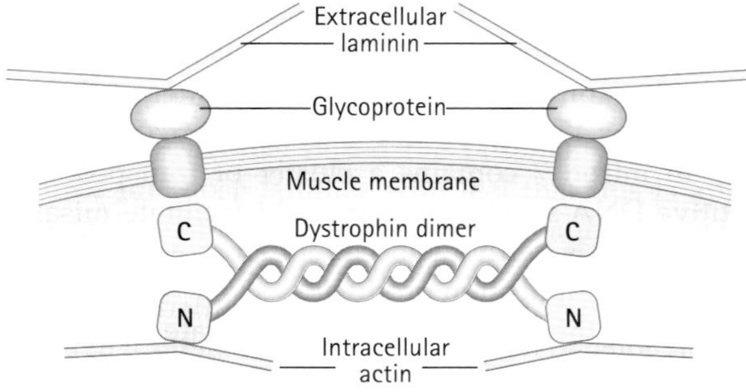


**Fig. 19.11**
Probable structure of the dystrophin protein molecule, which is depicted as a dimer linking intracellular actin with extracellular laminin. (Adapted from Ervasti J M, Campbell K P 1991 Membrane organization of the dystrophin–glycoprotein complex. Cell 66:1121–1131.)

## PROSPECTS FOR TREATMENT

At present, there is no cure for DMD or BMD, although physiotherapy is beneficial for maintaining mobility and preventing muscle spasm and joint contractures.

Gene therapy offers the only realistic hope of a cure in the short to medium term. Several approaches have been tried experimentally in transgenic and naturally occurring mutant mice with dystrophin-negative MD. These include direct injection of recombinant DNA, myoblast implantation, and transfection with retroviral or adenoviral vectors carrying a dystrophin minigene containing only those sequences which code for the important functional domains. The fact that mice with dystrophin-negative MD can show spontaneous muscle repair indicates that there could be a way of switching on an alternative compensatory protein such as *utrophin*. This is expressed in the fetus instead of dystrophin, with which it shares a large degree of homology. Genetically engineered mice that are deficient for both dystrophin and utrophin develop a typical Duchenne-like form of MD. If the utrophin gene could be reactivated as in the dystrophin-negative mouse, this could have a striking beneficial therapeutic effect in affected boys.

## HEMOPHILIA

There are two forms of hemophilia-A and B. Hemophilia A is the most common severe inherited coagulation disorder, with an incidence of 1 in 5000 males. It is caused by a deficiency of factor VIII, which, together with factor IX, plays a critical role in the intrinsic pathway activation of prothrombin to thrombin. Thrombin then converts fibrinogen to fibrin, which forms the structural framework of clotted blood. The existence of hemophilia was recognized in the Talmud and the tendency for males to

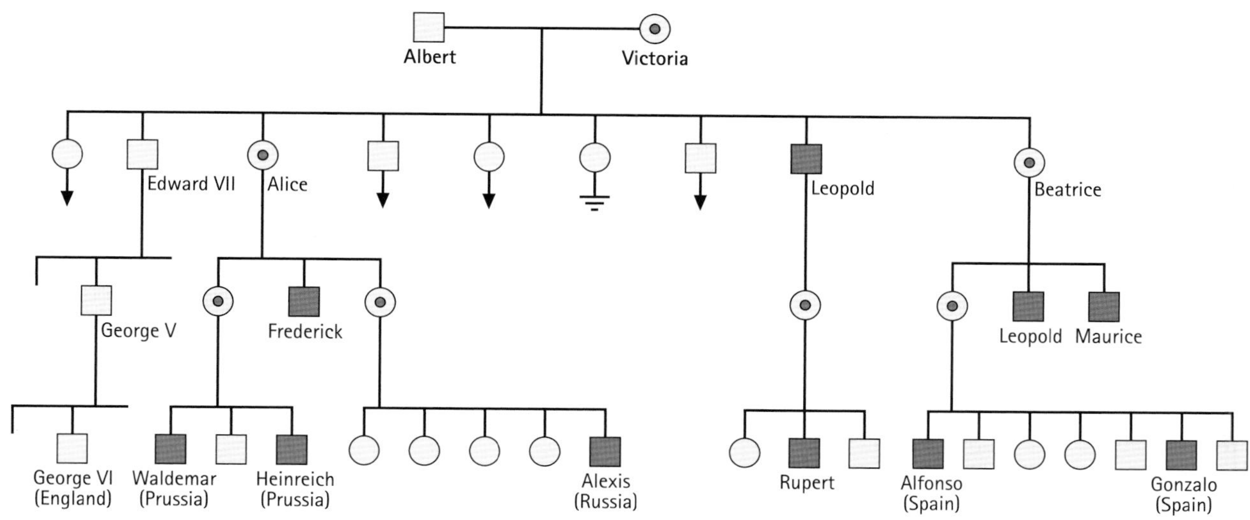


**Fig. 19.12**
Pedigree showing the segregation of hemophilia among Queen Victoria's descendants.

be affected much more often than females was acknowledged by the Jewish authorities 2000 years ago when they excused from circumcision the sons of the sisters of a mother who had an affected son. Queen Victoria was a carrier and as well as having an affected son, Leopold Duke of Albany, she transmitted the disorder through two of her daughters to most of the royal families of Europe (Fig. 19.12).

Hemophilia B affects approximately 1 in 40 000 males and is caused by deficiency of factor IX. It is also known as Christmas disease, whereas hemophilia A is sometimes referred to as 'classic hemophilia'.

## CLINICAL FEATURES

These are similar in both forms of hemophilia and vary from mild bleeding following major trauma or surgery to spontaneous hemorrhage into muscles and joints. The degree of severity shows a close correlation with the reduction in factor VIII or IX activity. Levels below 1% are usually associated with a severe hemorrhagic tendency dating from birth. Hemorrhage into joints causes severe pain and swelling which, if recurrent, causes a progressive arthropathy with severe disability (Fig. 19.13). Affected family members generally show the same degree of severity.

## GENETICS

Both forms of hemophilia show sex-linked recessive inheritance. The loci lie close together near the distal end of the long arm of the X chromosome.

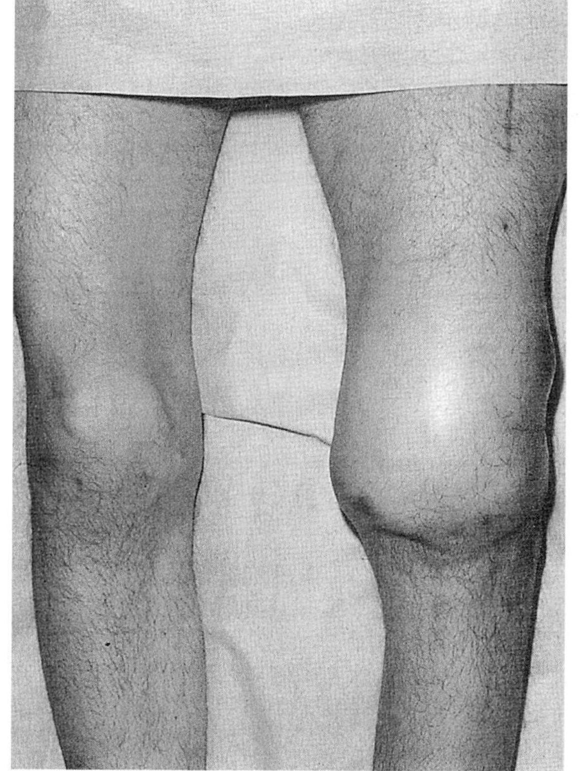

**Fig. 19.13**
The lower limbs of a male with hemophilia showing the effect of recurrent hemorrhage into the knees. (Courtesy of Dr G Dolan, University Hospital, Nottingham.)

## Hemophilia A

The factor VIII gene is relatively large, spanning 186 kb with 26 exons and a 9 kb mRNA transcript. Deletions account for 5% of all cases and usually cause complete absence of factor VIII expression. Frameshift, nonsense and missense mutations have also been described, as have insertions and a 'flip' inversion, which represented a new form of mutation when first identified in hemophilia A in 1993. These inversions account for 50% of all severe cases, i.e. those cases with less than 1% factor VIII activity. They are caused by recombination between a small gene called A located within intron 22 of the factor VIII gene and other copies of the A gene, which are located upstream near the telomere (Fig. 19.14). This inversion results in disruption of the factor VIII gene and very low factor VIII activity. It can be detected relatively simply by PCR, in contrast to the numerous other heterogeneous mutations that require more complex methods of mutation scanning.

Recent studies have shown that, as in DMD, point mutations usually originate in male germ cells whereas deletions arise mainly in the female, probably as a consequence of unequal crossing over. The 'flip' inversions show a greater than tenfold higher mutation rate in male than in female germ cells. This is probably because the long arm of the X chromosome does not pair with a homologous chromosome in male meiosis, so that there is much greater opportunity for intra-chromosomal recombination to occur via looping of the distal end of the long arm (Fig. 19.14).

Because the mean factor VIII concentration is about half normal, a substantial proportion of female carriers are predisposed to a bleeding tendency. Carrier detection used to be based on assay of the ratio of factor VIII coagulant activity to the level of factor VIII antigen, but, as with creatine kinase estimation in DMD, this does not always provide clear discrimination between carriers and non-carriers. This approach has been superseded by linkage analysis, using polymorphic intragenic markers, and specific mutation analysis. Prenatal diagnosis is sometimes requested in families with severe hemophilia A. This can usually be achieved by mutation or linkage analysis.

## Hemophilia B

The gene for factor IX is 34 kb long and contains eight exons. Over 800 different point mutations, deletions and insertions have been reported, for which a complete international database is maintained in a central registry. By analyzing only 2.2 kb of the gene it is possible to detect the mutation in 96% of all patients. The remaining mutations can be identified by sequencing the rest of the gene.

A rare variant form known as hemophilia B Leyden shows the extremely unusual characteristic of age-dependent expression. During childhood the disease is

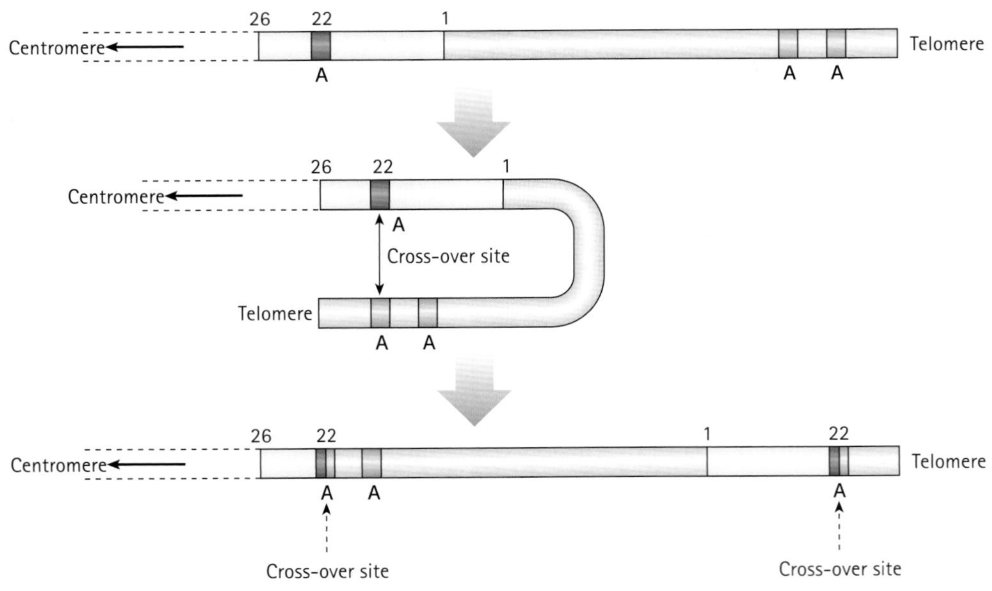


Fig. 19.14
How intrachromosomal recombination causes the 'flip' inversion, which is the most common mutation found in severe hemophilia A. (Adapted from Lakich D, Kazazian H H, Antonarakis S E, Gitschier J 1993 Inversions disrupting the factor VIII gene are a common cause of severe hemophilia A. Nature Genet 5: 236–241.)

very severe, with factor IX levels of less than 1%. After puberty these levels rise to around 50% of normal and the condition resolves to become asymptomatic. Hemophilia B Leyden has been shown to be caused by mutations in the promoter region.

Factor IX levels are now rarely used in carrier detection and prenatal diagnosis, both of which are achieved much more reliably by linkage analysis or direct mutation analysis.

## TREATMENT

Both forms of hemophilia have been treated successfully for many years using plasma-derived factor VIII or factor IX. Factor VIII is concentrated in the cryoprecipitate fraction of plasma and has been used widely for replacement therapy. It has a half-life of 8 hours, so that repeated infusions are necessary for elective surgery or major trauma.

Two major disadvantages emerged using this approach. The first was that the purification process for preparation of cryoprecipitate did not prevent transmission of viral infection such as hepatitis B and HIV, with the inevitable disastrous consequence that many males with hemophilia contracted AIDS. This problem of viral contamination was overcome by better purification and screening processes. In addition, recombinant factor VIII became available in 1994, although expense has been a limiting factor in its widespread introduction.

The second disadvantage was that around 10% of patients with both forms of hemophilia developed inhibitory antibodies to the relevant factor that their immune systems recognized as a foreign agent. This problem can sometimes be overcome using porcine factor VIII or by immunosuppression.

Hemophilia A and B are excellent candidates for gene therapy as only a slight increase in the plasma level of the relevant factor is of major clinical benefit. Studies in dogs and mice with hemophilia B have shown encouraging results using an adeno-associated viral vector expressing factor IX, which is injected into skeletal muscle. The early results of similar studies in severely affected humans were encouraging, with evidence that severe disease might be converted to a milder form. However, the small increases seen in factor levels was not sustained long term; nevertheless, hemophilia remains a prime target for gene therapy.

## FURTHER READING


Biros I, Forrest S 1999 Spinal muscular atrophy: untangling the knot? J Med Genet 36: 1–8
*A contemporary account of current understanding of the genetic basis of childhood spinal muscular atrophy.*

Bolton-Maggs P H B, Pasi K J 2003 Haemophilias A and B. The Lancet 361: 1801–1809
*An excellent recent review.*

Brown T, Schwind E L 1999 Update and review: cystic fibrosis. J Genet Counseling 8: 137–162
*A useful review of recent genetic developments in cystic fibrosis.*

Collinge J 1997 Human prion diseases and bovine spongiform encephalopathy (BSE). Hum Mol Genet 6: 1699–1705
*A clear account of human prion diseases and their known causes with particular reference to BSE.*

De Paepe A, Devereux R B, Hennekam R C M, et al 1996 Revised diagnostic criteria for the Marfan syndrome. Am J Med Genet 62: 417–426
*Essential reading for those required to make a diagnosis of Marfan syndrome.*

Emery A E H 1993 Duchenne muscular dystrophy, 2nd edn. Oxford University Press, Oxford.
*A detailed monograph reviewing the history, clinical features and genetics of Duchenne and Becker muscular dystrophy.*

Harper P S 1996 Huntington's disease, 2nd edn. W B Saunders, London
*A comprehensive review of the clinical and genetic aspects of Huntington disease.*

Harper P S 2001 Myotonic dystrophy, 3rd edn. W B Saunders, London
*A comprehensive review of the clinical and genetic aspects of myotonic dystrophy.*

Huson S M, Hughes R A C (eds) 1994 The neurofibromatoses. Chapman & Hall, London
*A very thorough description of the different types of neurofibromatosis. Includes a chapter on the 'Elephant Man'.*

Karpati G, Pari G, Molnar M J 1999 Molecular therapy for genetic muscle diseases – status 1999. Clin Genet 55: 1–8
*An optimistic review of possible approaches to gene therapy for inherited muscle disorders such as Duchenne muscular dystrophy.*

Kay M A, Manno C S, Ragni, M V et al 2000 Evidence for gene transfer and expression of factor IX in haemophilia B patients treated with an AV vector. Nature Genet 24: 257–261
*Report of provisional encouraging results of gene therapy in patients with hemophilia B.*

Lakich D, Kazazian H H, Antonarakis S E, Gitschier J 1993 Inversions disrupting the factor VIII gene are a common cause of severe haemophilia A. Nature Genet 5: 236–241
*The first report showing how the common 'flip' inversion is generated.*

## ELEMENTS

1. Huntington disease is an autosomal dominant disorder characterized by choreiform movements and progressive dementia. The disease locus has been mapped to the short arm of chromosome 4 and the mutational basis involves expansion of a CAG triple repeat sequence. Meiotic instability is greater in the male than in the female, which probably explains why the severe 'juvenile'-onset form is almost always inherited from a more mildly affected father.

2. Myotonic dystrophy shows autosomal dominant inheritance and is characterized by slowly progressive weakness and myotonia. The disease locus has been mapped to chromosome 19 and the mutational basis involves expansion of an unstable CTG triple repeat sequence. The range of meiotic expansion is greater in the female than in the male, which almost certainly accounts for the almost exclusive maternal inheritance of the severe 'congenital' form.

3. Hereditary motor and sensory neuropathy (HMSN) includes several clinically and genetically heterogeneous disorders characterized by slowly progressive distal muscle weakness and wasting. HMSN Ia has been mapped to chromosome 17 and is usually caused by duplication of a gene (*PMP-22*) which encodes a protein present in the myelin membrane of peripheral nerve. The reciprocal deletion product of the unequal cross-over event that generates a duplication causes a mild disorder known as hereditary liability to pressure palsies.

4. Neurofibromatosis type I (NF1) shows autosomal dominant inheritance with complete penetrance and variable expression. The NF1 gene has been mapped to chromosome 17, where it encodes a protein known as *neurofibromin*. This normally acts as a tumor suppressor by inactivating the RAS-mediated signal transduction of mitogenic signaling.

5. Cystic fibrosis (CF) shows autosomal recessive inheritance and is characterized by recurrent chest infection and malabsorption. The CF locus has been mapped to chromosome 7, where the gene (*CFTR*) encodes the CF transmembrane receptor protein. This acts as a chloride channel and controls the level of intracellular sodium chloride, which in turn influences the viscosity of mucous secretions.

6. The childhood forms of spinal muscular atrophy (SMA) are characterized by hypotonia and progressive muscle weakness. They show autosomal recessive inheritance and the disease locus has been mapped to chromosome 5q13. This region shows a high incidence of instability, with duplication of a 500 kb fragment containing two genes (*SMN, NAIP*) that are deleted in a high proportion of patients.

7. Duchenne muscular dystrophy (DMD) shows X-linked recessive inheritance, with most carriers being entirely healthy. The DMD locus has been mapped to chromosome Xp21 and is the largest known in humans. The gene product, dystrophin, links intracellular actin with extracellular laminin. The commonest mutational mechanism is a deletion that disturbs the translational reading frame. Deletions that maintain the reading frame cause the milder Becker form of MD.

8. Hemophilia A is the most common severe inherited coagulation disorder in humans. It shows X-linked recessive inheritance and is caused by a deficiency of factor VIII. The most common mutation in severe hemophilia A is caused by a 'flip' inversion that disrupts the factor VIII gene at intron 22. Treatment with factor VIII replacement therapy is very effective and the results of gene therapy in animal models offer hope that this will soon be possible in humans.

CHAPTER 20

# Screening for genetic disease

Genetic disease affects individuals and their families dramatically but every person, and every couple having children, is at some risk of seeing a disorder with a genetic component suddenly appearing. Our concepts and approaches to screening reflect the different burdens that these two realities impose. Firstly, there is screening of individuals and couples known to be at significant or high risk because of a positive family history – sometimes referred to as *targeted*, or *family*, screening because it focuses on those most likely to benefit. This includes *carrier*, or *heterozygote*, screening, as well as *presymptomatic* testing. Secondly, there is the screening offered to the general population, who are at low risk – this is sometimes referred to as *community genetics*. Population screening involves the offer of genetic testing on an equitable basis to all relevant individuals in a defined population. Its primary objective is to enhance autonomy by enabling individuals to be better informed about genetic risks and reproductive options. A secondary goal is the prevention of morbidity due to genetic disease and alleviation of the suffering that this would impose.

## SCREENING THOSE AT HIGH RISK

Here we focus on the very wide range of general genetic disease as opposed to screening in the field of cancer genetics, which is addressed in Chapter 14 (p. 220). Prenatal screening is also covered in more detail in the next chapter. If it was easy to recognize carriers of autosomal and X-linked recessive disorders and persons who are heterozygous for autosomal dominant disorders which show reduced penetrance or a late age of onset, much doubt and uncertainty would be removed when providing information in genetic counseling. Increasingly, mutation analysis in genes that cause these disorders is indeed making the task easier. Where this is not possible, either because no gene test is available or the molecular pathology cannot be detected in a gene known to be associated with the disorder in question, a number of strategies and types of analysis are available to detect carriers for autosomal and X-linked recessive disorders, and for presymptomatic diagnosis of heterozygotes for autosomal dominant disorders.

## CARRIER TESTING FOR AUTOSOMAL RECESSIVE AND X-LINKED DISORDERS

In a number of autosomal recessive disorders, such as some of the inborn errors of metabolism, e.g. Tay–Sachs disease (p. 173), and the hemoglobinopathies, e.g. sickle-cell disease (p. 154), carriers can be recognized with a high degree of certainty using biochemical or hematological techniques such that DNA analysis is not necessary. In other single-gene disorders, it is possible to detect or confirm carrier status by biochemical means in only a proportion of carriers, e.g. the presence of abnormal coagulation studies in a woman at risk of being a carrier for hemophilia (p. 312). A significant proportion of obligate carriers of hemophilia will have normal coagulation, however, so that a normal result in a woman at risk does not exclude her from being a carrier.

There are several possible ways in which carriers of genetic diseases can be recognized.

### CLINICAL MANIFESTATIONS IN CARRIERS

Occasionally, carriers for certain disorders can have mild clinical manifestations of the disease (Table 20.1), particularly with some of the X-linked disorders. These manifestations are usually so slight that they will only be apparent on careful clinical examination. Such manifestations, even though minimal, are unmistakably pathological, e.g. the mosaic pattern of retinal pigmentation seen in manifesting female carriers of X-linked ocular albinism. Unfortunately, in most autosomal and X-linked recessive disorders there are either no manifestations at all in carriers, or they overlap with variation seen in the general population. An example would be female carriers of hemophilia, who have a tendency to bruise easily. This would not, however, be a reliable sign of carrier time a younger sister of a male with DMD seeks advice about her carrier status, the affected male will no longer be alive. If the family structure is suitable, e.g. there are one or more unaffected males in the pedigree, it is often possible to 'reconstruct' the likely alleles of the linked polymorphic DNA markers in the affected male. This will, however, affect the risk estimation in the pedigree as the phase of the marker in the affected male cannot be known with certainty (p. 347).

### *Polymorphic variation*

Another problem that can be encountered in the use of linked DNA markers is whether the family possesses the necessary variation in a linked marker to be what is known as *informative*. This is now very rare with the large number of different types of DNA sequence variants in the human genome available, especially the variable number tandem repeat sequences such as CA dinucleotide repeats (p. 18). It will also become less of a problem as specific mutational analysis becomes available for an increasingly greater number of single-gene disorders.

### *Locus heterogeneity*

Polymorphic DNA markers can be extremely reliable if the disease in question is caused by mutations in only one gene in the entire genome. In infantile polycystic kidney disease, for example, an autosomal recessive disorder, there is no evidence for a locus other than that on chromosome 6p21. In the overwhelming majority of cases it is a lethal condition in early postnatal life and the pathology is characteristic. For couples who have had one affected child in whom the diagnosis is confidently made, and from whom DNA is available, linked DNA markers can be used for prenatal diagnosis in subsequent pregnancies, providing the markers are informative. In many other conditions, however, mutations in more than one gene can give rise to the same basic phenotype. This is true for sensorineural hearing impairment and retinitis pigmentosa, limb girdle muscular dystrophy, Bardet–Biedl syndrome, and many others that demonstrate enormous *locus heterogeneity*. It is usually not practical to use DNA polymorphic markers in conditions such as these because of the high chance of false-positive results.

## PRESYMPTOMATIC DIAGNOSIS OF AUTOSOMAL DOMINANT DISORDERS

Many autosomal dominant single-gene disorders either have a delayed age of onset (p. 343) or exhibit reduced penetrance (p. 108). The results of clinical examination, specialist investigations, biochemical studies and family DNA studies can allow one to predict whether a person has inherited the gene before the onset of symptoms or signs. This is known as *presymptomatic diagnosis* or *predictive testing*.

## CLINICAL EXAMINATION

In a number of dominantly inherited disorders simple clinical means can be used for presymptomatic diagnosis, taking into account possible pleiotropic effects of a gene (p. 107). For example, persons with the dominantly inherited disorder neurofibromatosis type I (NF1) can have a number of different clinical features (p. 298). It is not unusual to examine an apparently unaffected relative of someone with NF1 who has had no medical problems, only to discover that they have sufficient numbers of a diagnostic feature, such as café-au-lait spots or cutaneous *neurofibromas*, to confirm that they are affected. However, NF1 is a relatively rare example of a dominantly inherited disorder that is virtually 100% penetrant by the age of 5 or 6 years, with visible external features. With many other disorders clinical examination presents greater challenges.

In tuberous sclerosis (TSC) a number of body systems may be involved and the external manifestations, such as the facial rash of angiokeratoma (Ch. 7, Fig. 7.5) may not be present. Similarly, seizures and learning difficulties are not inevitable. In autosomal dominant polycystic kidney disease, which is extremely variable and may have a delayed age of onset, there may be no suspicion of the condition from routine examination and hypertension may be borderline without raising suspicions of a serious underlying disease. Reaching a diagnosis in Marfan syndrome (p. 301) can be notoriously difficult because of the variable features and the overlap with other joint hypermobility disorders, even though very detailed diagnostic criteria have been established.

## SPECIALIST INVESTIGATION

In conditions where clinical assessment leaves diagnostic doubt or ambiguity, special investigations of relevant body systems can serve to clarify status and presymptomatic diagnosis. In TSC imaging studies of the brain by CT scan to look for intracranial calcification (Fig. 20.3) is a more or less routine investigation, as well renal ultrasound to identify the cysts known as angiomyolipoma(ta) (Fig. 20.4). Use of these relatively non-invasive tests in relatives of persons with TSC can detect evidence of the condition in asymptomatic persons.

Similarly, assessment for Marfan syndrome involves ophthalmic examination for evidence of ectopia lentis, echocardiography for measurement of the aortic root

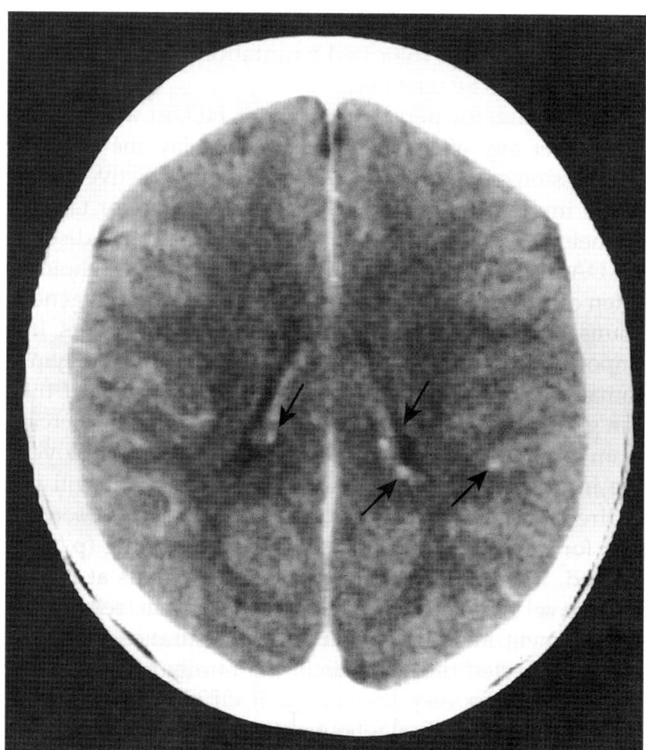

Fig. 20.3
Intracranial calcification (arrowed) in an asymptomatic person with tuberous sclerosis.

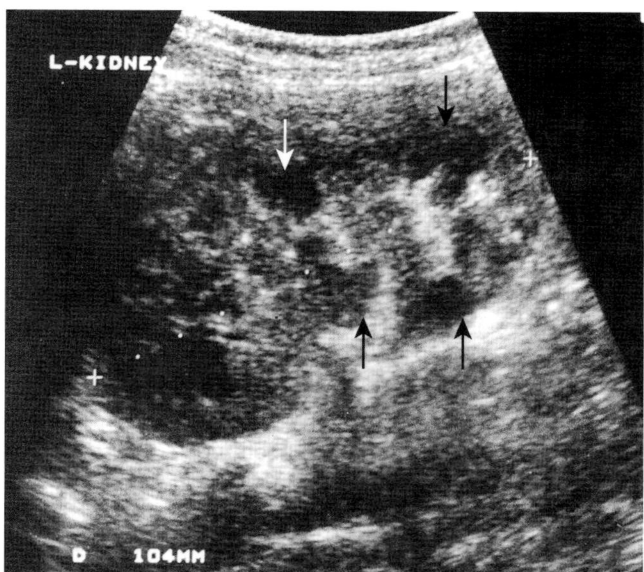


Fig. 20.4
Renal ultrasound of an asymptomatic person with tuberous sclerosis showing abnormal echogenicity due to presumed angiomyolipomata (arrowed).

diameter, and sometimes an MRI scan of the lumbar spine to look for evidence of dural ectasia – all of these features counting as major criteria in the disorder.

It is important to point out, however, that the absence of these findings on clinical or specialist investigation does not always exclude the diagnosis of the disorder being tested for but does reduce the likelihood of the person concerned having inherited the gene. If the relative frequencies of such findings in persons with the disorder and in persons from the general population are known, it is possible to give the person at risk a residual relative likelihood of having inherited the gene. This information can be used in conjunction with other information, such as the pedigree risk, in genetic counseling.

## BIOCHEMICAL TESTS

In a number of autosomal dominant disorders biochemical tests can determine whether or not a person at risk has inherited a gene. Examples include the use of serum cholesterol levels in persons at risk for familial hypercholesterolemia (p. 170) and assay of the appropriate urinary porphyrins or the specific enzyme deficiency in the various dominant porphyrias (p. 175).

## LINKED DNA MARKERS

Linked DNA polymorphic markers can be used in presymptomatic diagnosis of dominantly inherited disorders and all the principles and pitfalls discussed earlier in this chapter apply. A common difficulty in dominantly inherited conditions is that of informativity because often a key individual is deceased or unavailable for some other reason. Despite this, the availability of linked DNA markers has found widespread use in presymptomatic or predictive testing for a number of single-gene disorders inherited in an autosomal dominant manner. Increasingly, however, the cloning of the gene responsible means that direct mutational analysis, for example the Huntington disease (HD) gene, has begun to replace the use of linked polymorphic DNA markers. For relatively common disorders, for example NF1, TSC and Marfan syndrome, mutation analysis is expensive, time-consuming, and not guaranteed to be successful in identifying the causative mutation in the affected individual in the family, even though the diagnosis is certain. This problem is frequently seen in familial breast cancer. In such situations judicious use of linked DNA markers can be very helpful, particularly NF1, which demonstrates virtually 100% penetrance and no locus heterogeneity. Table 20.2 lists some of the more common conditions in which DNA analysis is regularly used to offer presymptomatic diagnosis, but there are of course many more.

entirely voluntary in the case of prenatal programs, but the ethical principles are more complex in neonatal screening for conditions where early treatment is essential and effective in preventing morbidity. In these situations the principles of *beneficience* (doing good) and *non-maleficence* (not doing harm) are relevant (p. 369). Easily understood information and well-informed counseling should both be readily available.

It is often stated that the cost of a screening program should be reasonable and affordable. This does not mean that the potential savings gained through a reduction in the number of affected cases requiring treatment should exceed or even balance the cost of screening, although this is an argument which is popular with health administrators and planners who have to fund the program. It is reasonable to point out that cost–benefit analyses also have to take into account non-tangible factors such as the emotional costs of human suffering borne by both the affected individuals and those who care for them.

**Table 20.7 Conditions for which neonatal screening can be undertaken**

| Disorder | Test/method |
|---|---|
| **Widely applied** | |
| Phenylketonuria | Guthrie* or automated fluorometric assay |
| Congenital hypothyroidism | Thyroxine or thyroid stimulating hormone |
| **Other inborn errors** | |
| Biotidinase deficiency | Specific enzyme assay |
| Galactosemia | Modified Guthrie |
| Homocystinuria | Modified Guthrie |
| Maple syrup urine disease | Modified Guthrie |
| Tyrosinemia | Modified Guthrie |
| **Miscellaneous** | |
| Congenital adrenal hyperplasia | 17-Hydroxyprogesterone assay |
| Cystic fibrosis | Immunoreactive trypsin and DNA analysis |
| Duchenne muscular dystrophy | Creatine kinase |
| Sickle-cell disease | Hemoglobin electrophoresis |

*The Guthrie test is based on reversal of bacterial growth inhibition by a high level of phenylalanine

## NEONATAL SCREENING

Newborn screening programs have been introduced on a widespread basis for phenylketonuria, galactosemia and congenital hypothyroidism. In all of these disorders early treatment can prevent the development of learning disabilities. Screening for several other disorders is carried out more selectively in different centres (Table 20.7). For most of these conditions the rationale is to try to prevent subsequent morbidity. The importance of adhering to the principle of screening for a disorder that needs to be treated early is illustrated by the Swedish experience of neonatal screening for $\alpha_1$-antitrypsin deficiency. In this condition neonatal complications occur in up to 10% but for most cases the morbidity is seen in adult life, and the main message on diagnosing the disorder is avoidance of smoking. During 1972–74 200 000 newborns were screened and follow-up studies showed that considerable anxiety was generated when the information was conveyed to parents, who perceived their children to be at risk of a serious, life-threatening disorder. The case of newborn screening for Duchenne muscular dystrophy (p. 308) also deviates from the screening paradigm because there is no effective treatment. In this situation the indication is to try to identify families for whom genetic counseling could be offered with a view to alerting relevant females to their possible carrier status. Here again, parental reaction has not been uniformly favorable.

### PHENYLKETONURIA

Routine biochemical screening of newborn infants for phenylketonuria was recommended by the Ministry of Health in the UK in 1969 after it had been shown that a low-phenylalanine diet could prevent the severe learning disabilities that previously had been a hallmark of this condition (p. 161). The screening test, which is sometimes known as the *Guthrie test*, is carried out on a small sample of blood obtained by heel-prick at age 7 days. An abnormal test result is further investigated by repeat analysis of phenylalanine levels in a venous blood sample. A low-phenylalanine diet is extremely effective in preventing learning disabilities, and, although it is not particularly palatable, most affected children can be persuaded to adhere to it until early adult life when it can be relaxed. Any woman with phenylketonuria who is contemplating pregnancy should adhere to a strict low-phenylalanine diet both before and during pregnancy to minimize the risk of brain damage to her unborn child (pp. 165, 260). Without strict dietary control this risk is very high.

### GALACTOSEMIA

Classic galactosemia affects approximately 1 in 50 000 newborn infants and usually presents with vomiting, lethargy and severe metabolic collapse within the first 2 or 3 weeks of life. Newborn screening is based on a modification of the Guthrie test with subsequent confirmation by specific enzyme assay. The early introduction of appropriate dietary restriction can prevent the development of serious complications such as cataracts, liver failure and learning disabilities.

## CONGENITAL HYPOTHYROIDISM

Screening for congenital hypothyroidism was first introduced in the USA in 1974 and is now undertaken in most parts of the developed world. The test is based on assay of either *thyroxine* or *thyroid stimulating hormone*. This disorder is particularly suitable for screening as it is relatively common, with an incidence of approximately 1 in 4000, and treatment with life-long thyroxine replacement is extremely effective in preventing the severe developmental problems associated with the classic picture of 'cretinism'. The most common cause of congenital hypothyroidism is absence of the thyroid gland rather than an inborn error of metabolism (p. 164). Congenital absence of the thyroid gland is usually not caused by genetic factors.

## CYSTIC FIBROSIS

Newborn screening for cystic fibrosis has been introduced in several countries with a significant population of northern European origin. It is based on the detection of an elevated blood level of *immunoreactive trypsin* (IRT), which is a consequence of blockage of pancreatic ducts in utero, supplemented by DNA analysis (p. 304). The rationale for screening is that it is hoped that early treatment with physiotherapy and antibiotics will improve the long-term prognosis. Initial results are encouraging but absolute confirmation of long-term benefit has not yet been forthcoming. Despite this, it is now policy in the England to introduce screening for all newborns from 2004.

## SICKLE-CELL DISEASE AND THALASSEMIA

Newborn screening based on *hemoglobin electrophoresis* is undertaken in many countries with a significant Afro-Caribbean community. As with cystic fibrosis, it is hoped that early prophylaxis will reduce morbidity and mortality, thereby improving the long-term outlook. In the case of sickle-cell disease, treatment involves the use of oral penicillin to reduce the risk of pneumococcal infection resulting from immune deficiency secondary to splenic infarction (p. 154). Even in Western countries with good medical facilities, a significant proportion of sickle-cell homozygotes, possibly as many as 15%, die as a result of infection in early childhood. In the case of thalassemia, early diagnosis makes it possible to optimize transfusion regimens and iron-chelation therapy from an early stage. Linked antenatal and neonatal screening programs for both these hemoglobinopathies are due to be implemented in the UK by 2005.

**Table 20.8 Autosomal recessive disorders suitable for population carrier screening**

| Disorder | Ethnic group or community | Test |
|---|---|---|
| α-Thalassemia | China and eastern Asia | Mean corpuscular hemoglobin and hemoglobin electrophoresis |
| β-Thalassemia | Indian subcontinent and Mediterranean countries | Mean corpuscular hemoglobin and hemoglobin electrophoresis |
| Sickle-cell disease | Afro-Caribbeans | Sickle test and hemoglobin electrophoresis |
| Cystic fibrosis | Western European Caucasians | Common mutation analysis |
| Tay–Sachs disease | Ashkenazi Jews | Hexosaminidase A |

## POPULATION CARRIER SCREENING

Widespread screening for carriers of autosomal recessive disorders in high-incidence populations was first introduced for the hemoglobinopathies (p. 152) and has been extended to several other disorders (Table 20.8). The rationale behind these programs is that carrier detection can be supported by genetic counseling so that carrier couples can be forewarned of the 1 in 4 risk that each of their children could be affected.

Experience with the two common hemoglobinopathies, thalassemia and sickle-cell disease, illustrates the extremes of success and failure that can result from well- or poorly planned screening programs.

### THALASSEMIA

α- and β-thalassemia are caused by abnormal globin chain synthesis due to mutations involving the α- and β-globin genes or their promoter regions (p. 155). Both disorders show autosomal recessive inheritance, and both are extremely common in certain parts of the world, notably China (α-thalassemia) and Cyprus, Italy and the Indian subcontinent (β-thalassemia).

In Cyprus in 1974 the birth incidence of β-thalassemia was 1 in 250 (carrier frequency 1 in 8). Following the introduction of a comprehensive screening program to determine the carrier status of young adults, which had the support of the Greek Orthodox Church, the incidence of affected babies declined by over 95% within 10 years. Similar programs in Greece and Italy have seen a drop in the incidence of affected homozygotes of over 50%.

If it is acceptable to judge the outcome of these screening programs on the basis of a reduction in the births of affected babies, then they have been very successful, due largely to the efforts of highly motivated staff interacting with a well-informed target population that has usually opted not to have affected children.

## SICKLE-CELL DISEASE

In contrast to the Cypriot response to β-thalassemia screening, early attempts to introduce sickle-cell carrier detection in the black population of North America were disastrous. Information pamphlets tended to confuse the sickle-cell carrier state, or trait, which is usually harmless, with the homozygous disease, which conveys significant morbidity (p. 154). Several US states passed legislation making sickle-cell screening in black people mandatory, and sickle-cell carriers began to be discriminated against by employers and insurance companies. It is not surprising that public criticism was aroused, leading to abandonment of the screening programs and amendment of the ill-conceived legislation.

This experience with sickle-cell carrier screening emphasizes the importance of ensuring voluntary participation and providing adequate and appropriate information and counseling. More recent pilot studies in the USA and in Cuba have shown that individuals of Afro-Caribbean origin are perfectly receptive to well-planned non-directive sickle-cell screening programs.

## CYSTIC FIBROSIS

The discovery in 1989 that the ΔF508 deletion/mutation accounts for a high proportion of all cystic fibrosis heterozygotes soon led to the suggestion that screening programs could be implemented for carrier detection on a population basis. In the white population of the UK, the cystic fibrosis carrier frequency is approximately 1 in 25 and the ΔF508 mutation accounts for 75–80% of all heterozygotes. A further 10–15% of carriers can be detected relatively easily and cheaply using a multiplex PCR analytical procedure.

Initial studies of attitudes to cystic fibrosis carrier detection yielded quite divergent results. A casual written invitation generates a poor take-up response of around 10%, whereas personal contact during early pregnancy, whether mediated through general practice or the antenatal clinic, results in uptake rates of over 80%. Further studies are under way to explore attitudes to cystic fibrosis screening among specific groups, such as school leavers and women in early pregnancy.

Two approaches for screening pregnant women have been considered. The first is referred to as *two-step* and involves testing pregnant mothers at the antenatal clinic. Those who test positive for a common mutation, i.e. approximately 85% of all cystic fibrosis carriers, are informed of the result and invited to bring their partners for testing – hence 'two-step' testing. If both partners are found to be carriers then an offer of prenatal diagnosis is made. This approach has the advantage that all carriers detected are informed of their result and further family studies-*cascade screening* can be initiated. The disadvantages are that those women whose partners are subsequently found to have a normal result experience considerable unnecessary anxiety that creates a need for counseling and support.

The second approach is referred to as *couple screening*. This involves testing both partners simultaneously and only disclosing positive results if both partners are found to be carriers. In this way much less anxiety is generated but the opportunity for offering tests to the extended family when only one partner is a carrier is lost. At present it is not clear which, if either, of these approaches will be recommended for widespread implementation. The results of pilot studies indicate that these 'two-step' and 'couple screening' approaches are equally acceptable to pregnant mothers, with take-up rates of approximately 70%.

## POSITIVE AND NEGATIVE ASPECTS OF POPULATION SCREENING

Well-planned population screening enhances informed choice and offers the prospect of a significant reduction in the incidence of disabling genetic disorders. These potential advantages have to be weighed against the potential disadvantages that can arise from the overenthusiastic pursuit of a poorly planned or ill-judged screening program (Table 20.9). Experience to date indicates that in relatively small well-informed groups, such as the Greek Cypriots and American Ashkenazi Jews, community screening is welcomed. When screening is offered to larger populations the outcome is less certain.

A 3-year follow-up of almost 750 individuals screened for cystic fibrosis carrier status in the UK revealed that a positive test result had not caused undue anxiety, although some carriers did have a relatively poor perception of their own general health. A more worrying outcome was that almost 50% of the individuals tested could not accurately recall or interpret their results. This emphasizes the importance of pretest counseling and the provision of accurate information that can be easily processed and fully understood.

# GENETIC REGISTERS

Most clinical genetic units maintain what is known as a *genetic register* of families and individuals who are either affected by, or at risk of developing, a serious hereditary

**Table 20.9 Potential advantages and disadvantages of genetic screening**

| |
|---|
| **Advantages** |
| Informed choice |
| Improved understanding |
| Early treatment when available |
| Reduction in births of affected homozygotes |
| **Disadvantages and hazards** |
| Pressure to participate causing mistrust and suspicion |
| Stigmatization of carriers (social, insurance and employment) |
| Inappropriate anxiety in carriers |
| Inappropriate reassurance if test is not 100% sensitive |

**Table 20.10 Roles of a genetic register**

| |
|---|
| To maintain an informal two-way communication process between the family and the genetics unit |
| To offer carrier detection to relevant family members as they reach adult life |
| To coordinate presymptomatic and prenatal diagnosis when requested |
| To coordinate multidisciplinary management of patients with complex hereditary conditions such as the familial cancer syndromes |
| To ensure effective implementation of new technology and treatment |
| To provide a long-term source of information and support |

disorder. The primary purpose of a genetic register is to maintain two-way contact between a genetics unit and relevant family members (Table 20.10). This permits investigations to be offered as appropriate and ensures that families do not feel abandoned or excluded from a source of information and support.

Entry on to a genetic register should be entirely voluntary and it is essential that confidentiality is not breached. Information is never revealed to outside agencies without the consent of the relevant individual.

Genetic registers are most appropriate for conditions that are relatively common, have potentially serious effects, convey high risks to other family members, and in which complications can be treated or prevented (Table 20.11). They are particularly valuable for conditions that show a delayed age of onset or for which unaffected carriers could be at high risk of having seriously affected children.

Well-organized genetic registers can also play a key role in coordinating a multidisciplinary approach to the management of patients with conditions such as the familial cancer-predisposing syndromes (p. 218). The management of such patients often involves the interpretation of molecular investigations and the organization of regular visits to other hospital departments where screening for early signs of malignancy can be undertaken (p. 222). Programs of this nature are much appreciated by family members and can make a major contribution to improving the quality of life for individuals and families

**Table 20.11 Disorders suitable for a genetics register**

| Disorder |
|---|
| ***Autosomal dominant*** |
| Adult-onset polycystic kidney disease |
| Familial adenomatous polyposis |
| Familial hypercholesterolemia |
| Huntington disease |
| Multiple endocrine neoplasia types 1 and 2 |
| Myotonic dystrophy |
| Neurofibromatosis types I and II |
| Retinoblastoma |
| Von Hippel–Lindau syndrome |
| ***Autosomal recessive*** |
| Cystic fibrosis |
| Sickle-cell disease |
| Thalassemia |
| ***X-linked*** |
| Duchenne/Becker muscular dystrophy |
| Fragile X syndrome |
| Hemophilia |
| Retinitis pigmentosa |
| ***Chromosomal*** |
| Deletions/insertions |
| Inversions |
| Translocations |

at risk of developing serious genetic disease. Genetic registers will prove to be particularly valuable when effective methods of gene therapy have been developed for the common single-gene disorders.

## FURTHER READING


Axworthy D, Brock D J H, Bobrow M, Marteau T M 1996 Psychological impact of population-based carrier testing for cystic fibrosis: 3-year follow-up. Lancet 347: 1443–1446

*A review of the impact of carrier testing for cystic fibrosis on over 700 individuals.*

Brock D J H, Rodeck C H, Ferguson Smith M A (eds) 1992 Prenatal diagnosis and screening. Churchill Livingstone, Edinburgh

*A huge multiauthor textbook with excellent chapters on all aspects of genetic screening.*

Cunningham G C, Tompkinson D G 1999 Cost and effectiveness of the California triple marker prenatal screening program. Genet Med 1: 199–206

*A detailed review of the impact of triple test screening over a 10-year period in California.*

Genetic screening ethical issues 1993 Nuffield Council on Bioethics, London

*The report of a working party on genetic screening on the associated ethical and societal issues.*

Harper P S 1998 Practical genetic counselling, 5th edn. Butterworth-Heinemann, Oxford

*As the title suggests, a practical book which serves as a good starting point in almost every aspect of genetic counseling, including carrier testing.*

Marteau T, Richards M (eds.) 1996 The troubled helix. Cambridge University Press, Cambridge

*Perspectives on the social and psychological implications of genetic testing and screening.*

Modell B, Modell M 1992 Towards a healthy baby. Oxford University Press, Oxford

*A clearly written and easily understood guide to genetic counseling and community genetics.*

Pauli R, Motulsky A G 1981 Risk counselling in autosomal dominant disorders with undetermined penetrance. J Med Genet 18: 340–343

*A paper that considers the problem of counseling for autosomal dominant disorders with reduced penetrance.*

Pembrey M E, Davies K E, Winter R M, Elles R G, Williamson R, Fazzone T E, Walker C 1984 Clinical use of DNA markers linked to the gene for Duchenne muscular dystrophy. Arch Dis Child 59: 208–216

*A useful discussion of how DNA markers can be used for carrier detection in Duchenne muscular dystrophy.*

## ELEMENTS

1. Determination of carrier status for autosomal recessive and X-linked disorders can involve detailed clinical examination looking for specific minor features, specialist clinical investigations, biochemical tests or family studies using linked biochemical, blood group or DNA polymorphic markers.

2. Presymptomatic or predictive testing for persons at risk for autosomal dominant disorders with reduced penetrance or a delayed age of onset can also be carried out by detailed clinical examination for specific features, specialist investigations, biochemical testing and the use of linked biochemical or DNA polymorphisms.

3. Consideration should be given to the advantages and disadvantages of presymptomatic or predictive testing both from a practical and an ethical point of view.

4. Population screening involves the offer of genetic testing to all members of a particular population, with the primary objective being the enhancement of informed personal choice.

5. Participation should be voluntary and each program should be widely available, equitably distributed, acceptable to the target population and supported by full information and counseling.

6. Prenatal screening is now offered routinely for neural tube defects, by assay of maternal serum $\alpha$-fetoprotein, and for chromosome abnormalities by assay of three or four biochemical markers, constituting either the 'triple' or the 'quadruple' test.

7. Neonatal screening is widely available for phenylketonuria, galactosemia and congenital hypothyroidism. Other conditions are screened for in specific populations.

8. Population screening programs for carriers of $\beta$-thalassemia have resulted in a major fall in the births of affected homozygotes. Similar programs could be equally effective for sickle-cell disease and cystic fibrosis if care is taken to ensure that they are acceptable to their target populations.

9. Well-organized genetic registers provide an effective means of maintaining two-way contact between genetics centres and families with hereditary disease.

CHAPTER

# 21 Prenatal testing and reproductive genetics

*"The more alternatives, the more difficult the choice."*
Abbe D'Allainval

Until recently, couples at high risk of having a child with a genetic disorder had to choose between taking the risk or considering other reproductive options, such as long-term contraception, sterilization and termination of all pregnancies. Other alternatives included adoption, long-term fostering and donor insemination (DI).

Over the last three decades prenatal diagnosis – the ability to detect abnormalities in an unborn child – has been widely used. While it is never easy for a couple to decide to pursue prenatal diagnosis because of the possibility of subsequently having to consider termination of pregnancy, prenatal diagnosis is an option that is chosen by many couples at high risk of having a child with a serious hereditary disorder.

The ethical issues surrounding prenatal diagnosis and selective termination of pregnancy are both complex and emotive, and are considered more fully in Chapter 24 (p. 370). In this chapter we shall focus on the practical aspects of prenatal testing and diagnosis, including prenatal screening, as well as some aspects of reproductive genetics.

**Table 21.1 Standard techniques used in prenatal diagnosis**

| Technique | Optimal time (in weeks) | Disorders diagnosed |
|---|---|---|
| **Non-invasive** | | |
| *Maternal serum screening* | | |
| α-Fetoprotein | 16 | Neural tube defects |
| Triple test | 16 | Down syndrome |
| Ultrasound | 18 | Structural abnormalities, e.g. CNS, heart, kidneys and limbs |
| **Invasive** | | |
| *Amniocentesis* | 16 | |
| Fluid | | Neural tube defects |
| Cells | | Chromosome abnormalities, metabolic disorders, molecular defects |
| *Chorionic villus sampling* | 10–12 | Chromosome abnormalities, metabolic disorders, molecular defects |
| *Fetoscopy* | | |
| Blood (cordocentesis) | | Chromosome abnormalities, hematological disorders, congenital infection |
| Liver | | Metabolic disorders, e.g. ornithine transcarbamylase deficiency |
| Skin | | Hereditary skin disorders, e.g. epidermolysis bullosa |

## TECHNIQUES USED IN PRENATAL DIAGNOSIS

There are several techniques that can be utilized for the prenatal diagnosis of hereditary disorders and structural abnormalities (Table 21.1).

### AMNIOCENTESIS

Amniocentesis involves the aspiration of 10–20 ml of amniotic fluid through the abdominal wall under ultrasound guidance (Fig. 21.1). This is usually performed around the 16th week of gestation. The sample is spun down to yield a pellet of cells and supernatant fluid. The fluid can be used in the prenatal diagnosis of neural tube defects by assay of α-fetoprotein (p. 330). The cell pellet is resuspended in culture medium with fetal calf serum, which stimulates cell growth. While most of these cells in the amniotic fluid that have been shed from the amnion, fetal skin and urinary tract epithelium will be non-viable, a small proportion will grow. After approximately 14 days there are usually sufficient cells for chromosome analysis, although a longer period is usually needed before enough cells are obtained for biochemical or DNA studies. The availability of PCR has meant that direct DNA analysis is usually possible without the need for culture.

When a couple is considering amniocentesis as an option they should be informed of the 0.5–1% risk of miscarriage associated with the procedure, and that if the result is abnormal they will be facing the possibility of having to consider a late mid-trimester termination of pregnancy that involves an induction of labor.

Trials carrying out amniocentesis earlier in pregnancy, at 12–14 weeks gestation, yielded comparable rates of

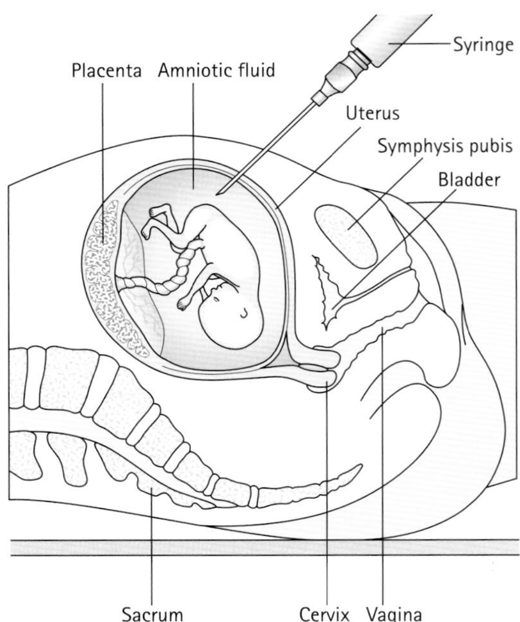


Fig. 21.1
A diagram of the technique of amniocentesis.

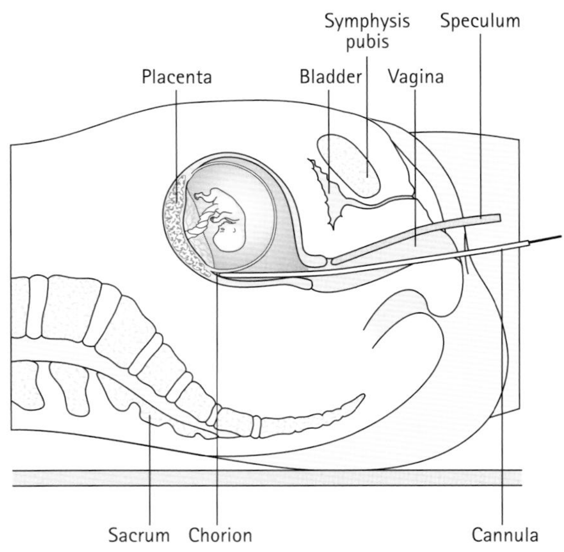


Fig. 21.2
A diagram of the technique of transvaginal chorionic villus sampling.

success in obtaining results with a similar risk of miscarriage. However, concerns have been expressed regarding the reduction in amniotic fluid at this early stage of pregnancy and early amniocentesis is not widely practiced. Although it has the advantage of allowing a result to be given earlier in the pregnancy, it will usually still require a mid-trimester termination of pregnancy if the fetus is found to be affected.

## CHORIONIC VILLUS SAMPLING

In contrast to amniocentesis, chorionic villus sampling (CVS), which was first developed in China, enables prenatal diagnosis to be undertaken during the first trimester. This procedure is usually carried out at 11–12 weeks gestation under ultrasound guidance by either transcervical or, more usually, transabdominal aspiration of chorionic villi (Fig. 21.2). These are fetal in origin, being derived from the outer cell layer of the blastocyst, i.e. the trophoblast. Maternal decidua, normally present in the biopsy sample, must be removed before the sample is analyzed. Placental biopsy is the term used if the procedure is carried out at later stages of pregnancy.

Chromosome analysis can be undertaken on chorionic villi either directly, looking at metaphase spreads from actively dividing cells, or following culture. Direct chromosomal analysis of chorionic villi usually allows a provisional result to be given within 24 h. Confirmation by analysis of cultured chorionic villi is required in order to obtain good-quality banded chromosomal analysis. For single-gene disorders, sufficient tissue is usually obtained to allow prenatal diagnosis by biochemical assay or DNA analysis using uncultured villi.

The major advantage of CVS sampling is that it offers first-trimester prenatal diagnosis, although it has the disadvantage that even in experienced hands this procedure conveys a 1–2% risk of causing miscarriage. There is also evidence that this technique can cause limb abnormalities in the embryo if carried out before 9–10 weeks gestation – for this reason CVS is not now performed before 11 weeks gestation.

## ULTRASOUND

Ultrasound offers a valuable means of prenatal diagnosis. It can be used not only for obstetric indications, such as placental localization and the diagnosis of multiple pregnancies, but also for the prenatal diagnosis of structural abnormalities that are not associated with known chromosomal, biochemical or molecular defects. Ultrasound is particularly valuable because it is non-invasive and conveys no known risk to the fetus or to the mother. It does, however, require specialized expensive equipment and a skilled and experienced operator. For example, a search can be made for polydactyly as a diagnostic feature of a multiple abnormality syndrome, such as one of the autosomal recessive short-limb polydactyly syndromes that are associated with severe pulmonary hypoplasia and are invariably lethal (Fig. 21.3). Similarly, a scan can reveal that the fetus has a small jaw, which can be associated with a posterior cleft palate and other more serious abnormalities in several single-gene syndromes (Fig. 21.4).

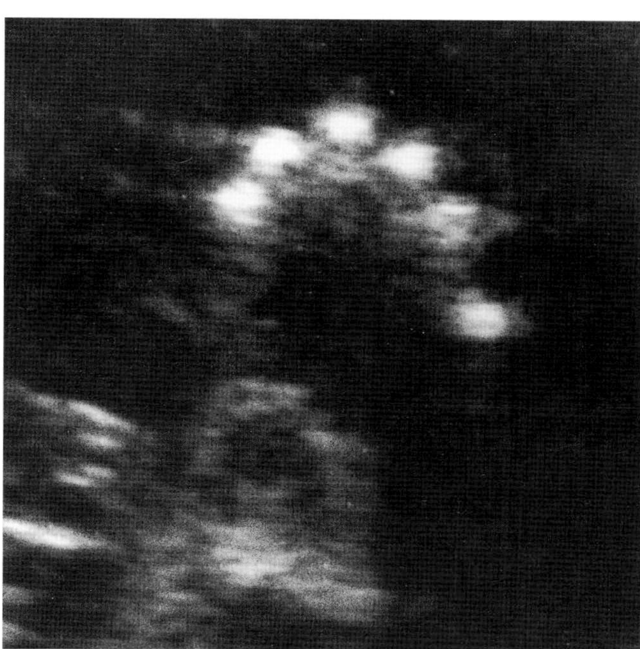

Fig. 21.3
Ultrasound image of a transverse section of the hand of a fetus showing polydactyly.

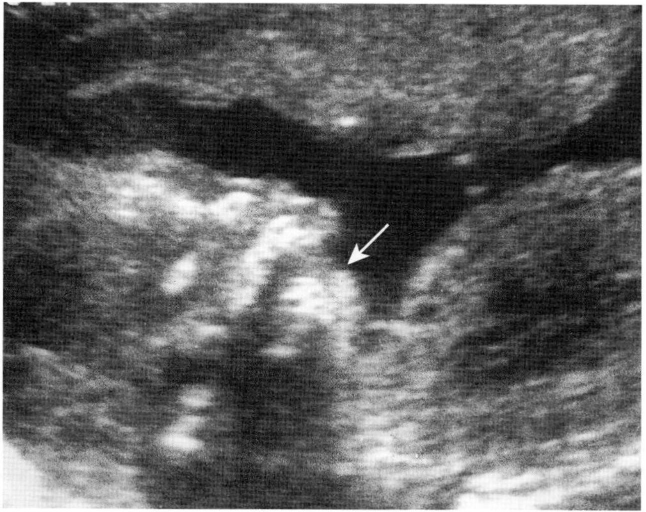

Fig. 21.4
Longitudinal sagittal ultrasound image of the head and upper chest of a fetus showing micrognathia (small jaw) (arrowed).

Until recently, detailed ultrasound scanning for structural abnormalities was offered only to couples who had a child with a genetic disorder or syndrome for which there was no chromosomal, biochemical or molecular marker. Increasingly, however, detailed 'fetal anomaly' scanning is being offered routinely to all pregnant women at around 18 weeks gestation as a screening procedure for structural abnormalities such as neural tube defects or cardiac anomalies. This technique can also identify features that suggest the presence of an underlying chromosomal abnormality (p. 331). Such a finding would lead to an offer of amniocentesis or placental biopsy for definitive chromosome analysis.

### Nuchal translucency

In addition, the observation that increased nuchal translucency (NT) is seen in fetuses who are subsequently born with Down syndrome, has resulted in the introduction of measurements of nuchal pad thickness in the first and second trimesters as a screening test for Down syndrome (p. 331).

## FETOSCOPY

Fetoscopy involves visualization of the fetus by means of an endoscope. Increasingly, this technique is being superseded by detailed ultrasound scanning, although occasionally fetoscopy is still undertaken during the second trimester to try to detect the presence of subtle structural abnormalities that would point to a serious underlying diagnosis.

Fetoscopy has also been used to obtain samples of tissue from the fetus that can be analyzed as a means of achieving the prenatal diagnosis of several rare disorders. These have included inherited skin disorders such as epidermolysis bullosa and, before DNA testing became available, metabolic disorders in which the enzyme is expressed only in certain tissues or organs, such as the liver, e.g. ornithine transcarbamylase deficiency (p. 167).

Unfortunately, fetoscopy is associated with a 3–5% risk of miscarriage. This relatively high risk, coupled with the increasing sensitivity of ultrasound scanning and the availability of either linked DNA markers or specific mutation analysis, means that fetoscopy is used only infrequently and in highly specialized prenatal diagnostic centers.

## CORDOCENTESIS

Although fetoscopy can also be used to obtain a small sample of fetal blood from one of the umbilical cord vessels in the procedure known as cordocentesis, improvements in ultrasound have enabled visualization of the vessels in the umbilical cord, allowing transabdominal percutaneous fetal blood sampling. Fetal blood sampling is routinely used in the management of rhesus isoimmunization (p. 199) and can be used to obtain samples for chromosome analysis to resolve problems associated with possible chromosomal mosaicism in chorionic villus or amniocentesis samples.

## RADIOGRAPHY

The fetal skeleton can be visualized by radiography from 10 weeks onwards and this technique has been used in the past to diagnose inherited skeletal dysplasias. It is now rarely if ever employed because of the dangers of radiography to the fetus (p. 27) and the widespread availability of detailed ultrasound scanning.

# PRENATAL SCREENING

## MATERNAL SERUM SCREENING

It has been government policy in the UK since 2001 that antenatal Down syndrome screening will be available to all women. Whilst this has almost been realized it is still not universally available in the country. Where it is standard practice, maternal serum screening is offered for neural tube defects and Down syndrome using a blood sample obtained from the mother at 16 weeks gestation. In this way up to 75% of all cases of open neural tube defects and 60–70% of all cases of Down syndrome can be detected.

## NEURAL TUBE DEFECTS

In 1972 it was recognized that many pregnancies in which the baby had an open neural tube defect (NTD) (p. 256) could be detected at 16 weeks' gestation by assay of a protein in maternal serum known as α-fetoprotein (αFP). αFP is the fetal equivalent of albumin and is the major protein in fetal blood. If the fetus has an open NTD, the level of αFP is elevated in both the amniotic fluid and maternal serum as a result of leakage from the open defect. Open NTDs fulfil the criterion of being serious disorders, as anencephaly is invariably fatal, and between 80% and 90% of the small proportion of babies who survive with an open lumbo-sacral lesion are severely handicapped.

Unfortunately maternal serum αFP screening for NTDs is neither 100% sensitive nor 100% specific. The curves for the levels of maternal serum αFP in normal and affected pregnancies overlap (Fig. 21.5), so that in practice an arbitrary cut-off level has to be introduced below which no further action is taken. This is usually either the 95th centile or 2.5 multiples of the median (MoM), and as a result around 75% of screened open spina bifida cases are detected. Those pregnant women with results that lie above this arbitrary cut-off level are offered further investigations, such as detailed ultrasonography and possibly also amniocentesis, which gives a clearer distinction between the levels of αFP in normal and affected pregnancies.

Lack of specificity results from the elevation in maternal serum αFP that can occur for reasons other than an open NTD (Table 21.2), such as a threatened miscarriage, a twin pregnancy, or a fetal abnormality such as exomphalos, in which there is a protrusion of abdominal contents through the umbilicus.

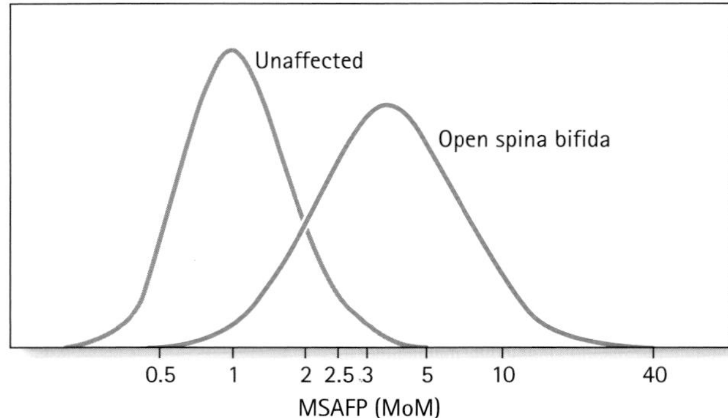


**Fig. 21.5**
Maternal serum aFP levels at 16 weeks' gestation plotted on a logarithmic scale as multiples of the median (MoMs). Women with a value on or above 2.5 multiples of the median are offered further investigations. (Adapted from Brock D J H, Rodeck C H, Ferguson-Smith M A (eds) 1992 Prenatal diagnosis and screening. Churchill Livingstone, Edinburgh.)

| Table 21.2 Causes of elevated maternal serum αFP |
|---|
| Anencephaly |
| Open spina bifida |
| Incorrect gestational age |
| Intra-uterine fetal bleed |
| Threatened miscarriage |
| Multiple pregnancy |
| Congenital nephrotic syndrome |
| Abdominal wall defect |

Despite these limitations prenatal maternal serum αFP screening has been widely implemented and is one of the main factors that have led to a striking decline in the incidence of open NTDs in liveborn and stillborn babies. Other contributory factors are a general improvement in diet and the introduction of periconceptional folic acid supplementation (p. 257). In England and Wales the combined incidence of anencephaly and spina bifida in liveborn and stillborn babies fell from 1 in 250 in 1973 to 1 in 6250 in 1993.

## DOWN SYNDROME AND OTHER CHROMOSOME ABNORMALITIES

### The triple test

Confirmation of a chromosome abnormality in an unborn baby requires cytogenetic studies using material obtained by an invasive procedure such as chorionic villus sampling or amniocentesis (p. 327). However, chromosome abnormalities, and in particular Down syndrome, can be

**Table 21.3 Maternal risk factors for Down syndrome**

| Advanced age (35 years or over) | |
|---|---|
| Maternal serum | MoM* |
| α-Fetoprotein (αFP) | (0.75) |
| Unconjugated estriol (μE3) | (0.73) |
| Human chorionic gonadotrophin (hCG) | (2.05) |
| Inhibin-A | (2.10) |

*Numbers in brackets refer to the mean values in affected pregnancies, expressed as multiples of the median (MoMs) in normal pregnancies

screened for in pregnancy by taking into account risk factors such as maternal age and the levels of three biochemical markers in maternal serum (Table 21.3).

This latter approach is based on the discovery that, at 16 weeks gestation, maternal serum αFP and unconjugated estriol levels tend to be lower in Down syndrome pregnancies than in normal pregnancies, whereas the level of maternal serum human chorionic gonadotropin is usually elevated. None of these parameters gives absolute discrimination, but taken together they provide a means of modifying a woman's prior age-related risk to give an overall probability that the unborn baby is affected. When this probability exceeds 1 in 250, invasive testing in the form of amniocentesis or placental biopsy is offered.

Using age alone as a screening parameter, if all pregnant women aged 35 years and over opt for fetal chromosome analysis approximately 35% of all Down syndrome pregnancies will be detected (Table 21.4A). If the aforementioned three biochemical markers are also included, this being the so-called triple test, 60% of all Down syndrome pregnancies will be detected, using a risk of 1 in 250 or greater as the criterion for offering amniocentesis. This approach will also result in the detection of approximately 50% of all cases of trisomy 18 (p. 274). In the latter condition *all* the biochemical parameters are low, including hCG.

It has recently been shown that another biochemical marker, inhibin-A, is also increased in maternal serum in Down syndrome pregnancies. If this fourth marker is used as part of a 'quadruple' serum screening test, the proportion of Down syndrome pregnancies detected rises from 60% to 75% if amniocentesis is offered to the 5% of mothers tested who have the highest risk.

Published results from California provide a useful indication of the outcome of a triple-test prenatal screening program. California has a population of 32 million and all pregnant women are offered triple-test screening. This was accepted by 67% of all eligible women, of whom 2.6% went on to have amniocentesis, resulting in the detection of 41% of all cases of Down syndrome. These

**Table 21.4A Detection rates using different Down syndrome screening strategies**

| Screening modalities | % of all pregnancies tested | % of Down syndrome cases detected |
|---|---|---|
| Age alone | | |
| 40 years and over | 1.5 | 15 |
| 35 years and over | 7 | 35 |
| Age + αFP | 5 | 34 |
| Age + αFP, μE3 + hCG | 5 | 61 |
| Age + aFP, μE3, hCG + inhibin-A | 5 | 75 |

**Table 21.4B**

| Screening modalities | % of all pregnancies tested | % of Down syndrome cases detected |
|---|---|---|
| NT alone | 5 | 61 |
| NT + age | 5 | 69 |
| hCG, αFP + age | 5 | 73 |
| NT + αFP, hCG + age | 5 | 86 |

figures are similar to those observed in other studies and serve to illustrate the discrepancy between what is possible in theory (i.e. a detection rate of 60%) and what actually happens in practice.

## Ultrasonography

Almost all pregnant women are routinely offered a 'dating' scan at around 12 weeks gestation. In recent years it has been shown that at around this time there is a strong association between chromosome abnormalities and the abnormal accumulation of fluid behind the baby's neck – increased fetal nuchal translucency (NT). This applies to Down syndrome, the other autosomal trisomy syndromes, i.e. trisomy 13 and trisomy 18 (p. 274), Turner syndrome, triploidy, as well as a wide range of other fetal abnormalities and rare syndromes. The risk of Down syndrome correlates with absolute values of NT as well as maternal age (Fig. 21.6) but, as NT also increases with gestational age, it more usual now to relate the risk to the centile value for any given gestational age. In one study, 80% of Down syndrome fetuses had NT above the 95th centile. By combining information on maternal age with the results of fetal NT thickness measurements, together with maternal serum markers, it is possible to detect more than 80% of fetuses with trisomy 21 if invasive testing is offered to the 5% of pregnant women with the highest risk (Table 21.4B).

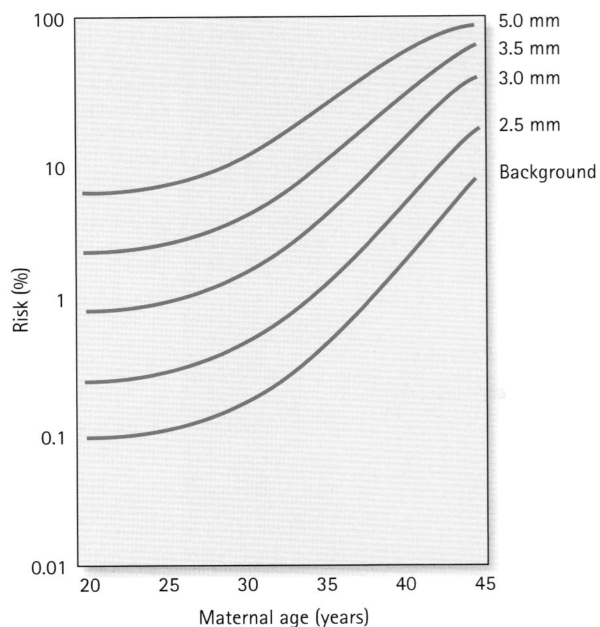


Fig. 21.6
The risk for trisomy 21 (Down syndrome) with maternal age, for different absolute values of nuchal translucency (NT) at 12 weeks gestation.

In many centers it is also standard practice to offer a detailed 'fetal anomaly' scan to all pregnant women at 18 weeks. Although chromosome abnormalities cannot be diagnosed directly, their presence can be suspected by the detection of an abnormality such as exomphalos (Fig. 21.7) or a rocker-bottom foot (Fig. 21.8A, B) (Table 21.5). A chromosome abnormality is found in 50% of fetuses with an exomphalos identified at 18 weeks, and a rocker-bottom foot is a very characteristic finding in babies with trisomy 18 (p. 274), who are also invariably growth retarded. The use of other ultrasound 'soft markers' in identifying chromosome abnormalities in pregnancy is discussed in Chapter 21 (p. 328).

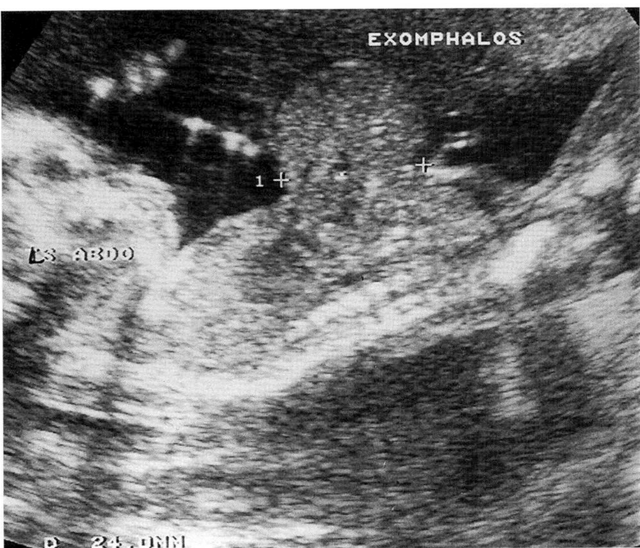


Fig. 21.7
Ultrasound scan at 18 weeks showing exomphalos. (Courtesy of Dr D. Rose, City Hospital, Nottingham.)

**Table 21.5 Prenatal ultrasound findings suggestive of a chromosome abnormality**

| Feature | Chromosome abnormality |
|---|---|
| Cardiac defect (especially common atrio-ventricular canal) | Trisomy 13, 18, 21 |
| Clenched overlapping fingers | Trisomy 18 |
| Cystic hygroma or fetal hydrops | Trisomy 13, 18, 21, 45, X (Turner syndrome) |
| Duodenal atresia | Trisomy 21 |
| Exomphalos | Trisomy 13, 18 |
| Rocker-bottom foot | Trisomy 18 |

## INDICATIONS FOR PRENATAL DIAGNOSIS

There are numerous indications for offering prenatal diagnosis. Ideally, couples at high prior risk of having a baby with an abnormality should be identified and assessed before embarking upon a pregnancy so that they can be counseled and come to a decision about which options they wish to pursue at their leisure. A less satisfactory alternative is that such couples be identified early in pregnancy so that they still have an opportunity to consider all available prenatal diagnostic options as soon as possible in the pregnancy. Unfortunately, many couples at an increased risk, because of their family history or previous reproductive history, are still not referred until mid-pregnancy, when it can be too late to offer the most appropriate forms of prenatal diagnosis.

### ADVANCED MATERNAL AGE

This has been the most common indication for offering prenatal diagnosis. There is a well-recognized association of advanced maternal age with increased risk of having a child with Down syndrome (Table 18.4, p. 272) and the other autosomal trisomy syndromes. No standard criterion exists for determining at what age a mother should be offered the option of an invasive prenatal diagnostic technique for fetal chromosome analysis. Most centers routinely offer amniocentesis or CVS to women aged 37 years or over, and the option is often discussed with women from the age of 35 years onwards. These

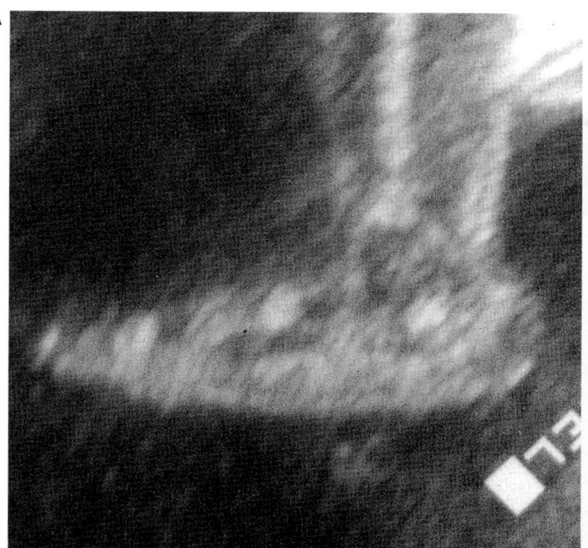


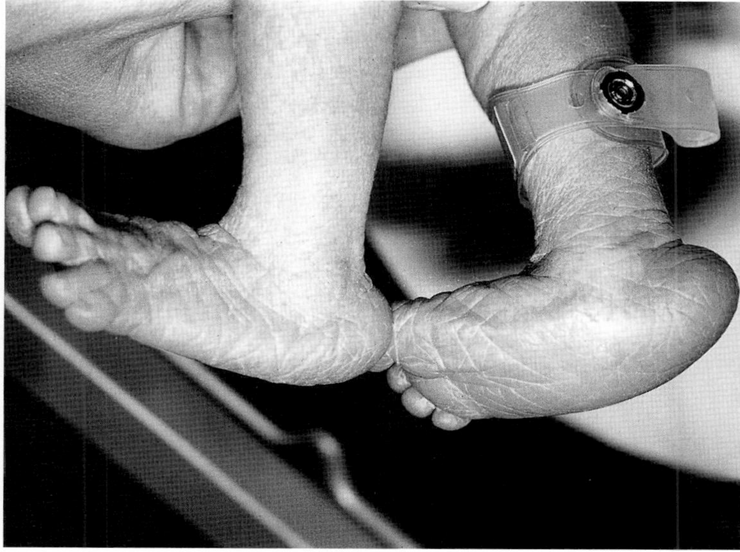


Fig. 21.8
(A) Ultrasound scan at 18 weeks showing a rocker-bottom foot in a fetus subsequently found to have trisomy 18, together with (B) a photograph of the feet of a newborn with trisomy 18. (Courtesy of Dr D Rose, City Hospital, Nottingham.)

risk figures relate to the maternal age at the expected date of delivery. The risk figures for Down syndrome at the time of CVS, amniocentesis and delivery differ (Fig. 18.1, p. 271) because a proportion of pregnancies with trisomy 21 are lost spontaneously during the first and second trimesters.

## PREVIOUS CHILD WITH A CHROMOSOME ABNORMALITY

Although there are a number of series with slightly different recurrence risk figures, for couples who have had a child with Down syndrome due to non-disjunction or a de novo unbalanced Robertsonian translocation, the risk in a subsequent pregnancy is usually given as the mother's age-related risk plus approximately 0.5%. If one of the parents has been found to carry a balanced chromosomal rearrangement, such as a chromosomal translocation (p. 49) or pericentric inversion (p. 53), which has caused a previous child to be born with serious problems due to an unbalanced chromosome abnormality, then the recurrence risk is likely to be between 1–2% and 15–20%. The precise risk will depend on the nature of the parental rearrangement and the specific segments of the individual chromosomes involved (p. 54).

## FAMILY HISTORY OF A CHROMOSOME ABNORMALITY

Couples are often referred for prenatal diagnosis because of a family history of a chromosome abnormality, most commonly Down syndrome. For most couples there will usually be no increase in risk compared to the general population, since most cases of trisomy 21 and other chromosomal disorders will have arisen as a result of non-disjunction rather than as a result of a familial chromosomal rearrangement. However, each situation should be carefully evaluated, either by confirming the nature of the chromosome abnormality in the affected individual or, if this is not possible, by urgent chromosome analysis of blood from the relevant parent at risk. The results of parental chromosomal analysis can usually be obtained within 3–4 days; if normal, an invasive prenatal diagnostic procedure is not then appropriate since the risk is no greater than that for the general population.

## FAMILY HISTORY OF A SINGLE-GENE DISORDER

If prospective parents have already had an affected child, or if one of the parents is affected or has a positive family history of a single-gene disorder that conveys a significant risk to offspring, then the option of prenatal diagnosis should be discussed with them. Prenatal diagnosis is available for a large and ever-increasing number of single-gene disorders by either biochemical or DNA analysis.

## FAMILY HISTORY OF A NEURAL TUBE DEFECT

Careful evaluation of the pedigree is necessary to determine the risk that applies to each pregnancy. Risks can be determined based on empiric data (p. 349). In high-risk situations amniocentesis with assay of the chemical α-fetoprotein has been used for prenatal diagnosis in the past. Ultrasound examination of the fetus in conjunction with assay of maternal serum α-fetoprotein has proved equally reliable. Even with the best possible equipment and an experienced ultrasonographer, small closed neural tube defect can still be missed. Fortunately the latter type of neural tube defects are not usually associated with the serious problems seen with large open neural tube defects (p. 256).

## FAMILY HISTORY OF OTHER CONGENITAL STRUCTURAL ABNORMALITIES

As with neural tube defects, evaluation of the family pedigree should enable the provision of a risk derived from the results of empiric studies. If the risk to a pregnancy is increased, detailed ultrasound examination looking for the specific structural abnormality can be offered at around 16–18 weeks gestation. Mid-trimester ultrasound will detect most serious cranial, cardiac, renal and limb malformations. Some couples request detailed ultrasound scanning, not because they wish to pursue the option of termination of pregnancy but because they wish to prepare themselves if the baby is found to be affected.

## ABNORMALITIES IDENTIFIED IN PREGNANCY

The widespread introduction of prenatal diagnostic screening procedures, such as triple testing and fetal anomaly scanning, has meant that many couples unexpectedly present with diagnostic uncertainty during the pregnancy that can only be resolved by an invasive procedure such as amniocentesis or CVS. Other factors, such as poor fetal growth, can also be an indication for prenatal chromosome analysis, as confirmation of a serious and non-viable chromosome abnormality, such as trisomy 18 or triploidy (p. 48), can influence subsequent management of the pregnancy and mode of delivery.

## OTHER HIGH-RISK FACTORS

These include parental consanguinity, a poor obstetric history and certain maternal illnesses. Parental consanguinity conveys an increased risk that a child will have a hereditary disorder or congenital abnormality (p. 267). Consequently, if the parents are concerned, it is appropriate to offer detailed ultrasonography to try to exclude a serious structural abnormality. A poor obstetric history, such as recurrent miscarriages or a previous unexplained stillbirth, could indicate an increased risk of problems in a future pregnancy and would be an indication for detailed ultrasound monitoring. A history of three or more unexplained miscarriages should be investigated by parental chromosome studies to exclude a chromosomal rearrangement such as a translocation or inversion (p. 289). Maternal illnesses, such as poorly controlled insulin-dependent diabetes mellitus (p. 260) or epilepsy treated with anticonvulsant medications such as sodium valproate (p. 260), would also be indications for detailed ultrasonography. Both of these factors convey an increased risk of structural abnormality in a fetus.

## SPECIAL PROBLEMS IN PRENATAL DIAGNOSIS

While the significance of the result of a prenatal diagnostic investigation is usually clear-cut, situations can arise that pose major problems of interpretation. Problems also occur if the diagnostic investigation is unsuccessful or if an unexpected result is obtained.

### FAILURE TO OBTAIN A SAMPLE OR CULTURE FAILURE

It is important that every woman undergoing one of these invasive procedures is alerted to the possibility that, on occasion, it can prove impossible to obtain a suitable sample or the cells obtained subsequently fail to grow. Fortunately, the risk of either of these events occurring is less than 1%.

### AN AMBIGUOUS CHROMOSOME RESULT

In approximately 1% of cases, CVS shows evidence of apparent chromosome mosaicism, i.e. the presence of two or more cell lines with different chromosome constitutions (p. 54). This can occur for several reasons:

1. The sample is *contaminated* by maternal cells. This is more likely to be seen when using cultured cells than with direct preparations.
2. The mosaicism is a *culture artifact*. Usually several separate cell cultures are routinely established at the time of the procedure because of this possibility in order to help resolve this problem rapidly. If mosaicism is present in only one culture then it is probably an artifact and does not reflect the true fetal karyotype.
3. The mosaicism is limited to a portion of the placenta, or what is known as *confined placental mosaicism*. This arises due to an error in mitosis during the formation and development of the trophoblast and is of no consequence to the fetus.
4. There is *true fetal mosaicism*.

In the case of amniocentesis, in most laboratories it is routine for the sample to be split and for two or three separate cultures to be established. If a single abnormal cell is identified in only one culture this is assumed to be a culture artifact, or what is termed *level 1 mosaicism* or *pseudomosaicism*. If the mosaicism extends to two or more cells in two or more cultures this is taken as evidence of true mosaicism, or what is known as level 3 mosaicism. The most difficult situation to interpret is when mosaicism is present in two or more cells in only one culture, which is termed level 2 mosaicism. This is most likely to represent a culture artifact but, there is up to a 20% chance that the mosaicism is real and will be present in the fetus.

In order to resolve the uncertainty generated by the finding of mosaicism with chromosomal analysis of chorionic villus samples it can be necessary to proceed to amniocentesis. If the latter test yields a normal chromosomal result then it is concluded that the result obtained from chorionic villi was not a true indication of the fetal karyotype.

Counseling couples in this situation is always extremely difficult. Even if true mosaicism is confirmed, it can be impossible to predict the probable phenotypic outcome for the baby. An attempt can be made to resolve ambiguous findings by proceeding to fetal blood sampling for urgent karyotype analysis. Whatever option the parents choose, it is important that tissue (blood, skin or placenta) is obtained at the time of delivery, whether the couple elect to terminate or continue with the pregnancy, in order to resolve the significance of the prenatal findings.

## AN UNEXPECTED CHROMOSOME RESULT

Three different unexpected chromosome results can be given to couples, each of which usually necessitates specialized detailed genetic counseling.

### A different numerical chromosomal abnormality

Although most invasive prenatal diagnostic procedures, such as chorionic villus sampling and amniocentesis, are carried out because of an increased risk of trisomy 21 through increased maternal age or as a result of increased risk through the triple test or nuchal pad screening (p. 329), a chromosomal abnormality other than trisomy 21 can be found, e.g. one of the other autosomal trisomies (trisomy 13 or 18) or one of the sex chromosome aneuploidies (45,X, 47,XXX, 47,XXY or 47,XYY). While the implication for the outcome of the pregnancy with one of the autosomal trisomies is reasonably straightforward, it is not so clear-cut with the sex chromosomal aneuploidies. Ideally, all women undergoing amniocentesis should be alerted to this possibility before the test is carried out, although in practice this is rarely done. When a diagnosis such as Turner syndrome (45,X) or Klinefelter syndrome (47,XXY) is obtained it is essential that the parents be given full details of the nature and consequences of the diagnosis. Recent studies have shown that when objective and informed counseling is available, less than 50% of the parents of a fetus with an 'incidental' diagnosis of a sex chromosome abnormality opt for termination of pregnancy.

### A structural chromosomal rearrangement

A second difficult situation not infrequently encountered when providing prenatal diagnosis by amniocentesis or CVS is the discovery of an apparently balanced chromosome rearrangement in the fetus, such as an inversion or translocation. If analysis of parental chromosomes shows that one of the parents has the same structural chromosomal rearrangement, then the parents can be reassured that it is very unlikely that this will cause any problems in the fetus. If, however, the apparently balanced chromosomal rearrangement has occurred as a de novo event in the fetus, then there is between a 5% and 10% chance that the fetus will have physical abnormalities and/or subsequently show developmental delay. This is likely to reflect a subtle chromosomal imbalance that cannot be detected using conventional cytogenetic techniques, or damage to a critical gene at one or both of the rearrangement break-points. It is not surprising that couples in this situation can have great difficulty in deciding what to do. Detailed ultrasonography, if normal, can provide some, but not complete, reassurance. The opportunity should, in due course, be taken to investigate the extended family if the rearrangement is found to be present in one of the parents.

### The presence of a marker chromosome

A third situation that presents difficulty in counseling is the discovery in the amniocentesis or CVS sample of a small additional chromosome known as a marker chromosome, i.e. a small chromosomal fragment the specific identity of which cannot be determined by conventional cytogenetic techniques (p. 33). If this is found to be present in one of the parents, then it is unlikely that it will be of any significance to the fetus. If, on the other hand, it is a de novo finding, there is up to a 15% chance that the fetus will be phenotypically abnormal. The risk is lower if the marker chromosome contains satellite material (p. 32), or is largely made up of heterochromatin (p. 32), than if it does not have satellites and is mostly made up of euchromatin (p. 32). The availability of fluorescent in situ hybridization (p. 35) means that the origin of the marker chromosome can often be more specifically determined so that it is often possible to give more precise prognostic information.

## ULTRASOUND 'SOFT' MARKERS

The increasing sophistication of mid-trimester ultrasonography has resulted in the identification of subtle

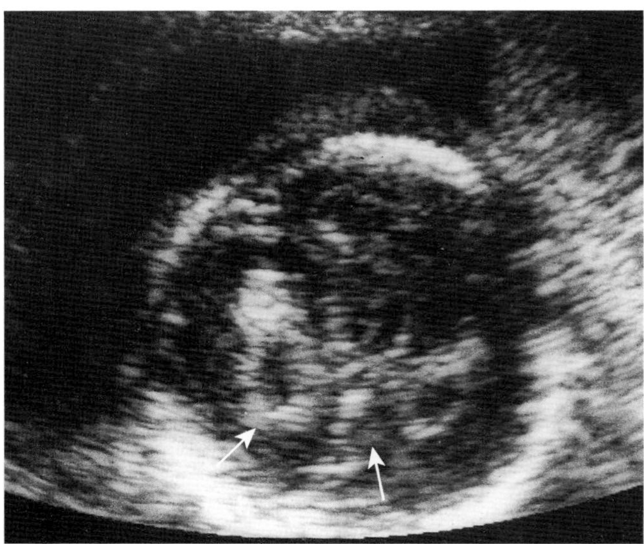

Fig. 21.9
Ultrasound scan of a fetal brain showing bilateral choroid plexus cysts (arrowed).

anomalies in the fetus, the significance of which is not always clear. For example, choroid plexus cysts are sometimes seen in the developing cerebral ventricles in mid-trimester (Fig. 21.9). Initially, it was thought that these were invariably associated with the fetus having trisomy 18. It is now known that choroid plexus cysts occur frequently in normal fetuses, although if they are very large and do not disappear spontaneously they can be indicative of a chromosome abnormality.

More recently, increased echogenicity of the fetal bowel has been reported as being associated with the baby subsequently having cystic fibrosis. It is presumed that this is the prenatal equivalent of meconium ileus (p. 303). Although initial reports suggested that the finding of 'echogenic bowel' could convey a risk as high as 10% for the fetus having cystic fibrosis, it is now clear that this risk is probably no greater than 1–2%. These types of novel ultrasound findings associated with possible fetal abnormalities are often called *soft markers*.

The difficulty in distinguishing normal from abnormal variation, coupled with lack of knowledge of the natural history of other commonly observed findings, emphasizes the importance of viewing reports of ultrasound soft markers and their possible association with abnormality in the fetus with great caution!

## TERMINATION OF PREGNANCY

The presence of a serious abnormality in a fetus in the majority of developed countries is an acceptable legal indication for termination of pregnancy. This does not mean, however, that this is an easy choice for a couple to make. It is essential that all couples undergoing any form of prenatal diagnostic investigation, whether invasive or non-invasive, be provided with information about the practical aspects of termination of pregnancy before the prenatal diagnostic procedure is carried out. This should include a practical explanation that termination in the first trimester is carried out by surgical means under general anesthetic, whereas a woman undergoing a mid-trimester termination will have to experience labor and delivery.

## PREIMPLANTATION GENETIC DIAGNOSIS

For many couples prenatal diagnosis on an established pregnancy, with a view to possible termination, is too difficult to contemplate. For some of these couples *preimplantation genetic diagnosis* (PGD) provides an acceptable alternative. The second largest group of PGD users are those with sub- or infertility who wish to combine assisted reproduction with genetic testing of the early embryo. In the procedure the female partner is given hormones to induce hyperovulation, and oocytes are then harvested transcervically, under sedation, with ultrasound guidance. Motile sperm from a semen sample are added to the oocytes in culture (*in-vitro fertilization* (IVF) – the same technique as developed for infertility) and incubated to allow fertilization to occur. If genetic analysis is to be undertaken on DNA from a single cell (blastomere) from the early embryo (blastocyst) at the eight-cell stage on the third day, fertilization is achieved using *intracytoplasmic sperm injection* (ICSI) of a single sperm to avoid the presence of extraneous sperm.

At the eight-cell stage the early embryo is biopsied and one, sometimes two, cells are removed for analysis. Whatever genetic analysis is undertaken, it essential that this is a practical possibility on genomic material from a single cell. From the embryos tested, two that are both healthy and unaffected by the disorder from which they are at risk, are re-introduced into the mother's uterus. Implantation must then occur for a successful pregnancy and this is a major hurdle – the success rate for the procedure is only about 25% per cycle of treatment even in the best centers. A variation of the technique is removal of the first, and often second, polar bodies from the unfertilized oocyte, which lie under the zona pellucida. As the first polar body degenerates quite rapidly analysis is necessary within 6 h of retrieval. Analysis of polar bodies is an indirect method of genotyping because the oocyte and first polar body divide from each other during meiosis I and, therefore, contain different members of each pair of homologous chromosomes.

**Table 21.6 Some of the conditions for which PGD has been used and is available**

| Mode of inheritance | Disease |
|---|---|
| Autosomal dominant | Charcot–Marie–Tooth<br>FAP<br>HD<br>Marfan syndrome<br>Myotonic dystrophy<br>Neurofibromatosis<br>Osteogenesis imperfecta<br>Tuberous sclerosis |
| Autosomal recessive | β-Thalassemia<br>Cystic fibrosis<br>Epidermolysis bullosa<br>Gaucher disease<br>Sickle-cell disease |
| Spinal muscular atrophy | |
| | Tay–Sach disease |
| X-linked | Alport syndrome<br>Duchenne muscular dystrophy (DMD)<br>Hunter syndrome<br>Kennedy syndrome<br>Fragile-X syndrome |
| X-linked – sexing only | DMD<br>Ornithine transcarbamylase deficiency<br>Incontinentia pigmenti<br>Other serious disorders |
| Mitochondrial | MELAS |
| Chromosomal | Robertsonian translocations<br>Reciprocal translocations<br>Aneuploidy screening<br>Inversions, deletions |

There are four licensed centres for PGD in the UK and practice is strictly regulated by the Human Fertilization and Embryology Authority (HFEA). In numerical terms the impact of PGD has been small to date, but a wide range of genetic conditions have now been tested (Table 21.6). The most common referral reasons for single-gene disorders are cystic fibrosis, myotonic dystrophy, Huntington disease, β-thalassemia, spinal muscular atrophy and Fragile X syndrome. The technique to identify normal and abnormal alleles in these conditions, and DNA linkage analysis where appropriate, is PCR (p. 62). Sex selection in the case of serious X-linked conditions is available where single-gene analysis is not possible. The biggest group of referrals for PGD, however, is chromosome abnormalities – reciprocal and Robertsonian translocations in particular (pp. 49, 51). Genetic analysis in these cases uses FISH technology (p. 35) and substantial work has to be undertaken for the couple prior to treatment because of the unique nature of many translocations.

Recently there have been a very small number of high profile cases whereby PGD has been used not only to select embryos unaffected for the genetic disorder for which the pregnancy is at risk, but also to provide an HLA tissue type match so that the new child can function as a stem cell donor for the couple's child affected with Fanconi anemia. The ethical debate surrounding these cases has been strongly argued on both sides, and is discussed further in Chapter 24.

A further development using micromanipulation methods also attracted a lot of attention recently. In order to circumvent the problem of genetic disease due to mutation in the mitochondrial genome the nucleus of the oocyte from the genetic mother (who carried the mitochondrial mutation) was removed and inserted into a donor oocyte from which the nucleus had been removed. This is cell nuclear replacement (CNR) technology, similar to that used in reproductive cloning experiments in animals ('Dolly' the sheep – see p. 376). The resulting fertilization led to the headline that the fetus had three genetic parents. The technique has also been used in other situations where the oocytes are generally of poor quality, but there is disquiet about the procedure due to the failure rate and its use in the future is in question.

## ASSISTED CONCEPTION AND IMPLICATIONS FOR GENETIC DISEASE

### IN VITRO FERTILIZATION

Many thousands of babies worldwide have been born by *in vitro fertilization* (IVF) over the last 25 years since the technique was first successful. The indication for the treatment in most cases is subfertility – which now affects 1 in 7 couples. For most of this time the accumulated data suggested that the risk of congenital abnormalities was basically the same as for the general population conceiving in the normal way. However, concern has begun to emerge that there might be a small but abnormal increase in the incidence of conditions due to defective genomic imprinting (p. 118). In particular, there appear to have been an unusual number of cases of mild Beckwith–Wiedemann syndrome. The true extent of the problem has yet to be determined, and the possible mechanisms are unclear.

### INTRACYTOPLASMIC SPERM INJECTION

As mentioned, this technique is employed as part of IVF when combined with PGD but the main indication for directly injecting the sperm into the egg is male subfertility due to low sperm count, poor sperm motility, abnormal sperm morphology, or mechanical blockage to the passage of sperm along the vas deferens. Chromosomal abnormalities or rearrangements have been found in about 5% of men for whom *intracytoplasmic sperm injection* (ICSI) is suitable, and 10–12% in those with azoospermia or severe oligospermia. Examples include the Robertsonian 13:14 translocation and Y chromosome deletions. For men with azoospermia or severe oligospermia the karyotype should be checked, including the application of molecular techniques looking for submicroscopic Y deletions. In those with mechanical blockage due to congenital bilateral absence of the vas deferens (CBAVD) a significant proportion have cystic fibrosis mutations, either as heterozygotes or compound heterozygotes. ICSI offers hope to men with CBAVD, as well as those with Klinefelter syndrome, following testicular aspiration of sperm.

Some of the chromosomal abnormalities in the men may be heritable – especially involving the sex chromosomes – and there is a small but definite increase in chromosomal abnormalities in the offspring (1.6%).

## DONOR INSEMINATION

As a means of assisted conception to treat male infertility or the risk of a genetic disease, *donor insemination* (DI) has been around for about half a century. Only relatively recently, however, has awareness of medical genetic issues been incorporated into practice. Following cases of children conceived by DI who were subsequently discovered to have balanced or unbalanced chromosome disorders, or in some cases cystic fibrosis (indicating that the sperm donor was a carrier for cystic fibrosis), screening of sperm donors for cystic fibrosis mutations and chromosome rearrangements has become routine practice in many countries. This was recommended only as recently as 2000 by the British Andrology Society in the UK. In the Netherlands a donor whose sperm was used to father 18 offspring developed an autosomal dominant late-onset neurodegenerative disorder – one of the spinocerebellar ataxias – thus indicating that all 18 offspring were conceived at 50% risk. This has led to a ruling that the sperm from one donor should be used no more than 10 times, as against 25 prior to this experience. In the UK men over 40 cannot be donors, due to the small but increasing risk of new germline mutations arising in sperm with advancing paternal age.

Of course, it is not possible to screen the donor for all eventualities but these cases have served to highlight the potential conflict between treating infertility (or genetic disease) by DI and maintaining a high level of concern for the welfare of the child conceived. More high profile in this respect is the ongoing debate about how much information DI children should be allowed about their genetic fathers, and the law varies across the world.

Naturally, all of these issues apply in an equivalent way to women who wish to be egg donors.

## ASSISTED CONCEPTION AND THE LAW

In the USA no federal law exists to regulate the practice of assisted conception other than the requirement that outcomes of IVF and ICSI must be reported. In the UK strict regulation operates through the HFEA based on the Human Fertilization and Embryology Act of 1990. The HFEA has 18 members, reports to the Secretary of State for Health, issues licences, and arranges inspections of the centers to which licences are granted. The different licences granted are for *treatment* (Table 21.7), *storage* (gametes and embryos), and *research* (on human embryos in vitro). A register of all treatment cycles and children born by IVF or use of donated gametes must be kept. The research permitted under licence covers treatment of infertility, increase in knowledge regarding birth defects, miscarriage, genetic testing in embryos, the development of the early embryo, and potential treatment of serious disease.

**Table 21.7 Assisted conception treatments requiring a licence from the HFEA**

| |
|---|
| In vitro fertilization |
| Intracytoplasmic sperm injection |
| Preimplantation genetic diagnosis |
| Sperm donation |
| Egg donation |
| Embryo donation |
| Surrogacy |

## DETECTION OF FETAL CELLS IN THE MATERNAL CIRCULATION

Finally, it is possible that an entirely non-invasive means of prenatal diagnosis for chromosome and DNA abnormalities could become available. Using antibodies raised to antigens specific to the fetal trophoblast, there is evidence that cells of fetal origin are present in the maternal circulation in the first trimester. The validity of these claims has been substantiated by the use of PCR to detect the presence of paternally derived DNA markers in blood taken from women during early pregnancy. Although immunological techniques using antibodies to fetal trophoblast antigens can be used to enrich for fetal cells in the maternal circulation, problems can be encountered in excluding the possibility of significant maternal cell contamination in the sample being analyzed. This technique has been used in a limited number of disorders, e.g. to predict the rhesus status of the fetus in couples where the mother is Rh-negative and the father is heterozygous to try to determine which pregnancies need monitoring for rhesus isoimmunization. More recently, the fact that fetal red blood cells are nucleated has been used to enrich for cells of fetal origin. Although this technique allows a couple to conceive naturally, it is important to remember that, unlike PGD, use of this approach still requires a couple to consider termination of pregnancy as a possible option if the fetus is found to be affected.

## PRENATAL TREATMENT

So far this chapter has focused on prenatal diagnosis and screening for abnormalities with the subsequent option of termination of pregnancy, as well as other techniques designed to prevent genetic disease. While these are the only options in most situations, there is cautious optimism that prenatal diagnosis will, in time, lead to the possibility of effective treatment in utero.

A possible model for successful prenatal treatment is provided by the autosomal recessive disorder congenital adrenal hyperplasia (CAH) (pp. 168). Affected female infants are born with virilization of the external genitalia. There is evidence that in a proportion of cases the virilization can be prevented if the mother takes a powerful steroid known as dexamethasone in a very small dose from 4 to 5 weeks gestation onwards. Specific prenatal diagnosis of CAH can be achieved by DNA analysis of chorionic villi. If this procedure confirms that the fetus is both female and affected, then the mother continues to take low doses of dexamethasone throughout pregnancy, which suppresses the fetal pituitary–adrenal axis and can prevent virilization of the female fetus. If the fetus is male and affected or unaffected, the mother ceases to take dexamethasone and the pregnancy can proceed uneventfully.

More recently, in utero treatment of a fetus affected with severe combined immunodeficiency (p. 197) has been reported. The immunological tolerance of the fetus to foreign antigens introduced in utero means that the transfused stem cells are recognized as 'self', with the prospect of good long-term results.

When gene therapy (p. 355 ) has been proved to be both safe and effective, the immunological tolerance of the fetus should make it easier to commence such therapy before birth rather than afterwards. This will have the added advantage of reducing the period in which irreversible damage can occur in organs such as the central nervous system, which can be affected by progressive neurodegenerative disorders.

## FURTHER READING


Abramsky L, Chapple J (eds) 2003 Prenatal diagnosis: the human side. Nelson Thornes, Cheltenham, UK

*Dealing with the legal, emotional and ethical issues, this still contains a lot of medical information in a very readable format with interesting case studies.*

Brock D J H, Rodeck C H, Ferguson Smith M A (eds) 1992 Prenatal diagnosis and screening. Churchill Livingstone, Edinburgh

*A very comprehensive multiauthor textbook covering all aspects of prenatal diagnosis.*

Drife J O, Donnai D (eds) 1991 Antenatal diagnosis of fetal abnormalities. Springer-Verlag, London

*The proceedings of a workshop on the practical aspects of prenatal diagnosis.*

ESHRE PGD Steering Committee 2002 ESHRE Preimplantation Genetic Diagnosis Consortium: data collection III (May 2001). Human Reproduction 17: 233–246

*An up-to-date appraisal of the use of PGD.*

Lilford R J (ed) 1990 Prenatal diagnosis and prognosis. Butterworth–Heinemann, Oxford

*Provides useful information on recurrence risks for Down's syndrome, the prognosis for abnormalities detected by ultrasound, and decision analysis.*

Stranc L C, Evans J A, Hamerton J L 1997 Chorionic villus sampling and amniocentesis for prenatal diagnosis. Lancet 349: 711–714

*A good review of the practical and ethical aspects of the two main prenatal invasive diagnostic techniques.*

Whittle M J, Connor J M (eds) 1989 Prenatal diagnosis in obstetric practice. Blackwell, Oxford

*Describes prenatal diagnostic techniques and the types of abnormalities identified.*


## ELEMENTS

1. Prenatal diagnosis can be carried out by non-invasive procedures such as maternal serum α-fetoprotein screening for neural tube defects, the triple test and nuchal pad screening for Down syndrome, and ultrasonography for structural abnormalities.

2. Specific prenatal diagnosis of chromosome and single-gene disorders usually requires an invasive technique such as amniocentesis or chorionic villus sampling by which material of fetal origin can be obtained for analysis.

3. Invasive prenatal diagnostic procedures convey small risks for causing miscarriage, e.g. amniocentesis 0.5–1%, cordocentesis 1–2%, chorionic villus sampling 2–3%, fetoscopy 3–5%.

4. The commonest indication for prenatal diagnosis is advanced maternal age. Other indications include a family history of a chromosome, single-gene or structural abnormality, or an increased risk predicted on the result of a screening test.

5. While the significance of most prenatal diagnostic findings is clear, situations can arise in which the implications for the fetus are very difficult to predict. When this occurs the parents should be offered specialized genetic counseling.

CHAPTER

22

# Risk calculation

*"As far as the laws of mathematics refer to reality, they are not certain; and as far as they are certain, they do not refer to reality."*

Albert Einstein

One of the most important aspects of genetic counseling is the provision of a risk figure. This is often referred to as a recurrence risk. Estimation of the recurrence risk will usually require careful consideration and take into account:

1. the diagnosis and its mode of inheritance
2. analysis of the family pedigree
3. the results of tests that can include linkage studies using DNA markers.

Sometimes the provision of a risk figure can be quite easy, but in a surprisingly large number of situations complicating factors arise that can make the calculation very difficult. For example, the mother of a boy who is an isolated case of a sex-linked recessive disorder could very reasonably wish to know the recurrence risk for her next child. This is a very simple question, but the solution is far from straightforward, as will become clear later in this chapter.

Before proceeding any further, it is necessary to clarify what we mean by probability and review the different ways in which it can be expressed. The probability of an outcome can be defined as the number or, more correctly, the *proportion* of times it occurs in a large series of events. Conventionally, probability is indicated as a proportion of 1, so that a probability of 0 implies that an outcome will never be observed, whereas a probability of one implies that it will always be observed. Therefore a probability of 0.25 indicates that, on average, a particular outcome or event will be observed on 1 in 4 or 25% of occasions. The probability that the outcome will not occur is 0.75, which can also be expressed as 3 chances out of 4, or 75%. Alternatively, this probability could be expressed as odds of 3 to 1 against or 1 to 3 in favor of this particular outcome being observed. In this chapter fractions will be used where possible as these tend to be more easily understood than proportions of 1 expressed as decimals.

## PROBABILITY THEORY

In order to calculate genetic risks it is necessary to have a basic understanding of probability theory. This will be discussed in so far as it is relevant to the skills required for genetic counseling.

### LAWS OF ADDITION AND MULTIPLICATION

When considering the probability of two different events or outcomes, it is essential to clarify whether they are mutually exclusive or independent. If the events are mutually exclusive then the probability that *either* one or the other will occur equals the sum of their individual probabilities. This is known as the *law of addition*.

If, however, two or more events or outcomes are independent, then the probability that *both* the first and the second will occur equals the product of their individual probabilities. This is known as the law of multiplication.

As a simple illustration of these laws consider parents who have embarked upon their first pregnancy. The probability that the baby will be *either* a boy *or* a girl equals 1, i.e. $\frac{1}{2} + \frac{1}{2}$. If the mother is found on ultrasound scan to be carrying twins who are non-identical, then the probability that *both* the first *and* the second twin will be boys equals $\frac{1}{4}$, i.e. $\frac{1}{2} \times \frac{1}{2}$.

### BAYES' THEOREM

*Bayes' theorem*, which was first devised by the Reverend Bayes and published after his death in 1763, is widely used in genetic counseling. Essentially it provides a very valuable method for determining the overall probability of an event or outcome, such as carrier status, by considering all initial possibilities, e.g. carrier or non-carrier, and then modifying or 'conditioning' these by incorporating information, such as test results, that indicates which is the more likely.

The initial probability of each event is known as its *prior probability*, which is based on ancestral or *anterior information*. The observations that modify these prior

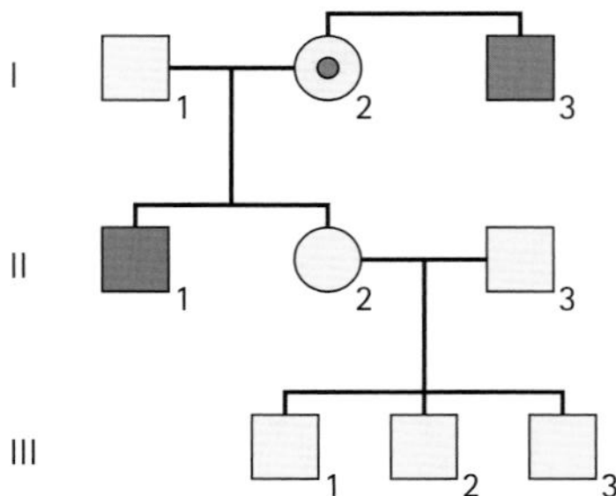


Fig. 22.1
A pedigree showing sex-linked recessive inheritance. When calculating the probability that $II_2$ is a carrier it is necessary to take into account her three unaffected sons.

**Table 22.1 Bayesian calculation for $II_2$ in Figure 22.1**

| Probability | $II_2$ is a carrier | $II_2$ is not a carrier |
|---|---|---|
| **Prior** | $\frac{1}{2}$ | $\frac{1}{2}$ |
| **Conditional** | | |
| Three healthy sons | $(\frac{1}{2})^3 = \frac{1}{8}$ | $(1)^3 = 1$ |
| **Joint** | $\frac{1}{6}$ | $\frac{1}{2}(= \frac{8}{16})$ |
| Expressed as odd | 1 to | 8 |
| **Posterior** | $\frac{1}{9}$ | $\frac{8}{9}$ |

probabilities allow *conditional probabilities* to be determined. In genetic counseling these are usually based on numbers of offspring and/or the results of tests. This is *posterior information*. The resulting probability for each event or outcome is known as its *joint probability*. The final probability for each event is known as its *posterior* or *relative probability* and is obtained by dividing the joint probability for that event by the sum of all the joint probabilities.

This is not an easy concept to grasp! To try to make it a little more comprehensible, consider a pedigree with two males, $I_3$ and $II_1$, who have a sex-linked recessive disorder (Fig. 22.1). The sister, $II_2$, of one of these men wishes to know the probability that she is a carrier. Her mother, $I_2$, must be a carrier as she has both an affected brother and an affected son, i.e. she is an obligate carrier. Therefore the prior probability that $II_2$ is a carrier equals $\frac{1}{2}$. Similarly, the prior probability that $II_2$ is not a carrier equals $\frac{1}{2}$.

The fact that $II_2$ already has three healthy sons must be taken into consideration, as intuitively this makes it rather unlikely that she is a carrier. Bayes' theorem provides a way to quantify this intuition. These three healthy sons provide posterior information. The conditional probability that $II_2$ would have three healthy sons if she is a carrier equals $\frac{1}{2} \times \frac{1}{2} \times \frac{1}{2}$, which equals $\frac{1}{8}$. These values of are multiplied as they are independent events in that the health of one son is not influenced by the health of his brother(s). The conditional probability that $II_2$ would have three healthy sons if she is not a carrier equals 1.

This information is now incorporated into a Bayesian calculation (Table 22.1). From this table the posterior probability that $II_2$ is a carrier equals $\frac{1}{16}/(\frac{1}{16} + \frac{1}{2})$, which reduces to $\frac{1}{9}$. Similarly the posterior probability that $II_2$ is not a carrier equals $\frac{1}{2}/(\frac{1}{16} + \frac{1}{2})$, which reduces to $\frac{8}{9}$. Another way to obtain these results is to consider that the odds for $II_2$ being a carrier versus not being a carrier are $\frac{1}{16}$ to $\frac{1}{2}$, i.e. 1 to 8, which equals 1 in 9. Thus by taking into account the fact that $II_2$ has three healthy sons, we have been able to reduce her risk of being a carrier from 1 in 2 to 1 in 9.

Perhaps by now the use of Bayes' theorem will be a little more clear. Try to remember that the basic approach is to draw up a table showing all of the possibilities (e.g. carrier, not a carrier), then establish the background (prior) risk for each possibility, next determine the chance (conditional possibility) that certain observed events (e.g. healthy children) would have happened if each possibility is true, then work out the combined (joint) likelihood for each possibility, and finally weigh up each of the joint probabilities to calculate the exact (posterior) probability for each of the original possibilities. If this is still confusing some of the following worked examples may bring a little more clarity!

## AUTOSOMAL DOMINANT INHERITANCE

For someone with an autosomal dominant disorder, the risk that each of his or her children will inherit the mutant gene equals 1 in 2. This will apply whether the affected individual inherited the disorder from a parent or developed the condition as the result of a new mutation. Therefore the provision of risks for disorders showing autosomal dominant inheritance is usually straightforward as long as there is a clear family history, the condition is characterized by being fully penetrant, and there is a reliable means of diagnosing heterozygotes. However, if penetrance is incomplete or if there is a delay in the age of onset so that heterozygotes cannot always be diagnosed, then risk calculation becomes more complicated. Two examples will be discussed to illustrate the sort of problem that can arise.

### REDUCED PENETRANCE

A disorder is said to show *reduced penetrance* when it has clearly been demonstrated that individuals who must possess the abnormal gene, who by pedigree analysis must be obligate heterozygotes, show absolutely no manifestations of the condition (p. 108). For example, if someone who was completely unaffected had both a parent and a child with the same autosomal dominant

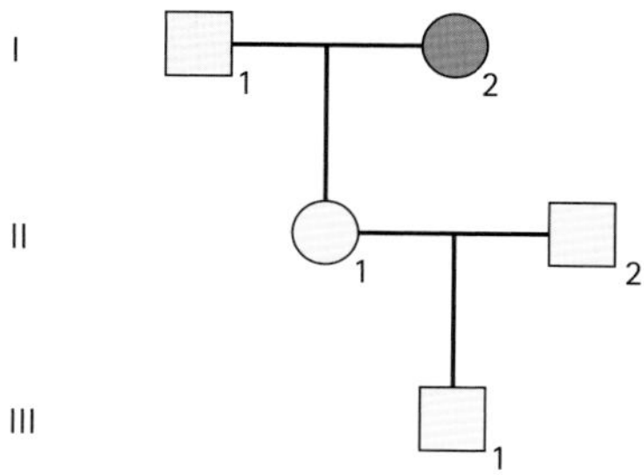


Fig. 22.2
$I_2$ has an autosomal dominant disorder which shows reduced penetrance. The probability that $III_1$ will be affected has to take into account the possibility that his mother ($II_1$) is a non-penetrant heterozygote.

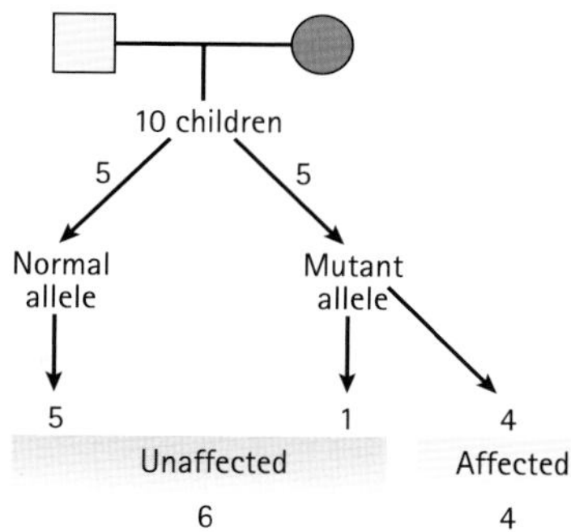


Fig. 22.3
The expected genotypes and phenotypes in ten children born to an individual with an autosomal dominant disorder with penetrance equal to 0.8.

disorder, then this would be an example of *non-penetrance*. Penetrance is usually quoted as a percentage, e.g. 80%, or as a proportion of 1, e.g. 0.8. This would imply that 80% of all heterozygotes express the condition in some way.

For a condition showing reduced penetrance, the risk that the child of an affected individual will be affected equals $\frac{1}{2}$, i.e. the probability that the child will inherit the mutant allele, × P, the proportion of heterozygotes who are affected. Therefore, for a disorder such as hereditary retinoblastoma, an embryonic eye tumor (p. 209), which shows dominant inheritance in some families with a penetrance of P = 0.8, the risk that the child of an affected parent will develop a tumor equals $\frac{1}{2} \times 0.8$, which equals 0.4.

A more difficult calculation arises when a risk is sought for the future child of someone who is healthy but whose parent has or had an autosomal dominant disorder showing reduced penetrance (Fig. 22.2).

Let us assume that the penetrance, P, equals 0.8. Calculation of the risk that $III_1$ will be affected can be approached in two ways. The first simply involves a little logic. The second utilizes Bayes' theorem.

1. Imagine that $I_2$ has 10 children. On average five children will inherit the gene but as P = 0.8 only four will be affected (Fig. 22.3). Therefore, six out of the 10 children will be unaffected, one of whom has the mutant allele with the remaining five having the normal allele. $II_1$ is unaffected so that there is therefore a probability of 1 in 6 that she is, in fact, a heterozygote. Consequently the probability that $III_1$ will both inherit the mutant gene and be affected equals $\frac{1}{6} \times \frac{1}{2} \times P$, which equals $\frac{1}{15}$ if P is 0.8.
2. Now consider $II_1$ in Figure 22.2. The prior probability that she is a heterozygote equals $\frac{1}{2}$. Similarly the prior probability that she is not a heterozygote equals $\frac{1}{2}$. Now a Bayesian table can be constructed to determine how these prior probabilities are modified by the fact that $II_1$ is not affected.

**Table 22.2 Bayesian calculation for $II_1$ in Figure 22.2**

| Probability | $II_1$ is heterozygous | $II_1$ is not heterozygous |
|---|---|---|
| **Prior** | $\frac{1}{2}$ | $\frac{1}{2}$ |
| **Conditional** | | |
| Not affected | 1 – P | 1 |
| **Joint** | $\frac{1}{2}(1 - P)$ | $\frac{1}{2}$ |

The posterior probability that $II_1$ is a heterozygote equals $\frac{1}{2}(1 - P)/[\frac{1}{2}(1 - P) + \frac{1}{2}]$, which reduces to $\frac{1-P}{2-P}$. Therefore, the risk that $III_1$ will both inherit the mutant allele and be affected equals $(\frac{1-P}{2-P}) \times \frac{1}{2} \times P$, which reduces to $\frac{(P-P^2)}{(4-2P)}$. If P equals 0.8, this expression equals $\frac{1}{15}$ or 0.067.

By substituting different values of P in the above expression, it can be shown that the maximum risk for $III_1$ being affected equals 0.086, approximately $\frac{1}{12}$, which is obtained when P equals 0.6. This maximal risk figure can be used when counseling persons at risk for late-onset autosomal disorders with reduced penetrance who have an affected grandparent and unaffected parents.

## DELAYED AGE OF ONSET

Many autosomal dominant disorders do not present until well into adult life. Healthy members of families in which these disorders are segregating often wish to know whether they themselves will develop the condition and/or pass it on to their children. Risks for these individuals can be calculated in the following way.

Consider someone who has died with a confirmed diagnosis of Huntington disease (Fig. 22.4). This is a late-onset autosomal dominant disorder. The son of $I_2$ is entirely healthy at age 50 years and wishes to know the probability that his 10-year-old daughter, $III_1$, will develop Huntington disease in later life. In this condition the first

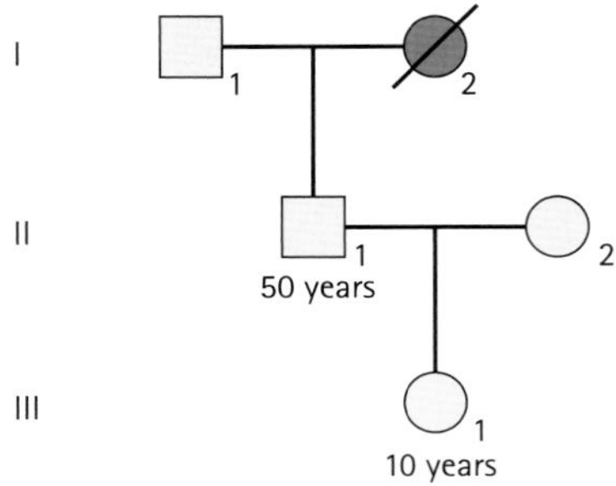


Fig. 22.4
$I_2$ had an autosomal dominant disorder showing delayed age of onset. When calculating the probability that $III_1$ will develop the disorder it is necessary to determine the probability that $II_1$ is a heterozygote who is not yet clinically affected.

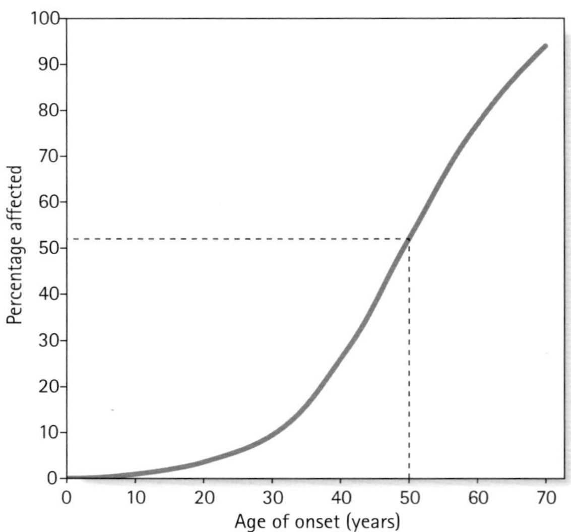


Fig. 22.5
Graph showing age of onset in years of clinical expression in Huntington disease heterozygotes. Approximately 50% show clinical signs or symptoms by age 50 years. (Data from Newcombe R G 1981 A life table for onset of Huntington's chorea. Ann Hum Genet 45: 375–385.)

signs usually appear between the ages of 30 and 60 years, and approximately 50% of all heterozygotes have shown signs by the age of 50 years (Fig. 22.5).

To answer the question about the risk to $III_1$ it is first necessary to calculate the risk for $II_1$ (if $III_1$ was asking about her own risk, her father might be referred to as the *dummy consultand*). The probability that $II_1$ has inherited the gene, given that he shows no signs of the condition, can be determined by a simple Bayesian calculation (Table 22.3).

The posterior probability that $II_1$ is heterozygous equals $\frac{1}{4}/(\frac{1}{4}+\frac{1}{2})$, which equals $\frac{1}{3}$. Therefore the prior probability that his daughter $III_1$ will have inherited the disorder equals $\frac{1}{3} \times \frac{1}{2}$, or $\frac{1}{6}$.

**Table 22.3 Bayesian calculation for $II_1$ in Figure 22.4**

| Probability | $II_1$ is heterozygous | $II_1$ is not heterozygous |
|---|---|---|
| Prior | $\frac{1}{2}$ | $\frac{1}{2}$ |
| Conditional | | |
| Unaffected at age 50 years | $\frac{1}{2}$ | 1 |
| Joint | $\frac{1}{4}$ | $\frac{1}{2}$ |

There is a temptation when doing calculations such as this to conclude that the overall risk for $II_1$ being a heterozygote simply equals $\frac{1}{2} \times \frac{1}{2}$, i.e. the prior probability that he will have inherited the mutant gene times the probability that a heterozygote will be unaffected at age 50 years, giving a risk of $\frac{1}{4}$. This is correct in as much as it gives the joint probability for this possible outcome, but it does not take into account the possibility that $II_1$ is not a heterozygote. Consider the possibility that $I_2$ has four children. On average two will inherit the mutant allele, one of whom will be affected by the age of 50 years. The remaining two children will not inherit the mutant allele. By the time these children have grown up and reached the age of 50 years, on average one will be affected and three will not. Therefore, on average one-third of the healthy 50-year-old offspring of $I_2$ will be heterozygotes. Hence the correct risk for $II_1$ is $\frac{1}{3}$ and not $\frac{1}{4}$.

## AUTOSOMAL RECESSIVE INHERITANCE

With an autosomal recessive condition, the *biological* parents of an affected child are both heterozygotes. Apart from undisclosed non-paternity and donor insemination, there are two possible exceptions, both of which are very rare. These arise when only one parent is a heterozygote, in which case a child can be affected if either a new mutation occurs on the gamete inherited from the other parent, or uniparental disomy occurs resulting in the child inheriting two copies of the heterozygous parent's mutant allele (p. 117). For practical purposes it is usually assumed that both parents of an affected child are carriers.

### CARRIER RISKS FOR THE EXTENDED FAMILY

When both parents are heterozygotes, the risk that each of their children will be affected equals 1 in 4. On average three of their four children will be unaffected, of whom, on average, two will be carriers (Fig. 22.6). Therefore the probability that the healthy sibling of someone with an autosomal recessive disorder will be a carrier equals $\frac{2}{3}$.

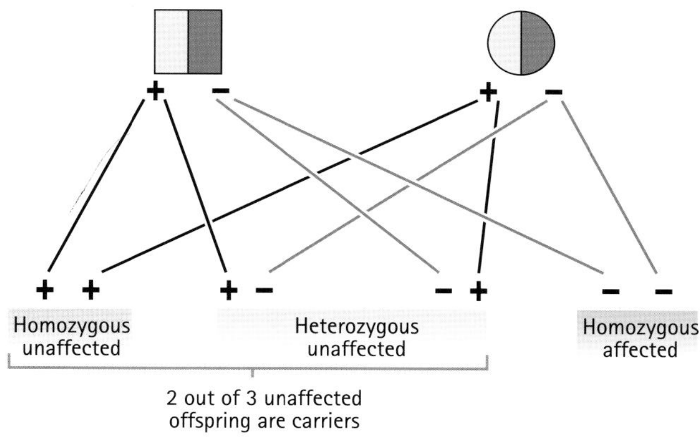


Fig. 22.6
The possible genotypes and phenotypes in the offspring of parents who are both carriers of an autosomal recessive disorder. On average two out of three healthy offspring are carriers.

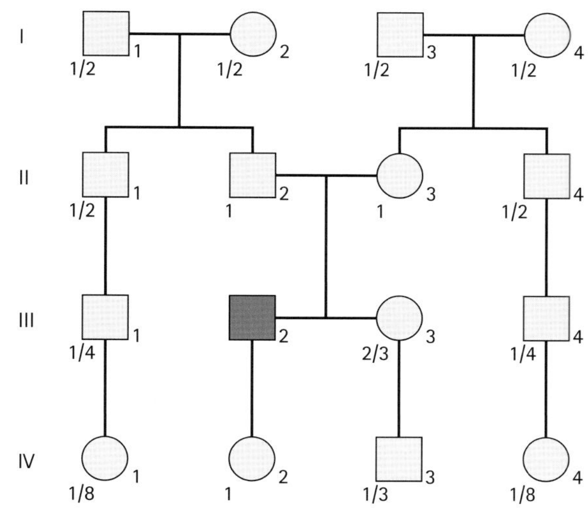


Fig. 22.7
Autosomal recessive inheritance. The probabilities that various family members are carriers are indicated as fractions.

Carrier risks can be derived for other family members, starting with the assumption that both parents of an affected child are carriers (Fig. 22.7).

When calculating risks in autosomal recessive inheritance the underlying principle is to establish the probability that each prospective parent is a carrier, and then multiply the product of these probabilities by $\frac{1}{4}$, this being the risk that any child born to two carriers will be affected. Therefore, in Figure 22.7, if the sister, $III_3$, of the affected boy was to marry her first cousin, $III_4$, then the probability that their first baby would be affected would equal $\frac{2}{3} \times \frac{1}{4} \times \frac{1}{4}$, i.e. the probability that $III_3$ is a carrier times the probability that $III_4$ is a carrier times the probability that a child of two carriers will be affected. This gives a total risk of $\frac{1}{24}$.

If this same sister, $III_3$, was to marry a healthy unrelated individual, the probability that their first child would be affected would equal $\frac{2}{3} \times 2pq \times \frac{1}{4}$, i.e. the probability that $III_3$ is a carrier times the carrier frequency in the general population (p. 126) times the probability that a child of two carriers will be affected. For a condition such as cystic fibrosis, with a disease incidence of approximately 1 in 5000, $q^2 = \frac{1}{2500}$ and therefore $q = \frac{1}{50}$ and thus $2pq = \frac{1}{25}$. Therefore, the final risk would be $\frac{2}{3} \times \frac{1}{25} \times \frac{1}{4}$ or 1 in 150.

## MODIFYING A CARRIER RISK BY MUTATION ANALYSIS

Population screening for cystic fibrosis is currently being introduced in the UK following a number of pilot studies (p. 324). More than 1300 different mutations have been identified in the cystic fibrosis gene, so that carrier detection by DNA mutation analysis is not straightforward. However, a relatively simple test has been developed for the most common mutations that enables about 90% of all carriers of Western European origin to be detected. What is the probability that a healthy individual who has no family history of cystic fibrosis and who tests negative on the common mutation screen is a carrier?

**Table 22.4 Bayesian table for cystic fibrosis carrier risk if common mutation screen is negative**

| Probability | Carrier | Not a carrier |
|---|---|---|
| **Prior** | $\frac{1}{25}$ | $\frac{24}{25}$ |
| **Conditional** | | |
| Normal result on common mutation screening | 0.10 | 1 |
| **Joint** | $\frac{1}{250}$ | $\frac{24}{25}$ |

The answer is obtained once again by drawing up a simple Bayesian table (Table 22.4). The prior probability that this healthy member of the general population is a carrier equals $\frac{1}{25}$; therefore the prior probability that he or she is not a carrier equals $\frac{24}{25}$. If this individual is a carrier, then the probability that the common mutation test will be normal is 0.10 as only 10% of carriers do not have a common mutation. The probability that someone who is not a carrier will have a normal common mutation test result is 1.

This gives a joint probability for being a carrier of 1/250 and for not being a carrier of $\frac{24}{25}$. Therefore the posterior probability that this individual is a carrier equals $\frac{1}{250}/\frac{1}{250} + \frac{24}{25}$, which equals $\frac{1}{241}$. Thus the normal result on common mutation testing has reduced the carrier risk from $\frac{1}{25}$ to $\frac{1}{241}$.

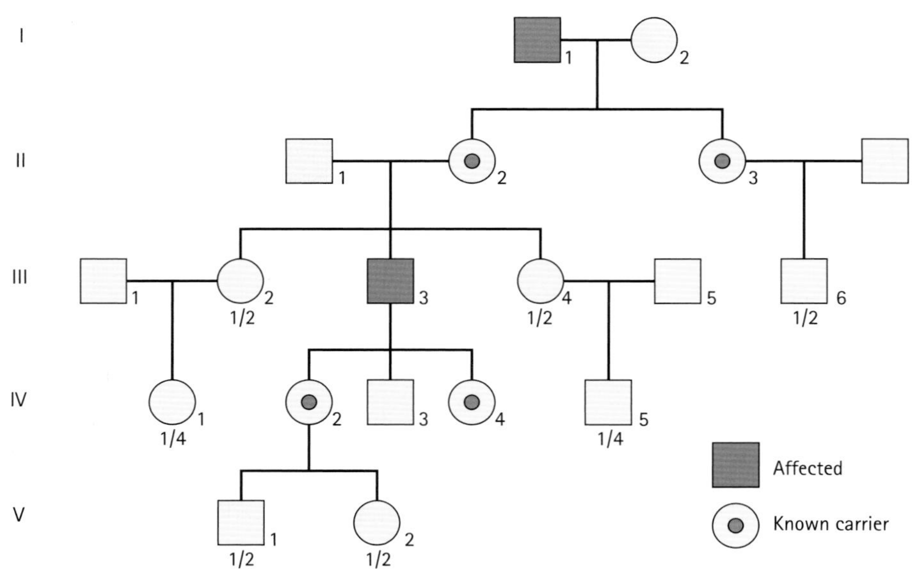


**Fig. 22.8**
The probabilities of male relatives being affected and female relatives being carriers of an X-linked recessive disorder. All the daughters of an affected male are obligate carriers.

## SEX-LINKED RECESSIVE INHERITANCE

This pattern of inheritance tends to generate the most complicated risk calculations when counseling for Mendelian disorders. In severe sex-linked conditions, affected males are often unable to have their own children. Consequently, these conditions are usually transmitted only by healthy female carriers. The carrier of a sex-linked recessive disorder transmits the gene on average to half of her daughters, who are therefore carriers, and to half of her sons who will thus be affected. If an affected male does have children, then he will transmit his Y chromosome to all of his sons, who will be unaffected, and his X chromosome to all of his daughters, who will be carriers (Fig. 22.8).

An example of how the birth of unaffected sons to a possible carrier of a sex-linked disorder results in a reduction of her carrier risk has already been discussed in the introductory section on Bayes' theorem (p. 341). In this section we shall consider two further factors that can complicate risk calculation in sex-linked recessive disorders.

### THE ISOLATED CASE

If a woman has only one affected son, then in the absence of a positive family history there are three possible ways in which this can have occurred:

1. The woman is a carrier of the mutant allele, in which case there is a risk of $\frac{1}{2}$ that any future son will be affected.
2. The disorder in the son arose as a new mutation that occurred during meiosis in the gamete that led to his conception. The recurrence risk in this situation is negligible.
3. The woman is a *gonadal mosaic* for the mutation that occurred in an early mitotic division during her own embryonic development. The recurrence risk will be equal to the proportion of ova that carry the mutant allele, i.e. between 0% and 50%.

In practice it is often very difficult to distinguish between these three possibilities unless reliable tests are available for carrier detection. If a woman is found to be a carrier then risk calculation is straightforward. If the tests indicate that she is not a carrier, then the recurrence risk is probably low, but not negligible because of the possibility of *gonadal mosaicism*.

For example, in Duchenne muscular dystrophy it has been estimated that among the mothers of isolated cases approximately two-thirds are carriers, 5–10% are gonadal mosaics, and in the remaining 25–30% the disorder has arisen as a new mutation in meiosis.

Leaving aside the complicating factor of gonadal mosaicism, risk calculation in the context of an isolated case (Fig. 22.9) is possible but may require calculating the risk for a *dummy consultand* within the pedigree as well as taking account of the *mutation rate*, or $\mu$. For a fuller understanding of $\mu$ the student is referred to one of the more detailed texts listed at the end of the chapter.

### INCORPORATING CARRIER TEST RESULTS

Several biochemical tests are available for detecting carriers of sex-linked recessive disorders. Unfortunately, there is often overlap in the values obtained for controls and women known to be carriers, i.e. obligate carriers. Although an abnormal result in a potential carrier would suggest that she is likely to be a carrier, a normal test result does not exclude a woman being a carrier. While

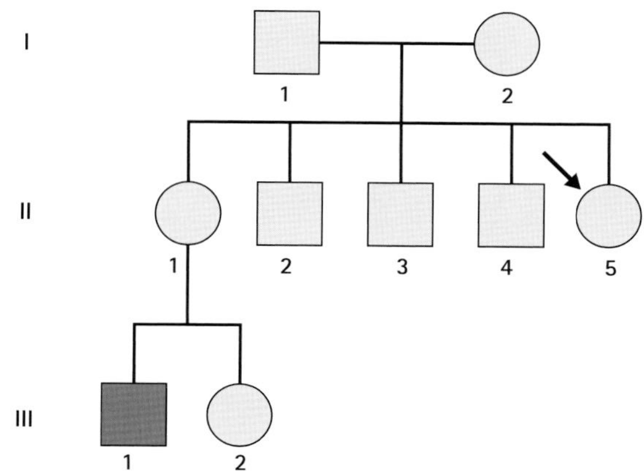


Fig. 22.9
In this pedigree $III_1$ is affected by Duchenne muscular dystrophy and is an isolated case, i.e. there is no history of the condition in the wider family. The consultand, $II_5$ (arrowed), wishes to know whether she is at risk of having affected sons. To calculate her risk, the risk that her mother, I.2, is a carrier is first calculated, which requires consideration of the mutation rate, μ.1.2 is the *dummy consultand* in this scenario.

**Table 22.5 Bayesian calculation for $II_2$ in Figure 22.1**

| Probability | $II_2$ is a carrier | $II_2$ is not a carrier |
|---|---|---|
| **Prior** | $\frac{1}{2}$ | $\frac{1}{2}$ |
| **Conditional** | | |
| Three healthy sons | $\frac{1}{8}$ | 1 |
| Normal creatine kinase | $\frac{1}{3}$ | 1 |
| **Joint** | $\frac{1}{48}$ | $\frac{1}{2}$ |

for many sex-linked recessive disorders this problem can be overcome by using linked DNA markers (pp. 73, 317), the difficulties presented by overlapping biochemical test results arise sufficiently often to justify further consideration.

For example, in Duchenne muscular dystrophy, serum creatine kinase is elevated in approximately two out of three obligate carriers (Fig. 20.1, p. 316). Therefore, if a possible carrier such as $II_2$ in Figure 22.1 is found to have a normal level of creatine kinase, this would provide further support for her not being a carrier. The test result therefore provides a conditional probability, which is included in a new Bayesian calculation (Table 22.5).

The posterior probability that $II_2$ is a carrier equals $\frac{1}{48}/(\frac{1}{48} + \frac{1}{2})$ or $\frac{1}{25}$. Consequently, by taking into account firstly this woman's three healthy sons and secondly her normal creatine kinase test result it has been possible to reduce her carrier risk from 1 in 2 to 1 in 9 and then to 1 in 25.

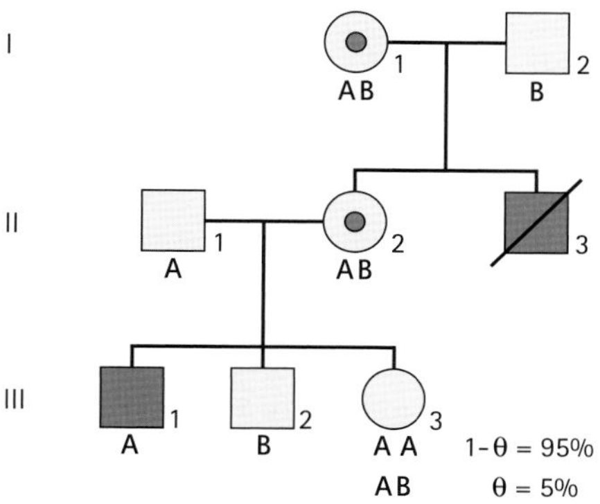


Fig. 22.10
A pedigree showing sex-linked recessive inheritance. A and B represent alleles at a locus closely linked to the disease locus.

## THE USE OF LINKED MARKERS

As a result of the developments which have taken place in molecular biology over the last 15 years, most of the more common single-gene disorders have been mapped to the human genome (p. 79). For many conditions the gene has been isolated and characterized so that specific mutation analysis is available.

This now applies to disorders such as Huntington disease and cystic fibrosis, and is also the case for many families in which Duchenne muscular dystrophy is present. However, in conditions such as Duchenne muscular dystrophy in which each family usually has its own unique mutation, direct mutation analysis is not always possible if, for example, there are no surviving affected males. In these families DNA markers at a locus closely linked to the disease locus can be used to assist in carrier detection.

As an illustration of the potential value of this approach, consider the sister of a boy affected with Duchenne muscular dystrophy, whose mother is an obligate carrier as she herself had an affected brother (Fig. 22.10).

A DNA marker with alleles A and B is available and is known to be closely linked to the DMD disease locus with a recombination fraction (θ) equal to 0.05 (p. 132). The disease allele must be in coupling with the A marker allele in $II_2$ as this woman has inherited both the A allele and the DMD allele on the X chromosome from her mother (she must have inherited the B allele from her father, so the A allele must have come from her mother). Therefore, if $III_3$ inherits this A allele from her mother, the probability that she will also inherit the disease allele and be a carrier equals 1 – θ, i.e. the probability that a crossover will not have occurred between the disease and marker loci in the meiosis of the ova that resulted in her conception. For a value of θ equal to 0.05 this gives a carrier risk of 0.95 or 95%. Similarly, the probability that

$III_3$ will be a carrier if she inherits the B allele from her mother equals 0.05 or 5%.

Closely linked DNA markers are now available for most single-gene disorders, and these are widely used in genetic counseling for carrier detection and prenatal diagnosis when direct mutation testing is not available. The smaller the value of θ, then the smaller the likelihood of a predictive error. If DNA markers are available that 'bridge' or 'flank' the disease locus, this greatly reduces the risk of a predictive error as only a double crossover will go undetected, and the probability of a double crossover is extremely low.

## BAYES' THEOREM AND PRENATAL SCREENING

As a further illustration of the potential value of Bayes' theorem in risk calculation and genetic counseling, an example from prenatal screening will be given. Consider the situation that arises when a woman aged 20 years presents at 13 weeks gestation with a fetus that has been shown on ultrasound scanning to have significant nuchal translucency (NT). NT may be present in about 75% of fetuses with Down syndrome (p. 331). In contrast the incidence in babies not affected with Down syndrome is approximately 5%. In other words NT is 15 times more common in Down syndrome than in unaffected babies.

Question. Does this mean that the odds are 15 to 1 that this unborn baby has Down syndrome? No! This risk, or more precisely *odds ratio*, would only be correct if the prior probabilities that the baby would be affected or unaffected were equal. In reality the prior probability that the baby will be unaffected is much greater than the prior probability that it will have Down syndrome.

Actual values for these prior probabilities can be obtained by reference to a table showing maternal age specific risks for Down syndrome (Table 18.4, p. 272). For a woman aged 20 years the incidence of Down syndrome is approximately 1 in 1500: hence the prior probability that the baby will be unaffected equals $\frac{1499}{1500}$. If these prior probability values are used in a Bayesian calculation then it can be shown that the posterior probability that the unborn baby will have Down syndrome is approximately 1 in 100 (Table 22.6). Obviously, this is much lower than the conditional odds of 15 to 1 in favor of the baby being affected.

In practice the demonstration of NT on ultrasound in a fetus would usually prompt an offer of definitive chromosome analysis by placental biopsy, amniocentesis or fetal blood sampling (Ch. 21). This example of NT has been used to emphasize that an observed conditional probability ratio should always be combined with a knowledge of the prior probabilities to obtain a correct indication of the actual risk.

**Table 22.6 Bayesian calculation to show the posterior probability that a fetus with nuchal translucency conceived by a 20-year-old mother will have Down syndrome**

| Probability | Fetus unaffected | Fetus affected |
|---|---|---|
| **Prior** | $\frac{1499}{1500}$ | $\frac{1}{1500}$ |
| **Conditional** | | |
| Nuchal translucency | 1 | 15 |
| **Joint** | $\frac{1499}{1500} = 1$ | $\frac{1}{100}$ |
| Expressed as odds | 100 to | 1 |
| Posterior | $\frac{100}{101}$ | $\frac{1}{101}$ |

## EMPIRIC RISKS

Up to this point risks have been calculated for single-gene disorders using knowledge of basic Mendelian genetics and applied probability theory. In many counseling situations it is not possible to arrive at an accurate risk figure in this way, either because the disorder in question does not show single-gene inheritance or because the clinical diagnosis with which the family has been referred shows causal heterogeneity (p. 109). In these situations it is usually necessary to resort to the use of observed or *empiric risks*. These are based on observations derived from family studies rather than theoretical calculations.

### MULTIFACTORIAL DISORDERS

One of the basic principles of multifactorial inheritance is that the risk of recurrence in first-degree relatives, siblings and offspring, equals the square root of the incidence of the disease in the general population (p. 140), i.e. $P^{\frac{1}{2}}$, where P equals the general population incidence. For example, if the general population incidence equals $\frac{1}{1000}$, then the theoretical risk to a first-degree relative equals the square root of $\frac{1}{1000}$, which approximates to 1 in 32 or 3%. The theoretical risks for second- and third-degree relatives can be shown to approximate to $P^{\frac{3}{4}}$ and $P^{\frac{7}{8}}$ respectively. Therefore, if there is strong support for multifactorial inheritance, it is reasonable to use these theoretical risks when counseling close family relatives.

However, when using this approach it is important to remember that the confirmation of multifactorial inheritance will often have been based on the study of observed recurrence risks. Consequently it is generally more appropriate to refer back to the original family studies and counsel on the basis of the risks derived in these (Table 22.7).

**Table 22.7 Empiric recurrence risks for common multifactorial disorders**

| Disorder | Incidence (per 1000) | Sex ratio (M:F) | Unaffected parents having a second affected child (%) | Affected parents having an affected child (%) |
|---|---|---|---|---|
| Cleft lip ± cleft palate | 1–2 | 3:2 | 4 | 4 |
| Club foot (talipes) | 1–2 | 2:1 | 3 | 3 |
| Congenital heart defects | 8 | 1:1 | 1–4 | 2 (father affected)<br>6 (mother affected) |
| Congenital dislocation of the hip | 1 | 1:6 | 6 | 12 |
| Hypospadias (in males) | 2 | – | 10 | 10 |
| Manic–depressive psychosis | 4 | 2:3 | 10–15 | 10–15 |
| Neural tube defects | | | | |
| Anencephaly | 1.5 | 1:2 | 4–5 | – |
| Spina bifida | 2.5 | 2:3 | 4–5 | 4 |
| Pyloric stenosis | | | | |
| Male index | 2.5 | – | 2 | 4 |
| Female index | 0.5 | – | 10 | 17 |
| Schizophrenia | 10 | 1:1 | 10 | 14 |

**Table 22.8 Empiric recurrence risks for conditions showing causal heterogeneity**

| Disorder | Incidence (per 1000) | Sex ratio (M:F) | Unaffected parents having a second affected child (%) | Affected parents having an affected child (%) |
|---|---|---|---|---|
| Autism | 0:2 | 4:1 | 2–3 | – |
| Epilepsy (idiopathic) | 5 | 1:1 | 5 | 5 |
| Hydrocephalus | 0.5 | 1:1 | 3 | – |
| Mental retardation (idiopathic) | 3 | 1:1 | 3–5 | 10 |
| Profound childhood sensorineural deafness | 1 | 1:1 | 10–15 | 5–10 |

Ideally, reference should be made to local studies as recurrence risks can differ quite substantially in different communities, ethnic groups, and geographical locations. For example, the recurrence risk for neural tube defects in siblings is quoted as 4%. This is essentially an average risk. The actual risk varies from 2 to 3% in south-east England up to 8% in Northern Ireland, and also shows an inverse relationship with the family's socioeconomic status, being greatest for mothers in poorest circumstances.

Unfortunately empiric risks are rarely available for families in which there are several affected family members or for disorders with variable severity or different sex incidences. A computer program has been devised that allows theoretical estimates to be made in many of these more complex situations.

## CONDITIONS SHOWING CAUSAL HETEROGENEITY

Many referrals to genetic clinics relate to a clinical phenotype rather than to a precise underlying diagnosis (Table 22.8). In these situations great care must be taken to ensure that all appropriate diagnostic investigations have been undertaken before resorting to the use of empiric risk data (p. 263).

It is worth emphasizing that the use of empiric risks for conditions such as sensorineural hearing loss in childhood is at best a compromise, as the figure quoted to an individual family will rarely be the correct one for their particular diagnosis. Severe sensorineural hearing loss in a young child is usually caused by either single-gene inheritance, most commonly autosomal recessive but occasionally autosomal dominant or sex-linked recessive, or by an environmental condition such as rubella embryopathy. Therefore, for most families the correct risk of recurrence will be either 25% or 0%. In practice it is often not possible to establish the precise cause so that the only option available is to offer the family an empiric or 'average' risk.

## FURTHER READING


Bayes T 1958 An essay towards solving a problem in the doctrine of chances. Biometrika 45: 296–315
*A reproduction of the Reverend Bayes' original essay on probability theory that was first published, posthumously, in 1763.*

Emery A E H 1986 Methodology in medical genetics, 2nd edn. Churchill Livingstone, Edinburgh
*An introduction to statistical methods of analysis in human and medical genetics.*

Murphy E A, Chase G A 1975 Principles of genetic counseling. Year Book Medical Publications, Chicago
*A very thorough explanation of the use of Bayes' theorem in genetic counseling.*

Young I D 1999 Introduction to risk calculation in genetic counselling, 2nd edn. Oxford University Press, Oxford
*A short introductory guide to all aspects of risk calculation in genetic counseling. Highly recommended!*


## ELEMENTS

1. Risk calculation in genetic counseling requires a knowledge and understanding of basic probability theory. Bayes' theorem enables initial background 'prior' risks to be modified by 'conditional' information to give an overall probability or risk for a particular event such as carrier status.

2. For disorders showing autosomal dominant inheritance it is often necessary to consider factors such as reduced penetrance and delayed age of onset. For disorders showing autosomal recessive inheritance, risks to offspring are determined by calculating the probability that each parent is a carrier and then multiplying the product of these probabilities by $\frac{1}{4}$.

3. In sex-linked recessive inheritance a particular problem arises if only one male in a family is affected. The results of carrier tests that show overlap between carriers and non-carriers can be incorporated in a Bayesian calculation.

4. Polymorphic DNA markers linked to the disease locus can be used in many single-gene disorders for carrier detection, preclinical diagnosis and prenatal diagnosis.

5. Empiric (observed) risks are available for multifactorial disorders and for etiologically heterogeneous conditions such as non-syndromal sensorineural hearing loss.

CHAPTER 23

# The Human Genome Project, treatment of genetic disease and gene therapy

*"So little done. So much to do."*

Alexander Graham Bell

## THE HUMAN GENOME PROJECT

### BEGINNING AND ORGANIZATION OF THE HUMAN GENOME PROJECT

The concept of a map of the human genome was proposed as long ago as 1969 by Victor McKusick (Fig. 1.5, p. 7), one of the founding fathers of medical genetics. Human gene mapping workshops were held regularly from 1973 to collate the mapping data. The human genome project as an entity in its own right had its beginnings in a workshop held in Alta, Utah, under the auspices of the US Department of Energy (DOE) in 1984. The involvement of the DOE might at first appearance seem odd, but they had historically been interested in the detection of mutations in DNA to assess the effects of exposure to radiation and chemicals. A subsequent report on the technologies involved in detecting mutations in DNA and a further international meeting organized by the DOE held in 1986 at Sante Fe, New Mexico, led to the idea of a dedicated human genome project. The DOE in the following year produced a report on the Human Genome Initiative outlining the major objectives.

In the subsequent year the United States Congress approved a 15-year US Human Genome Project, which started in 1991 with an estimated budget of 200 million US dollars per annum. Other nations, notably France, the UK and Japan, soon followed with their own major national human genome programs and have subsequently been joined by a number of other countries. These individual national projects are all coordinated by the Human Genome Organization (HUGO). which has three centers, one for the Americas based in Bethesda, Maryland, one for Europe located in London, and one for the Pacific in Tokyo.

The US Human Genome Project (HGP) is run jointly under the auspices of the National Institute of Health's National Center for Human Genome Research (NCHGR), initially headed by James Watson, who was succeeded by Francis Collins, and the DOE through the National Laboratories at Lawrence Livermore, Lawrence Berkeley and Los Alamos.

### OBJECTIVES OF THE HUMAN GENOME PROJECT

Many persons, particularly the general public, have the impression that the only objective of the Human Genome Project is to sequence all $3\times10^9$ base pairs of the human genome. This is, however, only one of the six main objectives/areas of work of the Human Genome Project.

#### Human gene maps and mapping of human inherited diseases

Designated genome mapping centers with earmarked funding were involved in the coordination and production of genetic or recombination and physical maps of the human genome. The genetic maps initially involved the production of fairly low-level resolution index, skeleton or framework maps, which were based on polymorphic variable number di-, tri- and tetranucleotide tandem repeats (p. 18) spaced at approximately 10 cM intervals throughout the genome. The most recent high-level resolution maps have polymorphic markers that are, on average, spaced at intervals of less than 1 cM.

The mapping information from these genetic maps has been integrated with high-resolution physical maps (Fig. 23.1). The information for the latter maps comes from a variety of sources using a number of different technologies that include fluorescent in situ hybridization

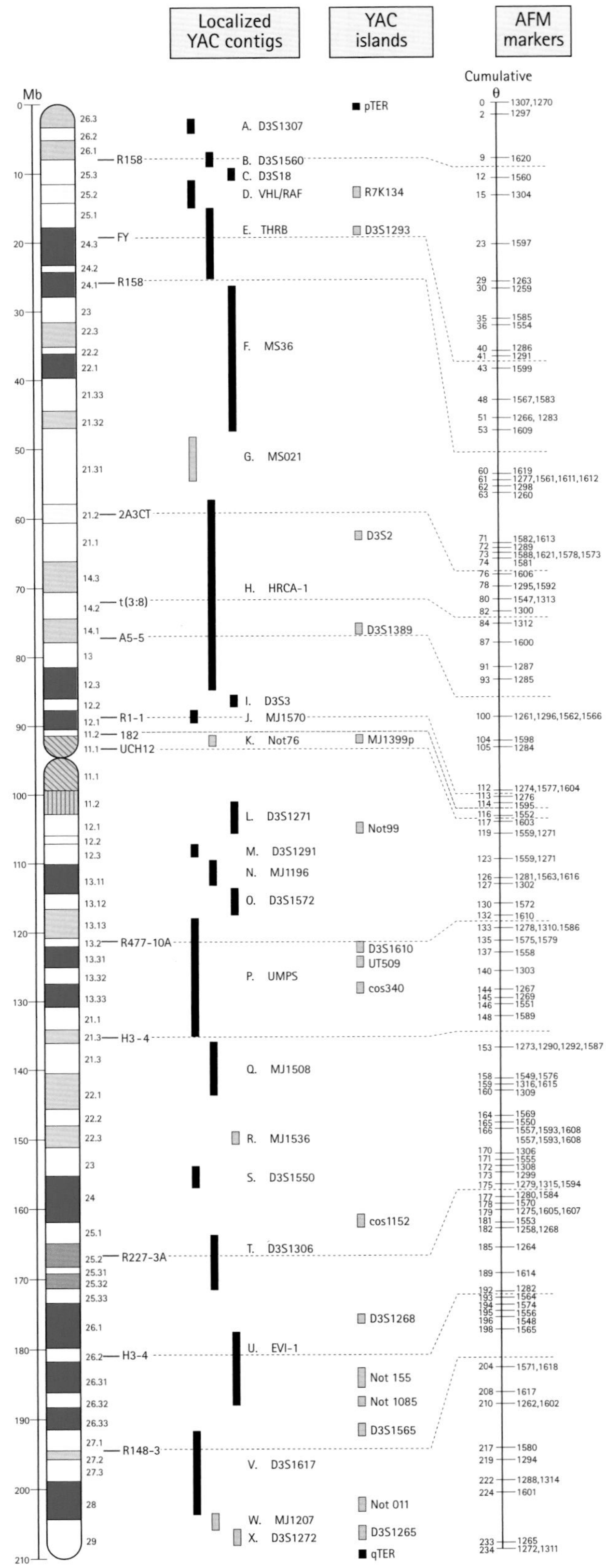


Fig. 23.1
A summary map of human chromosome 3, estimated to be 210 Mb in size, which integrates physical mapping data covered by 24 YAC contigs and the Genethon genetic map with cumulative map distances. (From Gemmill R M, Chumakov I, Scott P et al 1995 A second-generation YAC contig map of human chromosome 3. Nature 377: 299–319, with permission.)

(FISH) (p. 35), somatic cell and radiation hybrids (p. 75), and YAC or cosmid contigs (p. 76). Access to the detailed information from these high-resolution genetic and physical maps allows individual research groups, often interested in a specific or particular inherited disease or group of diseases, to rapidly and precisely localize or map a disease gene to a specific region of a chromosome. The presence of CpG islands (p. 77), exon trapping (p. 77) and/or expressed sequence tags (ESTs) (p. 77) can be used to identify coding sequences in the region involved. Along with the known genes or ESTs, which map to the region, these can then serve as positional candidate genes (p. 81) for analysis to determine whether they are responsible for an inherited disorder.

## Development of new DNA technologies

A second major objective is the development of new DNA technologies for human genome research. For example, at the outset of the Human Genome Project, the technology involved in DNA sequencing was very time consuming, laborious and relatively expensive. The development of high-throughput automated capillary sequencers and robust fluorescent sequencing kits has helped transform the ease and cost of large-scale DNA sequencing projects. Future developments in the use of DNA microarray technology are likely to further revolutionize analytical applications of the information from the Human Genome Sequence Project.

## Sequencing of the human genome

While sequencing the entire human genome would have been seen to be the obvious main focus of the Human Genome Project, it was not initially the straightforward proposal it seemed. The human genome contains large sections of repetitive DNA (p. 18) that are often technically difficult to clone and sequence. In addition, it would seem a waste of time to collect sequence data on the entire genome when only a small proportion is made up of expressed sequences or genes, the latter being most likely to be the regions of greatest medical and biological importance. Furthermore, the sheer magnitude of the prospect of sequencing all $3 \times 10^9$ base pairs of the human genome seemed overwhelming. With conventional sequencing technology, as was carried out in the early 1990s, it was estimated that a single laboratory worker could sequence up to approximately 2000 base pairs per day. This would mean that it would have taken $1.5 \times 10^6$ person-days to sequence the whole of the human genome!

Projects involving sequencing of other organisms with smaller genomes have shown how much work is involved as well as how the rate of producing sequence data has increased with the development of new DNA technologies. For example, initial efforts at producing genome sequence data for yeast took an international collaboration involving 35 laboratories in 17 countries from when it was started in 1989 until 1995 to sequence just 315 000 base pairs of chromosome 3, one of the 16 chromosomes which make up the 14 million base pairs of the yeast genome. Advances in the DNA technologies meant, however, that by the middle of 1995 more than one-half of the yeast genome had been sequenced, with the complete genomic sequence being reported the following year.

Further advances in DNA sequencing technology have resulted in the reporting of the full sequence of the nematode *C. elegans* in 1998, the 50 million base pairs of the DNA sequence of human chromosome 22 at the end of 1999, and the sequence of the 125 million base pairs of the fruit fly in early 2000, the latter some 3 years ahead of schedule. As a consequence of these technical developments, the 'working draft' sequence covering 90% of the human genome was announced on 26 June 2000, followed by publication in *Nature* in February 2001. The finished sequence (>99% coverage) was announced more than 2 years ahead of schedule in April 2003, the 50th anniversary of the discovery of the DNA double helix. Researchers now have access to the full catalog of approximately 30 000 genes and the human genome sequence will underpin biomedical research for decades to come.

This portion of the Human Genome Project has been associated with much controversy. Substantial sums of public money have been dedicated to the sequencing of the human genome, with involvement of a number of centers and the sequence information generated being freely available to the scientific community. The strategy being used was to carry out the DNA sequencing on an ordered modular basis, i.e. different groups concentrating on specific chromosomes, with the sequencing being carried on a clone-by-clone basis using the mapping information previously generated.

The approach of the commercial sector to the sequencing of the human genome has been, perhaps not surprisingly, different. Rather than the modular approach, they suggested it was simpler and more efficient just to 'shotgun' sequence the whole of the human genome at random and then to take the sequence information generated and assemble it by means of a computer program that recognizes overlapping DNA sequences. This approach was assisted by information deposited in the public domain databases that allowed the sequences to be positioned on the map. In addition, although the commercial sector originally indicated that they would release the DNA sequence information they generated into the public domain (Appendix: GenBank), they have maintained that they have the right to release this information on a 'non-redistribution' basis, i.e. that they should have the right to sell the human genome sequence information they generated. They argue that it is reasonable for them to expect commercial returns on their investment, which would be likely to result from the identification of novel genes that would allow elucidation of the role of their gene products in biological pathways involved in health and disease, with the potential for the development of diagnostic tools and pharmacological therapeutic interventions. This is an area of controversy that also involves ethical and social aspects and will not easily be resolved. Meanwhile the human genome sequence is freely available within public domain databases.

Although the Human Genome Sequencing Project is complete, a number of new projects have been initiated as a direct consequence, including the Cancer Genome Project and the HapMap Project. The goal of the International HapMap Project is to develop a haplotype map of the human genome, the HapMap, which will describe the common DNA sequence variants present in 270 individuals from various populations. The HapMap is expected to provide a key resource for research into genes affecting health, disease and response to drugs.

## Development of bioinformatics

Essential to the overall success of the Human Genome Project is what is known as bioinformatics – the establishment of facilities for collecting, storing, organizing, interpreting, analyzing and communicating the data from the project, which can be widely shared by the scientific community at large. It is vital for anyone involved in any aspect of the Human Genome Project to have rapid and easy access to the data/information arising from it. This dissemination of information has been met by the establishment of a large number of electronic databases available on the World Wide Web (WWW) on the Internet (Appendix). These include protein and DNA sequence databases (for example GenBank and EMBL), databases of genetic maps for humans (such as the GDB, Genethon, CEPH, CHLC and the Whitehead Institute sites) and other species (the Mouse Genome Database and the *Caenorhabditis elegans* database), linkage analysis programs (e.g. the Rockefeller University website), annotated genome data (Ensembl and UCSC Genome Bioinformatics) and the catalog of inherited diseases in humans (Online Mendelian Inheritance in Man, or OMIM). The latter was first set up as a computer-based information system by Victor McKusick more than 30 years ago.

These developments in bioinformatics now allow the prospect of identifying coding sequences and determining their likely function(s) from homologies to known genes, leading to the prospect of identifying a new gene without the need for any laboratory experimental work, or what has been called 'cloning in silico'.

### Comparative genomics

In addition to the Human Genome Project, there are separate genome projects for a number of other species, for what are known as 'model organisms'. These include various prokaryotic organisms such as the bacteria *Escherichia coli* and *Haemophilus influenzae*, as well as eukaryotic organisms such as *Saccharomyces cerevisiae* (yeast), *Caenorhabditis elegans* (flatworm), *Drosophila melanogaster* (fruit fly), *Mus musculus* (mouse), *Rattus norvegicus* (rat), *Fugu rubripes rupripes* (puffer fish), mosquito and zebrafish. While the impact of what is called *comparative genomics* is not necessarily immediately obvious, it is of vital importance in the Human Genome Project.

For example, the availability of the total genome sequence of yeast revealed it to contain a total of approximately 6000 genes, only some 2300 of which had been previously identified from traditional genetic studies in yeast. In addition, of the 3700 new genes identified by the sequencing project, only approximately 2300 shared significant sequence homology with any known genes from any other organism, i.e. they are novel genes whose functions are unknown. The sequencing of the fruit fly has also revealed so far some 13 000 genes, half of whose functions are unknown. Mapping of the human homologs of these newly identified genes from other species provides new 'candidate' genes for inherited diseases in humans.

### Functional genomics

The second major way in which model organisms are proving to be invaluable in the Human Genome Project is to provide the means to follow the expression of genes and the function of their protein products in normal development as well as their dysfunction in inherited disorders. This is referred to as *functional genomics*, or what has also been called *post-genomic genetics*.

The ability to introduce targeted mutations in specific genes, along with the production of transgenic animals (p. 81), for example in the mouse, allows the production of animal models to study the pathodevelopmental basis for inherited human disorders as well as serve as a test system for the safety and efficacy of gene therapy and other treatment modalities (p. 362). Strategies using different model organisms in a complementary fashion, taking into account factors, such as the ease/complexity of producing transgenic organisms and the generation times of different species, allow the possibility of relatively rapid analysis of gene expression, function and interactions in providing an understanding of the complex pathobiology of inherited diseases in humans.

In addition, in the last few years the development of *microarrays* has provided a useful tool for the analysis of the pattern of gene expression in health and disease. This technique, which has come out of the developments in DNA microarray technology (p. 67), involves use of robotic automated miniaturized microscopic spots of aliquots of cDNAs or oligonucleotides from specific genes in a standardized high-density gridded arrangement on glass (Fig. 23.2). This allows large-scale analysis of the pattern of gene expression by analysis of RNA species looking at differences between tissues, at different times of development and differentiation, as well as under a variety of different conditions, e.g. exposure to hormones, drugs, and so on.

Microarray gene expression analysis has an enormous potential, allowing whole genome expression screening, offering the prospect of being able to move from the 'anatomy' of the genes of the human genome in the form of DNA sequence information to its 'function', through what has been termed *proteomics*. This is the identification of the respective proteins and the elucidation of their involvement in the biological pathways and interactions in development, differentiation, health and disease.

## ETHICAL, LEGAL AND SOCIAL ISSUES OF THE HUMAN GENOME PROJECT

The rapid advances in the science and application of developments from the Human Genome Project present complex ethical issues for both the individual and society. Five per cent of the budget from the Department of Energy and the National Institutes of Health in the USA for the Human Genome Project is devoted to the study of the ethical, legal and social issues (ELSI) surrounding the availability of genetic information. These issues include ones of immediate practical relevance, such as who owns and should control genetic information with respect to privacy and confidentiality; who is entitled to access to it and how; whether it should be used by employers, schools, etc.; the psychological impact and potential stigmatization of persons positive for genetic testing; and the use of genetic testing in reproductive decision making. Other issues that will be increasingly important in future as developments from the Human Genome Project become more widespread are the concept of disability/differences that have a genetic basis in relation to the treatment of genetic disorders/diseases by gene therapy and the

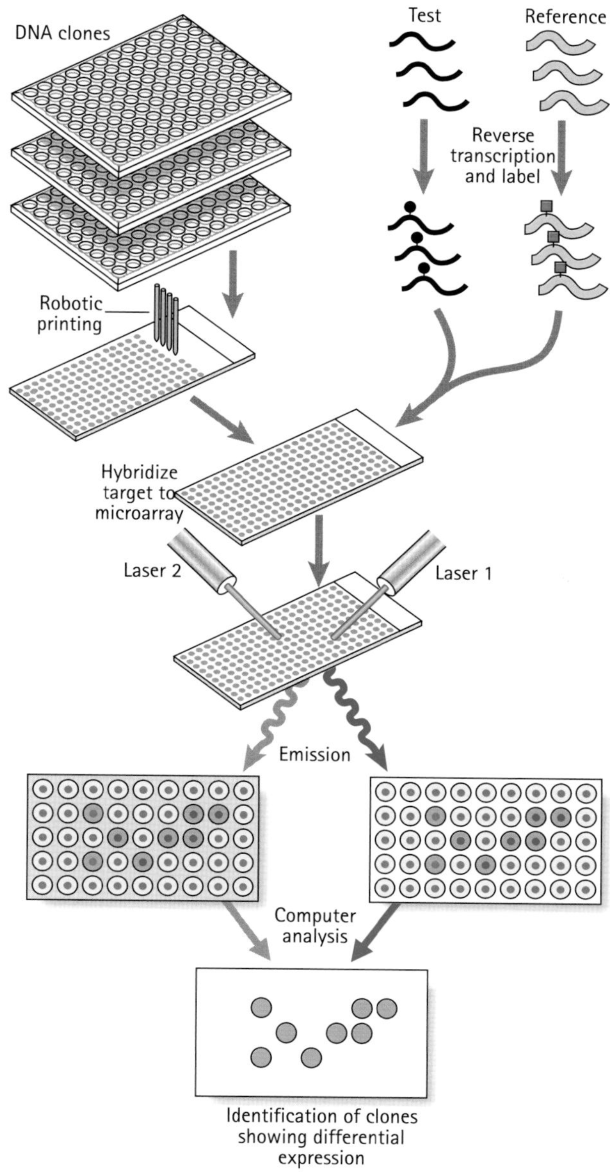


Fig. 23.2
Diagrammatic representation of a cDNA microarray. Aliquots of cDNAs of interest are gridded on a glass template using a computer-controlled robot. The test and reference RNA samples that are labeled with differently colored fluorochromes by reverse transcription are mixed and allowed to hybridize with the cDNAs on the microarray. The templates are exposed to laser light and the excitation pattern generated is compared, identifying genes that show differences in expression between the reference and test samples.

possibility of genetic enhancement, i.e. using gene therapy to supply certain characteristics, such as height. Lastly, issues need to be resolved with regard to the appropriateness and fairness of the use of the genetic technologies that come out of the Human Genome Project, with prioritization of the use of public resources and commercial involvement and property rights, especially with regard to patenting. It is probably fair to say that, although the public debate is appropriate and much overdue, a quick and simple resolution of many of these complex issues is unlikely.

## PROS AND CONS OF THE HUMAN GENOME PROJECT

Opponents of the Human Genome Project argue that an expenditure likely to exceed the planned total of $3 billion over the 15 years of the project could be better used in other medical and scientific research. Many such critics have often mistakenly viewed the Human Genome Project as a mindless sequencing exercise that will be devoid of any intrinsic biological interest. Others, through a misunderstanding of the normal interaction that takes place between genetic make-up and environmental factors in the development of the characteristics and health of an individual, cite the danger of what is commonly called biological or genetic determinism, i.e. that we will be able to precisely predict the intelligence or characteristics of a person, or when and what they will die of. Persons with such concerns often feel it is a short step to raise the potential dangers of the misuse of this information in the form of positive or negative eugenics.

Supporters of the Human Genome Project maintained that it would be of major benefit to humankind by improving our understanding and development of new strategies for the prevention and treatment of inherited disease. While it is obvious that the information and understanding gained by the Human Genome Project will be of enormous benefit and importance to those individuals and families with, or at risk of, inherited diseases, there should be genuine and real concern that the same developments could be misused, for example by employers or insurance companies, to discriminate against the same such individuals. The right of ownership of this information and its confidentiality are vital concerns for any developed and caring society (p. 369).

## TREATMENT OF GENETIC DISEASE

Many genetic disorders are characterized by progressive disability or chronic ill-health for which there is, at present, no effective treatment. Consequently one of the most exciting aspects of the developments in biotechnology is the prospect of successful gene therapy. It is important, however, to keep a perspective on the limitations of gene therapy for the immediate future and to consider, in the first instance, conventional approaches to the treatment of genetic disease.

## CONVENTIONAL APPROACHES TO TREATMENT OF GENETIC DISEASE

Most genetic disorders cannot be cured or even ameliorated using conventional methods of treatment. Sometimes this is because the underlying gene and gene product have not been identified so that there is little, if any, understanding of the basic metabolic or molecular defect. If, however, this is understood then dietary restriction, as in phenylketonuria (p. 161), or hormone replacement, as in congenital adrenal hyperplasia (p. 168), can be used very successfully in the treatment of the disorder. In a few disorders, such as homocystinuria (p. 166) and some of the organic acidurias (p. 176), supplementation with a vitamin or coenzyme can increase the activity of the defective enzyme with beneficial effect (Table 23.1).

### Protein/enzyme replacement

If a genetic disorder is found to be the result of a deficiency of or an abnormality in a specific enzyme or protein then, in theory, treatment could involve replacement of the deficient or defective enzyme or protein. An obviously

**Table 23.1 Examples of various methods for treating genetic disease**

| Treatment | Disorder |
|---|---|
| **Enzyme induction by drugs** | |
| Phenobarbitone | Congenital non-hemolytic jaundice |
| **Replacement of deficient enzyme/protein** | |
| Blood transfusion | SCID due to adenosine deaminase deficiency |
| **Bone marrow transplantation** | Mucopolysaccharidoses |
| **Enzyme/protein preparations** | |
| Trypsin | Trypsinogen deficiency |
| $\alpha_1$-Antitrypsin | $\alpha_1$-Antitrypsin deficiency |
| Cryoprecipitate/factor VIII | Hemophilia A |
| β-Glucosidase | Gaucher disease |
| **Replacement of deficient vitamin or coenzyme** | |
| $B_6$ | Homocystinuria |
| $B_{12}$ | Methylmalonic acidemia |
| Biotin | Propionic acidemia |
| D | Vitamin D-resistant rickets |
| **Replacement of deficient product** | |
| Cortisone | Congenital adrenal hyperplasia |
| Thyroxine | Congenital hypothyroidism |
| **Substrate restriction in diet** | |
| **Amino acids** | |
| Phenylalanine | Phenylketonuria |
| Leucine, isoleucine, valine | Maple syrup urine disease |
| **Carbohydrate** | |
| Galactose | Galactosemia |
| **Lipid** | |
| Cholesterol | Familial hypercholesterolemia |
| **Protein** | **Urea cycle disorders** |
| **Drug therapy** | |
| Aminocaproic acid | Angioneurotic edema |
| Dantrolene | Malignant hyperthermia |
| Cholestyramine | Familial hypercholesterolemia |
| Pancreatic enzymes | Cystic fibrosis |
| Penicillamine | Wilson disease, cystinuria |
| **Drug/dietary avoidance** | |
| Sulphonamides | G6PD deficiency |
| Barbiturates | Porphyria |
| **Replacement of diseased tissue** | |
| Kidney transplantation | Adult-onset polycystic kidney disease, Fabry disease |
| Bone marrow transplantation | X-linked SCID, Wiskott–Aldrich syndrome |
| **Removal of diseased tissue** | |
| Colectomy | Familial adenomatous polyposis |
| Splenectomy | Hereditary spherocytosis |

successful example of this is the use of factor VIII concentrate in the treatment of hemophilia A (p. 310).

In most of the inborn errors of metabolism in which an enzyme deficiency has been identified, although recombinant DNA techniques may be used to biosynthesize the missing or defective gene product, injection of the enzyme or protein may not be successful if the metabolic processes involved are carried out within cells and the protein or enzyme is not normally transported into the cell. Artificial delivery systems, such as liposomes, allow proteins to cross the cell membrane. Liposomes are artificially prepared cell-like structures in which one or more bimolecular layers of phospholipid enclose one or more aqueous compartments, which can include specific proteins. Although, in theory, it was thought liposomes would work, they have met with limited success in the treatment of genetic disorders such as the mucopolysaccharidoses. In some instances, however, biochemical modification of the protein or enzyme allows utilization of normal cellular transport mechanisms to target the enzyme to its normal location within the cell. For example, modifications in β-glucosidase as used in the treatment of Gaucher's disease enable it to enter the lysosomes, resulting in an effective form of treatment (p. 174). Another example is the modification of adenosine deaminase (ADA) by an inert polymer, polyethylene glycol (PEG), to generate a replacement enzyme which is less immunogenic and has an extended half-life.

## Drug treatment

In some genetic disorders drug therapy is possible, e.g. certain drugs can help lower cholesterol levels in familial hypercholesterolemia (p. 170). In others, avoidance of certain drugs or foods can prevent the manifestation of the disorder, e.g. sulphonamides and fava beans in glucose-6-phosphate dehydrogenase (G6PD) deficiency (p. 183). Drug therapy might also be directed at a subset of patients according to their molecular defect. A recent example is a trial where gentamicin was administered via nasal drops to patients with cystic fibrosis. Aminoglycoside antibiotics such as gentamicin cause readthrough of premature stop codons in vitro and only patients with nonsense mutations (p. 26) showed evidence of expression of full-length CFTR protein in the nasal epithelium.

## Transplantation

This may involve transplantation of organs, particular cell types or stem cells (undifferentiated precursor cells).

### *Tissue transplantation*

Replacement of defective tissue is another option that became available with the advent of tissue typing (p. 194), e.g. renal transplantation in adult polycystic kidney disease or lung transplantation in patients with cystic fibrosis.

An exciting new treatment for insulin-dependent diabetes mellitus is islet transplantation. Islet cells are prepared from donated pancreases (usually two per patient) and injected into the liver of the recipient. The 'Edmonton' protocol has proved very successful: 3 years post transplant over 80% of patients are still producing their own insulin.

### *Stem-cell transplantation*

Bone-marrow transplantation can be an effective treatment for patients with a number of genetic disorders, including ADA deficiency, severe-combined immunodefficiency (SCID), lysosomal storage diseases and Fanconi anemia. The main limitation is the lack of a suitable bone-marrow donor, but it is hoped that the use of stem cells derived from cord blood may overcome this problem in the future.

Transplantation of stem cells (e.g. pluripotent hematopoietic stem cells) *in utero* offers the prospect of a novel mode of treatment for genetic disorders with a congenital onset. The immaturity of the fetal immune system means that the fetus will be tolerant of foreign cells so that there is no need to match the donor cells with those of the fetus. Trials of *in utero* stem cell transplantation are under way for a number of disorders that include severe combined immunodeficiency (SCID), α- and β-thalassemia and sickle-cell disease.

Embryonic stem cells can differentiate into any type of cell and hence the potential applications of embryonic stem-cell therapy are vast. For example, it is possible to culture mouse embryonic stem cells to generate dopamine-producing neurons. When these neural cells were transplanted into a mouse model for Parkinson disease, the dopamine-producing neurons showed long-term survival and ultimately corrected the phenotype. This is described as 'therapeutic cloning' and the ethics of its use in humans is currently a topic of hot debate (p. 376).

# THERAPEUTIC APPLICATIONS OF RECOMBINANT DNA TECHNOLOGY

The advent of recombinant DNA technology has also led to rapid progress in the availability of biosynthetic gene products for the treatment of certain inherited diseases.

## Biosynthesis of gene products

Insulin used in the treatment of diabetes mellitus was, until recently, obtained from pig pancreases. This had to be very carefully purified for use, and even then it occasionally produced sensitivity reactions in patients.

**Table 23.2 Proteins produced biosynthetically using recombinant DNA technology**

| Protein | Disease |
|---|---|
| Insulin | Diabetes mellitus |
| Growth hormone | Short stature due to growth hormone deficiency |
| Factor VIII | Hemophilia A |
| Factor IX | Hemophilia B |
| Erythropoietin | Anemia |
| α-Galactosidase A | Fabry disease (XL lysosomal storage disorder) |
| β-interferon | Multiple sclerosis |

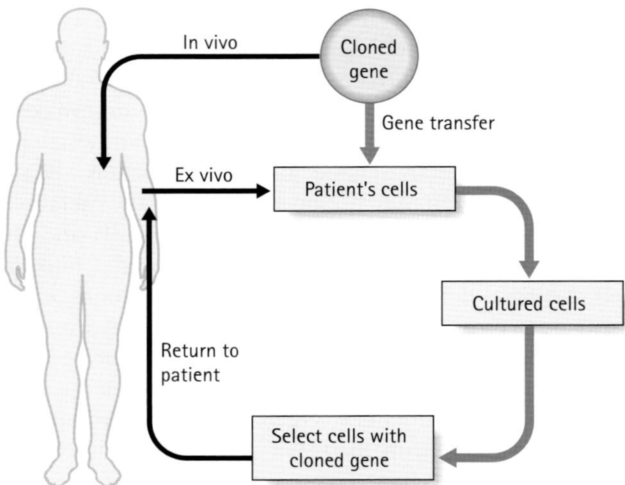


**Fig. 23.3**
In vivo and ex vivo gene therapy. In vivo gene therapy delivers genetically modified cells directly to the patient. An example is *CFTR* gene therapy using liposomes or adenovirus via nasal sprays. Ex vivo gene therapy removes cells from the patient which are modified in vitro and then returned to the patient. An example is the treatment of fibroblasts from patients with hemophilia B by the addition of the factor IX gene. Modified fibroblasts are then injected into the stomach cavity.

However, with recombinant DNA technology, microorganisms can be used to synthesize insulin from the human insulin gene. This is inserted, along with appropriate sequences to ensure efficient transcription and translation, into a recombinant DNA vector such as a plasmid and cloned in a microorganism, such as *E. coli*. In this way large quantities of insulin can be made. An artificial gene that is not identical with the natural gene needs to be constructed for this purpose, however, because synthetically produced genes cannot contain the non-coding intervening sequences, or introns (p. 17), found in the majority of structural genes in eukaryotic organisms, since microorganisms such as *E. coli* do not possess a means for splicing of the mRNA after transcription.

Recombinant DNA technology is being employed in the production of a number of other biosynthetic products (Table 23.2). The biosynthesis of medically important peptides in this way is usually more expensive than obtaining the product from conventional sources because of the research and development involved. However, biosynthetically derived products have the dual advantages of providing a pure product that is unlikely to induce a sensitivity reaction and one that is free of the risk of chemical or biological contamination. In the past, the use of growth hormone from human cadaver pituitaries has been associated with the transmission of Creutzfeldt–Jakob disease, and HIV has been a contaminant in cryoprecipitate containing factor VIII used in the treatment of hemophilia A (p. 310).

## GENE THERAPY

Gene therapy can be defined as the replacement of a deficient gene product or correction of an abnormal gene. Gene therapy can be carried out either ex vivo by treatment of cells or tissue from an affected individual in culture, with reintroduction into the affected individual, or in vivo if cells cannot be cultured or be replaced in the affected individual (Fig. 23.3).

Advances in molecular biology leading to the identification of many important human disease genes and their protein products have raised the prospect of gene therapy for many genetic and non-genetic disorders. The first human gene therapy trial began in 1990, but it is important to emphasize that, although it is often presented as the new panacea in medicine, progress to date has been limited and there are many practical difficulties to overcome before gene therapy can deliver its promise.

### REGULATORY REQUIREMENTS

There has been much publicity about the potential uses and abuses of gene therapy. Regulatory bodies have been established in several countries to oversee the technical, therapeutic and safety aspects of gene therapy programs (p. 375). There is universal agreement that *germ-line gene therapy*, in which genetic changes could be distributed to both somatic and germ cells and therefore be transmitted to future generations, is morally and ethically unacceptable. Therefore all programs are focusing only on *somatic cell gene therapy*, in which the alteration in genetic information is targeted to specific cells, tissues or organs in which the disorder is manifest.

In the United States the Human Gene Therapy Subcommittee of the National Institutes of Health has produced guidelines for protocols of trials of gene therapy that must be submitted for approval to both the Food and Drug Administration and the Recombinant DNA Advisory Committee, along with their institutional review boards (IRBs). In the UK the Gene Therapy Advisory Committee (GTAC) advises on the ethical acceptibility of proposals for gene therapy research in humans, taking account of the scientific merits, and the potential benefits and risks.

Over 300 clinical trials of gene therapy have been approved for children and adults for a variety of genetic and non-genetic disorders. For the most part these appear to be proceeding without event, but the unexpected death of a patient in one trial in 1999 and the development of leukemia in two children who received gene therapy for X-linked SCID (p. 198) has highlighted the risks of gene therapy.

## TECHNICAL ASPECTS

Before a gene therapy trial is possible, there are a number of technical aspects that must be addressed.

### Gene characterization

One of the basic prerequisites of gene therapy is that the gene involved should have been cloned. This should include not only the structural gene but also the DNA sequences involved in the control and regulation of expression of that gene.

### Target cells/tissue/organ

The specific cells, tissue or organ affected which is to be treated must be identified and accessible. Again this seems obvious. Some of the early attempts at treating the inherited disorders of hemoglobin, such as β-thalassemia, involved removing bone marrow from affected individuals, treating it in vitro, and then returning it to the patient by transfusion. While in principle this could have worked, in order to have any likelihood of success the particular cells that needed to be targeted were the small number of bone-marrow stem cells from which the immature red blood cells, or reticulocytes, develop.

### Vector system

The means by which a foreign gene is introduced needs to be both efficient and safe. If gene therapy is to be considered as a realistic alternative to conventional treatments, there should be unequivocal evidence from trials of gene therapy carried out in animal models that the inserted gene functions adequately with appropriate regulatory, promoter and enhancer sequences. In addition, it needs to be shown that the treated tissue or cell population has a reasonable life span, that the gene product continues to be expressed and that the body does not react adversely to the gene product, e.g. by producing antibodies to the protein product. Lastly, it is essential to demonstrate that introduction of the foreign gene or DNA sequence has no deleterious effects, such as inadvertently leading to a malignancy or a mutagenic effect on either the somatic or the germ cell lines, e.g. through mistakes arising as a result of the insertion of the gene or DNA sequence into the host DNA, or what is known as insertional mutagenesis. In both patients who developed leukemia after gene therapy for XL-SCID, the retrovirus used to deliver the γ-c (*IL2RG*) gene had inserted into the *LMO-2* oncogene on chromosome 11, which plays a role in some forms of childhood leukemia.

## METHODS OF GENE THERAPY

These can be divided into two main types, viral and non-viral methods.

### Viral agents

A number of different viruses can be used to transport foreign genetic material into cells. Each of these has its own particular advantages and disadvantages (Table 23.3).

#### *Oncoretroviruses*

These are RNA viruses that can integrate into the host DNA by making a copy of their RNA molecule using the enzyme reverse transcriptase (p. 205). The provirus so formed is the template for the production of the mRNAs for the various viral gene products and the new genomic RNA of the virus. If the provirus is stably integrated into dividing stem cells, all subsequent progeny cells will inherit a copy of the viral genome.

One of the disadvantages associated with the use of retroviruses as a vector system in gene therapy is that only a relatively small DNA sequence can be introduced into the target cells – usually less than 7 kb – which limits their use. For example, even if all of the introns were removed from the dystrophin gene (p. 308) for use in gene therapy of Duchenne muscular dystrophy, the gene would still be much too large to be incorporated into a retroviral vector. Attempts have been made to overcome this by inserting a modified dystrophin gene in which a large amount of the gene has been deleted, but which still has relatively normal function. This is known as a minidystrophin gene (p. 310).

A second disadvantage of using retroviruses as vectors in gene therapy is that they can only integrate into cells that divide shortly after infection. This limits their potential use, as few cell types are continually dividing, although they may be beneficial for targeting cancers within non-dividing cells.

**Table 23.3 Methods of gene transfer**

| Features | Oncoretrovirus | Adenovirus | Adeno-associated virus | Lentivirus | Herpes virus | Liposome | Gene repair |
|---|---|---|---|---|---|---|---|
| Maximum insert size | 7 kb | 36 kb | 5 kb | 7 kb | 20 kb | Unlimited | n/a |
| Chromosomal integration | Yes | No | Yes/No | Yes | No | No | n/a |
| Duration of expression | Short | Short | Long | Long | Short | Short | Long |
| Host immune response | Unlikely | Possible | Possible | Unlikely | Possible | None | None |
| Safety | Possibility of insertional mutagenesis | Toxicity | Toxicity | Possibility of insertional mutagenesis | Toxicity | None | Possibility of non-specific events |

### *Lentiviruses*

The lentivirus family includes HIV (human immunodeficiency virus). Lentiviruses are complex viruses that infect macrophages and lymphocytes, but unlike oncoretroviruses they can be integrated into non-dividing cells. They may, therefore, be useful in the treatment of neurological conditions.

### *Adenoviruses*

Adenoviruses can be used as vectors in gene therapy since they infect a wide variety of cell types. They have advantages over oncoretroviruses in that they are stable and can be easily purified to produce high titers for infection. Unlike retroviruses, they can infect non-dividing cells and carry up to 36 kb of foreign DNA. In addition, they are suitable for targeted treatment of specific tissues such as the respiratory tract and have been extensively used in gene therapy trials for treatment of cystic fibrosis.

Adenoviruses do not integrate into the host genome, which avoids the possibility of insertional mutagenesis but has the disadvantage that expression of the introduced gene is usually unstable and often transient. In addition, by virtue of their infectivity, they can produce adverse effects secondary to infection and by stimulating the host immune response. Lastly, adenoviruses contain genes known to be involved in the process of malignant transformation, so that there is a potential risk that they could inadvertently induce malignancy.

### *Adeno-associated viruses*

Adeno-associated viruses are non-pathogenic parvoviruses in humans that require coinfection with helper adenoviruses or certain members of the herpes virus family to achieve infection. In the absence of the helper virus the adeno-associated virus DNA integrates into chromosomal DNA at a specific site on the long arm of chromosome 19 (19q13.3-qter). Subsequent infection with an adenovirus activates the integrated adeno-associated viral DNA-producing virions. They have the advantages of being able to infect a wide variety of cell types, exhibiting long-term gene expression and lack of generation of an immune response to transduced cells. The safety of adeno-associated viruses as vectors occurs by virtue of their site-specific integration but, unfortunately, this is often impaired with the inclusion of foreign DNA in the virus. The disadvantages of adeno-associated viruses include the fact that they can be activated by any adenovirus infection and that, although 95% of the vector genome is removed, they can only take inserts of foreign DNA up to 5 kb in size.

Some of the more recent developments of the adeno-associated viruses as vectors for gene therapy allow the prospect of the introduction of pharmacologically controlled induction of the expression of transduced genes.

### *Herpes virus*

Herpes viruses are neurotropic, i.e. infect nervous tissue, and, if suitably modified, could be used to target gene therapy to the central nervous system, for the treatment of neurological disorders such as Parkinson disease. An immediate disadvantage of using herpes viruses as a vector system is their direct toxic effects on nerve cells as well as the consequent immune response, although recent modifications of this potential neurotropic vector have been produced that are devoid of viral expression and neurotoxicity. Herpes viruses, however, do not integrate into the host genome, and therefore it is likely that the expression of introduced genes would be temporary and unstable.

## Non-viral methods

There are a number of different non-viral methods of gene therapy. These have the theoretical advantage of not eliciting an immune response and being safer and simpler to use, as well as allowing large-scale production, but differ in their efficacy.

### *Naked DNA*

Direct injection of DNA into cells has been used in gene therapy, e.g. the minidystrophin gene into myoblasts in the mouse model for Duchenne muscular dystrophy (p. 308). While success has been reported in terms of evidence of localized gene expression, clearly this approach has a limited place except for the possibility of the expression of hormones or proteins for which small amounts will result in a significant clinical effect, e.g. erythropoietin or factor VIII.

### *Liposome-mediated DNA transfer*

Liposomes are lipid bilayers surrounding an aqueous vesicle that can facilitate the introduction of foreign DNA into a target cell (Fig. 23.4). A disadvantage of liposomes is that they are not very efficient in gene transfer and the expression of the foreign gene is transient, so that the treatment has to be repeated. An advantage of liposome-mediated gene transfer is that a much larger DNA sequence can be introduced into the target cells or tissues than with viral vector systems. This can be as large as an artificially constructed minichromosome which, in addition to a specific structural gene, can include elements involved in the regulation of gene expression in a physiologically controlled fashion, as well as centromeric and telomeric sequences that will allow replication of the foreign DNA in mitotic divisions. Recent modifications of cationic lipid/DNA complexes have been developed that enhance the efficacy of gene transduction.

#### Receptor-mediated endocytosis

A variation of liposome-mediated gene transfer is to target the DNA to specific receptors on the surfaces of cells. A complex is made between plasmid DNA containing the foreign gene or DNA sequence and specific polypeptide ligands for which the cell has a receptor on its surface. For example, DNA complexed to a glycoprotein containing galactose will be recognized by receptors on the surface of liver cells that are specific to glycoproteins with a terminal galactose. This results in internalization of the complex into endocytic vesicles, which are then transported to the lysosomes where the complex is degraded. In order for the foreign gene to then be expressed, it has to escape from the lysosome. The rate at which it escapes from the lysosomes can be increased by inclusion of adenovirus or influenza gene products.

### *Repair of mutations in situ through the cellular DNA repair machinery*

A promising new approach is the use of chimeric double-stranded DNA/RNA oligonucleotides to repair genes in situ through the cellular DNA repair machinery (p. 29). Proof of principle has been demonstrated in an animal model of Pompe disease, where the point mutation was shown to be repaired at the DNA level and normal enzyme activity restored.

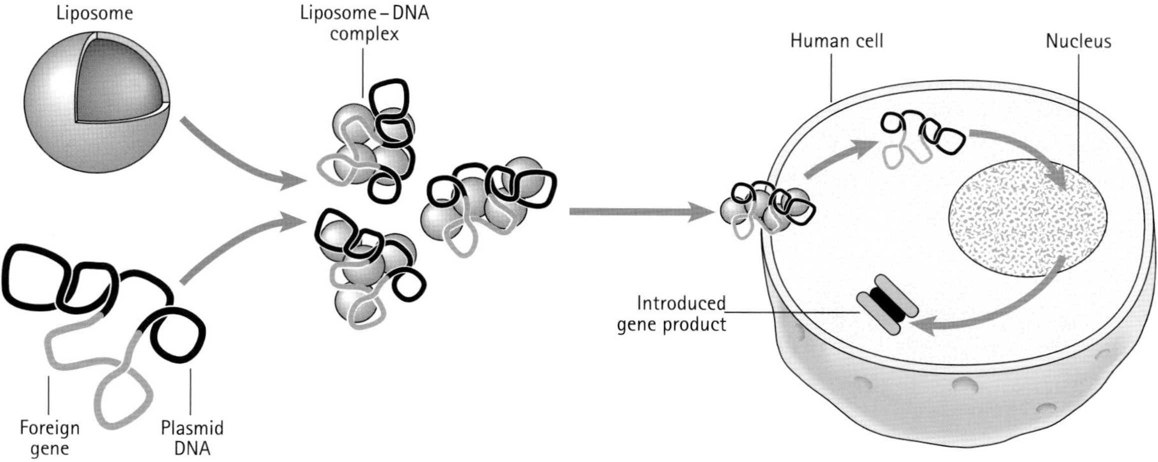


Fig. 23.4
Diagrammatic representation of liposome-mediated gene therapy.

### *Antisense-induced exon splicing*

The recent identification of exon-splicing enhancer (ESE) sequences (p. 26) has increased our understanding of the process of exon splicing. If an ESE is mutated, the exon is more likely to be spliced out. Some proteins with in-frame whole exon deletions retain some residual activity, e.g. dystrophin mutations in Becker muscular dystrophy (p. 309). In an in vitro experiment using muscle cells from two patients with Duchenne muscular dystrophy, it was possible to block an ESE with an antisense oligonucleotide (a short synthetic DNA fragment complementary in sequence to the mRNA). The reading frame was restored and the detection of significant levels of dystrophin protein in the muscle cells confirmed the therapeutic potential of this approach.

### *In utero fetal gene therapy*

The report of successful adenovirus vector-mediated in utero gene therapy in a cystic fibrosis mouse model in 1997 means that fetal gene therapy in utero may be possible in humans. At present it is considered unacceptable because of the possibility of inadvertent germ cell modification. The use of stem cells genetically modified ex vivo should reduce this risk. However, in utero stem-cell transplantation without genetic modification currently offers the best prospects for the successful treatment of serious neurodegenerative disorders with a very early onset, such as Krabbe disease or Hurler syndrome (p. 171).

## Animal models

One of the basic prerequisites for assessing the suitability of gene therapy trials in humans is the existence of an animal model. While there are naturally occurring animal models for some inherited human diseases, for most there is no animal counterpart. The techniques used to generate animal models for human disease are outside the scope of this book, but much effort has focused upon the production of animal models that faithfully recreate disease phenotypes. Animal models for cystic fibrosis, Duchenne muscular dystrophy, Huntington disease, and Friedreich ataxia have been generated and provide just a few examples that may be used to evaluate gene therapy before trials in humans.

## Target organs

In many instances gene therapy will need to be and should be directed or limited to a particular organ, tissue or body system.

### *Liver*

Viral vectors for gene therapy of inherited hepatic disorders have been of limited use due to the lack of vectors that specifically target hepatocytes. Although liver cells are refractory to retroviruses in vivo, they are, somewhat surprisingly, susceptible to transfection by retroviruses in vitro. Cells removed from the liver by partial hepatectomy can be treated in vitro and then reinjected via the portal venous system, from which they seed in the liver. The effectiveness of this approach has been demonstrated by the lowering of cholesterol levels in a rabbit animal model with a defect in the low-density lipoprotein (LDL) receptor. The injection of the hepatocytes into the portal venous system is, however, associated with a significant risk of thrombosis of the portal venous system that can lead to the complication of portal hypertension. Nevertheless, because of the serious outlook for homozygotes with mutations in the LDL receptor (p. 170), gene therapy by this means has been attempted in a woman homozygous for an LDL receptor defect. This has led, in the short term, to a reduction of LDL levels, although the long-term benefit is, as yet, undetermined. Other disorders affecting or involving the liver in which a similar approach could be considered are phenylketonuria, $\alpha_1$-antitrypsin deficiency and hemophilia A.

### *CNS*

CNS-directed vector systems are being developed in which replication-defective neurotropic adenoviruses lacking the so-called E1 region can be produced and then be made infective by growing them in cells engineered to express the E1 genes. In addition, lentiviruses could be used for the treatment of central nervous system disorders, such as Parkinson and Alzheimer diseases, because they integrate into the host genome of non-dividing cells and could, therefore, act as a delivery system for stable expression.

Another approach which has been suggested in genetic disorders affecting the CNS is to transplant cells that have been genetically modified in vitro into specific regions of the brain, such as the caudate nucleus in persons with or at risk of Huntington disease.

### *Muscle*

Unlike other tissues, direct injection of foreign DNA into muscle has met with some success in terms of retention and expression of the foreign gene in the treated muscle. Alternatively, injection of myoblasts into muscle results in their incorporation into recipient muscle bundles. Although animal model work showed some promise of efficacy, this approach has met with difficulties in humans. Direct DNA injection has, however, been used to express the protein products of genes, transferred in vitro into myoblasts, which are unrelated to muscle function, such as human growth hormone and factor VIII. Other primary cell types, such as fibroblasts treated in vitro, could also be transplanted back as skin grafts to deliver circulating gene products.

### *Bone marrow*

In the treatment of disorders affecting the bone marrow, problems arise due to the small numbers of stem cells, which need to be transduced if there is to be more than a transient response with gene therapy. Stem cells often constitute less than 1% of the total cells present. Pretreatment of the bone marrow to expand the number of stem cells has been tried for certain inherited immunological disorders by the use of growth factors such as the granulocyte colony-stimulating factor (G-CSF) and the cytotoxic agent 5-fluorouracil. Reliable identification of specific stem cell types would enable them to be enriched for, thereby increasing the likelihood of success.

## DISEASES SUITABLE FOR TREATMENT USING GENE THERAPY

The disorders that are possible candidates for gene therapy include both genetic and non-genetic diseases (Table 23.4).

### Genetic disorders

There are a number of single-gene diseases that are obvious candidates for gene therapy.

### *Adenosine deaminase deficiency*

One of the first diseases for which gene therapy has been attempted in humans is the inherited immunodeficiency disorder caused by adenosine deaminase (ADA) deficiency (p. 175). The most successful conventional treatment for ADA deficiency is bone-marrow transplantation, but in the absence of a compatible donor, patients may be treated with PWG-conjugated ADA. In 1990 the first gene therapy trial enrolled 10 patients with ADA-SCID. Although no adverse events were reported, none of the patients were 'cured', probably due to the low efficiency of gene transfer from the retroviral vector. In addition, the continuing treatment of these patients with PEG-ADA is thought to have diminished any selective growth advantage of transduced cells. A trial is now under way where patients are not be treated with PEG-ADA, but

**Table 23.4 Genetic and non-genetic diseases that can potentially be treated by gene therapy**

| Genetic disorder | Defect |
|---|---|
| Immune deficiency | Adenosine deaminase deficiency<br>Purine nucleoside phosphorylase deficiency<br>Chronic granulomatous disease |
| Hypercholesterolemia | Low-density lipoprotein receptor abnormalities |
| Hemophilia | Factor VIII deficiency (A)<br>Factor IX deficiency (B) |
| Gaucher disease | Glucocerebrosidase deficiency |
| Mucopolysaccharidosis VII | β-Glucuronidase deficiency |
| Emphysema | $\alpha_1$-Antitrypsin deficiency |
| Cystic fibrosis | *CFTR* mutations |
| Phenylketonuria | Phenylalanine hydroxylase deficiency |
| **Urea cycle abnormalities**<br>Hyperammonemia<br>Citrullinemia<br>Muscular dystrophy<br>Thalassemia/sickle-cell | <br>Ornithine transcarbamylase deficiency<br>Argininosuccinate synthetase deficiency<br>Dystrophin mutations<br>α- and β-globin mutations disease |
| **Cancer**<br>Malignant melanoma<br>Ovarian cancer<br>Brain tumors<br>Neuroblastoma<br>Renal cancer<br>Lung cancer<br>Acquired immune deficiency syndrome (AIDS)<br>Cardiovascular diseases<br>Rheumatoid arthritis | |

receive mild chemotherapy prior to ex vivo treatment of their bone marrow cells with a novel retroviral vector. The chemotherapy aims to kill off diseased cells and enhance the selective growth advantage of the modified cells. Two patients have been successfully treated using this approach.

### *Hemoglobinopathies*

Attempts at treating β-thalassemia and sickle-cell disease by gene therapy have not been effective as yet, primarily because the numbers of α- and β-globin chains must be equal (p. 149). Gene therapy must, therefore, be dose specific, and this is not possible at the present time.

### *Cystic fibrosis*

Double-blind trials are being carried out in the UK and the USA treating cystic fibrosis patients using either a liposome-gene complex or an adeno-associated virus vector sprayed into the nasal passages. Studies of their efficacy and safety involve looking for the presence of the introduced *CFTR* gene in biopsies of the nasal epithelium and measurement of ion transport in nasal epithelial cells. Reports to date of trials of gene therapy in cystic fibrosis have shown that it is not obviously harmful, although there is very limited evidence of efficacy.

### *Hemophilia A and B*

Hemophilia A and B are excellent candidates for gene therapy as a modest increase in the level of factor VIII or IX, respectively, will be of major clinical benefit. Recent trials have used direct intramuscular injection of adeno-associated virus expressing factor VIII or ex vivo treatment of fibroblasts with plasmid-borne factor IX followed by injection into the stomach cavity. The results are encouraging, with some patients able to reduce their usage of exogenous clotting factors.

### *Duchenne muscular dystrophy*

The main difficulty with gene therapy for Duchenne muscular dystrophy is the sheer size of the dystrophin gene (the cDNA is 14 kb). A trial is in progress using plasmid vectors that can accommodate the large cDNA, but delivery to the muscle is inefficient. An alternative strategy is to use antisense oligonucleotides to force exon skipping and convert out-of-frame deletions that cause DMD to in-frame deletions usually associated with the milder Becker muscular dystrophy phenotype. This approach may be successful for up to 75% of DMD patients. There is also the possibility of upregulating a dystrophin homolog, utrophin. Immune rejection is not a problem and studies in the *mdx* mouse have shown significant improvement in muscle function. Research is now under way to find a pharmacological compound that will upregulate utrophin expression.

## Common multifactorial diseases

In the majority of human diseases in which there is a genetic etiology, both genes and environmental factors are involved (p. 139). Gene therapy will have a much more widespread impact in medicine if it can be used in this group of disorders. It is important, however, to remember that for most of the common multifactorial diseases in humans, the identification and subsequent avoidance of causative environmental factors is likely to be much more effective than gene therapy at present or in the near future.

### *Cancer*

In contrast to the limited number of gene therapy trials for single-gene disorders, numerous cancer-gene therapy trials have been initiated. Gene therapy for cancer aims to selectively kill cancer cells either directly through the use of toxins targeted at cancer cells, or by enhancing the body's immune response.

**Supply tumor suppressor genes**
It has been proposed that the targeted introduction of recognized tumor suppressor genes (p. 209), such as *Tp53*, to cancer cells could result in control of their growth. More detailed knowledge of the biology of cancer will be needed before this approach can be reliable and safe.

**Inhibit oncogenic proteins**
Imatinib (also known as STI-571 or Glivec) is a protein tyrosine kinase inhibitor used to treat chronic myeloid leukemia. It is a very effective treatment that works by binding the Bcr-Abl fusion protein resulting from the t(9;22) translocation. This is an example of effective drug design resulting from knowledge of the molecular etiology.

**Stimulate natural killing of tumor cells**
Mitogens, such as interleukin-2, introduced in vitro into melanosomes, which have been removed from patients with malignant melanoma and then reintroduced into the patient, could be used to activate the patient's immune response. The use of liposome-bound plasmid DNA containing foreign histocompatibility genes to transduce tumor cells to enhance the immune response has also been proposed as a possible form of gene therapy in

cancer. Again, a better understanding of the malignant process and the body's immune response to malignancy will be necessary before this form of gene therapy can be effective.

**Introduce genes that selectively damage cancer cells**

The introduction of the tumor necrosis factor gene into tumor-infiltrating lymphocytes, which can then be returned to the patient, has been promoted as another approach for gene therapy in cancer. More recently, a proposal has been made to introduce what have been called conditionally toxic or suicide genes into cancer cells. An example is the thymidine kinase gene of the herpes simplex virus, which allows the metabolism of the substance gancyclovir by cellular kinases into the triphosphate form that inhibits DNA polymerase, resulting in the death of the cancer cells as well as surrounding cells through a 'bystander' effect. It has also been proposed that 'antiangiogenic' genes could be used to compromise the circulatory supply of tumors. An example, is the inhibition of the angiogenic vascular endothelial growth factor (VEGF).

### *Coronary artery disease*

VEGF is also a target for gene therapy in coronary artery disease where patients cannot be treated by angioplasty or coronary artery by-pass grafting. The aim is to over-express VEGF and increase angiogenesis.

### *Peripheral vascular disease*

A number of different trials of gene therapy in persons with peripheral arterial vascular disease are under way, involving introduction of genes which lead to proliferation of new vessels (e.g. VEGF) and the production of anticlotting agents.

### *Autoimmune disorders*

The use of gene therapy in autoimmune disorders to restore immune homeostasis has been suggested. Interleukin-1 (IL-1) is an immune system signal which triggers inflammation. For example, it has been proposed that gene therapy could be used to introduce genes for the IL-1 receptor antagonist protein into synovial cells in persons with rheumatoid arthritis, in which the inflammatory process is believed to play a key etiological role.

## Other modalities

New therapeutic modalities include the use of antisense oligonucleotides, RNA interference and intrabodies that may be used in the treatment of cancer and viral infections. They may also be used to target polyglutamine expansions seen in neurodegenerative diseases, including Huntington disease.

### *Antisense oligonucleotides*

Antisense therapy may be used to modulate the expression of genes associated with malignancies and other genetic disorders. The principle of antisense technology is the sequence-specific binding of an antisense oligonucleotide to a target mRNA which results in inhibition of gene expression at the protein level. They can be delivered to the cell by liposomes, but the folding of mRNAs or interaction with proteins may prevent binding of an antisense oligonucleotide to its target. Nevertheless, one compound has already been approved for treatment of cytomegalovirus-induced retinitis, and a number of other trials are ongoing.

### *RNA interference*

This technique also has broad therapeutic application as any gene may be a potential target for silencing by RNA interference. In contrast to antisense oligonucleotide therapy, as a result of RNA interference the target mRNA is cleaved rather than just bound, and it is estimated to be up to 1000-fold more active. RNA interference works through the targeted degradation of mRNAs containing homologous sequences to synthetic double-stranded RNA molecules known as small interfering RNAs (siRNA – see Fig. 23.5). The siRNA may be delivered in drug form using strategies developed to stabilize antisense oligonucleotides, or from plasmids or viral vectors. In vitro, siRNAs have been shown to reduce in vitro expression of Bcr-Abl and Bcl2 targets in cancer, viral infections including HIV, and polyglutamine repeat sequences in neurodegenerative disorders. RNA interference has been shown to be successful in mice; the next step is a human pilot study.

### *Intrabodies*

Intracellular antibodies, or intrabodies, are designed to mimic antibody–antigen binding, but within the cell. Intrabodies are derived from the V (variable) regions of the heavy and light chains (p. 191) in order to harness the affinity of the parent antibody. The therapeutic applications are broad and include treatment of cancer, viral infections, automimmune, inflammatory and neurodegenerative disorders. Intrabodies are promising tools, but are still at an early stage of development.

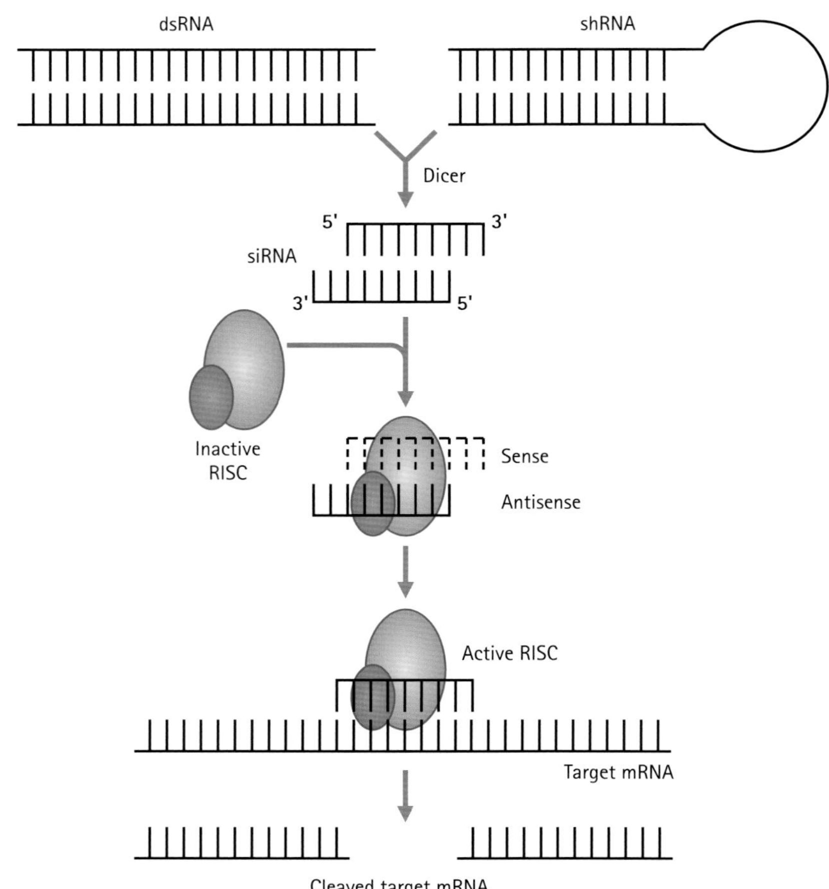


**Fig. 23.5**
Mechanism of RNA interference. Double-stranded (ds) RNA are processed by Dicer, in an ATP-dependent process, to produce small interfering RNAs (siRNA) of ~21–23 nucleotides in length with two-nucleotide overhangs at each end. Short hairpin (sh) RNAs, either produced endogenously or expressed from viral vectors, are also processed by Dicer into siRNA. An ATP-dependent helicase is required to unwind the dsRNA, allowing one strand to bind to the RNA-induced silencing complex (RISC). Binding of the antisense RNA strand activates the RISC to cleave mRNAs containing a homologous sequence. (From Lieberman J et al 2003 Trends in molecular medicine 9: 397–403 with permission).

## ELEMENTS

1. The Human Genome Project aimed to sequence the human genome in order to track down the genes responsible for inherited disease in humans. The sequencing was completed by an international consortium in 2003, and this research is likely to pay dividends in our understanding of both genetic and non-genetic diseases.

2. Treatment of genetic disease by conventional means requires identification of the gene product and an understanding of the pathophysiology of the disease process. Therapeutic options can include dietary restriction or supplementation, drug therapy, replacement of an abnormal or deficient protein or enzyme and replacement or removal of an abnormal tissue.

3. Recombinant DNA technology has enabled human-derived biosynthetic gene products such as human insulin and growth hormone to be produced for the treatment of human disease.

4. Before a trial of gene therapy is carried out in humans, the gene involved must be characterized, the particular cell type or tissue to be targeted must be identified, an efficient, reliable and safe vector system that results in stable continued expression of the introduced gene has to be developed, and the safety and effectiveness of the particular modality of gene therapy has to be demonstrated in an animal model.

5. Germ-line gene therapy is universally viewed as ethically unacceptable, while somatic cell gene therapy is generally viewed as being acceptable, as this is seen as similar to existing treatments such as organ transplantation.

## FURTHER READING


Adams M D, Celniker S E, Holt R A et al 2000 The genome sequence of the *Drosophila melanogaster*. Science 287: 2185–2195

*The sequence of the fruit fly, one of the first 'model' organisms in genetics.*

Anderson W F 1992 Human gene therapy. Science 256: 808–813

*A consideration of gene therapy by one of its main proponents.*

Dunham I, Shimizu N, Roe B A et al 1999 The DNA sequence of chromosome 22. Nature 402: 489–95

*The first report of the DNA sequence of a human chromosome.*

International Human Genome Sequencing Consortium 2001 Initial sequencing and analysis of the human genome. Nature 409: 860–921

*The report describing the working draft of the human genome sequence.*

Lieberman J, Song E, Lee S-K et al 2003 Interfering with disease: opportunities and roadblocks to harnessing RNA interference. Trends Molec Med 9: 397–403

*Article describing the potential applications of RNA interference.*

Müller-Hill B 1993 The shadow of genetic injustice. Nature 362: 491–492

*A brief commentary urging caution against being caught up in the enthusiasm for the Human Genome Project.*

Van Deutekom J C T and van Ommen G-J B 2003 Advances in Duchenne muscular dystrophy gene therapy. Nature Rev Genet 4: 774–783

*A recent review of gene therapy for DMD that includes a good overview of different strategies.*

CHAPTER

# 24 Ethical issues in medical genetics

*"The mere existence of the complete reference map and DNA sequence down to the last nucleotide may lead to the absurdity of* reductionism *– the misconception that we know everything it means to be human – or to the absurdity of* determinism *– that what we are is a direct and inevitable consequence of what our genome is."*

Victor McKusick (1991)

Ethics is the branch of knowledge that deals with moral principles, which in turn relates to principles of right and wrong and standards of behavior. Traditionally, the reference points are based on a synthesis of the philosophical and religious views of well-informed, respected, thinking members of society. In this way a code of practice evolves that is seen as reasonable and acceptable by a majority and that often forms the basis for professional guidelines or regulations.

Ethical issues arise in all branches of medicine but are particularly prominent in genetics because of the way this subject impinges not just on an individual, but also on the extended family and on society in general. In the minds of the general public, clinical genetics and genetic counseling can easily be confused with eugenics – defined as the science of 'improving' a species through breeding. It is important to stress that the modern specialty of clinical genetics has absolutely nothing in common with the totally unacceptable eugenic philosophies that were practiced in Nazi Germany and, to a much lesser extent, elsewhere in Europe and in the USA between the two world wars. Emphasis has already been placed on the fundamental principle that genetic counseling is a *non-directive* and *non-judgmental* communication process whereby factual knowledge is imparted to facilitate informed personal choice (Ch. 17). Indeed, clinical geneticists have been pioneers in recent times in practicing and promoting non-paternalistic medicine, and 5% of the original budget for the Human Genome Project was set aside for funding studies into the ethical and social implications of the knowledge gained from the project. Coercion and eugenics certainly have no place in modern medical genetics.

Nevertheless, this is a subject that lends itself to ethical debate, not least because of the new challenges and opportunities provided by discoveries in molecular genetics. In this chapter some of the more controversial and difficult areas will be considered. It will soon become apparent that for many of these issues there is no clear right or wrong approach and individual views will vary widely. Sometimes in a clinical setting the best that can be hoped for is to arrive at a mutually acceptable compromise, with an explicit agreement that opposing views are respected and, personal conscience permitting, a patient's expressed wishes are carried out.

## GENERAL PRINCIPLES

The principles of medical ethics that command wide consensus are listed in Table 24.1. These principles provide an acceptable framework, though close scrutiny of many difficult dilemmas highlights limitations in these principles and apparent conflicts between them. Everyone involved in clinical genetics will sooner or later be confronted by complex and challenging ethical situations, some of which pose particularly difficult problems with no obvious solution, and certainly no perfect one. Just as patients need to balance risks when making a decision about a treatment option, so the clinician/counselor may need to balance these principles one against the other. A particular difficulty in medical genetics can be the principle of *autonomy*, given that we all share our genes with our biological relatives. Individual autonomy needs

**Table 24.1 Fundamental ethical principles**

| |
|---|
| AUTONOMY – incorporating respect for the individual, privacy, the importance of informed consent and confidentiality |
| BENEFICENCE – the principle of seeking to do good and therefore acting in the best interests of the patient |
| NON-MALEFICENCE – the principle of seeking, overall, not to harm, i.e. not to leave the patient in a worse condition than pre-treatment |
| JUSTICE – incorporating fairness for the patient in the context of the resources available, equity of access and opportunity |

sometimes to be weighed against the principle of doing good, and doing no harm, to close family members.

In practice, the issues that commonly arise in the genetic clinic during any patient contact are outlined below.

## AUTONOMY

The patient should be in charge when it comes to decisions that have to be made. The degree to which this is possible is a function of the quality of information given. Sometimes patients are still seeking some form of guidance in order to give them confidence in the decision they reach, and it will require the judgment of the clinician/counselor as to how much guidance is appropriate in a given situation. The patient should feel comfortable to proceed no further, and opt out if they wish, at any stage of the process, which applies particularly in the context of predictive genetic testing.

## INFORMED CHOICE

The patient is entitled to full information about all options available in a given situation, including the option of not participating. Potential consequences of each decision option should be discussed. No duress should be applied and the clinician/counselor should not have a vested interest in the patient pursuing any particular course of action.

## INFORMED CONSENT

A patient is entitled to an honest and full explanation before any procedure or test is undertaken. Information should include details of the risks, limitations, implications and possible outcomes of each procedure. In the current climate, with respect to full information and the doctor–patient contract, some form of *signed* consent is increasingly being obtained for every action that exposes the patient – access to medical records, clinical photography, genetic testing and storage of DNA. In clinical genetics many patients having genetic tests are children or individuals with learning difficulties who lack the capacity to grant informed consent. Furthermore, the test result has only a small chance of directly benefiting the patient, but is potentially very important for members of the wider family. Decisions must take into account not only the 'best interests' of the patient but also the wider interests.

## CONFIDENTIALITY

A patient has a right to complete confidentiality, and there are clearly many issues relating to genetic disease which a patient, or a couple, would wish to keep totally private. Stigmatization and guilt may still accompany the concept of hereditary illness. Traditionally, confidentiality should only be breached under extreme circumstances, for example when it is deemed that an individual's behavior could convey a high risk of harm to self or to others. In trying to help some patients in the genetic clinic, however, it may be desirable to have a sample of DNA from a key family member, in which case some disclosure of detail is necessary. There is the difficult area of sharing information and results between different regional genetic services. This is a complex area in the context of genetic disease.

# ETHICAL DILEMMAS

## PRENATAL DIAGNOSIS

Many methods are now widely available for diagnosing structural abnormalities and genetic disorders during the first and second trimesters (Ch. 21). The last 20–30 years have seen the first real availability of *choice* in the context of pregnancy in human history. Not surprisingly, the issue of prenatal diagnosis and subsequent offer of termination of pregnancy raises many difficult issues for individuals and families, and raises serious questions about the way in which society views and cares for both children and adults with disability. In the UK termination of pregnancy is permitted up to and beyond 24 weeks gestation if the fetus has a lethal condition such as anencephaly, or if there is a serious risk of major physical or mental handicap. Terms such as 'serious' are not defined in the relevant legislation.

The difficulties surrounding prenatal diagnosis can be illustrated by considering some of the general principles that have already been discussed. At the top of the list comes informed consent. In the UK approximately 70% of all pregnancies are monitored for the presence of a neural tube defect by measurement of $\alpha$-fetoprotein in maternal serum at approximately 16 weeks gestation (p. 327). In theory all women undergoing this test should have a full understanding of its potential implications. This also applies to every woman who is offered a detailed ultrasound scan to assess fetal anatomy at around 18 weeks gestation (p. 328). For fully informed consent to be obtained in these situations it is essential that pregnant women should have access to detailed counseling by unhurried staff who are well informed, experienced and sympathetic. In practice it is unlikely that this always applies; indeed, there is evidence that the quality of information provided varies widely.

The most difficult problems in prenatal diagnosis are those involving autonomy and individual choice. This relates particularly to disease severity and who should make the decision that termination is justified. This can be illustrated by considering the following situations. First of all, parents whose first child, a boy, has autism are expecting another baby. They have read that autism is more common in boys than girls, so they request sexing of the fetus with a view to terminating a male fetus but continuing if the sex is female. Overall, however, the risk of having another child with autism is only about 5%. Such a request presents the clinician and counselor with a challenge. There is general agreement in the medical genetics community that sex selection for purely social reasons is not justified as grounds for termination of pregnancy (nor indeed for embryo selection by PGD, though in the USA it is permissible to perform sex selection by PGD for 'family balancing'). In the UK the general public, through a public consultation process overseen by the HFEA, has overwhelmingly expressed the view that sex selection for social reasons and family balancing is not acceptable – children should be considered as gifts, not consumer commodities. But what about this situation, when the risk of a second child having autism is low, and it cannot be guaranteed that a daughter would not be affected?

Next, consider the unusual but not unprecedented dilemma that arises when parents with an inherited condition indicate that they only wish to continue with a pregnancy if tests show that their unborn baby *is also affected*. Examples of conditions that could generate a request of this nature include achondroplasia and congenital sensorineural hearing loss. If the family's autonomy and right to choose is to be respected then their request should be granted. Many readers of this chapter will be very uncomfortable with the suggestion that an unaffected pregnancy should be terminated. This particular scenario illustrates the difficulty of defining what is normal.

The issue of autonomy and individual choice can also arise when a fetus is found to have a relatively mild abnormality, such as a non-syndromal cleft lip and palate, for which surgical correction usually achieves an excellent outcome. For some parents, particularly those who themselves have had an unhappy childhood because of being stigmatized for a similar problem, the prospect of having a similarly affected child can be unacceptable. Understandably, medical and nursing staff may feel very uneasy about complying with a request for termination of pregnancy in this situation.

It is inevitable that a subject as emotive as termination of pregnancy will generate controversy and the ethical dilemmas that arise are not easily resolved. Proponents of choice argue that selective termination should be available, particularly if the alternative involves a lifetime of pain and suffering. More often than not prenatal diagnostic techniques provide reassurance and their availability allows many couples to embark upon a pregnancy who would otherwise have been deterred. When viewed in the context of abortion in general, termination on the grounds of fetal abnormality constitutes less than 2% of the total of nearly 200 000 abortions carried out each year in the UK.

Those who hold opposing views argue on religious, moral or ethical grounds that selective termination is little less than legalized infanticide. Key to the ethical issue here are views on the status and rights of the embryo and fetus, and for those who believe that the fertilized egg constitutes full human status PGD and embryo research are unacceptable. Indeed, logically, all IVF programs are unacceptable by virtue of generating thousands of spare human embryos to be kept in freezers, most never used. There is also concern that prenatal diagnostic screening programs could lead to a devaluing of handicapped individuals in society, with a possible shift of resources away from their care to the funding of programs aimed at 'preventing' their birth. The debate about the ethics of prenatal diagnosis is a fierce one that will become even more difficult when genes are identified for common multifactorial disorders such as depression and schizophrenia. Mutations or polymorphisms in such genes are likely to confer a *risk* that the fetus will develop the condition as an adult, not that the individual will definitely be affected. A technology likely to stoke the ethical debate is the development of DNA microarrays and automated mutation detection methods. This could open up the possibility of affordable, wide-ranging genetic screening that might be offered antenatally.

Current indications from public consultation exercises conducted by the Advisory Committee on Genetic Testing (now subsumed into the Human Genetics Commission) and the Human Fertilization and Embryology Authority are reasonably reassuring. The views expressed support the applications of genetics in prenatal testing for *serious* disorders but concern over wider applications of the techniques. Similarly, research published by the British Social Attitudes survey, in the context of genetic research and gene manipulation for the detection of disease, suggests that the public supports these activities in general but expresses deep reservations for application of the technologies for *genetic enhancement*. Genetic enhancement, through manipulation of embryos or gametes, strikes at the very heart of what it means to have one's own identity through natural laws of chance. This, it seems, is a powerful undercurrent in the understanding of who we are as individuals and as a species.

## PREDICTIVE TESTING IN CHILDHOOD

Understandably, parents sometimes wish to know whether or not a child has inherited the gene for an adult-onset autosomal dominant disorder that runs in the family. It could be argued that this knowledge will help the parents guide their child towards the most appropriate educational and career opportunities and that to refuse their request is a denial of their rights as parents.

Similarly, parents sometimes request information about the carrier status of young healthy siblings of a child with a recessive disorder such as cystic fibrosis. Sometimes this information will have become available as a result of prenatal diagnostic testing for the homozygous affected state.

The problem with agreeing to this type of request is that it is a clear infringement of the child's own future autonomy. Increasingly, it is felt that testing should be delayed until the child reaches an age when he or she can make his or her own informed decision. There is also concern about the possible deleterious effects on a child of growing up with the certain knowledge of developing a serious adult-onset hereditary disorder or being a carrier of a recessive disorder, particularly if the tests have proved negative in the child's other siblings. Such a situation could raise a very real possibility of stigmatization. However, although there is consensus among geneticists that children should not be tested for carrier status, the evidence that such testing causes emotional or psychological harm is weak.

The situation is very different if predictive testing could be of direct medical benefit to the child. This applies to conditions such as familial hypercholesterolemia (p. 170) for which early dietary management can be introduced, and also to some of the familial cancer-predisposing syndromes (p. 218) for which early screening, sometimes prophylactic surgery, is indicated. Generally, it is felt that in these situations genetic testing is acceptable at around the time when other screening tests or preventive measures would be initiated.

One of the arguments for not testing children for adult-onset disorders is that parents might view their child differently, perhaps prejudicially, in some way. This type of argument has been voiced in relation to the PGD cases that have selected embryos not only for their negative affection status for Fanconi anemia but also in order to be a potential stem cell donor for their affected child. Those objecting to this use of technology cite a *utilitarian*, or *instrumental*, attitude towards the child created in this way. Furthermore, the child so created has no choice about whether to be a tissue-matched donor for the sick sibling. Will the child eventually feel 'used' by the parents, and how might it feel if the treatment fails and the sick sibling dies? At present these questions are imponderables because the children created for this purpose are too young to tell how they feel, and the numbers of such children will be very small for the foreseeable future.

## IMPLICATIONS FOR THE IMMEDIATE FAMILY (INADVERTENT TESTING OR TESTING BY 'PROXY')

A positive test result in an individual can have major implications for close antecedent relatives who themselves do not wish to be informed of their disease status. For example, consider Huntington disease (HD), for which direct mutational analysis is now available (p. 293). A young man aged 20 years requests predictive testing prior to starting his family; his fears are based on a confirmed diagnosis in his 65-year-old paternal grandfather. Predictive testing would be relatively straightforward were it not for the fact that his father, who is obviously at a prior risk of 1 in 2, specifically does not wish to know whether he will develop the disease.

Thus the young man has raised the difficult question of how to comply with his request without inadvertently carrying out a predictive test on his father. A negative result in the young man leaves scope for doubt; in principle no harm would be done. A positive result in the son, however, would be difficult to conceal from an observant father, who will be alert to his son's subsequent behavior. Clearly a positive result in the son would indicate that the father must be heterozygous for the HD gene – and would, therefore, be expected to develop the disease if he has not done so already.

There is no easy solution to this particular problem. In the guidelines drawn up in 1994 for predictive testing in HD it was concluded that 'every effort should be made by the counselors and the persons concerned to come to a satisfactory solution' with the rider that 'if no consensus can be reached the right of the adult child to know should have priority over the right of the parent not to know'.

## IMPLICATIONS FOR THE EXTENDED FAMILY

It is widely agreed that the identification of a condition that could have implications for other family members should lead to the offer of tests for the extended family. This applies particularly to balanced translocations and serious X-linked recessive disorders. In the case of translocations this is sometimes referred to as translocation 'chasing'. For an autosomal recessive disorder such as cystic fibrosis the term 'cascade screening' is applied (p. 324).

The main ethical problem which arises here is that of confidentiality. A carrier of a translocation or serious X-linked recessive disorder is usually urged to alert close family relatives to the possibility that they could also be carriers and therefore be at risk of having affected children. Alternatively, permission can be sought for members of the genetics team to make these approaches. Occasionally a patient, for whatever reason, will refuse to allow this information to be disseminated.

Faced with this situation, what should the clinical geneticist do? In practice most clinical geneticists would try to convince their patient of the importance of offering information and tests to relatives, possibly by providing an explanation of the consequences and ill-feeling that could arise in the future if a relative was to have an affected child whose birth could have been predicted and perhaps avoided. In most cases skilled and sensitive counseling will lead to a satisfactory solution. Ultimately, however, many clinical geneticists would opt to respect their patient's confidentiality rather than break the trust that forms a cornerstone of the traditional doctor–patient relationship. Not all would agree, and where the application of this standard could result in damage or morbidity to other family members the clinician might seek to *persuade* the individual to disclose the medical/genetic information, and this view is backed up by the statements of authoritative working parties, such as the Nuffield Council on Bioethics. Sometimes it is possible to draw the issue to the attention of the general practitioner who looks after the family member believed to be at risk – the general practitioner might be well placed to open the issue up in a sensitive way.

## INFORMED CONSENT IN GENETIC RESEARCH

All individuals who agree to undergo genetic testing in a service context are obviously entitled to a full and clear explanation of what the test involves and how the results could have implications for both themselves and other family members. Vigorous efforts are usually made to ensure that these basic principles are adhered to, particularly when predictive testing for serious late-onset genetic disorders is being undertaken.

The issues relating to informed consent when participating in genetic research are just as complex. Many people are perfectly willing to hold out their arm for a blood test 'which might help others', particularly if they have personal experience of a serious disorder in their own family. However, few will have given any serious thought to the possible ramifications of their simple act of altruism. For example, it is unlikely that they will ever have considered whether their sample will be tested anonymously, who will be informed of the result, or whether other tests will be carried out on stored DNA in the future as new techniques are developed. These concerns, among others (Table 24.2), have prompted the NIH Office of Protection from Research Risks to draw up proposals on the steps that should be taken to try to ensure that all aspects of informed consent are addressed when samples are collected for genetic research. Just as signed consent for genetic testing and storage of DNA is becoming quite routine in the service setting, similar procedures should be adhered to in a research setting.

**Table 24.2 Issues of disclosure and consent in genetic research**

| The nature of the study |
|---|
| Who is doing the study and where is it being carried out? |
| Availability of results and their implications for the individual and extended family regarding health, employment and insurance |
| Anonymity of testing and confidentiality of results |
| Long-term storage of DNA and its possible use in other research projects |
| Potential commercial applications and profit |

## ETHICAL DILEMMAS IN A WIDER CONTEXT

Recent progress in genetics, most notably in the area of molecular testing, has brought the ethical debate into a much wider public arena. Topics such as insurance and DNA databases, patenting, gene therapy, population screening, cloning and stem-cell research are now rightly viewed as being of major societal, commercial and political importance, and perhaps not surprisingly they feature prominently in media discussion. All of these subjects impact on the specialty of medical genetics and each of these will now be considered in turn.

## GENETICS AND INSURANCE

The availability of predictive tests for disorders of adult onset that convey a risk for chronic ill health with the possibility of a reduction in life expectancy has generated widespread concern about the extent to which the results of these tests should be revealed to outside agencies. Chief among these are the life insurance companies. In countries with only limited welfare medical services this is also an issue for private health care insurance, including critical illness and disability income. In addition, if either life or health insurance is arranged through an employer, then in theory there could also be implications for long-term career prospects as a positive predictive genetic test could lead to withdrawal of an offer of employment.

The life insurance industry is competitive and profit driven. Private insurance is based on the concept of 'mutuality', whereby risks are pooled for individuals in similar circumstances. In contrast public health services are based on the principle of 'solidarity', whereby health provision for everyone is funded from general taxation. It is understandable that the life insurance industry is concerned that individuals who receive a positive result from a predictive test will take out large policies without revealing their true risk status. This is referred to as 'antiselection' or 'adverse selection'. On the other hand, there is a very real fear among the genetics community that individuals who test positive will find themselves victims of discrimination, possibly to the extent that they become uninsurable. This concern also extends to those who have a family history of a late-onset disorder who might be refused insurance unless they undergo predictive testing.

Concerns about this very real possibility that DNA testing will create an uninsurable 'genetic underclass' have led to the introduction of legislation in many parts of the USA aimed at limiting the use of genetic information by health insurers. This culminated in 1996 in President Clinton signing The Health Insurance Portability and Accountability Act, which expressly prevents employer-based health plans refusing coverage on genetic grounds when a person changes employment. In the UK this whole area was considered in 1995 by the House of Commons Science and Technology Committee, which recommended that a Human Genetics Advisory Commission be established to overview developments in human genetics. In 1997 this Advisory Commission (now subsumed into the Human Genetics Commission) recommended that applicants for life insurance should not have to disclose the results of any genetic test to a prospective insurer and that a moratorium on disclosure of genetic test results should last for at least 2 years until genetic testing had been carefully evaluated.

To the disappointment of the genetics community, the UK government opted not to accept the recommendation of this advisory body, preferring instead to allow the recommendations of the Association of British Insurers (ABI) to prevail. Some of the key points in these recommendations are listed in Table 24.3. In the 1999 revision of its Code of Practice, the ABI reiterated its view that applicants should not be asked to undergo genetic testing and that existing genetic test results need not be disclosed in applications for mortgage-related life assurance up to a total of £100 000.

In the UK the Genetics and Insurance Committee has been established with a broad membership drawn from the insurance industry, the medical community and interested public bodies. One of the chief remits of this committee is to evaluate genetic tests as they are developed, and the ABI has stated in its code of practice that genetic test results should not be taken into account until each specific test is fully validated.

**Table 24.3 Key points in the Association of British Insurers (ABI) Code of Practice for genetic testing (1999)**

| |
|---|
| Applicants must not be asked to undergo genetic testing* |
| Results of genetic tests that have been undertaken should be disclosed |
| Only test results that have been validated should be taken into account |
| Existing genetic test results need not be disclosed in applications for mortgage-related life assurance up to a total of £100 000. |
| The results of genetic tests undertaken by an applicant will not be taken into account when assessing an application from another individual and vice versa |

*A genetic test is defined as 'an examination of the chromosome, DNA or RNA to find out if there is an otherwise undetectable related genotype, which may indicate an increased chance of that individual developing a specific disease in the future'

The issues involved in genetic testing and the insurance industry are not going to be easily resolved. If 'polygenes' conveying susceptibility to common disorders of adult life are identified, then almost the entire population could find itself at the mercy of a profit-driven commercially focused insurance industry. Among the genetics community there is a strong view that legislation is urgently needed to ensure that those who are genetically disadvantaged, through no fault of their own, do not face discrimination when seeking health-care or long-term life insurance. These are powerful arguments favoring retention of the principles of the NHS.

The possibility of government-controlled DNA databases for the population has also brought the insurance debate into focus. The use of DNA matching (fingerprinting) in criminal investigations is now so sophisticated that there is a natural desire on the part of law enforcers to be able to identify the DNA fingerprint for anyone in the general population. The existing database in the UK, which once contained material solely from sentenced offenders, is being expanded. In certain types of crime whole sections of a community are invited to come forward to give a sample of DNA so that they can be eliminated from enquiries. By the summer of 2003 one in 30 people in the UK already featured on the database. Large numbers of samples have been, or will be, collected as part of big population studies such as ALSPAC (Avon Longitudinal Study of Parents and Children) or the UK Biobank project. Clearly, there is a need for safeguards to be built into the use that is made of DNA collections like these, and access to them. Debate will certainly continue on the use and misuse of personal genetic data.

## GENE PATENTING AND THE HUMAN GENOME PROJECT

The controversy surrounding the patenting of naturally occurring human DNA sequences, be they complete genes or ESTs, neatly encapsulates the conflict between harsh commercial realism and altruistic academic idealism. On the one hand biotechnology companies that have invested heavily in molecular research can argue with conviction that both they and their shareholders are entitled to benefit from the fruits of their labors. Biotechnology research is indeed expensive, and it can reasonably be argued that any commercial company is entitled to a fair return on its investments. Those who embrace a more idealistic view have argued that the human genome represents mankind's 'common heritage' and that information gained through the Human Genome Project, or other molecular research, should be freely available for the benefit of everyone. Proponents of this latter view frequently cite alleged exploitation of patients and communities who have donated their blood samples for research, little realizing that their generosity could be exploited for financial gain. This is amply illustrated by the furore surrounding the proposed use (or abuse) of a centralized medical database of the entire Icelandic population to help identify 'polygenes' for potential commercial gain (p. 142).

Given the complexity of the legal issues involved it is not surprising that the international community has struggled to identify satisfactory solutions. With the exception of the USA, most international regulatory bodies prohibit payment for the procurement of human genetic material, but their views on patenting are much less well defined. In the new millennium, the reality is that many important human genes have been patented, and companies such as Myriad Genetics in the USA have clearly indicated that they intend to exercise their exclusive licence for genetic testing for *BRCA1* and *BRCA2* (p. 217). In the short term the impact of gene patents will be mainly on single-gene disorders, and clearly if excessive costs are imposed this will raise a direct challenge to the fundamental ethical principle of equity of access. In the longer term gene patenting could impinge directly on testing for common polygenic disorders and for treating both genetic and non-genetic problems, such as baldness and obesity, using gene therapy. As illustrations of the prevailing levels of investment it is worth noting that the rights to one gene associated with obesity were sold in 1995 for $70 million, while in 1997 DeCODE, the Icelandic genomics company at the centre of the controversy regarding national assent, sold the potential rights to 12 genes, possibly associated with common complex diseases, to Hoffman-La Roche for $200 million.

## GENE THERAPY

One of the most exciting aspects of recent progress in molecular biology is the prospect of successful gene therapy (p. 358), although it is obviously disappointing that this potential has not as yet been realized. It is understandable that both the general public and the health-care professions should be concerned about the possible side-effects and its abuse. Frequent reference has been made to the 'slippery slope' argument, whereby it is claimed that one innocent concession will lead inevitably to uncontrolled experimentation. To address these anxieties, advisory or regulatory committees have been established in several countries to assess the practical and ethical aspects of gene therapy research program.

Concern centers around two fundamental issues. The first relates to the practical aspects of ensuring informed consent on the part of patients who wish to participate in gene therapy research. Adult patients and parents of affected children could well be desperate to participate in gene therapy research, particularly if their disease is otherwise incurable. Consequently they could be tempted to disregard the possible hazards of what is essentially a new, untried and unproven therapeutic approach. In the UK, the Committee on the Ethics of Gene Therapy has recommended that until this is shown to be safe, all gene therapy program should be subjected to careful scrutiny by local hospital research ethical committees. In addition, a national supervisory body, the Gene Therapy Advisory Committee, has been established to review all proposals to conduct gene therapy in humans and to monitor and record complications in ongoing gene therapy trials. In this way it is anticipated that the rights of individual patients in terms of both consent and confidentiality will be safeguarded.

The second aspect of gene therapy that generates concern is the possibility that it could be used for eugenic purposes. On this point the British committee has recommended that genetic modification involving the germ line (p. 358) should not be attempted. Therefore, by limiting gene therapy to somatic cells it should not be possible for newly modified genes to be transmitted to future generations. This committee has also recommended that somatic cell gene therapy should only be used to try to treat serious diseases, and should not be used to alter human characteristics such as intelligence or athletic prowess, nor used in any sense that could be construed as cosmetic.

The potential benefits of gene therapy are enormous and, although it is disappointing that initial success has been very limited, it is inevitable that both somatic and germ-line gene therapy will continue to be the focus of intense research activity. The degree of caution exercised by national committees overseeing the ethics of gene therapy illustrates the care that is being taken by medical and governing bodies to ensure that human gene manipulation will not be abused. This is demonstrated by the halting of gene therapy trials at an American institute following the death of a young man who was being treated for ornithine decarboxylase deficiency. The US Food and Drug Administration promptly suspended this particular study and halted all others pending further investigations.

## POPULATION SCREENING

Population screening programs offering carrier detection for common autosomal recessive disorders have been in operation for many years (p. 322). These have been well received for thalassemia and Tay–Sachs disease, for which screening has been carefully planned using well-informed and highly motivated target populations. In contrast, early efforts to introduce sickle-cell carrier detection in North America were largely unsuccessful because of misinformation, discrimination and stigmatization. Pilot studies assessing the responses to cystic fibrosis carrier screening in Caucasian populations have yielded conflicting results (p. 323).

The differing receptions to these various screening programs illustrate the importance of informed consent and the difficulties of ensuring both autonomy and informed choice. For example, it is now UK government policy for cystic fibrosis screening to be introduced into the neonatal screening program. Whilst aimed at identifying babies with CF the screening will inevitably detect a proportion who are simply carriers. It has also been suggested that screening for CF carrier status be introduced as an option for all school children at age 16 years. Clearly newborn infants cannot make an informed choice and it is doubtful whether all 16-year-olds are sufficiently mature to make a fully reasoned decision for themselves.

Consequently, many pilot studies have focused on adults and their responses to the offer of carrier testing, either from their general practitioner or at the antenatal clinic. This has raised the vexed question of whether an offer from a respected family doctor could be interpreted as an implicit recommendation to participate that cannot be easily refused. A personal 'opportunistic' invitation to participate from a general practitioner yields a much higher acceptance rate than a casual written invitation to attend for screening at a future date. This difference in rates of uptake could simply be a reflection of inertia, but could also indicate that individuals feel pressurized to agree to a test which they do not necessarily want.

It is, therefore, important that even the most well-intended offer of carrier detection should be worded carefully so as to ensure that participation is entirely voluntary. Full counseling in the event of a positive result is also essential to minimize the risk of any feeling of stigmatization or genetic inferiority.

In population screening confidentiality is also important. Many will not wish their carrier status to be known by classmates or colleagues at work. The issue of confidentiality will become particularly difficult for individuals who are found to be genetically susceptible to a potential industrial hazard such as smoke or dust. There is concern that such individuals will be discriminated against by potential employers (p. 187), and doctors could find themselves in the invidious position of having to provide information that jeopardizes their patient's employment prospects.

These anxieties led in 1995 to the Equal Employment Opportunity Commission in the USA issuing a guideline that allows for anyone denied employment because of a disease susceptibility to claim protection under the Americans with Disabilities Act.

## CLONING AND STEM CELL RESEARCH

'Dolly' the sheep, born in July 1996 near Edinburgh, was the first mammal cloned from an adult cell, and when her existence was announced about 6 months later the world suddenly became intensely interested in cloning. Dolly was 'conceived' by fusing individual mammary gland cells with unfertilized eggs from which the nucleus had been removed, and 277 attempts failed before a successful pregnancy ensued. It was immediately assumed that the technology would sooner or later lead to a cloned human being and there have been some unsubstantiated, almost certainly bogus, claims to this effect. In fact, there has been widespread rejection of any desirability for human *reproductive* cloning, with strong statements emanating from politicians, religious leaders, and scientists. Experiments with animals have continued to have a very poor success rate and for this reason alone no rational person is advocating 'experiments' in humans. In some cloned animals the features have suggested possible defects in genomic imprinting. Dolly died prematurely of lung disease in February 2003 and she had a number of characteristics suggesting she was not biologically normal.

Lessons have been learned from Dolly in relation to cell nuclear replacement (CNR) technology and this has, potentially, opened the door to understanding more about cell differentiation. The focus has therefore shifted to *therapeutic* cloning using stem cells, and the prospects this holds with respect to human disease. If stem cells were subjected to nuclear transfer from a patient in need, these might be stimulated to grow into any tissue, perhaps in unlimited quantities and genetically identical to the patient, thus avoiding rejection. The potential possibilities are legion, and one can envisage novel treatment for Parkinson or Alzheimer disease, myocardial infarction, osteoporosis or severe burns, to name but a few. The main ethical difficulty arises in relation to the source of stem cells. Currently, the best source is believed to be *embryonic* stem cells, and the UK Parliament moved swiftly to approve an extension to research on early human embryos for this purpose. Research on human embryos up to 14 days of age was already permitted under the 1990 Human Fertilisation and Embryology Act.

Those who object to the use of embryonic stem cells believe it could be the first step towards reproductive cloning and some consider it unethical because it treats the embryo with disrespect and as a means to an end. The research envisaged would probably be performed on human embryos surplus to requirements from IVF clinics, but there is understandable concern that embryos would be deliberately created for research purposes. In fact, the HFE Act of 1990 permits the creation of human embryos for research, but only about 100 have been created since the HFEA began granting licences. Those who object have further pointed out that significant advances are being made on adult stem cells. If these could be harvested and manipulated to the same potential as embryonic stem cells, those objecting to embryo research would be satisfied. Clearly, this remains a contentious and hotly debated ethical issue.

## CONCLUSION

It is clear that ethical issues are of major importance in medical genetics. Each new discovery brings new challenges and raises new dilemmas for which there are usually no easy answers. On a global scale the computerization of medical records, together with the widespread introduction of genetic testing, makes it essential that safeguards are introduced to ensure that fundamental principles such as privacy and confidentiality are maintained. Members of the medical genetics community will continue to play a pivotal role in trying to balance the needs of their patients and families with the demands of an increasingly cost-conscious society and a commercially driven biotechnology industry. Cost–benefit arguments can be persuasive in cold financial terms but take no account of the fundamental human and social issues that are often involved. Increasingly, it will fall upon the shoulders of the medical genetics community to try to ensure that the interests of their patients and families take precedence, and towards that end it is hoped that this chapter, and, indeed, the rest of this textbook, can make a positive contribution.

## FURTHER READING


American Society of Human Genetics Report 1996 Statement on informed consent for genetic research. Am J Hum Genet 59: 471–474

*The statement of the American Society of Human Genetics Board of Directors on the issues relating to informed consent in genetic research.*

Association of British Insurers 1999 Genetic testing. ABI code of practice. ABI, London

*A formal statement of the principles and practice adopted by the British insurance industry with regard to genetic testing.*

British Medical Association 1998 Human genetics. Choice and responsibility. Oxford University Press, Oxford

*A comprehensive wide ranging report produced by a BMA medical ethics committee steering group on the ethical issues raised by genetics in clinical practice.*

Bryant J, Baggott la Velle L, Searle J (eds) 2002 Bioethics for scientists. John Wiley & Sons, Chichester, England

*A multi-author text of wide scope with many contributions relevant to medical genetics.*

Clarke A (ed) 1997 The genetic testing of children. Bios Scientific Publishers, Oxford

*A comprehensive multi-author text dealing with this important subject.*

Collins F S 1999 Shattuck lecture – medical and societal consequences of the human genome project. New Engl J Med 341: 28–37

*A contemporary overview of the human genome project with due emphasis on its possible ethical and social implications.*

Harper P S, Clarke A J 1997 Genetics society and clinical practice. Bios Scientific, Oxford

*A thoughtful account of the important ethical and social aspects of recent developments in clinical genetics.*

Human Genetics Commission 2002 Inside information: balancing interests in the use of personal genetic data. Department of Health, London

*A detailed working party report by the Human Genetics Commission covering the use and abuse of personal genetic information.*

Knoppers B M 1999 Status, sale and patenting of human genetic material: an international survey. Nature Genet 22: 23–26

*An overview of current international policies on gene patenting.*

McInnis M G 1999 The assent of a nation: genethics and Iceland. Clin Genet 55: 234–239

*A critical review of the complex ethical issues raised by the decision of the Icelandic government to collaborate in genetic research with a biotechnology company.*

Nuffiield Council on Bioethics 1993 Genetic screening: ethical issues. Nuffield Council on Bioethics, London

*A very helpful document for professional guidance.*

Nuffiield Council on Bioethics 1998 Mental disorders and genetics: the ethical context. Nuffield Council on Bioethics, London

*A further detailed document dealing with genetic issues in the context of mental health.*

Pokorski R J 1997 Insurance underwriting in the genetic era. Am J Hum Genet 60: 205–216

*A detailed account of the issues surrounding the use of genetic tests by the insurance industry.*

Report of the Committee on the Ethics of Gene Therapy 1992 HMSO, London

*The recommendations of the committee chaired by Sir Cecil Clothier on the ethical aspects of somatic cell and germ-line gene therapy.*


## ELEMENTS

1. Ethical considerations impinge on almost every aspect of clinical genetics. In a wider context developments in molecular biology have important ethical implications for society at large.

2. Subjects that can generate particularly difficult problems in clinical genetics include prenatal diagnosis, predictive testing in childhood and genetic testing in the extended family.

3. Possible applications of molecular genetics of importance on a wider scale include the use of genetic test results by the insurance industry, gene patenting, gene therapy and population screening.

4. There are no easy or correct solutions for many of the difficult ethical problems that arise in clinical genetics. It is important that guidelines and regulations are established that recognize each individual's fundamental entitlement to respect for autonomy, informed choice and consent, privacy and confidentiality.

APPENDIX

# WEBSITES AND CLINICAL DATABASES

## CLINICAL GENETICS SERVICES WEBSITES

The rate of generation of information about human, medical and clinical genetics and the Human Genome Project means that access to current information is vital to both the student and the doctor, particularly since patients and families often come to the clinic armed with the same information!

There are a number of general websites that students will find useful as entry points with a wealth of links to other sites for 'surfing'. Other specialized websites may be of interest, in relation to specific interests.

Clinical geneticists regularly use a number of expert databases to assist in the diagnosis of genetic disorders and diseases, some of which are listed. Some clinical genetics services have websites describing their service, as well as education aspects and other useful links.

Lastly, students may find it of interest and value to see the range of material available for teaching and learning medical genetics in medical schools throughout the world.

## GENERAL GENETIC WEBSITES

Online Mendelian Inheritance in Man (OMIM)
http://www3.ncbi.nlm.nih.gov/omim/
*Online access to McKusick's catalogue, an invaluable resource for clinical genetic information with a wealth of links to many other resources.*
Genetic Interest Group
http://www.gig.org.uk/
*Website for alliance of organizations supporting people affected with genetic disorders.*
Gene tests
http://www.genetests.org/
*Includes useful reviews of genetic disorders.*

## HUMAN GENOME WEBSITES

Research Program on Ethical, Legal and Social Implications of Human Genome Project
http://www.nhgri.nih.gov./PolicyEthics/
*Site about ethical, legal and social implications of the Human Genome Project.*
Genome Database
http://www.gdb.org/
*An encyclopedia of the current state of knowledge of the human genome.*
Ensembl Genome Browser
http://www.ensembl.org/
*Joint project between the European Bioinformatics Society and the Sanger Institute to provide annotated eukaryotic genomes.*
UCSC Genome Bioinformatics
http://genome.ucsc.edu/
*University of California at Santa Cruz genome browser.*
Human Genome Organization
http://www.gene.ucl.ac.uk/hugo/
*The website of the international organization of scientists involved in the Human Genome Project.*
International HapMap Project
http://www.hapmap.org/
*The website of the project to map common DNA variants.*

## SPECIALIZED WEBSITES

Human Gene Mutation Database
http://www.uwcm.ac.uk/uwcm/mg/hgmd0.html
*A database of the reported mutations in human genes.*
Whitehead Institute for Biomedical Research/MIT Center for Genome Research
http://www-genome.wi.mit.edu/
*Human gene map, sequencing and software programs.*
The Rockefeller University Genetic Linkage Analysis Resources
http://linkage.rockefeller.edu/
*Linkage analysis and marker mapping programs.*
Mammalian Genetics Unit and Mouse Genome Centre
*http://www.mgu.har.mrc.ac.uk/*
*Mouse genome site.*
Drosophila melanogaster Genome Database
http://flybase.bio.indiana.edu:82/
*A comprehensive database for information on the genetics and molecular biology of* D. melanogaster, *including the genome sequence.*
Caenorhabditis Elegans Genetics and Genomics
http://elegans.swmed.edu/genome.shtml

C. elegans *genome project information.*
Yeast Genome Project
http://mips.gsf.de/genre/proj/yeast/index.jsp
*Yeast genome project information.*

## UNIVERSITY AND MEDICAL SCHOOL HUMAN/MEDICAL GENETICS WEBSITES

Louisiana State University
http://www.sh.lsumc.edu/pediatrics/genetics/tableof.htm
*Course material, assignments and answers, case studies.*
University of California, San Diego
http://www.biology.ucsd.edu/classes/CBB-Genetics/CBB1997A.html
*Syllabus, lecture outline and links.*
Robert Wood Johnson Medical School of the University of Medicine and Dentistry, NJ
http://www2.umdnj.edu/~genetics/hg-1.htm
*Course outline, syllabus.*
George Mason University
http://www.ncc.gmu.edu/dna/
*Tutorial on DNA structure, replication, transcription and translation.*
Dolan DNA Learning Centre at Cold Spring Harbor Laboratory
http://www.dnalc.org/
*Information about genes in education.*

## CLINICAL GENETICS SERVICES WEBSITES

University of South Dakota School of Medicine
http://www.kumc.edu/gec/prof/guide_sd.html
*Clinical genetics: a self-study guide.*
Tulane University
http://www.tmc.tulane.edu/departments/human_genetics/main.htm
*Clinical genetics services.*
Vanderbilt University Medical School
http://peds.mc.vanderbilt.edu/VCHWEB_1/Medical-Genetics.html
*Links to teaching resources.*

## CLINICAL DATABASES

London Dysmorphology Database (LDDB) Winter R M, Baraitser M. Oxford Medical, Oxford University Press, Oxford
*A diagnostic database that contains a detailed list of clinical features and references for each of the syndrome entries along with an abstract.*
Pictures of Standard Syndromes and Undiagnosed Malformations (POSSUM) Bankier A. The Murdoch Institute for Research into Birth Defects, PO Box 1100, Parkville 3052, Melbourne, Australia
*A database for the diagnosis of dysmorphic syndromes with description of the syndrome, clinical features, references, photographs and video sequences.*
The Human Cytogenetic Database (HCDB) Schinzel A. Oxford Medical, Oxford University Press, Oxford
*A diagnostic database with features and references on 1200 chromosomal abnormalities.*
London Neurological Database (LNDB) Winter R M, Baraitser M. Oxford Medical, Oxford University Press, Oxford
*A database for the diagnosis of neurogenetic syndromes or disorders containing an abstract and information about clinical features and references.*
A Radiological Electronic Atlas of Malformation Syndromes and Skeletal Dysplasias (REAMS). Hall C, Washbrook J. Oxford University Press, Oxford
*A database for the diagnosis of skeletal dysplasias and malformation syndromes to assist with diagnosis.*
Program Listing Abnormalities in Prenatal Ultrasound (Platypus) Benzie R J (ed) Toikinnoin, Inc., Ottawa, Canada
*A reference source demonstrating real-time images of 337 fetal anomalies with a diagnostic search facility and information and references on 3500 associated syndromes.*

# Glossary

**A.** Abbreviation for adenine.
**Acentric.** Lacking a centromere.
**Acetylation.** The introduction of an acetyl group into a molecule; often used by the body to help eliminate substances by the liver.
**Acrocentric.** Term used to describe a chromosome where the centromere is near one end and the short arm usually consists of satellite material.
**Acute phase proteins.** A number of proteins involved in innate immunity produced in reaction to infection which include C-reactive protein, mannose binding protein and serum amyloid P component.
**Adenine.** A purine base in DNA and RNA.
**Adenomatous polyposis coli (APC).** See Familial adenomatous polyposis.
**AIDS.** Acquired immunodeficiency syndrome.
**Allele (= allelomorph).** Alternative form of a gene found at the same locus on homologous chromosomes.
**Allograft.** A tissue graft between non-identical individuals.
**Allotypes.** Genetically determined variants of antibodies.
**Alpha (α)-thalassemia.** Inherited disorder of hemoglobin involving underproduction of the α-globin chains occurring most commonly in persons from South-East Asia.
**Alternative pathway.** One of the two pathways of the activation of complement which, in this instance, involves cell membranes of microorganisms.
**Alu repeat.** Short repeated DNA sequences which appear to have homology with transposable elements in other organisms.
**Am**. The group of genetic variants associated with the IgA heavy chain.
**Amino acid.** An organic compound containing both carboxyl (—COOH) and amino groups (—$NH_2$).
**Amniocentesis.** Procedure for obtaining amniotic fluid and cells for prenatal diagnosis.
**Amorph.** A mutation which leads to complete loss of function.
**Anaphase.** The stage of cell division when the chromosomes leave the equatorial plate and migrate to opposite poles of the spindle.
**Anaphase lag.** Loss of a chromosome as it moves to the pole of the cell during anaphase which can lead to monosomy.
**Aneuploid.** A chromosome number which is not an exact multiple of the haploid number, i.e. 2N – 1 or 2N + 1 where N is the haploid number of chromosomes.
**Anterior information.** Information previously known which leads to the prior probability.
**Antibody (= immunoglobulin).** A serum protein which is formed in response to an antigenic stimulus and reacts specifically with that antigen.
**Anticipation.** The tendency for some autosomal dominant diseases to manifest at an earlier age and/or to increase in severity with each succeeding generation.
**Anticodon.** The complementary triplet of the tRNA molecule which binds to it with a particular amino acid.
**Antigen.** A substance which elicits the synthesis of antibody with which it specifically reacts.
**Antigen binding fragment (Fab).** The fragment of the antibody molecule produced by papain digestion responsible for antigen binding.
**Antiparallel.** Opposite orientation of the two strands of a DNA duplex, one runs in the 3′ to 5′ direction, the other in the 5′ to 3′ direction.
**Antisense oligonucleotide.** A short oligonucleotide synthesized to bind to a particular RNA or DNA sequence to block its expression.
**Antisense strand.** The template strand of DNA.
**Apical ectodermal ridge.** Area of ectoderm in the developing limb bud which produces growth factors.
**Apolipoproteins.** A number of different proteins which are involved in lipid transportation in the circulation.
**Apoptosis.** Programmed involution or cell death of a developing tissue or organ of the body.
**Artificial insemination by donor (AID).** Use of semen from a male donor as a reproductive option for couples at high risk of transmitting a genetic disorder.
**Ascertainment.** The finding and selection of families with a hereditary disorder.
**Association.** The occurrence of a particular allele in a group of patients more often than can be accounted for by chance.
**Assortative mating (= non-random mating).** The preferential selection of a spouse with a particular phenotype.
**Atherosclerosis.** The fatty degenerative plaque which accumulates in the intimal wall of blood vessels.
**Autoimmune diseases.** Diseases which are thought to be caused by the body not recognizing its own antigens.
**Autonomous replication sequences.** DNA sequences which are necessary for accurate replication within yeast.
**Autoradiography.** Detection of radioactively labeled molecules on an X-ray film.
**Autosomal dominant.** A gene on one of the non-sex chromosomes which manifests in the heterozygous state.
**Autosomal inheritance.** The pattern of inheritance shown by a disorder or trait determined by a gene on one of the non-sex chromosomes.
**Autosomal recessive.** A gene located on one of the non-sex chromosomes which manifests in the homozygous state.
**Autosome.** Any of the 22 non-sex chromosomes.
**Autozygosity.** Homozygosity as a result of identity by descent from a common ancestor.
**Azoospermia.** Absence of sperm in semen.
**B lymphocytes.** Antibody-producing lymphocytes involved in humoral immunity.
**Bacterial artificial chromosome (BAC).** An artificial chromosome created from modification of the fertility factor of plasmids which allows incorporation of up to 330 kb of foreign DNA.
**Bacteriophage (= phage).** A virus which infects bacteria.
**Balanced polymorphism.** Two different genetic variants which are stably present in a population, i.e. selective advantages and disadvantages cancel each other out.
**Balanced translocation.** See Reciprocal translocation.
**Bare lymphocyte syndrome.** A rare autosomal recessive form of severe combined immunodeficiency due to absence of the class II molecules of the major histocompatibility complex.
**Barr body.** The condensation of the inactive X chromosome seen in the nucleus of certain types of cells from females. See Sex chromatin.

**Base.** Short for the nitrogenous bases in nucleic acid molecules (A = adenine; T = thymine; U = uracil; C = cytosine, G = guanine).
**Base pair (bp).** A pair of complementary bases in DNA (A with T, G with C).
**Bayes' theorem.** Combining the prior and conditional probabilities of certain events or the results of specific tests to give a joint probability to derive the posterior or relative probability.
**Bence–Jones protein.** The antibody of a single species produced in large amounts by a person with multiple myeloma, a tumor of antibody-producing plasma cells.
**Beta (β)-thalassemia.** Inherited disorder of hemoglobin involving underproduction of the β-globin chain, occurring most commonly in persons from the Mediterranean region and Indian subcontinent.
**Bias of ascertainment.** An artifact which must be taken into account in family studies when looking at segregation ratios, caused by families coming to attention because they have affected individual(s).
**Biochemical disorder.** An inherited disorder involving a metabolic pathway, i.e. an inborn error of metabolism.
**Biological or genetic determinism.** The premise that our genetic make-up is the only factor determining all aspects of our health and disease.
**Biosynthesis.** Use of recombinant DNA techniques to produce molecules of biological and medical importance in the laboratory or commercially.
**Bipolar illness.** Affective manic–depressive illness.
**Bivalent.** A pair of synapsed homologous chromosomes.
**Blastocyst.** Early embryo consisting of embryoblast and trophoblast.
**Blastomere.** A single cell of the early fertilized conceptus.
**Blood chimera.** A mixture of cells of different genetic origin present in twins as a result of an exchange of cells via the placenta between non-identical twins in utero.
**Boundary elements.** Short sequences of DNA, usually 500 bp to 3 kb in size, which block or inhibit the influence of regulatory elements of adjacent genes.
**Break-point cluster (bcr).** Region of chromosome 22 involved in the translocation seen in the majority of persons with chronic myeloid leukemia.
**C.** Abbreviation for cytosine.
**CAAT box.** A conserved, non-coding, so-called 'promoter' sequence about 80 bp upstream from the start of transcription.
**Cancer family syndrome.** A term used to describe the clustering in certain families of particular types of cancers, in which it has been proposed that the different types of malignancy could be due to a single dominant gene, specifically Lynch type II.
**Cancer genetics.** The study of the genetic causes of cancer.
**Candidate gene.** A gene whose function or location suggests that it is likely to be responsible for a particular genetic disease or disorder.
**5′ Cap.** Modification of the nascent mRNA by the addition of a methylated guanine nucleotide to the 5′ end of the molecule by an unusual 5′ to 5′ triphosphate linkage.
**CA repeat.** A short dinucleotide sequence present as tandem repeats at multiple sites in the human genome, producing microsatellite polymorphisms.
**Carrier.** Person heterozygous for a recessive gene, male or female for autosomal genes or female for X-linked genes.
**Cascade screening.** Identification within a family of carriers for an autosomal recessive disorder or persons with an autosomal dominant gene following ascertainment of an index case.
**Cell-mediated immunity.** Immunity which involves the T lymphocytes to fight intracellular infection and is involved in transplantation rejection and delayed hypersensitivity.
**Cellular oncogene.** See Proto-oncogene.
**CentiMorgan (cM).** Unit used to measure map distances, equivalent to a 1% chance of recombination (crossing over).
**Central dogma.** The concept that genetic information is usually only transmitted from DNA to RNA to protein.
**Centric fusion.** The fusion of the centromeres of two acrocentric chromosomes to form a Robertsonian translocation.
**Centriole.** The cellular structure from which microtubules radiate in the mitotic spindle involved in the separation of chromosomes in mitosis.
**Centromere (= kinetochore).** The point at which the two chromatids of a chromosome are joined, and the region of the chromosome which becomes attached to the spindle during cell division.
**Chemotaxis.** The attraction of phagocytes to the site of infection by components of complement.
**Chiasmat**a. Cross-overs between chromosomes in meiosis.
**Chimera.** An individual composed of two populations of cells with different genotypes.
**Chorion.** Layer of cells covering a fertilized ovum some of which, the chorion frondosum, will later form the placenta.
**Chorionic villus sampling.** Procedure using ultrasound guidance to obtain chorionic villi from the chorion frondosum for prenatal diagnosis.
**Chromatid.** During cell division each chromosome divides longitudinally into two strands, or chromatids, which are held together by the centromere.
**Chromatin.** The tertiary coiling of the nucleosomes of the chromosomes with associated proteins.
**Chromatin fibre FISH.** Use of extended chromatin or DNA fibers with fluorescent in situ hybridization to physically order DNA clones or sequences.
**Chromosomal analysis.** The process of counting and analyzing the banding pattern of the chromosomes of an individual.
**Chromosomal fragments.** Acentric chromosomes that can arise as a result of segregation of a paracentric inversion and which are usually incapable of replication.
**Chromosome instability.** The presence of breaks and gaps in the chromosomes from persons with a number of disorders associated with an increased risk of neoplasia.
**Chromosome mapping.** Assigning a gene or DNA sequence to a specific chromosome or a particular region of a chromosome.
**Chromosome-mediated gene transfer.** The technique of transferring chromosomes or parts of chromosomes to somatic cell hybrids to enable more detailed chromosome mapping.
**Chromosome painting.** The hybridization in situ of fluorescent-labeled probes to a chromosome preparation to allow identification of a particular chromosome(s).
**Chromosome walking.** Using an ordered assembly of clones to extend from a known start point.
**Chromosomes.** Thread-like, darkly staining bodies within the nucleus composed of DNA and chromatin that carry the genetic information.
***Cis*-acting.** Regulatory elements in the promoter region which act on genes on the same chromosome.
**Class switching.** Term used for the normal change in antibody class from IgM to IgG in the immune response.
**Classic gene families.** Multigene families which show a high degree of sequence homology.
**Classic pathway.** One of the two ways of activation of complement, in this instance, involving antigen–antibody complexes.
**Clone.** A group of cells, all of which are derived from a single cell by repeated mitoses, all having the same genetic information.
**Clone contigs.** Assembly of clones that have been mapped and ordered to produce an overlapping array.
**Cloning in silico.** The use of a number of computer programs which can search genomic DNA sequence databases for sequence homology to known genes, as well as DNA sequences specific to all genes such as the conserved intron/exon splice junctions, promoter sequences, polyadenylation sites and stretches of open-reading frames (ORFs) to identify novel genes.
**cM.** Abbreviation for centiMorgan.
**Codominance.** When both alleles are expressed in the heterozygote.
**Codon.** A sequence of three adjacent nucleotides that codes for one amino acid or chain termination.
**Common cancers.** The cancers that occur commonly in humans, such as bowel and breast cancer.
**Common diseases.** The diseases that occur commonly in humans, e.g. cancer, coronary artery disease, diabetes, etc.
**Community genetics.** The branch of medical genetics concerned with screening and the prevention of genetic diseases on a population basis.

**Comparative genomics.** The identification of orthologous genes in different species.
**Competent.** Making bacterial cell membrane permeable to DNA by a variety of different methods, including exposure to certain salts or high voltage.
**Complement.** A series of at least 10 serum proteins in humans (and other vertebrates) that can be activated by either the 'classic' or the 'alternative' pathways and which interact in sequence to bring about the destruction of cellular antigens.
**Complementary DNA (cDNA).** DNA synthesized from mRNA by the enzyme reverse transcriptase.
**Complementary strands.** The specific pairing of the bases in the DNA of the purines adenine and guanine with thymine and cytosine.
**Complete ascertainment.** A term used in segregation analysis for a type of study which identifies all affected individuals in a population.
**Compound heterozygote.** An individual who is affected with an autosomal recessive disorder having two different mutations in homologous genes.
**Concordance.** When both members of a pair of twins exhibit the same trait they are said to be concordant. If only one twin has the trait they are said to be discordant.
**Conditional knockout.** A mutation that is only expressed under certain conditions, e.g. raised temperature.
**Conditional probability.** Observations or tests which can be used to modify prior probabilities using Bayesian calculation in risk estimations.
**Conditionally toxic or suicide gene.** Genes that are introduced in gene therapy and which, under certain conditions or after the introduction of a certain substance, will kill the cell.
**Confined placental mosaicism.** The occurrence of a chromosomal abnormality in chorionic villus samples obtained for first-trimester prenatal diagnosis in which the fetus has a normal chromosomal complement.
**Congenital.** Any abnormality, whether genetic or not, which is present at birth.
**Congenital hypertrophy of the retinal pigment epithelium (CHRPE).** Abnormal retinal pigmentation that, when present in persons at risk for familial adenomatous polyposis, is evidence of the heterozygous state.
**Conjugation.** A chemical process in which two molecules are joined, often used to describe the process by which certain drugs or chemicals can then be excreted by the body, e.g. acetylation of isoniazid by the liver.
**Consanguineous marriage.** A marriage between 'blood relatives', that is, between persons who have one or more ancestors in common, most frequently between first cousins.
**Consanguinity.** Relationship between blood relatives.
**Consensus sequence.** A GGGCGGG sequence promoter element to the 5′ side of genes in eukaryotes involved in the control of gene expression.
**Conservative substitution.** Single base pair substitution which, although resulting in the replacement by a different amino acid, if chemically similar, has no functional effect.
**Constant region.** The portion of the light and heavy chains of antibodies in which the amino acid sequence is relatively constant from molecule to molecule.
**Constitutional.** Present in the fertilized gamete.
**Constitutional heterozygosity.** The presence in an individual at the time of conception of obligate heterozygosity at a locus when the parents are homozygous at that locus for different alleles.
**Consultand.** The person presenting for genetic advice.
**Contigs.** Contiguous or overlapping DNA clones.
**Contiguous gene syndrome.** Disorder resulting from deletion of adjacent genes.
**Continuous trait.** A trait, such as height, for which there is a range of observations or findings, in contrast to traits which are all or none, cf. discontinuous, such as cleft lip and palate.
**Control gene.** A gene which can turn other genes on or off, i.e. regulate.
**Cordocentesis.** The procedure of obtaining fetal blood samples for prenatal diagnosis.
**Corona radiata.** Cellular layer surrounding the mature oocyte.
**Cor pulmonale.** Right-sided heart failure, which can occur after serious lung disease, such as in persons with cystic fibrosis.
**Correlation.** Statistical measure of the degree of association or resemblance between two parameters.
**Cosmid.** A plasmid that has had the maximum DNA removed to allow the largest possible insert for cloning but still has the DNA sequences necessary for in vitro packaging into an infective phage particle.
**Co-twins.** Both members of a twin pair, whether dizygotic or monozygotic.
**Counselee.** Person receiving genetic counseling.
**Coupling.** When a certain allele at a particular locus is on the same chromosome with a specific allele at a closely-linked locus.
**CpG dinucleotides.** The occurrence of the nucleotides cytosine and guanine together in genomic DNA, which is frequently methylated and which is associated with spontaneous deamination of cytosine converting it to thymine as a mechanism of mutation.
**CpG islands.** Clusters of unmethylated CpGs occur near the transcription sites of many genes.
**Cross-over (= recombination).** The exchange of genetic material between homologous chromosomes in meiosis.
**Cross-reacting material (CRM).** Immunologically detected protein or enzyme that is functionally inactive.
**Cryptic splice site.** A mutation in a gene leading to the creation of the sequence of a splice site which results in abnormal splicing of the mRNA.
**Cystic fibrosis transmembrane conductance regulator (CFTR).** The gene product of the cystic fibrosis gene responsible for chloride transport and mucin secretion.
**Cytogenetics.** The branch of genetics concerned principally with the study of chromosomes.
**Cytokinesis.** Division of the cytoplasm to form two daughter cells in meiosis and mitosis.
**Cytoplasm.** The ground substance of the cell, in which are situated the nucleus, endoplasmic reticulum and mitochondria, etc.
**Cytoplasmic inheritance.** See Mitochondrial inheritance.
**Cytosine.** A pyrimidine base in DNA and RNA.
**Cytosol.** The semi-soluble contents of the cytoplasm.
**Cytotoxic T cells.** A subclass of T lymphocytes sensitized to destroy cells bearing certain antigens.
**Cytotoxic T lymphocytes (= killer).** A group of T cells which specifically kill foreign or virus-infected vertebrate cells.
**Daltonism.** A term given in the past to X-linked inheritance, after John Dalton, who noted this pattern of inheritance in color blindness.
**Deformation.** A birth defect which results from an abnormal mechanical force which distorts an otherwise normal structure.
**Degeneracy.** Certain amino acids being coded for by more than one triplet codon of the genetic code.
**Deleted in colorectal carcinoma (DCC).** A region on the long arm of chromosome 18 often found to be deleted in colorectal carcinomas.
**Deletion.** A type of chromosomal aberration or mutation at the DNA level in which there is loss of part of a chromosome or one or more nucleotides.
**Delta-beta (δβ)-thalassemia.** A form of thalassemia in which there is reduced production of both the δ- and β-globin chains.
**De novo.** Literally 'from new', as opposed to inherited.
**Deoxyribonucleic acid.** See DNA.
**Desert hedgehog.** One of three mammalian homologs of the segment polarity hedgehog genes.
**Dicentric.** Possessing two centromeres.
**Dictyotene.** The stage in meiosis I in which primary oocytes are arrested in females until the time of ovulation.
**Digenic inheritance.** An inheritance mechanism resulting from the interaction of two non-homologous genes.
**Diploid.** The condition in which the cell contains two sets of chromosomes. Normal state of somatic cells in humans where the diploid number (2N) is 46.
**Discontinuous trait.** A trait which is all or none, e.g. cleft lip and palate, in contrast to continuous traits such as height.

**Discordant.** Differing phenotypic features between individuals, classically used in twin pairs.
**Disomy.** The normal state of an individual having two homologous chromosomes.
**Dispermic chimera.** Two separate sperm fertilize two separate ova and the resulting two zygotes fuse to form one embryo.
**Dispermy.** Fertilization of an oocyte by two sperm.
**Disruption.** An abnormal structure of an organ or tissue as a result of external factors disturbing the normal developmental process.
**Diversity region.** DNA sequences coding for the segments of the hypervariable regions of antibodies.
**Dizygotic twins (= fraternal).** Type of twins produced by fertilization of two ova by two sperm.
**DNA (= deoxyribonucleic acid).** The nucleic acid in chromosomes in which genetic information is coded.
**DNA chip.** DNA microarrays which, with the appropriate computerized software allow rapid, automated high-throughput DNA sequencing and mutation detection.
**DNA fingerprint.** Pattern of hypervariable tandem DNA repeats of a core sequence which is unique to an individual.
**DNA haplotype.** The pattern of DNA sequence polymorphisms flanking a DNA sequence or gene of interest.
**DNA library.** A collection of recombinant DNA molecules from a particular source, e.g. genomic or cDNA.
**DNA ligase.** An enzyme which catalyses the formation of a phosphodiester bond between a 3′-hydroxyl and a 5′-phosphate group in DNA, thereby joining two DNA fragments.
**DNA mapping.** The physical relationships of flanking DNA sequence, polymorphisms and the detailed structure of a gene.
**DNA polymorphisms.** Inherited variation in the nucleotide sequence, usually of non-coding DNA.
**DNA probes.** A DNA sequence which is labeled, usually either radioactively or fluorescently, and used to identify a gene or DNA sequence, e.g. a cDNA or genomic probe.
**DNA repair.** DNA damaged through a variety of mechanisms can be removed and repaired by a complex set of processes.
**DNA replication.** The process of copying the nucleotide sequence of the genome from one generation to the next.
**DNA sequence amplification.** See Polymerase chain reaction.
**DNA sequence variants.** See DNA polymorphisms.
**DNA sequencing.** Analysis of the nucleotide sequence of a gene or DNA fragment.
**Dominant.** A trait which is expressed in individuals who are heterozygous for a particular allele.
**Dominant-negative mutation.** A mutant allele in the heterozygous state which results in the loss of activity/function of its mutant gene product as well as interfering with the function of the normal gene product of the corresponding allele.
**Dosage compensation.** The phenomenon in women who have two copies of genes on the X chromosome having the same level of the products of those genes as males who have a single X chromosome.
**Dosimetry.** The measurement of radiation exposure.
**Double heterozygote.** An individual who is heterozygous at two different loci.
**Double-minute chromosomes.** Amplified sequences of DNA in tumor cells which can occur as small extra chromosomes, as in neuroblastoma.
**Drift (= random genetic drift).** Fluctuations in gene frequencies which tend to occur in small isolated populations.
**Dynamic mutation.** See Unstable mutation.
**Dysmorphology.** The study of the definition, recognition and etiology of multiple malformation syndromes.
**Dysplasia.** An abnormal organization of cells into tissue.
**Dystrophin.** The product of the Duchenne muscular dystrophy gene.
**Ecogenetics.** The study of genetically determined differences in susceptibility to the action of physical, chemical and infectious agents in the environment.
**Em.** The group of genetic variants of the IgE heavy chain of immunoglobulins.
**Embryoblast.** Cell layer of the blastocyst which forms the embryo.
**Embryonic stem cells.** A cell in the early embryo which is totipotent in terms of cellular fate.
**Empiric risks.** Advice given in recurrence risk counseling for multifactorially determined disorders based on observation and experience, in which the inherited contribution is due to a number of genes, i.e. polygenic.
**Endoplasmic reticulum.** A system of minute tubules within the cell involved in the biosynthesis of macromolecules.
**Endoreduplication.** Duplication of a haploid sperm chromosome set.
**Enhancer.** DNA sequence which increases transcription of a related gene.
**Enzyme.** A protein which acts as a catalyst in biological systems.
**Epidermal growth factor (EGF).** A growth factor which stimulates a variety of cell types including epidermal cells.
**Epistasis.** Interaction between non-allelic genes.
**Erythroblastosis fetalis.** See Hemolytic disease of the newborn.
**Essential hypertension.** Increased blood pressure for which there is no recognized primary cause.
**Euchromatin.** Genetically active regions of the chromosomes.
**Eugenics.** The 'science' which promotes the improvement of the hereditary qualities of a race or a species.
**Eukaryo**te. Higher organism with a well-defined nucleus.
**Exon (= expressed sequence).** Region of a gene which is not excised during transcription forming part of the mature mRNA and therefore specifying part of the primary structure of the gene product.
**Exon trapping.** A process by which a recombinant DNA vector which contains the DNA sequences of the splice site junctions is used to clone coding sequences or exons.
**Expansion**. Refers to the increase in the number of triplet repeat sequences in the various disorders due to dynamic or unstable mutations.
**Expressed sequence tags.** Sequence-specific primers from cDNA clones designed to identify sequences of expressed genes in the genome.
**Expressivity.** Variation in the severity of the phenotypic features of a particular gene.
**Extinguished.** Loss of one allelic variant at a locus due to random genetic drift.
**Extrinsic malformation.** Term previously used for disruption.
**Fab.** The two antigen binding fragments of an antibody molecule produced by digestion with the proteolytic enzyme papain.
**False-negative.** Affected cases missed by a diagnostic or screening test.
**False-positive.** Unaffected cases incorrectly diagnosed as affected by a screening or diagnostic test.
**Familial adenomatous polyposis.** A dominantly inherited cancer-predisposing syndrome characterized by the presence of a large number of polyps of the large bowel with a high risk of developing malignant changes.
**Familial cancer-predisposing syndrome.** One of a number of syndromes in which persons are at risk of developing one or more types of cancer.
**Favism.** A hemolytic crisis due to G6PD deficiency occurring after eating fava beans.
**Fc.** The complement binding fragment of an antibody molecule produced by digestion with the proteolytic enzyme papain.
**Fetoscopy.** Procedure used to visualize the fetus and often to take skin and/or blood samples from the fetus for prenatal diagnosis.
**Fetus.** The name given to the unborn infant during the final stage of in utero development, usually from 12 weeks' gestation to term.
**Filial.** Offspring.
**First-degree relatives.** Closest relatives, that is, parents, offspring, siblings, sharing on average 50% of their genes.
**Fitness (= biological fitness).** The number of offspring who reach reproductive age.
**Five-prime (5′) end.** The end of a DNA or RNA strand with a free 5′ phosphate group.
**Fixed.** The establishment of a single allelic variant at a locus due to random genetic drift.
**Fixed mutation.** See Stable mutation.
**Flanking DNA.** Nucleotide sequence adjacent to the DNA sequence being considered.

**Flanking markers.** Polymorphic markers which are located adjacent to a gene or DNA sequence of interest.
**Flow cytometry.** See Fluorescence-activated cell sorting.
**Flow karyotype.** A distribution histogram of chromosome size obtained using a fluorescence-activated cell sorter.
**Fluorescence-activated cell sorting (FACS).** A technique in which chromosomes are stained with a fluorescent dye which selectively binds to DNA; the differences in fluorescence of the various chromosomes allows them to be physically separated by a special laser.
**Fluorescent in situ hybridization (FISH).** Use of a single-stranded DNA sequence with a fluorescent label to hybridize with its complementary target sequence in the chromosomes, allowing it to be visualized under ultraviolet light.
**Foreign DNA.** A source of DNA incorporated into a vector in producing recombinant DNA molecules.
**Founder effect.** Certain genetic disorders can be relatively common in particular populations through all individuals being descended from a relatively small number of ancestors, one or a few of whom had a particular disorder.
**Fragile site.** A non-staining gap in a chromatid where breakage is liable to occur.
**Frameshift mutations.** Mutations, such as insertions or deletions, which change the reading frame of the codon triplets.
**Framework map.** A set of markers distributed at defined approximately evenly spaced intervals along the chromosomes in the human genome.
**Framework region.** Parts of the variable regions of antibodies which are not hypervariable.
**Fraternal twins.** Non-identical twins.
**Freemartin.** A chromosomally female twin calf with ambiguous genitalia due to gonadal chimerism.
**Frequency.** The number of times an event occurs in a period of time, e.g. 1000 cases per year.
**Full ascertainment.** See Complete ascertainment.
**Functional cloning.** Identification of a gene through its function, e.g. isolation of cDNAs expressed in a particular tissue in which a disease or disorder is manifest.
**Functional genomics.** The normal pattern of expression of genes in development and differentiation and the function of their protein products in normal development as well as their dysfunction in inherited disorders.
**Fusion polypeptide.** Genes which are physically near to each other and have DNA sequence homology can undergo a cross-over, leading to formation of a protein that has an amino acid sequence which is derived from both of the genes involved.
**G.** Abbreviation for the nucleotide guanine.
**Gain-of-function.** Mutations which in the heterozygote result in new functions.
**Gap mutant.** Developmental genes identified in *Drosophila* which delete groups of adjacent segments.
**Gastrulation.** The formation of the bi- then tri-laminar disc of the inner cell mass which becomes the early embyro.
**Gene.** A part of the DNA molecule of a chromosome which directs the synthesis of a specific polypeptide chain.
**Gene amplification.** Process in tumor cells of the production of multiple copies of certain genes, the visible evidence of which are homogeneously staining regions and double-minute chromosomes.
**Gene flow.** A term used to describe differences in allele frequencies between populations which reflect migration or contact between them.
**Gene superfamilies.** Multigene families which have limited sequence homology but are functionally related.
**Gene targeting.** The introduction of specific mutations into genes by homologous recombination in embryonic stem cells.
**Gene therapy.** Treatment of inherited disease by addition, insertion or replacement of a normal gene or genes.
**Genetic code.** The triplets of DNA nucleotides which code for the various amino acids of proteins.
**Genetic counseling.** The process of providing information about a genetic disorder which includes details about the diagnosis, its cause, the risk of recurrence and options available for prevention.
**Genetic heterogeneity.** The phenomenon that a disorder can be caused by different allelic or non-allelic mutations.
**Genetic isolates.** Groups which are isolated for geographical, religious or ethnic reasons that often show differences in allele frequencies.
**Genetic load.** The total of all kinds of harmful alleles in a population.
**Genetic register.** A list of families and individuals who are either affected by or at risk of developing a serious hereditary disorder.
**Genetic susceptibility.** An inherited predisposition to a disease or disorder which is not due to a single-gene cause and is usually the result of a complex interaction of the effects of multiple different genes, i.e. polygenic inheritance.
**Genocopy.** The same phenotype due to different genetic causes.
**Genome.** All the genes carried by a cell.
**Genomic DNA.** The total DNA content of the chromosomes.
**Genomic imprinting.** Differing expression of genetic material dependent on the sex of the transmitting parent.
**Genotype.** The genetic constitution of an individual.
**Genotype–phenotype correlation.** Correlation of certain mutations with particular phenotypic features.
**Germ cells.** The cells of the body which transmit genetic information to the next generation.
**Germ-line gene therapy.** The alteration or insertion of genetic material in the gametes.
**Germ-line mosaicism.** The presence in the germ line or gonadal tissue of two populations of cells which differ genetically.
**Germ-line mutation.** A mutation in a gamete.
**Gestational diabetes.** Onset of an abnormal glucose tolerance in pregnancy which usually reverts to normal after delivery.
**Gm.** Genetic variants of the heavy chain of IgG immunoglobulins.
**Goldberg–Hogness box.** See CAAT box.
**Gonad dose.** Term used in radiation dosimetry to describe the radiation exposure of an individual to a particular radiological investigation or exposure.
**Gonadal mosaicism.** See Germ-line mosaicism.
**Gray (Gy).** Equivalent to 100 rad.
**Growth factors.** A substance which must be present in culture medium to permit cell multiplication, or substances involved in promoting growth of certain cell types, tissues or parts of the body in development, e.g. fibroblast growth factor.
**Growth factor receptors.** Receptors on the surfaces of cells for a growth factor.
**Guanine.** A purine base in DNA and RNA.
**Haploid.** The condition in which the cell contains one set of chromosomes, i.e. 23. This is the chromosome number in a normal gamete.
**Haploinsufficiency.** Mutations in the heterozygous state which result in half normal levels of the gene product leading to phenotypic effects, i.e. are sensitive to gene dosage.
**Haplotype.** Conventionally used to refer to the particular alleles present at the four genes of the HLA complex on chromosome 6. The term is also used to describe DNA sequence variants on a particular chromosome adjacent to or closely flanking a locus of interest.
**Hardy–Weinberg equilibrium.** The maintenance of allele frequencies in a population with random mating and absence of selection.
**Hardy–Weinberg formula.** A simple binomial equation in population genetics which can be used to determine the frequency of the different genotypes from one of the phenotypes.
**Hardy–Weinberg principle.** The relative proportions of the different genotypes remain constant from one generation to the next.
**Hb Barts.** The tetramer of $\gamma$-globin chains found in the severe form of $\alpha$-thalassemia, which causes hydrops fetalis.
**Hb H.** Tetramer of the $\beta$-globin chains found in the less severe form of thalassemia.
**Hedgehog.** A group of morphogens produced by segment polarity genes.
**Helix–loop–helix.** DNA binding motif controlling gene expression.
**Helix–turn–helix proteins.** Proteins made up of two $\alpha$ helices connected by a short chain of amnio acids which make up a 'turn'.

**Helper lymphocytes.** A subclass of T lymphocytes necessary for the production of antibodies by B lymphocytes.
**Helper virus.** A retroviral provirus engineered to remove all but the sequences necessary to produce copies of the viral RNA sequences along with the sequences necessary for packaging of the viral genomic RNA in retroviral-mediated gene therapy.
**Heme.** The iron-containing group of hemoglobin.
**Hemizygous.** A term used when describing the genotype of a male with regard to an X-linked trait, since males have only one set of X-linked genes.
**Hemoglobinopathy.** An inherited disorder of hemoglobin.
**Hemolytic disease of the newborn.** Anemia due to antibody produced by an Rh-negative mother to the Rh-positive blood group of the fetus crossing the placenta and causing hemolysis. If this hemolytic process is severe, it can cause death of the fetus due to heart failure because of the anemia, or what is known as hemolytic disease of the newborn.
**Hereditary non-polyposis colorectal cancer (HNPCC).** A form of familial cancer in which persons are at risk of developing bowel cancer, not associated with a large number of polyps as in familial polyposis coli, in which the bowel cancer is usually proximal and right-sided.
**Hereditary persistence of fetal Hb (HPFH).** Persistence of the production of fetal hemoglobin into childhood and adult life.
**Heritability.** The proportion of the total variation of a character attributable to genetic as opposed to environmental factors.
**Hermaphrodite.** An individual with both male and female gonads, often in association with ambiguous external genitalia.
**Heterochromatin**. Genetically inert or inactive regions of the chromosomes.
**Heterogeneity.** The phenomenon of there being more than a single cause for what appears to be a single entity. See Genetic heterogeneity.
**Heteromorphism.** An inherited structural polymorphism of a chromosome.
**Heteroplasmy.** The mitochondria of an individual consisting of more than one population.
**Heteropyknotic.** Condensed darkly staining chromosomal material, e.g. the inactivated X chromosome in females.
**Heterozygote (= carrier).** An individual who possesses two different alleles at one particular locus on a pair of homologous chromosomes.
**Heterozygote advantage.** An increase in biological fitness seen in unaffected heterozygotes compared to unaffected homozygotes, e.g. sickle-cell trait and resistance to infection by the malarial parasite.
**Heterozygous.** The state of having different alleles at a locus on homologous chromosomes.
**High-resolution DNA mapping.** Detailed physical mapping at the level of restriction site polymorphisms, expressed sequence tags, etc.
**Histocompatibility.** Antigenic similarity of donor and recipient in organ transplantation.
**Histone.** Type of protein rich in lysine and arginine found in association with DNA in chromosomes.
**HIV.** Human immunodeficiency virus.
**HLA (human leukocyte antigen).** Antigens present on the cell surfaces of various tissues, including leukocytes.
**HLA complex.** The genes on chromosome 6 responsible for determining the cell-surface antigens important in organ transplantation.
**Hogness box (= TATA box).** A conserved, non-coding, so-called 'promoter' sequence about 30 bp upstream from the start of transcription.
**Holandric inheritance.** The pattern of inheritance of genes on the Y chromosome: only males are affected and the trait is transmitted by affected males to their sons but to none of their daughters.
**Homeobox.** A stretch of approximately 180 bp conserved in different homeotic genes.
**Homeotic gene.** Genes which are involved in controlling the development of a region or compartment of an organism producing proteins or factors which regulate gene expression by binding particular DNA sequences.
**Homogeneously staining regions (HSR).** Amplification of DNA sequences in tumor cells which can appear as extra or expanded areas of the chromosomes, which stain evenly.
**Homograft.** Graft between individuals of the same species but with different genotypes.
**Homologous chromosomes.** Chromosomes which pair during meiosis and contain identical loci.
**Homologous recombination.** The process by which a DNA sequence can be replaced by one with a similar sequence to determine the effect of changes in DNA sequence in the process of site-directed mutagenesis.
**Homoplasmy.** The mitochondria of an individual consisting of a single population.
**Homozygote.** An individual who possesses two identical alleles at one particular locus on a pair of homologous chromosomes.
**Homozygous.** The presence of two identical alleles at a particular locus on a pair of homologous chromosomes.
**Hormone nuclear receptors.** Intracellular receptors involved in the control of transcription.
**Housekeeping genes.** Genes which express proteins common to all cells, e.g. ribosomal, chromosomal and cytoskeletal proteins.
**HTF islands.** Methylation-free clusters of CpG dinucleotides found near transcription initiation sites at the 5′ end of many eukaryotic genes which can be detected by cutting with the restriction enzyme *Hpa*II, producing *t*iny DNA *f*ragments.
**Human Genome Project.** A major international collaborative effort to map and sequence the entire human genome.
**Humoral immunity.** Immunity which is due to circulating antibodies in the blood and other bodily fluids.
**Huntingtin.** The protein product of the Huntington disease gene.
**H-Y antigen.** A histocompatibility antigen originally detected in the mouse and thought to be located on the Y chromosome.
**Hydatidiform mole.** An abnormal conceptus which consists of abnormal tissues: a complete mole contains no fetus but can undergo malignant change and receives both sets of chromosomes from the father; a partial mole contains a chromosomally abnormal fetus with triploidy.
**Hydrops fetalis.** The most severe form of $\alpha$-thalassemia, resulting in death of the fetus in utero due to heart failure secondary to the severe anemia caused by hemolysis of the red cells.
**Hypervariable DNA length polymorphisms.** A number of different types of variation in DNA sequence which are highly polymorphic, e.g. variable number tandem repeats, mini- and microsatellites.
**Hypervariable minisatellite DNA.** Highly polymorphic DNA consisting of a 9–24 bp sequence often located near the telomeres.
**Hypervariable region.** A number of small regions present in the variable regions of the light and heavy chains of antibodies in which the majority of the variability in antibody sequence occurs.
**Hypomorph.** Loss-of-function mutations which result in either reduced activity or complete loss of the gene product due to either reduced activity or to decreased stability of the gene product.
**Identical twins.** See Monozygotic twins.
**Idiogram.** An idealized representation of an object, e.g. an idiogram of a karyotype.
**Immunoglobulin.** See Antibody.
**Immunoglobulin allotypes.** Genetically determined variants of the various antibody classes, e.g. the Gm system associated with the heavy chain of IgG.
**Immunoglobulin superfamily.** The multigene families primarily involved in the immune response with structural and DNA sequence homology.
**Immunological memory.** The ability of the immune system to 'remember' previous exposure to a foreign antigen or infectious agents, leading to the enhanced secondary immune response upon re-exposure.
**Imprinting.** The phenomenon of a gene or region of a chromosome showing different expression depending on the parent of origin.
**Inborn error of metabolism.** An inherited metabolic defect which results in deficient production or synthesis of an abnormal enzyme.
**Incest.** Union between first-degree relatives.

**Incestuous.** Description of a relationship between first-degree relatives.
**Incidence.** The rate at which new cases occur, e.g. 2 in 1000 births are affected by neural tube defects.
**Incompatibility.** A donor and host are incompatible if the latter rejects a graft from the former.
**Incomplete ascertainment.** A term used in segregation analysis to describe family studies in which complete ascertainment is not possible.
**Index case.** See Proband.
**Index map.** See Framework map.
**Indian hedgehog.** One of three mammalian homologs of the segment polarity hedgehog genes.
**Inducer.** Small molecule which interacts with a regulator protein and triggers gene transcription.
**Informative.** Variation in a marker system in a family which enables a gene or inherited disease to be followed in that family.
**Innate immunity.** A number of non-specific systems involved in immunity which do not require or involve prior contact with the infectious agent.
**Insertion.** Addition of chromosomal material or DNA sequence of one or more nucleotides within the genome.
**Insertional mutagenesis.** The introduction of mutations at specific sites to determine the effects of these changes.
**In situ hybridization.** Hybridization with a DNA probe carried out directly on a chromosome preparation or histological section.
**Insulin-dependent diabetes mellitus.** Diabetes requiring the use of insulin, usually of juvenile onset, now known as type 1 diabetes.
**Intermediate inheritance.** See Codominance.
**Interphase.** The stage between two successive cell divisions during which DNA replication occurs.
**Interphase cytogenetics.** The study of chromosomes during interphase, usually by FISH.
**Intersex.** An individual with external genitalia not clearly male or female.
**Interval cancer.** Developing cancer in the interval between repeated screening procedures.
**Intra-cytoplasmic sperm injection (ICSI).** A technique whereby a secondary spermatocyte or spermatozoon is removed from the testis and used to fertilize an egg.
**Intrinsic malformation.** A malformation due to an inherent abnormality in development.
**Intron (= intervening sequence).** Region of DNA which generates that part of precursor RNA which is spliced out during transcription and does not form mature mRNA and therefore does not specify the primary structure of the gene product.
**Inv.** The group of genetic variants of the κ light chains of immunoglobulins.
**Inversion.** A type of chromosomal aberration or mutation in which part of a chromosome or sequence of DNA is reversed in its order.
**Inversion loop.** The structure formed in meiosis I by a chromosome with either a para- or pericentric inversion.
**In vitro.** In the laboratory, literally 'in glass'.
**In vivo.** In the normal cell, literally 'in the living organism'.
**Ionizing radiation.** Electromagnetic waves of very short wavelength (X-rays and γ-rays), and high-energy particles (α particles, β particles and neutrons).
**Isochromosome.** A type of chromosomal aberration in which one of the arms of a particular chromosome is duplicated because the centromere divides transversely and not longitudinally as normal during cell division. The two arms of an isochromosome are therefore of equal length and contain the same set of genes.
**Isolate.** A term used to describe a population or group of individuals who for religious, cultural or geographical reasons have remained separate from other groups of persons.
**Isozymes.** Enzymes that exist in multiple molecular forms which can be distinguished by biochemical methods.
**Joining region.** Short conserved sequence of nucleotides involved in somatic recombinational events in the production of antibody diversity.
**Joint probability.** The product of the prior and conditional probability for two events.
**Karyogram.** Photomicrograph of chromosomes arranged in descending order of size.
**Karyotype.** The number, size and shape of the chromosomes of an individual. Also used for the photomicrograph of an individual's chromosomes arranged in a standard manner.
**Kb.** Abbreviation for kilobase.
**Killer lymphocytes.** See Cytotoxic T lymphocytes.
**Kilobase.** 1000 base pairs (bp).
**Km.** Genetic variants of the κ light chain of immunoglobulins.
**Knockout mutation.** Complete loss of function of a gene.
**Lagging strand.** One of the two strands created in DNA replication which is synthesized in the 3′ to 5′ direction made up of pieces synthesized in the 5′ to 3′ direction which are then joined together as a continuous strand by the enzyme DNA ligase.
**Law of addition.** If two or more events are mutually exclusive then the probability that either one or the other will occur equals the sum of their individual probabilities.
**Law of independent assortment.** Members of different gene pairs segregate to offspring independently of one another.
**Law of multiplication.** If two or more events or outcomes are independent, then the probability that both the first and the second will occur equals the product of their individual probabilities.
**Law of segregation.** Each individual possesses two genes for a particular characteristic, only one of which can be transmitted at any one time.
**Law of uniformity.** When two homozygotes with different alleles are crossed, all the offspring in the F1 generation are identical and heterozygous, i.e. the characteristics do not blend and can reappear in later generations.
**Leading strand.** The synthesis of one of the DNA strands created in DNA replication which occurs in the 5′ to 3′ direction synthesized as a continuous process.
**Lethal mutation.** A mutation which leads to the premature death of an individual or organism.
**Leucine zipper.** A DNA binding motif controlling gene expression.
**Liability.** A concept used in disorders which are multifactorially determined to take into account all possible causative factors.
**Library.** Set of cloned DNA fragments derived from a particular DNA source, e.g. a cDNA library from the transcript of particular tissue, or a genomic library.
**Ligase.** Enzyme used to join DNA molecules.
**Ligation.** Formation of phosphodiester bonds to link two nucleic acid molecules.
**Linkage.** Two loci situated close together on the same chromosome, the alleles at which are usually transmitted together in meiosis in gamete formation.
**Linkage disequilibrium.** The occurrence together of two or more alleles at closely linked loci more frequently than would be expected by chance.
**Liposomes.** Artificially prepared cell-like structures in which one or more bimolecular layers of phospholipid enclose one or more aqueous compartments, which can include proteins.
**Localization sequences.** Certain short amino acid sequences in newly synthesized proteins which result in their transport to specific cellular locations, e.g. the nucleus, or their secretion.
**Location score.** Diagrammatic representation of likelihood ratios used in multipoint linkage analysis.
**Locus.** The site of a gene on a chromosome.
**Locus control region (LCR).** A region near the β-like globin genes involved in the timing and tissue specificity of their expression in development.
**Locus heterogeneity.** The phenomenon of a disorder being due to mutations in more than one gene or locus.
**Lod score.** A mathematical score of the relative likelihood of two loci being linked.
**Long interspersed nuclear elements (LINEs).** 50000–100000 copies of a DNA sequence of approximately 6000 bp which occurs approximately once every 50 kb and encodes a reverse transcriptase.
**Long terminal repeat (LTR).** One of two long sections of double-stranded DNA synthesized by reverse transcriptase from the RNA of a retrovirus involved in regulating viral expression.

**Loss of constitutional heterozygosity (LOCH).** Loss of an allele inherited from a parent-frequently seen as evidence of a 'second hit' in tumorigenesis.
**Loss-of-function mutation.** Phenotypic features of a disorder due to reduced or absent activity of the gene.
**Low resolution mapping.** See Chromosome mapping.
**Lymphokines.** A group of glycoproteins released from T lymphocytes after contact with an antigen which act upon other cells of the host immune system.
**Lyonization.** The process of inactivation of one of the X chromosomes in females, originally proposed by the geneticist Mary Lyon.
**Major histocompatibility complex (MHC).** A multigene locus which codes for the histocompatibility antigens involved in organ transplantation.
**Malformation.** A primary structural defect of an organ or part of an organ which results from an inherent abnormality in development.
**Manifesting heterozygote or carrier.** The phenomenon of a female carrier for an X-linked disorder having symptoms or signs of that disorder due to non-random X-inactivation, e.g. muscular weakness in a carrier for Duchenne muscular dystrophy.
**Map unit.** See CentiMorgan.
**Marker.** A loose term used for a blood group, biochemical or DNA polymorphism which, if shown to be linked to a disease locus of interest, can be used in presymptomatic diagnosis, determining carrier status and prenatal diagnosis.
**Marker chromosome.** A small extra structurally abnormal chromosome.
**Maternal (matrilineal) inheritance.** Transmission of a disorder through females.
**Matrilineal inheritance.** See Maternal inheritance.
**Maximum likelihood method.** The calculation of the Lod score for various values of the recombination fraction θ to determine the best estimate of the recombination fraction.
**Meconium ileus.** Blockage of the small bowel in the newborn period due to inspissated meconium, a presenting feature of cystic fibrosis.
**Meiosis.** The type of cell division which occurs in gamete formation with halving of the somatic number of chromosomes, with the result that each gamete is haploid.
**Meiotic drive.** Preferential transmission of one of a pair of alleles during meiosis.
**Mendelian inheritance.** Inheritance which follows the laws of segregation and independent assortment as proposed by Mendel.
**Merlin.** The protein product of the neurofibromatosis type II gene.
**Messenger RNA (mRNA).** A single-stranded molecule complementary to one of the strands of double-stranded DNA which is synthesized during transcription and transmits the genetic information in the DNA to the ribosomes for protein synthesis.
**Metabolic disorder.** An inherited disorder involving a biochemical pathway, i.e. an inborn error of metabolism.
**Metacentric.** Term used to describe chromosomes in which the centromere is central with both arms being of approximately equal length.
**Metaphase.** The stage of cell division when the chromosomes line up on the equatorial plate and the nuclear membrane disappears.
**Metaphase spreads.** The preparation of chromosomes during the metaphase stage of mitosis in which they are condensed.
**Methemoglobin.** A hemoglobin molecule in which the iron is oxidized.
**Microdeletion.** A small chromosomal deletion detectable by high resolution prometaphase chromosomal analysis or FISH.
**Microdeletion syndrome.** The pattern of abnormalities caused by a chromosome microdeletion.
**Microsatellite DNA.** Polymorphic variation in DNA sequences due to a variable number of tandem repeats of the dinucleotide CA, tri- or tetranucleotides.
**Microsatellite instability.** The alteration of the size of microsatellite polymorphic markers compared to the constitutional markers of an individual with hereditary non-polyposis colorectal cancer due to mutations in the genes for the mismatch repair enzymes.
**Microtubules.** Long cylindrical tubes composed of bundles of small filaments which are an important part of the cytoskeleton.
**Minichromosomes.** Artificially constructed chromosomes which contain centromeric and telomeric elements that allow replication of foreign DNA as a separate entity.
**Minidystrophin.** A modified dystrophin gene in which a large amount of the gene has been deleted but which still has relatively normal function.
**Minigene.** A construct of a gene with the majority of the sequence removed which still remains functional, e.g. a dystrophin minigene.
**Minisatellite.** Polymorphic variation in DNA sequences due to a variable number of tandem repeats of a short DNA sequence.
**Mismatch repair genes.** Genes for the DNA proof-reading enzymes, mutations in which cause hereditary non-polyposis colorectal cancer.
**Missense mutation.** A point mutation which results in a change in an amino acid-specifying codon.
**Mitochondria.** Minute structures situated within the cytoplasm which are concerned with cell respiration.
**Mitochondrial DNA (mtDNA).** Mitochondria possess their own genetic material which codes for enzymes involved in energy-yielding reactions, mutations of which are associated with certain diseases in humans.
**Mitochondrial inheritance.** Transmission of a mitochondrial trait exclusively through maternal relatives.
**Mitosis.** The type of cell division which occurs in replication of somatic cells.
**Mixoploidy.** The presence of cell lines with a different genetic constitution in an individual.
**Modifier gene.** Phenotypic variability due to the consequence of interactions with other genes.
**Monosomy.** Loss of one member of a homologous pair of chromosomes so that there is one less than the diploid number of chromosomes (2N – 1).
**Monozygotic twins (= identical).** Type of twins derived from a single fertilized ovum.
**Morphogen.** A chemical or substance which determines a developmental process.
**Morphogenesis.** The evolution and development of form and shape.
**Morula.** The 12–16-cell stage of the early embryo at 3 days post conception.
**Mosaic.** An individual with two different cell lines derived from a single zygote.
**mRNA splicing.** The excision of intervening non-coding sequences or introns in the primary mRNA resulting in the non-contiguous exons being spliced together to form a shorter mature mRNA before its transportation to the ribosomes in the cytoplasm for translation.
**Mucoviscidosis.** An older term used for cystic fibrosis.
**Multifactorial inheritance.** Inheritance controlled by many genes with small additive effects (polygenic) plus the effects of the environment.
**Multigene families.** Genes with functional and/or sequence similarity.
**Multiple alleles.** The existence of more than two alleles at a particular locus in a population.
**Multiple myeoloma.** A cancer of antibody-producing B cells which leads to the production of a single species of an antibody in large quantities.
**Multipoint linkage analysis.** Analysis of the segregation of alleles at a number of closely adjacent loci.
**Mutagen.** Natural or artificial ionizing radiation, chemical or physical agents which can induce alterations in DNA.
**Mutant.** A gene which has undergone a change or mutation.
**Mutated in colorectal carcinoma (MCC).** A gene involved in colorectal cancer as evidenced by loss of constitutional heterozygosity at 5q21.
**Mutation.** A change in genetic material, either of a single gene, or in the number or structure of the chromosomes. A mutation which occurs in the gametes is inherited, a mutation which occurs in the somatic cells (somatic mutation) is not inherited.

**Mutation rate.** The number of mutations at any one particular locus which occur per gamete per generation.
**Mutational heterogeneity.** The occurrence of more than one mutation in a particular single-gene disorder.
**Mutator genes.** The equivalent in yeast to the DNA proof-reading enzymes which cause hereditary non-polyposis colorectal cancer.
**Myeloma.** A tumor of the plasma or antibody-producing cells.
**Natural killer cells.** Large granular lymphocytes which have carbohydrate binding receptors on their cell surface which recognize high molecular weight glycoproteins expressed on the cell surface of the infected cell as a result of the virus taking over the cellular replicative functions.
**Neurofibromin.** The protein product of the neurofibromatosis type I gene.
**Neutral gene.** A gene which appears to have no obvious effect on the likelihood of an individual's ability to survive.
**New mutation.** The occurrence of a change in a gene arising as a new event.
**Non-conservative substitution.** A mutation which codes for an amino acid which is chemically dissimilar, e.g. a different charge, will result in a protein the structure of which will be altered.
**Non-disjunction.** The failure of two members of a homologous chromosome pair to separate during cell division so that both pass to the same daughter cell.
**Non-identical twins.** See Dizygotic twins.
**Non-insulin-dependent diabetes mellitus.** Diabetes which can often be treated with diet and/or oral medication, now known as type 2 diabetes.
**Non-paternity.** The biological father is not as stated or believed.
**Non-penetrance.** The occurrence of an individual being heterozygous for an autosomal dominant gene but showing no signs of it.
**Non-random mating.** See Assortative mating.
**Nonsense mutation.** A mutation which results in one of the termination codons, which leads to premature termination of translation of a protein.
**Non-synonymous mutation.** A mutation which leads to an alteration in the encoded polypeptide.
**Northern blotting.** Electrophoretic separation of mRNA with subsequent transfer to a filter which can be localized with a radiolabeled probe.
**Nuclear envelope.** The membrane surrounding the nucleus separating it from the cytoplasm.
**Nuclear pores.** The gaps in the nuclear envelope which allow substances to pass from the nucleus to the cytoplasm and vice versa.
**Nucleolus.** A structure within the nucleus which contains high levels of RNA.
**Nucleosome.** DNA-histone subunit of a chromosome.
**Nucleotide.** Nucleic acid is made up of many nucleotides, each of which consists of a nitrogenous base, a pentose sugar and a phosphate group.
**Nucleus.** A structure within the cell which contains the chromosomes and nucleolus.
**Null allele.** See Amorph.
**Nullisomy.** Loss of both members of a homologous pair of chromosomes.
**Obligate carrier.** An individual who, by pedigree analysis, must carry a particular gene, e.g. parents of a child with an autosomal recessive disorder.
**Oligogene.** One of a relatively small number of genes which contribute to a disease phenotype.
**Oligonucleotide.** A chain of, literally, a few nucleotides.
**Oncogene.** A gene affecting cell growth or development which can cause cancer.
**Oncogenic.** Literally, 'cancer causing'.
**Opsonization.** The 'making ready' of an infectious agent in the production of an immune response.
**Origins of replication.** The points at which DNA replication commences.
**Orthologous.** Conserved genes or sequences between species.
**Ova.** Mature haploid female gametes.
**Oz.** The group of genetic variants of the λ light chain immunoglobulins.
**P1-derived artificial chromosomes (PACs).** Combination of the P1 and F-factor systems to incorporate foreign DNA inserts up to 150 kb.
**Pachytene quadrivalent.** The arrangement which the two pairs of chromosomes involved in a reciprocal translocation adopt in meiosis I when undergoing segregation.
**Packaging cell line.** A cell line which has been infected with a retrovirus in which the provirus is genetically engineered to lack the packaging sequence of the proviral DNA necessary to produce infectious viruses.
**Packaging sequence.** The DNA sequence of the proviral DNA of a retrovirus necessary for packaging of the retroviral RNA into an infectious virus.
**Paint.** Use of fluorescent labeled probes derived from a chromosome or region of a chromosome to hybridize with a chromosome in a metaphase spread.
**Pair-rule mutant.** Developmental genes identified in *Drosophila* which cause pattern deletions in alternating segments.
**Panmixis.** See Random mating.
**Paracentric inversion.** A chromosomal inversion which does not include the centromere.
**Paralogous.** Close resemblance of genes from different clusters, e.g. *HOXA13* and *HOXD13*.
**Parthenogenesis.** The development of an organism from an unfertilized oocyte.
**Partial sex-linkage.** A term used to describe genes on the homologous or pseudoautosomal portion of the X and Y chromosomes.
**Penetrance.** The proportion of heterozygotes for a dominant gene who express a trait, even if mildly.
**Peptide.** An amino acid, a portion of a protein.
**Pericentric inversion.** A chromosomal inversion which includes the centromere.
**Permissible dose.** An arbitrary safety limit which is probably very much less than that which would cause any significant effect on the frequency of harmful mutations within the population.
**Phage.** Abbreviation for bacteriophage.
**Pharmacogenetics.** The study of genetically determined variation in drug metabolism.
**Phase.** Assignment of the chromosome on which a particular allele is in relation to alleles at other closely linked marker loci.
**Phenocopy.** A condition which is due to environmental factors but resembles one which is genetic.
**Phenol enhanced reassociation technique (pERT).** Use of the chemical phenol to facilitate rehybridization of slightly differing sources of double-stranded DNA to enable isolation of sequences which are absent from one of the two sources.
**Phenotype.** The appearance (physical, biochemical and physiological) of an individual which results from the interaction of the environment and the genotype.
**Pink-eyed dilution.** Human homolog to mouse pink-eye gene for albinism.
**Plasma cells.** Mature antibody-producing B lymphocytes.
**Plasmid.** Small, circular DNA duplex capable of autonomous replication within a bacterium.
**Platelet-derived growth factor (PDGF).** A substance derived from platelets which stimulates growth of certain cell types.
**Pleiotropy.** The multiple effects of a gene.
**Point mutation.** A single base pair change.
**Polar body.** The daughter cell of gamete division in the female in meiosis I and II which does not go on to become a mature gamete.
**Poly(A) tail.** A sequence of 20–200 adenylic acid residues which is added to the 3′ end of most eukaryotic mRNAs, increasing its stability by making it resistant to nuclease digestion.
**Polygenes.** Genes which make a small additive contribution to a polygenic trait.
**Polygenic inheritance.** A term used to describe the genetic contribution to the etiology of disorders in which there are both environmental and genetic causative factors.
**Polymerase chain reaction (PCR).** The repeated serial reaction involving the use of oligonucleotide primers and DNA

polymerase which is used to amplify a particular DNA sequence of interest.
**Polymorphic information content (PIC).** The amount of variation at a particular site in the DNA.
**Polymorphism.** The occurrence in a population of two or more genetically determined forms in such frequencies that the rarest of them could not be maintained by mutation alone.
**Polypeptide.** An organic compound consisting of three or more amino acids.
**Polyploid.** Any multiple of the haploid number of chromosomes (e.g. 3N, 4N, etc.).
**Polyribosome.** See Polysome.
**Polysome (= polyribosome).** A group of ribosomes associated with the same molecule of mRNA.
**Population genetics.** The study of the distribution of alleles in populations.
**Positional candidate gene.** A gene which by virtue of its position to which a disorder maps becomes a possible gene responsible for the disorder.
**Positional cloning.** The mapping of a disorder to a particular region of a chromosome which then leads to the identification of the gene responsible.
**Posterior information.** Information available for risk calculation from the results of tests or analysis of offspring in pedigrees.
**Posterior probability.** The joint probability for a particular event divided by the sum of all possible joint probabilities.
**Post-genomic genomics.** See Functional genomics.
**Post-translational processing.** Various modifications of protein which occur after their synthesis, e.g. the addition of carbohydrate moieties.
**Predictive testing.** Presymptomatic testing, often used in relation to testing of persons at risk for Huntington disease.
**Preimplantation genetic diagnosis.** The ability to detect the presence of an inherited disorder in an in vitro fertilized conceptus before reimplantation.
**Premutation.** The existence of a gene in an unstable form which can undergo a further mutational event to cause a disease.
**Prenatal diagnosis.** The use of tests during a pregnancy to determine whether an unborn child is affected with a particular disorder.
**Presymptomatic diagnosis.** The use of tests to determine whether a person has inherited a gene for a disorder before he/she has any symptoms or signs.
**Prevalence.** At a point in time, the proportion of persons in a given population with a disorder or trait.
**Primary response.** The response to an infectious agent with an initial production of IgM, then subsequently IgG.
**Prion.** A proteinaceous infectious particle implicated in the cause of several rare neurodegenerative diseases.
**Prior probability.** The initial probability of an event.
**Probability.** The proportion of times an outcome occurs in a large series of events.
**Proband (= index case).** An affected individual (irrespective of sex) through whom a family comes to the attention of an investigator. Propositus if male; proposita if female.
**Probe.** A labeled, single-stranded DNA fragment which hybridizes with, and thereby detects and locates, complementary sequences among DNA fragments on, for example, a nitrocellulose filter.
**Processing.** Alterations of mRNA which occur during transcription including splicing, capping and polyadenylation.
**Progress zone.** The area of growth beneath the apical ectodermal ridge in the developing limb bud.
**Prokaryotes.** Lower organisms with no well-defined nucleus, e.g. bacteria.
**Prometaphase.** The stage of cell division when the nuclear membrane begins to disintegrate, allowing the chromosomes to spread, with each chromosome attached at its centromere to a microtubule of the mitotic spindle.
**Promoter.** Recognition sequence for the binding of RNA polymerase.
**Promoter elements.** DNA sequences which include the GGGCGGG consensus sequence, the AT-rich TATA or Hogness box, and the CAAT box which are in a 100–300 bp region located 5′ or upstream to the coding sequence of many structural genes in eukaryotic organisms and which control individual gene expression.
**Pronuclei.** The stage just after fertilization of the oocyte with the nucleus of the oocyte and sperm present.
**Prophase.** The first visible stage of cell division when the chromosomes are contracted.
**Proposita.** A female individual as the presenting person in a family.
**Propositus.** A male individual as the presenting person in a family.
**Protein.** A complex organic compound composed of hundreds or thousands of amino acids.
**Proto-oncogene.** DNA genomic sequences with homology to viral oncogenes, which are involved in regulating cell turnover.
**Pseudoautosomal.** A term used to describe genes which behave like autosomal genes as a result of being located on the homologous portions of the X and Y chromosomes.
**Pseudodominance.** The apparent dominant transmission of a disorder when an individual homozygous for a recessive gene has affected offspring through having children with an individual who is also a carrier.
**Pseudogene.** DNA sequence homologous with a known gene but is non-functional.
**Pseudohermaphrodite.** An individual with ambiguous genitalia or external genitalia opposite to the chromosomal sex in which there is gonadal tissue of only one type.
**Pseudohypertrophy.** Literally, false enlargement. Seen in the calf muscles of boys with Duchenne muscular dystrophy.
**Pseudomosaicism.** False mosaicism seen occasionally as an artifact with cells in culture.
**Pulsed field gel electrophoresis (PFGE).** A technique of DNA analysis using electrophoretic methods to separate large DNA fragments, up to 2 million base pairs in size, produced by digesting DNA with restriction enzymes with relatively long DNA recognition sequences which, as a consequence, cut DNA relatively infrequently.
**Purine.** A nitrogenous base with fused five- and six-member rings (adenine and guanine).
**Pyrimidine.** A nitrogenous base with a six-membered ring (cytosine, uracil, thymine).
**Quantitative inheritance.** See Polygenic inheritance.
**Radiation absorbed dose (rad).** A measure of the amount of any ionizing radiation which is absorbed by the tissues. 1 rad is equivalent to 100 erg of energy absorbed per gram of tissue.
**Radiation hybrids.** Cells exposed to radiation fragment their chromosomes which contain subchromosomal portions of a chromosome, enabling assignment of a particular gene or DNA sequence to a specific region.
**Random genetic drift.** The chance variation of allele frequencies from one generation to the next.
**Random mating (= panmixis).** Selection of a spouse regardless of the spouse's genotype.
**Reading frame.** The order of the triplets of nucleotides in the codons of a gene which are translated into the amino acids of the protein.
**Recessive.** A trait which is expressed in individuals who are homozygous for a particular allele but not in those who are heterozygous.
**Reciprocal translocation.** A structural rearrangement of the chromosomes in which material is exchanged between one homolog of each of two pairs of chromosomes. The rearrangement is balanced if there is no loss or gain of chromosome material.
**Recombinant DNA molecule.** A union of two different DNA sequences from two different sources, e.g. a vector containing a 'foreign' DNA sequence.
**Recombination.** Cross-over between two linked loci.
**Recombination fraction (θ).** A measure of the distance separating two loci determined by the likelihood that a cross-over will occur between them.
**Reduced penetrance.** A dominant gene which does not manifest itself in a proportion of heterozygotes.
**Relative probability.** See Posterior probability.
**Relative risk.** How frequently a disease occurs in an individual with a specific marker compared to those without the marker in the general population.

**Repetitive DNA.** DNA sequences of variable length which are repeated up to 100 000 (middle repetitive) or over 100 000 (highly repetitive) copies per genome.
**Replication.** The process of copying the double-stranded DNA of the chromosomes.
**Replication bubble.** The structure formed by coalescence of two adjacent replication forks in copying the DNA molecule of a chromosome.
**Replication error.** The phenomenon of microsatellite instability seen in hereditary non-polyposis colorectal cancer due to a mutation in one of the DNA proof-reading enzymes.
**Replication fork.** The structure formed at the site(s) of origin of replication of the double-stranded DNA molecule of chromosomes.
**Replication units.** Clusters of 20–80 sites of origin of DNA replication.
**Replicons.** A generic term for DNA vectors such as plasmids, phages and cosmids, which replicate in host bacterial cells.
**Repressor.** The product of the regulator gene of an operon which inhibits the operator gene.
**Repulsion.** When a certain allele at a locus is on the homologous chromosome for a specific allele at a closely linked locus.
**Response elements.** Regulatory sequences in the DNA to which signaling molecules bind, resulting in control of transcription.
**Restriction endonucleases or enzymes.** Group of enzymes each of which cleaves double-stranded DNA at a specific nucleotide sequence and so produces fragments of DNA of different lengths.
**Restriction fragment.** DNA fragment produced by a restriction endonuclease.
**Restriction fragment length polymorphism (RFLP).** Polymorphism due to the presence or absence of a particular restriction site.
**Restriction map.** Linear arrangement of restriction enzyme sites.
**Restriction site.** Base sequence recognized by a restriction endonuclease.
**Reticulocytes.** Immature red blood cells which still contain messenger RNA.
**Retrovirus.** RNA virus which replicates via conversion into a DNA provirus.
**Reverse genetics.** The process of identifying a protein or enzyme through its gene product.
**Reverse painting.** Amplification using PCR of an unidentified portion of chromosomal material, such as a small duplication or marker chromosome, which is then used as a probe for hybridization to a normal metaphase spread to identify its source of origin.
**Reverse transcriptase.** An enzyme which catalyses the synthesis of DNA from RNA.
**Reverse transriptase PCR (RT-PCR).** Using a special primer which contains a promoter and translation initiator from mRNA (for PCR) to make cDNA.
**Ribonucleic acid (RNA).** See RNA.
**Ribosomes.** Minute spherical structures in the cytoplasm, rich in RNA; the location of protein synthesis.
**Ring chromosome.** An abnormal chromosome caused by a break in both arms of the chromosome, the ends of which unite leading to the formation of a ring.
**RNA (= ribonucleic acid).** The nucleic acid which is found mainly in the nucleolus and ribosomes. Messenger RNA transfers genetic information from the nucleus to the ribosomes in the cytoplasm and also acts as a template for the synthesis of polypeptides. Transfer RNA transfers activated amino acids from the cytoplasm to messenger RNA.
**RNA-directed DNA synthesis.** An exception to the central dogma, a process utilized by many RNA viruses to produce DNA which can integrate with the host genome.
**Robertsonian translocation.** A translocation between two acrocentric chromosomes with loss of satellite material from their short arms.
**Roentgen equivalent for man (rem).** The dose of any radiation which has the same biological effect as 1 rad of X-rays.
**Satellite.** A distal portion of the chromosome separated from the remainder of the chromosome by a narrowed segment or stalk.
**Satellite DNA.** A class of DNA sequences which separates out on density gradient centrifugation as a shoulder or 'satellite' to the main peak of DNA and corresponds to 10–15% of the DNA of the human genome, consisting of short tandemly repeated DNA sequences which code for ribosomal and transfer RNAs.
**Screening.** The identification of persons from a population with a particular disorder, or who carry a gene for a particular disorder.
**Secondary hypertension.** Increased blood pressure which occurs as a result of another primary cause.
**Secondary oocyte or spermatocyte.** The intermediate stage of a female or male gamete in which the homologous duplicated chromosome pairs have separated.
**Secondary response.** The enhanced immune response seen after repeated exposure to an infectious organism or foreign antigen.
**Secretor locus.** A gene in humans which results in the secretion of the ABO blood group antigens in saliva and other body fluids.
**Secretor status.** The presence or absence of excretion of the ABO blood group antigens into various body fluids, e.g. saliva.
**Segment polarity mutants.** Developmental genes identified in *Drosophila* which cause pattern deletions in every segment.
**Segmental.** Limited area of involvement, e.g. a somatic mutation limited to one area of embryonic development.
**Segregation.** The separation of alleles during meiosis so that each gamete contains only one member of each pair of alleles.
**Segregation analysis.** Study of the way in which a disorder is transmitted in families to establish the mode of inheritance.
**Segregation ratio.** The proportion of affected to unaffected individuals in family studies.
**Selection.** The forces which affect biological fitness and therefore the frequency of a particular condition within a given population.
**Selfish DNA.** DNA sequences which appear to have little function and which, it has been proposed, preserve themselves as a result of selection within the genome.
**Semi-conservative.** The process in DNA replication in which only one strand of each resultant daughter molecule is newly synthesized.
**Sense strand.** Strand of genomic DNA to which the mRNA is identical.
**Sensitivity.** Refers to the proportion of cases which are detected. A measure of sensitivity can be made by determining the proportion of false-negative results, i.e. how many cases are missed.
**Sequence.** A stretch of DNA nucleotides. Also used in relation to birth defects or congenital abnormalities which occur as a consequence of a cascade of events intiated by a single primary factor, e.g. Potter's sequence, which occurs as a consequence of renal agenesis.
**Severe combined immunodeficiency.** A genetically heterogeneous lethal form of inherited immunodeficiency with abnormal B- and T-cell function leading to increased susceptibility to both viral and bacterial infections.
**Sex chromatin (= Barr body).** A darkly staining mass situated at the periphery of the nucleus during interphase which represents a single, inactive, condensed X chromosome. The number of sex chromatin masses is one less than the number of X chromosomes (e.g. none in normal males and in 45,X females, one in normal females and XXY males, etc.)
**Sex chromosomes.** The chromosomes responsible for sex determination (XX in women, XY in men).
**Sex-determining region of the Y (SRY).** The part of the Y chromosome which contains the testis-determining gene.
**Sex influence.** When a genetic trait is expressed more frequently in one sex than another. In the extreme when only one sex is affected this is called sex limitation.
**Sex limitation.** When a trait is only manifest in individuals of one sex.
**Sex linkage.** The pattern of inheritance shown by genes carried on the sex chromosomes. Since there are very few Mendelizing genes on the Y chromosome the term is often used synonymously for X-linkage.
**Sex-linked inheritance.** A disorder determined by a gene on one of the sex chromosomes.

**Sex ratio.** The number of male births divided by the number of female births.
**Short interspersed nuclear elements (SINEs).** 5% of the human genome consists of some 750 000 copies of DNA sequences of approximately 300 bp which have sequence similarity to a signal recognition particle involved in protein synthesis.
**Siamese twins.** Conjoined identical twins.
**Sib (= sibling).** Brother or sister.
**Sickle-cell crisis.** An acute hemolytic episode in persons with sickle-cell disease associated with a sudden onset of chest, back or limb pain, fever and dark urine due to the presence of free hemoglobin in the urine.
**Sickle-cell disease.** The homozygous state for hemoglobin S associated with anemia and the risk of sickle-cell crises.
**Sickle-cell trait.** The heterozygous state for hemoglobin S which is not associated with any significant medical risks under ordinary conditions.
**Sickling.** The process of distortion of red blood cell morphology under low oxygenation conditions in persons with sickle-cell disease.
**Sievert (Sv).** Equivalent to 100 rem.
**Signal transduction.** A complex multistep pathway from the cell membrane, through the cytoplasm to the nucleus, with positive and negative feedback loops for accurate cell proliferation and differentiation.
**Silencers.** A negative 'enhancer', the normal action of which is to repress gene expression.
**Silent mutation.** A point mutation in a codon which, due to the degeneracy of the genetic code, still results in the same amino acid in the protein.
**Single nucleotide polymorphisms (SNPs).** Single nucleotide DNA sequence variation which is polymorphic, occurring every 1/500 to 1/2000 base pairs.
**Single-stranded conformational polymorphism (SSCP).** A mutation detection system in which differences in the three-dimensional structure of single-stranded DNA result in differential gel electrophoresis mobility under special conditions.
**Sister chromatids.** Identical daughter chromatids derived from a single chromosome.
**Sister chromatid exchange.** Exchange (crossing-over) of genetic material between two chromatids of any particular chromosome in mitosis.
**Site-directed mutagenesis.** The ability to alter or modify DNA sequences or genes in a directed fashion by processes such as insertional mutagenesis or homologous recombination to determine the effect of these changes on their function.
**Skeleton map.** See Framework map.
**Skewed X-inactivation.** A non-random pattern of inactivation of one of the X chromosomes in a female which can arise through a variety of mechanisms, e.g. an X-autosome translocation.
**Slipped strand mispairing.** Incorrect pairing of the tandem repeats of the two complementary DNA strands during DNA replication which is thought to lead to variation in DNA microsatellite repeat number.
**Small nuclear RNA molecules.** RNA molecules involved in RNA splicing.
**Soft markers.** Minor structural ultrasound findings associated with the possibility of fetal abnormality.
**Solenoid model.** The complex model of the quarternary structure of chromosomes.
**Somatic cells.** The non-germ line cells of the body.
**Somatic cell gene therapy.** The alteration or replacement of a gene limited to the non-germ cells.
**Somatic cell hybrid.** A technique involving the fusion of cells from two different species which results in the loss of chromosomes from one of the cell types and which is used in assigning genes to particular chromosomes.
**Somatic mosaicism.** The occurrence of two different cell lines in a particular tissue or tissues which differ genetically.
**Somatic mutation.** A mutation limited to the non-germ cells.
**Sonic hedgehog.** One of three mammalian homologs of the segment polarity hedgehog genes.
**Southern blot.** Technique for transferring DNA fragments from an agarose gel to a nitrocellulose filter on which they can be hybridized to a radiolabeled single-stranded complementary DNA sequence or probe.
**Specific acquired or adaptive immunity.** A tailor-made immune response which occurs after exposure to an infectious agent.
**Specificity.** The extent to which a test detects only affected individuals. If unaffected persons are detected, these are referred to as false-positives.
**Spermatid.** Mature haploid male gamete.
**Spindle.** A structure responsible for the movement of the chromosomes during cell division.
**Splicing.** The removal of the introns and joining of exons in RNA during transcription, with introns being spliced out and exons being spliced together.
**Splicing branch site.** Intronic sequence involved in splicing of mRNA.
**Splicing consensus sequences.** DNA sequences surrounding splice sites.
**Spontaneous mutation.** A mutation which arises de novo, apparently not due to environmental factors such as mutagens.
**Sporadic.** When a disorder affects a single individual in a family.
**SRY (sex-reversed Y).** The sex-determining region of the Y chromosome which contains the testis-determining gene.
**Stable mutation.** A mutation which is transmitted unchanged.
**Stop codons.** One of three codons (UAG, UAA and UGA) which cause termination of protein synthesis.
**Subchromosomal mapping.** Mapping of a gene or DNA sequence of interest to a region of a chromosome.
**Submetacentric.** Term used to describe chromosomes in which the centromere is slightly off-center.
**Substitution.** A single base pair replaced by another nucleotide.
**Suppressor lymphocytes.** A subclass of T lymphocytes which regulates immune responses, particularly suppressing an immune response to 'self'.
**Switching.** Change in the type of β- or α-like globin chains produced in embryonic and fetal development.
**Synapsis.** The pairing of homologous chromosomes during meiosis.
**Synaptonemal complex.** A complex protein structure which forms between two homologous chromosomes which pair during meiosis.
**Syndrome.** The complex of symptoms and signs which occur together in any particular disorder.
**Synonymous mutation.** See Silent mutation.
**Syntenic genes.** Two genes at different loci on the same chromosome.
**T.** Abbreviation for thymine.
**TATA (Hogness) box.** See Hogness box.
**T cell surface antigen receptor.** Antigenic receptor on the cell surface of T lymphocytes.
**T lymphocytes.** Lymphocytes involved in the cellular immune response, 'thymus'-derived.
**Tandemly repeated DNA sequences.** DNA which consists of blocks of tandem repeats of non-coding DNA which can be either highly dispersed or restricted in their location in the genome.
**Target DNA.** The carrier or vector DNA to which foreign DNA is incorporated or attached to produce recombinant DNA.
**Telomere.** The distal portion of a chromosome arm.
**Telomeric DNA.** The terminal portion of the telomeres of the chromosomes contains 10–15 kb of tandem repeats of a 6 base pair DNA sequence.
**Telophase.** The stage of cell division when the chromosomes have completely separated into two groups and each group has become invested in a nuclear membrane.
**Template strand.** The strand of the DNA double helix which is transcribed into mRNA.
**Teratogen.** An agent which causes congenital abnormalities in the developing embryo or fetus.
**Teratogene.** A gene which can mutate to form a developmental abnormality.
**Terminator.** A sequence of nucleotides in DNA which codes for the termination of translation of mRNA.
**Tertiary trisomy.** The outcome when 3 to 1 segregation of a balanced reciprocal translocation results in the presence of an additional derivative chromosome.

**Tetraploidy.** Twice the normal diploid number of chromosomes (4N).
**Thalassemia intermedia.** A less severe form of β-thalassemia which requires less frequent transfusions.
**Thalassemia major.** An inherited disorder of human hemoglobin which is due to underproduction of one of the globin chains.
**Thalassemia minor.** See Thalassemia trait.
**Thalassemia trait.** The heterozygous state for β-thalassemia, associated with an asymptomatic mild microcytic, hypochromic anemia.
**Three-prime (3′) end.** The end of a DNA or RNA strand with a free 3′ hydroxyl group.
**Threshold.** A concept used in disorders which exhibit multifactorial inheritance to explain a discontinuous phenotype in a process or trait which is continuous, e.g. cleft lip as a result of disturbances in the process of facial development.
**Thymine.** A pyrimidine base in DNA.
**Tissue typing.** Cellular, serological and DNA testing to determine histocompatibility for organ transplantation.
**Trait.** Any detectable phenotypic property or character.
***Trans*-acting.** Transcription factors which act on genes at a distance, usually on both copies of a gene on each chromosome.
**Transcription.** The process whereby genetic information is transmitted from the DNA in the chromosomes to messenger RNA.
**Transcription factors.** Genes which include the Hox, Pax, and zinc finger-containing genes which control RNA transcription by binding to specific DNA regulatory sequences forming complexes which initiate transcription by RNA polymerase.
**Transfection.** The transformation of bacterial cells by infection with phage to produce infectious phage particles. Also the introduction of foreign DNA into eukaryotic cells in culture.
**Transfer RNA.** RNA molecule involved in transfer of amino acids in the process of translation.
**Transformation.** Genetic recombination in bacteria in which foreign DNA introduced into the bacterium is incorporated into the chromosome of the recipient bacterium. Also the change of a normal cell into a malignant cell, e.g. as results from infection of normal cells by oncogenic viruses.
**Transgenic animal model.** Use of techniques such as targeted gene replacement to introduce mutations into a particular gene in another animal species to study an inherited disorder in humans.
**Transient polymorphism.** Two different allelic variants present in a population whose relative frequencies are altering due to either selective advantage or disadvantage of one or the other.
**Transition.** A substitution involving replacement by the same type of nucleotide, i.e. a pyrimidine for a pyrimidine (C for T or vice versa) or a purine for a purine (A for a G or vice versa).
**Translation.** The process whereby genetic information from messenger RNA is translated into protein.
**Translocation.** The transfer of genetic material from one chromosome to another chromosome. If there is an exchange of genetic material between two chromosomes then this is referred to as a reciprocal translocation. A translocation between two acrocentric chromosomes by fusion at the centromeres is referred to as a Robertsonian translocation.
**Transposon.** Mobile genetic element able to replicate and insert a copy of itself at a new location in the genome.
**Transversion.** Substitution of a pyrimidine by a purine, or vice versa.
**Triple test.** The test which gives a risk for having a fetus with Down syndrome in mid-trimester as a function of age, serum α-fetoprotein, estriol and human chorionic gonadotropin levels.
**Triplet amplification or expansion.** Increase in the number of copies of triplet repeat sequences responsible for mutations in a number of single-gene disorders.
**Triplet code.** A series of three bases in the DNA or RNA molecule which codes for a specific amino acid.
**Triploid.** A cell with three times the haploid number of chromosomes, i.e. 3N.
**Trisomy.** The presence of a chromosome additional to the normal complement (i.e. 2N + 1) so that in each somatic nucleus one particular chromosome is represented three times rather than twice.
**Trophoblast.** The outer cell mass of the early embryo which gives rise to the placenta.
**Truncate ascertainment.** See Incomplete ascertainment.
**Tumor suppressor gene.** A term to describe genes which appear to prevent the development of certain types of tumor.
**Tyrosinase-negative albinism.** Form of oculocutaneous albinsim with no melanin production which can be tested for in vitro.
**Tyrosinase-positive albinism.** Form of oculocutaneous albinism with some melanin production which can be tested for in vitro.
**U.** Abbreviation for uracil.
**Ultrasound.** Use of ultrasonic soundwaves to image objects at a distance, e.g. the developing fetus in utero.
**Unbalanced translocation.** A translocation in which there is an overall loss or gain of chromosomal material, e.g. partial monosomy of one of the portions involved and partial trisomy of the other portion involved.
**Unifactorial (= Mendelizing).** Inheritance controlled by a single locus.
**Uniparental disomy.** When an individual inherits both chromosomes of a homologs pair from one parent.
**Uniparental heterodisomy.** Uniparental disomy due to inheritance of the two different homologs from one parent.
**Uniparental isodisomy.** Uniparental disomy due to inheritance of two copies of a single chromosome of a homologous pair from one parent.
**Unipolar illness.** Affective depressive illness.
**Universal donor.** A person of blood group O, Rh-negative, who can donate blood to any person irrespective of their blood group.
**Universal recipient.** A person of blood group AB, Rh-positive, who can receive blood from any donor irrespective of their blood group.
**Unstable mutation.** Mutation which, when transmitted, is passed on in altered form, e.g. triplet repeat mutations.
**Uracil.** A pyrimidine base in RNA.
**Utrophin.** A gene on chromosome 6 with homology to the dystrophin gene.
**Variable expressivity.** The variation in the severity of phenotypic features seen in persons with autosomal dominant disorders, e.g. variable number of café-au-lait spots or neurofibromata in neurofibromatosis type I.
**Variable region.** The portion of the light and heavy chains of immunoglobulins which differs between molecules and which helps to determine antibody specificity.
**Variants.** Alleles which occur less frequently than in 1% of the population.
**Vector.** A plasmid, phage or cosmid into which foreign DNA can be inserted for cloning.
**Virions.** Infectious viral particles.
**Virus.** A protein-covered DNA- or RNA-containing organism which is only capable of replication within bacterial or eukaryotic cells.
**Wingless.** A group of morphogens produced by segment polarity genes.
**X-chromatin.** See Barr body or Sex chromatin.
**X-inactivation.** See Lyonization.
**X-inactivation centre.** The part of the X chromosome responsible for the process of X-inactivation.
**X-linkage.** Genes carried on the X chromosome.
**X-linked dominant.** Genes on the X chromosome which manifest in heterozygous females.
**X-linked dominant lethals.** Disorders which are seen only in females and not in males, as they are thought to be incompatible with survival of the early embryo in hemizygous males, e.g. incontinentia pigmenti.
**X-linked recessive.** Genes which are carried by females and expressed in hemizygous males.
**Xanthomata.** Subcutaneous depositions of lipid, often around tendons; a physical sign associated with disordered lipid metabolism.
**Yeast artificial chromosome (YAC).** A plasmid-cloning vector which contains the DNA sequences for the centromere, telomere and autonomous chromosome replication sites that enable cloning of large DNA fragments up to 2–3 million base pairs in length.
**Y-linked inheritance.** See Holandric inheritance.

**Zinc finger.** A finger-like projection formed by amino acids positioned between two separated cysteine residues which form a complex with a zinc ion, found in genes which have important developmental regulatory roles.
**Zona pellucida.** Cellular layer surrounding the mature unfertilized oocyte.
**Zone of polarizing activity.** An area on the posterior margin of the developing limb bud which determines the antero-posterior axis.
**Zoo blot.** A Southern blot of DNA from a number of different species used to look for evidence of DNA sequences conserved during evolution.
**Zygote.** The fertilized ovum.

# Multiple-choice questions

## CHAPTER 2: THE CELLULAR AND MOLECULAR BASIS OF INHERITANCE

**1. Base substitutions:**

a. May result in nonsense mutations
b. Can affect splicing
c. Are always pathogenic
d. Can affect gene expression
e. Result in frameshift mutations

**2. Transcription:**

a. Describes the production of polypeptides from the mRNA template
b. Occurs in the nucleus
c. Produces single-stranded mRNA using the antisense DNA strand as a template
d. Is regulated by transcription factors that bind to the 3′ UTR
e. Precedes 5′ capping and polyadenylation

**3. The following are directly involved in DNA repair:**

a. Glycosylases
b. DNA polymerases
c. Ligases
d. Splicing
e. Ribosomes

**4. During DNA replication:**

a. DNA helicase separates the double-stranded DNA
b. DNA is synthesized in one direction
c. Okazaki fragments are synthesized
d. DNA is synthesized in a conservative manner
e. Uracil is inserted to pair with adenine

## CHAPTER 3: CHROMOSOMES AND CELL DIVISION

**1. Meiosis differs from mitosis in the following ways:**

a. Daughter cells are haploid, not diploid
b. Meiosis is restricted to the gametes and mitosis occurs only in somatic cells
c. In mitosis there is only one division
d. Meiosis generates genetic diversity
e. The prophase stage of mitosis is 1 step, in meiosis I there are 4 stages

**2. Chromosome abnormalities reliably detected by light microscopy include:**

a. Trisomy
b. Monosomy
c. Reciprocal translocation
d. Interstitial deletion
e. Robertsonian translocation

**3. Fluorescence in situ hybridization using whole chromosome (painting) or specific locus probes enables routine detection of:**

a. Gene amplification
b. Subtelomeric deletion
c. Trisomy
d. Supernumerary marker chromosomes
e. Reciprocal translocation

**4. Chemicals used in the preparation of metaphase chromosomes for analysis by light microscopy include:**

a. Colchicine
b. Phytohemagglutinin
c. Giemsa
d. Quinacrine
e. Hypotonic saline

## CHAPTER 4: DNA TECHNOLOGY AND APPLICATIONS

**1. The following statements apply to restriction enzymes:**

a. They can generate DNA fragments with 'sticky' ends
b. They are viral in origin
c. They are used to detect point mutations
d. They are used in Southern blotting
e. They are also called restriction exonucleases

**2. The following describe the polymerase chain reaction (PCR):**

a. A type of cell-free cloning
b. A process which uses a heat-labile DNA polymerase
c. A very sensitive method of amplifying DNA which can be prone to contamination
d. A technique that can routinely amplify up to 100 kb of DNA
e. A method of amplifying genes with no prior sequence knowledge required

**3. Types of nucleic acid hybridization include:**

a. Southern blotting
b. Microarray
c. Western blotting
d. Northern blotting
e. DNA fingerprinting

**4. The following techniques can be used to screen genes for unknown mutations:**

a. Sequencing
b. Single-stranded conformational polymorphism (SSCP)
c. Denaturing high-performance liquid chromatography (DHPLC)
d. Oligonucleotide ligation assay (OLA)
e. Real-time PCR

## CHAPTER 5: MAPPING AND IDENTIFYING GENES

**1. Genes can be mapped to subchromosomal regions using:**

a. Somatic cell hybridization
b. Fluorescence in situ hybridization (FISH)
c. Pulsed field gel electrophoresis (PFGE)
d. Radiation hybrid mapping
e. Fluorescence-activated chromosome sorting

**2. Methods of high-resolution physical mapping include:**

a. DNA sequencing
b. Pulsed field gel electrophoresis (PFGE)
c. Chromosome walking
d. Fiber FISH
e. DNA fingerprinting

**3. Positional cloning utilizes:**

a. Genetic databases
b. Knowledge of orthologous genes
c. Patients with chromosomal abnormalities
d. Candidate genes selected by biological knowledge
e. Microsatellite markers

**4. A candidate gene is likely to be a disease-associated gene if:**

a. A loss-of-function mutation causes the phenotype
b. An animal model with a mutation in the orthologous gene has the same phenotype
c. Multiple different mutations cause the phenotype
d. The pattern of expression of the gene is consistent with the phenotype
e. It is a pseudogene

## CHAPTER 6: DEVELOPMENTAL GENETICS

**1. In development, *HOX* genes:**

a. Function as transcription factors
b. When mutated have been shown to be associated with many malformation syndromes
c. Show very divergent structures across different species
d. Are functionally redundant in postnatal life
e. Individually, they can be important in the normal development of widely different body systems

**2.**

a. Gastrulation is the process leading to the formation of the 16-cell early embryo 3 days after fertilization
b. Organogenesis takes places between 8 and 12 weeks gestation
c. The notch signaling and sonic hedgehog pathways are important for ensuring normal development in diverse organs and tissues
d. Somites form in a caudo-rostral direction from the presomitic mesoderm
e. *TBX* genes appear to be crucial to normal limb development

**3.**

a. In mammalian development the jaw is formed from the second pharyngeal arch
b. Pharyngeal arch arteries ultimately become the great vessels around the heart
c. *TBX1* is a key gene in the defects associated with DiGeorge syndrome
d. Achondroplasia can be caused by a wide variety of mutations in the *FGFR3* gene
e. Loss-of-function mutations and gain-of-function mutations usually cause similar defects

4.

a. In most males with a karyotype of 46,XX the SRY gene is present and found on one of the X chromosomes
b. In Lyonization, or X chromosome inactivation, all the genes of one X are switched off
c. As a result of Lyonization, all females are X chromosome mosaics
d. Male fetal development is solely dependent on the SRY gene having normal functioning
e. X chromosome inactivation may be linked in some way to the monozygotic twinning process

**5. Transcription factors:**

a. Are RNA sequences that interfere with translation in the ribosomes
b. Their only function is to switch off genes in development
c. When mutated in *Drosophila* body segments may be completely reorganized
d. Are not involved in defects of laterality
e. Include genes that have a zinc finger motif

## CHAPTER 7: PATTERNS OF INHERITANCE

**1. Concerning autosomal recessive inheritance:**

a. Females are more likely to be affected than males
b. If both parents are carriers the risk at conception that any child might be a carrier is $\frac{3}{4}$
c. Diseases following this pattern of inheritance are more common in societies where cousin marriage is normal
d. Usually only a single generation has affected individuals
e. Angelman syndrome follows this pattern

**2. Concerning X-linked inheritance:**

a. The condition cannot be passed from an affected father to his son
b. When recessive, an affected man will not see the condition in his children but it may appear in his grandchildren
c. When dominant, females are usually as severely affected as males
d. When dominant, there are usually more affected females than affected males in a family
e. The risk of germline mosaicism does not need to be considered

3.

a. Heteroplasmy refers to the presence of more than one mutation in mitochondria
b. Mitochondrial genes mutate less often than nuclear genes
c. Mitochondrial conditions only affect muscle and nerve tissue
d. The risk of passing on a mitochondrial condition to the next generation may be as high as 100%
e. Mitochondrial diseases have nothing to do with nuclear genes

4.

a. Locus heterogeneity means the same disease can be caused by genes on different chromosomes
b. Pseudodominance refers to the risk to the offspring when both parents have the same dominantly inherited condition
c. If a condition demonstrates reduced penetrance it may skip generations
d. Variable expression characterizes diseases that demonstrate anticipation
e. Pleiotropy is simply a more striking form of variable expression

5.

a. An autosomal recessive condition can occasionally arise through uniparental disomy
b. Imprinted genes can be unmasked through uniparental disomy
c. Digenic inheritance is simply another way of referring to uniparental disomy
d. Hormonal factors may account for conditions demonstrating sex influence
e. Most of the human genome is subject to imprinting

## CHAPTER 8: MATHEMATICAL AND POPULATION GENETICS

**1. In applying the Hardy–Weinberg equilibrium the following assumptions are made:**

a. The population is small
b. There is no consanguinity
c. New mutations do not occur
d. No babies are born by donor insemination
e. There is no significant movement of population

**2. If the population incidence of a recessive disease is 1:10 000, the carrier frequency in the population is:**

a. 1 in 100
b. 1 in 200
c. 1 in 25
d. 1 in 50
e. 1 in 500

**3. Heterozygote advantage:**

a. May lead to an increased incidence of autosomal dominant disorders
b. Does not mean that biological fitness is increased in the homozygous state
c. May explain the worldwide distribution of sickle-cell disease and malaria
d. May lead to distortion of the Hardy–Weinberg equilibrium
e. Is very unlikely to be traced to a founder effect

4. **Polymorphic loci:**
a. Are defined as those loci at which there are at least two alleles, each with frequencies greater than 10%
b. Have been crucial to gene discoveries
c. Can be helpful in determining someone's genetic status in a family
d. Have nothing to do with calculating LOD scores
e. By themselves, have no consequence for genetically determined disease

5. **In population genetics:**
a. To calculate the mutation rate for a disorder it is only necessary to know the biological fitness for the condition
b. If medical treatment can improve biological fitness, the frequency of an autosomal dominant condition will increase far more rapidly than an autosomal recessive condition
c. Even when a large number of families are studied the calculated segregation ratio for a disorder might not yield the expected figures for a given pattern of inheritance
d. For X-linked disorders the frequency of affected males equals the frequency of the mutated allele
e. Autozygosity mapping is a useful strategy to look for the gene in any autosomal recessive condition

## CHAPTER 9: POLYGENIC AND MULTIFACTORIAL GENETICS

1. **Concerning autism:**
a. It is best classified as an inborn error of metabolism
b. The concordance rate in dizygotic twins is approximately 50%
c. Fragile-X syndrome is a major cause
d. The risk to the siblings of an affected person is approximately 5%
e. Girls are more frequently affected than boys

2. **Linkage analysis is more difficult in multifactorial conditions than in single-gene disorders because:**
a. Variants in more than one gene are likely to contribute to the disorder
b. The number of affected persons within in a family is likely to be fewer than for a single-gene disorder
c. The mode of inheritance is usually uncertain
d. Some multifactorial disorders are likely to have more than one etiology
e. Many multifactorial conditions have a late age of onset

3. **Association studies:**
a. Can give false positive results due to population stratification
b. Include the transmission disequilibrium test (TDT)
c. Positive association studies should be replicated
d. Are used to map genes in multifactorial disorders
e. Require closely matched control and patient groups

4. **Variants in genes which confer susceptibility to type 2 diabetes (T2DM) have been found:**
a. By linkage analysis using affected sibling pairs
b. Using animal models
c. By candidate gene studies from monogenic subtypes of diabetes
d. Through the study of biological candidates
e. In isolated populations

5. **Variants in the *NOD2/CARD15* gene:**
a. Are associated with Crohn disease and ulcerative colitis
b. Can result in a 40-fold increased risk of disease
c. Were identified after the gene was mapped to chromosome 16p12 by positional cloning
d. Has led to novel therapies
e. Are very rare in the general population

## CHAPTER 10: HEMOGLOBIN AND THE HEMOGLOBINOPATHIES

1.
a. The fetal hemoglobin chain, $\gamma$, resembles the adult $\beta$ chain
b. The Hb chains, $\alpha$, $\beta$ and $\gamma$ are all expressed throughout fetal life
c. In $\alpha$-thalassemia there are too many $\alpha$ chains
d. Hb Barts is a form of $\beta$-thalassemia
e. Carriers of $\beta$-thalassaemia frequently suffer from symptomatic anemia

2. **Regarding sickle-cell disease:**
a. The sickling effect of red blood corpuscles is the result of abnormal Hb binding with the red blood cell membrane
b. Life-threatening thrombosis can occur
c. Hb S differs from normal Hb A by a single amino-acid substitution
d. Splenic infarction may occur but this has little clinical consequence
e. Point (missense) mutations are the usual cause of abnormal Hb in the sickling disorders

3.
a. Many Hb variants are harmless
b. The types of mutation occurring in the hemoglobinopathies are very limited
c. In the thalassemias hypoplasia of the bone marrow occurs
d. In the thalassemias Hb demonstrates abnormal oxygen affinity
e. In some thalassemias increased red cell hemolysis occurs

**4.**

a. Persistence of fetal Hb into adult life is an acquired disorder
b. Throughout fetal life it is the liver that produces most of the body's Hb
c. The bone marrow is not involved in Hb production before birth
d. The liver continues to produce Hb into the second year of postnatal life
e. Persistence of fetal Hb into adult life is a benign condition

## CHAPTER 11: BIOCHEMICAL GENETICS

**1. In congenital adrenal hyperplasia (CAH):**

a. Females may show virilization and ambiguous genitalia
b. Males may show undermasculinization and ambiguous genitalia
c. Mineralocorticoid deficiency can be life threatening
d. Treatment is required during childhood but not usually in adult life
e. In affected females fertility is basically unaffected

**2. Phenylketonuria:**

a. Is the only cause of a raised phenylalanine in the neonatal period
b. Requires lifelong treatment
c. Is a cause of epilepsy and eczema
d. Results in reduced levels of melanin
e. Is part of the same pathway as cholesterol production

**3. Hepatomegaly is an important feature of:**

a. Hurler syndrome
b. Glycogen storage disorders
c. Abnormalities of porphyrin metabolism
d. Niemann–Pick disease
e. Galactosemia

**4. Concerning mitochondrial disorders:**

a. All follow matrilinear inheritance
b. Retinal pigmentation and diabetes can both be features
c. There are fewer than 50 gene products from the mitochondrial genome
d. Leigh disease is always caused by the same point mutation
e. The gene for Barth syndrome is known but the metabolic pathway is uncertain

**5.**

a. The carnitine cycle and long-chain fatty acids are linked
b. A single point mutation explains most cases of MCAD
c. Peroxisomal disorders include Menkes disease and Wilson disease
d. Inborn errors of metabolism may present with hypotonia and acidosis alone
e. X-rays are of no value in making a diagnosis of inborn errors of metabolism

## CHAPTER 12: PHARMACOGENETICS

**1. Thiopurine drugs used to treat leukemia:**

a. Include 6-mercaptopurine, 6-thioguanine and azathioprine
b. Are also used to suppress the immune system
c. May be toxic in 1–2% of patients
d. Can have serious side-effects
e. Are metabolized by thiopurine methyltransferase (TPMT)

**2. Liver enzymes which show genetic variation of expression and hence influence the response to drugs include:**

a. UDP-glucuronosyltransferase
b. *O*-acetyltransferase
c. Alcohol dehydrogenase
d. CYP2D6
e. CYP2C9

**3. The following have an increased risk of complications from anesthesia:**

a. First-degree relatives of patients affected with malignant hyperthermia
b. Patients with *RYR1* mutations
c. Patients with *G6DP* deficiency
d. Patients with *CHE1* mutations
e. Patients with elevated pseudocholinesterase levels

**4. Examples of diseases where treatment may be influenced by pharmacogenetics include:**

a. Maturity-onset diabetes of the young (MODY), subtype glucokinase
b. Maturity-onset diabetes of the young (MODY), subtype HNF-1$\alpha$
c. HIV
d. Epilepsy
e. Tuberculosis

## CHAPTER 13: IMMUNOGENETICS

**1.**

a. The complement cascade can only be activated by the binding of antibody and antigen
b. C1-inhibitor deficiency can result in complement activation through the classic pathway
c. C3 levels are reduced in hereditary angioneurotic edema
d. Complement helps directly in the attack on microorganisms
e. Complement is mainly found in the intracellular matrix

**2.**
a. The immunoglobulin molecule is made up of 6 polypeptide chains
b. The genes for the various light and heavy immunoglobulin chains are found close together in the human genome
c. Close relatives make the best organ donors because they are likely to share the same complement haplotypes
d. The DNA encoding the κ light chain contains four distinct regions
e. The diversity of T-cell surface antigen receptor can be compared to the process of immunoglobulin diversity

**3.**
a. Maternal transplacental mobility of antibodies gives infants protection for about 12 months
b. X-linked severe combined immunodeficiency (SCID) accounts for about 5–10% of the total of SCID
c. SCID, despite its name, is not always a severe condition
d. There is always a T-cell abnormality in the different forms of SCID
e. Chronic granulomatous disease (CGD) is a disorder of humoral immunity

**4.**
a. DiGeorge/Sedlácková syndrome is a primary disorder of immune function
b. Severe opportunistic bacterial infections are uncommon in DiGeorge syndrome
c. Genetic prenatal diagnosis is possible for common variable immune deficiency (CVID)
d. Autoimmune disorders follow autosomal dominant inheritance
e. Investigation of immune function should be considered in any child with failure to thrive (FTT)

## CHAPTER 14: CANCER GENETICS

**1.**
a. Chromosome translocations can lead to cancer through modification of oncogene activity
b. Oncogenes are the most common forms of genes predisposing to hereditary cancer syndromes
c. Defective apoptosis may lead to tumorigenesis
d. Loss of heterozygosity (LOH) is another term for a mutational event in an oncogene
e. A mutation in the *APC* gene is sufficient to cause colorectal cancer

**2.**
a. The two-hit hypothesis predicted that a tumor would develop when both copies of a critical gene were mutated
b. TP53 mutations are only found in Li–Fraumeni syndrome
c. The *RET* proto-oncogene is implicated in all forms of multiple endocrine neoplasia (MEN)
d. Individuals with familial adenomatous polyposis (FAP) should have screening of the upper GI tract
e. Endometrial cancer is a feature of hereditary non-polyposis colon cancer (HNPCC)

**3.**
a. Thyroid cancer is a risk in Bannayan–Riley–Ruvalcaba syndrome
b. Men with a germline mutation in *BRCA2* are at increased risk of prostate cancer
c. The genetic basis of all familial breast cancer is now well established
d. Familial breast cancer is usually fully penetrant
e. For men with prostate cancer, 3% of male first-degree relatives are similarly affected

**4.**
a. Medulloblastoma is a common tumor in von Hippel–Lindau (VHL) disease
b. Pheochromocytoma is frequently seen in Gorlin syndrome
c. There is a risk of ovarian cancer in Peutz–Jehgers syndrome and HNPCC
d. Cutaneous manifestations occur in Peutz–Jehgers syndrome, Gorlin syndrome and HNPCC
e. In two-thirds of HNPCC cases the predisposing gene is unknown

**5.**
a. Screening for renal cancer in VHL is recommended
b. Mammography detects breast cancer more easily in premenopausal women than postmenopausal
c. Screening for retinoblastoma should begin in the second year of life
d. Colorectal cancer in two close relatives is sufficient to indicate colonoscopy screening in other family members
e. Preventive surgery is strongly indicated in FAP and women positive for *BRCA1* mutations

## CHAPTER 15: GENETIC FACTORS IN COMMON DISEASES

1.

a. A genetic factor is believed to be present in 10% of epilepsy
b. Mutations in potassium channel genes predispose to epilepsy
c. Juvenile myoclonic epilepsy follows autosomal dominant inheritance
d. Epilepsy is common in deletion 1p36 syndrome
e. Unverricht–Lundborg disease is a benign form of Mendelian epilepsy

2.

a. There is a high risk of bipolar depressive illness in DiGeorge syndrome
b. The concordance rate for schizophrenia in monozygotic twins is approximately 80%
c. No mutations have so far been found in any gene to provide a cause for schizophrenia
d. Twin studies suggest a similar heritability for bipolar and unipolar illness
e. Analysis of APOE $\varepsilon 4$ is recommended as a screening procedure for Alzheimer's disease

3.

a. Susceptibility for Creutzfeldt–Jakob disease is conferred by homozygosity for a PRNP polymorphism
b. So far, three genes are known to cause autosomal dominant Alzheimer disease
c. Presenilin-1 is a low-penetrance gene for early-onset Alzheimer disease
d. Linkage studies are more important than twin studies in understanding the genetic contribution to bipolar illness
e. Persons with Down syndrome are at significant risk of Alzheimer disease

4. **Hemochromatosis:**

a. Is genetically heterogeneous
b. Affects more women than men
c. Can be treated by phlebotomy
d. Is fully penetrant
e. Is usually caused by a homozygous H63D mutation in the *HFE* gene

5. **The following statements about venous thrombosis are true:**

a. Factor V Leiden and the prothrombin G20210A variant are common causes of venous thrombosis
b. Testing for factor V Leiden and the prothrombin variant will change the management of a patient with venous thrombosis
c. The factor V Leiden mutation causes reduced expression of the factor V gene
d. The prothrombin variant causes increased expression of the prothrombin gene
e. Compound heterozygotes for factor V Leiden and the prothrombin variant have a 20-fold increased risk of venous thrombosis

## CHAPTER 16: CONGENITAL ABNORMALITIES AND DYSMORPHIC SYNDROMES

1.

a. Around 5% of all infant deaths are due to congenital abnormalities
b. At least half of all spontaneous miscarriages have a genetic basis
c. A major congenital abnormality affects approximately one newborn baby in every 100
d. Positional talipes is an example of a disruption to normal intrauterine development
e. Multiple abnormalities are sometimes the result of a sequence

2.

a. Down syndrome should more accurately be termed 'Down Association'
b. Sotos syndrome, like Down syndrome, is due to a chromosomal abnormality
c. Spina bifida affects approximately 2 per 1000 births
d. Infantile polycystic kidney disease is an example of a condition with different patterns of inheritance
e. Holoprosencephaly is an example of a condition with different patterns of inheritance

3.

a. Thalidomide embryopathy was an example of a disruption to normal intrauterine development
b. Talipes may be a consequence of renal agenesis
c. Limb defects are not caused by fetal exposure to sodium valproate
d. Symmetrical defects tend to feature in a dysplasia
e. Birth defects are unexplained in 20% of cases

**4.**

a. Congenital infection could lead to someone being both blind and deaf
b. The mid-trimester is the most dangerous time for a fetus to suffer from a maternal infection
c. Vertebral body defects can be a consequence of poorly treated diabetes mellitus in the first trimester
d. A polymorphism in the methylenetetrahydrofolate reductase (*MTHFR*) gene is always associated with an increased risk of neural tube defect
e. Pulmonary stenosis is a feature of Noonan syndrome and congenital rubella

**5.**

a. Cleft lip/palate occurs more frequently than 1:1000 births
b. Associations generally have a high recurrence risk
c. The recurrence risk for a multifactorial condition can usually be determined by looking at patient's family pedigree
d. One cause of holoprosencephaly is a metabolic defect
e. Congenital heart disease affects 1:1000 babies

## CHAPTER 17: GENETIC COUNSELING

**1.**

a. The individual who seeks genetic counseling is the proband
b. Retinitis pigmentosa is not genetically heterogeneous
c. Genetic counseling is all about recurrence risks
d. The counselor's own opinion about a difficult choice is always helpful
e. Good counseling should not be measured by the patient's/client's ability to remember genetic risks

**2.**

a. First-cousin partnerships are 10 times more likely to have babies with congenital abnormalities than the general population
b. On average, a grandparent and grandchild share $\frac{1}{4}$ of their genes
c. Incestuous relationships virtually always result in severe learning difficulties in the offspring
d. Consanguinity should be regarded as extremely abnormal
e. Consanguinity refers exclusively to cousin marriages/partnerships

**3.**

a. Genetic disorders are accidents of nature, so guilt feelings are rare
b. Clear genetic counseling changes patients' reproductive decisions in virtually all cases
c. The chance of first cousins having their first child affected with an autosomal recessive condition due to a deleterious gene inherited from a grandparent is 1:32
d. Far more genetic testing of children for adoption takes place than for children reared by their birth parents
e. Patient support groups have little value given that modern medical genetics is so technically complex

## CHAPTER 18: CHROMOSOME DISORDERS

**1.**

a. The chromosome number in man was discovered after the structure of DNA
b. The Turner syndrome karyotype is the most common single chromosome abnormality in spontaneous abortuses
c. The rate of miscarriage in Down syndrome is similar to the rate in karyotypically normal fetuses
d. Most Down syndrome babies are born to mothers aged less than 30 years
e. All Down syndrome children have to go to special school

**2.**

a. The life expectancy of children with trisomy 18 (Edwards syndrome) is about 2 years
b. 47,XYY males are fertile
c. The origin of Turner syndrome (45,X) can be in paternal meiosis
d. All cases of Angelman syndrome have a cytogenetically visible deletion on chromosome 15q
e. DiGeorge syndrome results from misaligned homologous recombination between flanking repeat gene clusters

**3.**

a. Premature vascular problems occur in adults with Williams syndrome
b. Congenital heart disease is a feature of Prader–Willi and Smith–Magenis syndromes
c. The Wilms tumor locus is on chromosome 13
d. Aniridia may be caused by either a gene mutation or a chromosome microdeletion
e. A child's behavior may help to make a diagnosis of a malformation syndrome

**4.**

a. Klinefelter syndrome affects approximately 1 in 10000 male live births
b. Learning difficulties are common in Klinefelter syndrome
c. Chromosome mosaicism is commonly seen in Turner syndrome
d. Females with a karyotype 47,XXX are infertile
e. Chromosome breakage syndromes can cause cancer

**5.**

a. In Fragile-X syndrome the triplet repeat does not change in size significantly when passed from father to daughter
b. Fragile-X syndrome is a single, well-defined condition
c. Girls with bilateral inguinal herniae should have their chromosomes tested
d. Normal karyotyping is a good way of diagnosing Fragile-X syndrome in girls
e. FISH analysis using multi-telomeric probes diagnose about 25% of non-specific learning difficulties

## CHAPTER 19: SINGLE-GENE DISORDERS

**1.**

a. In Huntington disease (HD) an earlier age of onset in the offspring is more likely if the gene is passed from an affected mother rather than an affected father
b. In HD, those homozygous for the mutation are no more severely affected than those who are heterozygous
c. From the onset of HD, the average duration of the illness until a terminal event is 25–30 years
d. In HD, non-penetrance of the disease may be associated with low repeat abnormal alleles
e. Anticipation is a feature of the inheritance of myotonic dystrophy

**2.**

a. Insomnia is a feature of myotonic dystrophy
b. Myotonic dystrophy is a cause of neonatal hypertonia
c. The clinical effects of myotonic dystrophy are mediated through RNA
d. Cardiac conduction defects are a feature of myotonic dystrophy and ion channelopathies
e. The diagnosis of cystic fibrosis (CF) may only come to light in the infertility clinic

**3.**

a. In CF the R117H mutation is the most common one in Northern Europe
b. In the *CFTR* gene a modifying intragenic polymorphism affects the phenotype
c. Hypertrophic cardiomyopathies are mostly due to mutations in ion channelopathy genes
d. Many different inherited muscular dystrophies can be linked to the complex that includes dystrophin (mutated in Duchenne and Becker muscular dystrophies)
e. Learning difficulties are part of spinal muscular atrophy

**4.**

a. Cystic fibrosis and hemophilia are unlikely candidates for gene therapy
b. An abnormal span:height ratio alone is a major feature of Marfan syndrome
c. Neurofibromatosis type 1 (NF1) sometimes 'skips generations'
d. Scoliosis can be a feature of both NF1 and Marfan syndrome
e. Cataracts can be a feature of NF1 but not NF2

**5.**

a. HMSN types I and II refer to a genetic classification
b. HMSN can follow all major patterns of inheritance
c. It is the nerve sheath, rather than the nerve itself, that is altered in the most common form of HMSN
d. Creatine kinase levels and factor VIII levels are good tests for identifying carriers of Duchenne dystrophy and hemophilia, respectively
e. Brugada syndrome is one of the varieties of spinal muscular atrophy

## CHAPTER 20: SCREENING FOR GENETIC DISEASE

**1.**

a. X-inactivation studies provide a useful means of identifying female carriers of some X-linked disorders
b. Reliable clinical signs to detect most carriers of X-linked disorders are lacking
c. DNA sequence variants are useful in targeted screening as long as they are not polymorphic
d. DNA markers are useful in targeted screening for retinitis pigmentosa
e. For the purposes of screening family members, opportunities should be taken for the banking of DNA from probands with lethal conditions

**2.**

a. Patients with presymptomatic tuberous sclerosis always have a characteristic facial rash
b. It is always possible to diagnose neurofibromatosis type 1 by age 2 years because it is a fully penetrant condition
c. Biochemical tests should not be considered as diagnostic genetic tests
d. An MRI scan of the lumbar spine may be useful in diagnosing Marfan syndrome
e. Predictive genetic testing must always be done by direct gene analysis

**3.**

a. Population screening programs should be legally enforced
b. Population screening programs should be offered if some form of treatment or prevention is available
c. The sensitivity of a test refers to the extent to which the test detects only affected individuals
d. The positive predictive value of a screening test refers to the proportion of positive tests that are true positives
e. If there is no effective treatment for a late-onset condition, predictive genetic testing should be undertaken with great care

**4.**

a. A high proportion of people who undergo carrier testing cannot remember their result properly
b. Carrier screening for cystic fibrosis is the most useful program among Greek Cypriots
c. The possibility of a screening test leading to employment discrimination is no major concern
d. Neonatal screening for Duchenne muscular dystrophy improves life expectancy
e. Neonatal screening for cystic fibrosis is a DNA-based test

**5.**

a. Newborn screening for hemochromatosis, the most common mutated gene in European populations, is a nationally managed program in the UK
b. The presymptomatic screening of children for adult-onset genetic disease is a decision made by the parents
c. Neonatal screening for phenylketonuria and congenital hypothyroidism are the longest-running screening programs
d. Screening for MCAD (medium-chain acyl-CoA dehydrogenase) deficiency is integrated into neonatal population screening
e. Genetic registers are mainly for research

## CHAPTER 21: PRENATAL TESTING AND REPRODUCTIVE GENETICS

**1.**

a. Amniocentesis is being routinely practiced earlier and earlier in pregnancy
b. The cells grown from amniocentesis are originate purely from fetal skin
c. The risk of miscarriage is higher from chorionic villus sampling (CVS) than from amniocentesis
d. CVS is a safe procedure at 9 weeks gestation
e. Fetal skin disorders can be diagnosed by ultrasound

**2.**

a. In Down syndrome pregnancies maternal serum human chorionic gonadotropin (hCG) is usually elevated
b. In Down syndrome pregnancies maternal serum α–fetoprotein (αFP) is usually reduced
c. In trisomy 18 pregnancies maternal serum markers behave in just the same way as in Down syndrome pregnancies
d. About 95% of Down syndrome pregnancies are picked up using maternal age, serum αFP and hCG, and fetal nuchal translucency
e. Twin pregnancy is a cause of elevated maternal serum αFP

**3.**

a. Chromosome mosaicism is detected in about 5% of CVS samples
b. Chromosome disorders are the main cause of abnormal nuchal translucency
c. Echogenic fetal bowel on ultrasound is a risk factor for cystic fibrosis
d. For a couple who have had one Down syndrome child, the risk in the next pregnancy is usually not greatly increased
e. Familial marker chromosomes are usually not clinically significant

**4.**

a. Donor insemination is a procedure not requiring a licence from the HFEA
b. Surrogacy is illegal in the UK
c. For preimplantation genetic diagnosis (PGD) fertilization of the egg is achieved by intracytoplasmic sperm injection (ICSI)
d. The success rate from IVF, in terms of taking home a baby, is only about 50%
e. The largest group of diseases being tested in PGD is single-gene conditions

**5.**

a. There is an increased risk of genetic conditions in the children conceived by ICSI
b. The sperm of one donor may only be used five times
c. Children conceived by donor insemination are entitled to as much information as adopted children about their biological parents
d. If prenatal diagnosis could be achieved by analyzing fetal cells in the maternal circulation, the couple would still have to consider termination of pregnancy
e. Infertility affects about 1 in 20 couples

## CHAPTER 22: RISK CALCULATION

**1.**

a. A probability of 0.5 is the same as a 50% risk
b. The probability of an event never exceeds unity
c. In a dizygotic twin pregnancy the probability that the babies will be the same sex equals 0.5
d. Bayes' theorem takes account of both prior probability and conditional information
e. In an autosomal dominant condition a penetrance of 0.7 means that 30% of heterozygotes will not manifest the disorder

**2. For an autosomal recessive condition the chance that the first cousin of an affected individual is a carrier is:**

a. 1 in 8
b. 1 in 2
c. 1 in 4
d. 1 in 10
e. 1 in 6

**3. In X-linked recessive inheritance:**

a. The sons of a female carrier have a 1 in 4 chance of being affected
b. The mother of an affected male is an obligate carrier
c. The gonadal mosaicism risk in Duchenne muscular dystrophy may be as high as 10%
d. For a woman who has an affected son, her chance of being a carrier is reduced if she goes on to have three unaffected sons
e. A dummy consultand refers to an individual in a pedigree who is ignored when it comes to calculating risk

**4. In autosomal recessive inheritance the risk that the nephew of an affected individual, born to the affected individual's healthy sibling, is a carrier is:**

a. 1 in 2
b. 1 in 4
c. 2 in 3
d. 1 in 3
e. 1 in 6

**5.**

a. In calculating risk, conditional information can include negative DNA data
b. In delayed onset of a dominantly inherited condition, calculating heterozygote risk requires clinical expression data
c. Calculating odds ratios does not require information about prior probabilities
d. Empiric risks derived from epidemiological studies have limited application to a particular situation
e. When using DNA marker data to predict risk the recombination fraction does not really matter

## CHAPTER 23: THE HUMAN GENOME PROJECT, TREATMENT OF GENETIC DISEASE AND GENE THERAPY

**1. Achievements of the Human Genome Project include:**

a. Draft sequence published in 2000
b. Sequencing completed in 2003
c. Development of bioinformatics tools
d. Identification of all disease-causing genes
e. Studies of ethical, legal and social issues

**2. Methods currently used to treat genetic disease include:**

a. Germ-cell gene therapy
b. Stem-cell transplantation
c. Enzyme/protein replacement
d. Dietary restriction
e. In situ repair of mutations by cellular DNA repair mechanism

**3. Gene therapy may be delivered by:**

a. Liposomes
b. Adeno-associated viruses
c. Antisense oligonucleotides
d. Lentiviruses
e. Injection of plasmid DNA

**4. Gene therapy has been used to successfully treat patients with the following diseases:**

a. Cystic fibrosis
b. Severe combined immunodeficiency (XL-SCID)
c. Sickle-cell disease
d. Hemophilia
e. Adenosine deaminase deficiency

**5. Potential gene therapy methods for cancer include:**

a. Inhibition of fusion proteins
b. Stimulation of the immune system
c. Increased expression of the angiogenic factors
d. RNA interference
e. Antisense oligonucleotides

# Case-based questions

## CHAPTER 6: DEVELOPMENTAL GENETICS

### Case 1

A $2\frac{1}{2}$-year-old child is referred to geneticists because of a large head circumference above the 97th centile, although it is growing parallel to the centile lines. The parents would like to have another child and are asking about the recurrence risk. The cerebral ventricles are dilated and there has been much discussion with the neurosurgeons about possible ventriculo-peritoneal shunting. On taking a full family history it emerges that the paternal grandmother is under review by dermatologists for skin lesions, some of which have been removed, and a paternal uncle has had some teeth cysts removed by a hospital dentist.

1. Is there a diagnosis that embraces the various features in these different family members?
2. What investigations would be appropriate for the child's father, and what is the answer to the couple's question about recurrence risk?

### Case 2

A 4-year-old girl is brought to a pediatrician because of behavioral difficulties, including problems with potty training. The pediatrician decides to test the child's chromosomes because he has previously seen a case of 47,XXX (triple X) syndrome where the girl had oppositional behavior. Somewhat to his surprise the chromosome result is 47,XY, i.e. the 'girl' is genetically 'male'.

1. What are the most important causes of sex reversal in a 4-year-old child who is phenotypically female and otherwise physically healthy?
2. What should the pediatrician tell the parents and which investigations should be performed?

## CHAPTER 7: PATTERNS OF INHERITANCE

### Case 1

A 34-year-old man has developed some spasticity of his legs in the past few years and his family have noted some memory problems and alteration in behavior. He has very brisk peripheral reflexes. He is seen with his mother in the genetic clinic and she is found to have significantly brisk peripheral reflexes on examination but has no health complaints. It emerges that her own father probably had problems similar to her son's in his thirties, but he was killed in the war.

1. Which patterns of inheritance need to be considered in this scenario?
2. What diagnostic possibilities should be considered?

### Case 2

A couple have a child who suffers a number of bone fractures during early childhood after minor trauma and they are told this is probably a mild form of osteogenesis imperfecta. The parents did not suffer childhood fractures themselves, and when they have another child who also develops fractures they are told the inheritance is autosomal recessive. This includes an explanation that the affected children should not see the condition occur in their offspring in the future.

1. Is the information given to the parents correct?
2. If not, what is the most likely pattern of inheritance and explanation for the sibling recurrence of fractures?

## CHAPTER 8: MATHEMATICAL AND POPULATION GENETICS

### Case 1

The incidence of a certain autosomal recessive disorder in population A is well established at approximately 1:10 000, whilst in population B the incidence of the same disorder is much higher at approximately 1:900. A man from the first population group and a woman from the second population group are planning to marry and start a family. Being aware of the relatively high incidence of the disorder in population B, they seek genetic counseling.

1. What essential question must be asked of each individual?
2. What is the risk of the disorder occurring in their first pregnancy, based on application of the Hardy–Weinberg equilibrium?

### Case 2

Neurofibromatosis type 1 is a relatively common Mendelian condition. In a population survey of 50 000 people in one town 12 cases are identified, of which eight all belong to one large affected family.

1. Based on these figures, what is the mutation rate in the neurofibromin gene?
2. Name some limitations to the validity of calculating the mutation rate from a survey like this.

## CHAPTER 9: POLYGENIC AND MULTIFACTORIAL INHERITANCE

### Case 1

A 16-year-old requests oral contraceptives from her GP. On taking a family history it emerges that her mother had a deep vein thrombosis at the age of 40 years and died following a pulmonary embolism aged 55 years. There is no other relevant family history.

1. What genetic testing is appropriate?
2. What are the limitations of testing in this situation?

### Case 2

A 35-year-old woman is diagnosed with diabetes and started on insulin treatment. She and her 29-year-old brother were adopted and have no contact with their birth parents. Her brother has no symptoms of hyperglycemia. Both have normal hearing and no other significant findings.

1. What possible subtypes of diabetes might she have and what are the modes of inheritance of these subtypes?
2. For each of these subtypes what is the risk of her brother developing diabetes?

## CHAPTER 10: HEMOGLOBIN AND THE HEMOGLOBINOPATHIES

### Case 1

A Chinese couple resident in the UK have had two pregnancies and the outcome in both was a stillborn, edematous baby (hydrops fetalis). These pregnancies occurred when they lived in Asia and they have no living children. They seek some genetic advice about the chances of this happening again but no medical records are available for the pregnancies.

1. What diagnostic possibilities should be considered?
2. What investigations are appropriate to this situation?

### Case 2

A young adolescent whose parents are of West Indian origin is admitted from A & E after presenting with severe abdominal pain and some fever. An acute abdomen is suspected and the patient undergoes laparotomy for possible appendicitis. However, no surgical pathology is identified. Subsequently the urine appears dark.

1. What other investigations might be appropriate at this stage?
2. What form of follow-up is appropriate?

## CHAPTER 11: BIOCHEMICAL GENETICS

### Case 1

A 2-year-old boy, who has a baby sister aged 4 months, is admitted to hospital with a vomiting illness and drowsiness. Despite his vomiting symptoms improving quite quickly with intravenous fluid support but his blood glucose remains low and IV fluids are required longer than might normally be expected. The parents say something like this happened before, though he recovered without seeing a doctor.

1. What does this history suggest?
2. What investigations are appropriate?



### Case 2

A 28-year-old woman has become aware over several years that she does not have the same energy as she did at the age of 20. She tires relatively easily on exertion and family members have noticed that she has developed slightly droopy eyelids as well as wondering if her hearing is deteriorating, which she vigorously denies.

1. How might a detailed family history help towards a diagnosis in this case?
2. What investigations should be performed?

## CHAPTER 13: IMMUNOGENETICS

### Case 1

A 32-year-old man has had low-back pain and stiffness for 2 years and recently developed some irritation in his eyes. X-rays are performed and a diagnosis of ankylosing spondylitis is made. He remembers his maternal grandfather having similar back problems as well as arthritis in other joints. He has three young children.

1. Is it likely that his grandfather also had ankylosing spondylitis?
2. What is the risk of passing the condition to his three children?

### Case 2

A 4-year-old girl suffers frequent upper respiratory infections with chest involvement, and each episode lasts longer than in her pre-school peers. Doctors have always assumed this is somehow a consequence of her stormy early months, when she had major heart surgery for tetralogy of Fallot. She also has nasal speech and in her neonatal record a radiologist commented on the small size of the thymus gland.

1. Is there another diagnosis that could explain her frequent and prolonged upper respiratory infections?
2. What further management of the family is indicated?

## CHAPTER 14: CANCER GENETICS

### Case 1

A 38-year-old woman, who recently had a mastectomy for breast cancer, requests a referral to the genetic service. Her father had some bowel polyps removed in his fifties and a cousin on the same side of the family had some form of thyroid cancer in her forties. The general practitioner consults a set of guidelines that suggest that a familial form of breast cancer is unlikely because she is the only one affected, even though quite young. He is reluctant to refer her.

1. Could the history suggest another familial condition and, if so, which one?
2. What other clinical features might give a clue to the diagnosis?

### Case 2

A 30-year-old is referred for genetic counseling because she is concerned about her risk of developing breast cancer. The consultand's mother has recently been diagnosed with breast cancer at the age of 55. Her brother's daughter (the consultand's cousin) had bilateral breast cancer diagnosed at 38 years and died 5 years ago from metastatic disease. The cousin had participated in a research study that identified a *BRCA2* gene mutation. The clinical geneticist suggests that the consultand's mother should be tested before predictive testing is offered to her daughter. They are surprised when a negative result is reported by the laboratory.

1. What are the possible explanations for this result?
2. What is the risk of the consultand's uncle developing breast cancer?

## CHAPTER 15: GENETIC FACTORS IN COMMON DISEASES

### Case 1

A 2-year-old girl presents with partial seizures. The episode is brief and unaccompanied by fever. As the child is well with no neurological deficit, a decision is made not to treat with an anticonvulsant drug. A year later she suffers a generalized seizure, again without fever. On this occasion her 30-year-old mother asks whether this might have anything to do with her own seizures that began at the age of 15 years, though she has had only two episodes since. She had undergone a brain CT scan and the doctors mentioned a condition whose name she could not remember. The child has an MRI brain scan that shows uncalcified nodules on the lateral ventricular walls.

1. The mother asks if the epilepsy is genetic and whether it could happen again if she has another child. What can she be told?
2. What diagnoses should be considered and can genetic testing be offered?

### Case 2

A 5-year-old child is admitted to hospital with an unexplained fever and found to have a raised blood glucose level. He makes a good recovery but 2 weeks later his fasting blood glucose level is shown to be elevated at 7 mmol/L. There is a strong family history of diabetes on his mother's side with his mother, maternal uncle and maternal grandfather all affected. His father has no symptoms of diabetes but his sister had gestational diabetes during her recent pregnancy. Molecular genetic testing identifies a heterozygous glucokinase gene mutation in the child.

1. The parents believe that their son's hyperglycemia is inherited from the mother's side of the family. Is this correct?
2. What are the consequences of finding a glucokinase gene mutation for this family?

## CHAPTER 16: CONGENITAL ABNORMALITIES AND DYSMORPHIC SYNDROMES

### Case 1

A young couple have just lost their first pregnancy through fetal abnormality. Polyhydramnios was diagnosed on ultrasound as well as a small fetal kidney on one side. Amniocentesis was performed and the karyotype showed a normal 46,XY pattern. The couple were unsure what to do but eventually elected for a termination of pregnancy at 21 weeks. They were very upset and did not want any further investigations performed, including a postmortem. They did agree to a whole body X-ray of the fetus and some of the upper thoracic vertebrae were misshapen.

1. The couple ask whether such a problem could recur - they do not feel they can go through this again. What can they be told?
2. What further investigations might have helped to inform the genetic risk?

### Case 2

On routine neonatal examination on the second day a baby is found to have a cleft palate. The pregnancy was uneventful with no exposure to potential teratogens, and the family history is negative. The pediatric registrar also wonders whether the limbs are slightly short. The baby's birth weight is on the 25$^{th}$ centile, length on the 2$^{nd}$ centile.

1. What diagnoses might be considered?
2. What are the management issues in a case like this?

## CHAPTER 17: GENETIC COUNSELING

### Case 1

A couple have a son with dysmorphic features, short stature and moderately severe developmental delay. On the second occasion when his karyotype is analyzed he is found to have a subtle chromosome translocation that was missed first time. The father is found to be a balanced translocation carrier. His family have always blamed the mother for the child's condition because of her past history of drug abuse, with the result that the couple no longer talk to his wider family. However, through friends he has learned that his sister is trying to start a family.

1. What are the important genetic issues?
2. What other issues does this case raise?

### Case 2

A couple have a child who is diagnosed with cystic fibrosis (CF) at the age of 18 months. The child is homozygous for the common ΔF508 mutation. They request prenatal diagnosis in the next pregnancy but DNA analysis shows that the father is not a carrier of ΔF508. It must be assumed he is not the biological father of the child with CF, and this is confirmed when further analysis shows that the child does not have a haplotype in common with him.

1. What medical issue does this information raise?
2. What counseling issues are raised by these results?

## CHAPTER 18: CHROMOSOME DISORDERS

### Case 1

A newborn baby girl looks a little dysmorphic, is diagnosed with an AVSD congenital heart, and the pediatricians consider this may be Down syndrome. This is discussed with the parents and a karyotype performed. The result comes back as normal – 46,XX. The baby is very 'good' during infancy with very little crying, and no further investigations are done. Subsequently the child shows global developmental delay, head-banging, wakes every night for about 3 h, and has mild brachydactyly. The pediatricians refer her to a geneticist for an opinion.

1. Does the history suggest a diagnosis?
2. What investigation should be requested?

**Case 2**

The parents of a 10-year-old girl seek a follow-up appointment in the genetic clinic. At the age of 4 years she had some behavioral problems and chromosomes were tested from a blood sample. The result came back as 47,XXX, and it was explained that these girls sometimes have behavioral problems, are usually tall, fertility is normal, and 'everything would be alright'. However, by 10 years she is the smallest girl in the class and still has the slightly webbed neck that was present at birth.

1. What diagnosis should be considered and what investigation should now be offered?
2. How are the genetic counseling and future management modified by the new diagnosis?

## CHAPTER 19: SINGLE-GENE DISORDERS

**Case 1**

A 31-year-old woman would like to start a family but is worried because her 39-year-old brother was diagnosed as having Becker muscular dystrophy nearly 30 years ago and she remembers having being told that the condition affects boys but the women pass it on. Her brother is still living but now quite disabled by his condition. There is no wider family history of muscular dystrophy.

1. Is the original diagnosis reliable?
2. What are the next steps in managing this situation?

**Case 2**

A middle-aged couple are devastated when their 21-year-old daughter collapses at a dance and cannot be resuscitated. At postmortem all toxicology tests are negative and no cause of death is found. The mother recalls that her father died suddenly in his fifties from what was presumed at the time to be a cardiac cause, and her sister has had some dizzy spells but has not thought it necessary to see her doctor. The couple have three other children who are young, sport-loving adults and wonder whether this could happen again.

1. What investigations are appropriate?
2. What advice should the family be given?

## CHAPTER 20: SCREENING FOR GENETIC DISEASE

**Case 1**

A 32-year-old man is tall and thin, and 20 years ago his father died suddenly aged 50. The GP wonders whether his patient has Marfan syndrome and refers him to a genetic clinic. He has some features of Marfan syndrome but, strictly speaking, would only meet the accepted criteria if the family history was definitely positive for the disorder. He has a brother of average height, and three young children who are in good health.

1. In terms of genetic testing, what are the limitations to screening if the diagnosis is Marfan syndrome?
2. What are the screening issues for the family?

**Case 2**

A screening test for cystic fibrosis (CF) is being evaluated on a population of 100 000 newborn babies. The test is positive in 805 babies, of whom 45 are eventually shown to have CF by a combination of DNA analysis and sweat testing. Of those babies whose screening test is negative, five subsequently develop symptoms and are diagnosed with CF.

1. What is the sensitivity and specificity of this screening test?
2. What is the positive predictive value of the screening test?

## CHAPTER 21: PRENATAL TESTING AND REPRODUCTIVE GENETICS

**Case 1**

A 36-year-old pregnant woman elects to undergo prenatal testing by chorionic villus biopsy after the finding of increased nuchal translucency on ultrasound scan. The initial result, using FISH probes, is good news – there is no evidence for trisomy 21 and she is greatly relieved. However, on the cultured cells more than 2 weeks later it emerges that there is mosiacism for trisomy 20. She undergoes amniocentesis a week later, and 3 weeks after that the result also shows some cells with trisomy 20.

1. Why was an amniocentesis performed in addition to the chorionic villus biopsy?
2. What else can be done following the amniocentesis result?

**Case 2**

A couple have two autistic sons and would very much like to have another child. They are prepared to do anything to ensure that the problem does not recur. They acquire a lot of information from websites and learn that boys are more commonly affected – the male:female sex ratio is approximately 4:1. As they see it, the simple solution to their problem is sex selection by preimplantation genetic diagnosis (PGD).

1. What investigations might be performed on the autistic sons?
2. If tests on the sons fail to identify a diagnosis, can the request of the couple for sex selection by PGD be supported by the geneticist?

## CHAPTER 22: RISK CALCULATION

**Case 1**

In the pedigree shown below two cousins have married and would like to start a family. However, their uncle died many years ago from Hurler syndrome, one of the mucopolysaccharidoses, an inborn error of metabolism following autosomal recessive inheritance. No tissue samples are available for genetic studies.

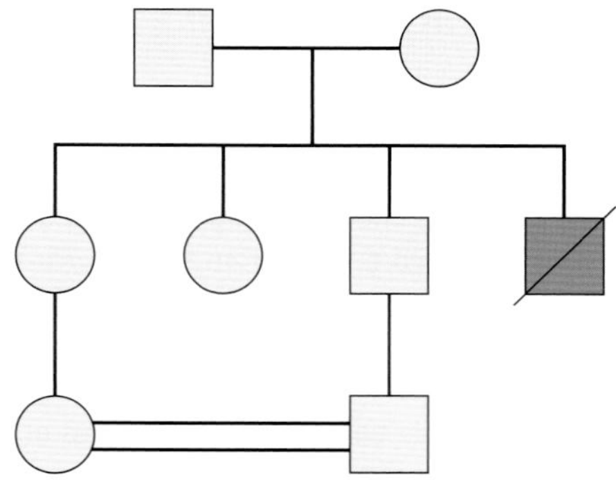

1. What is the risk that the couple's first child will be affected by Hurler syndrome?
2. Can the couple be offered anything more than a risk figure?

**Case 2**

A woman has a brother and a maternal uncle affected by hemophilia A. She herself has had two unaffected sons but would like more children. She is referred to a genetic clinic to discuss the risk and the options.

1. Purely on the basis of the information given, what is the woman's carrier risk for hemophilia A?
2. Can anything be done to modify her risk?

# Multiple-choice answers

## CHAPTER 2: THE CELLULAR AND MOLECULAR BASIS OF INHERITANCE

1. **Base substitutions:**
a. **True.** *When a stop codon replaces an amino acid*
b. **True.** *For example by mutation of conserved splice donor and acceptor sites*
c. **False.** *Silent mutations or substitutions in non-coding regions may not be pathogenic*
d. **True.** *For example promoter mutations may affect binding of transcription factors*
e. **False.** *Frameshifts are caused by the insertion or deletion of nucleotides*

2. **Transcription:**
a. **False.** *During transcription mRNA is produced from the DNA template*
b. **True.** *The mRNA product is then translocated to the cytoplasm*
c. **True.** *The mRNA is complementary to the antisense strand*
d. **False.** *Transcription factors bind to regulatory sequences within the promoter*
e. **True.** *The addition of the 5′ cap and 3′ polyA tail facilitates transport to the cytoplasm*

3. **The following are directly involved in DNA repair:**
a. **True.** *The DNA glycosylase MYH is involved in base excision repair (BER)*
b. **True.** *They incorporate the correct bases*
c. **True.** *They seal gaps after abnormal base excision and correct base insertion*
d. **False.** *Splicing removes introns during mRNA production*
e. **False.** *Ribosomes are involved in translation*

4. **During DNA replication:.**
a. **True.** *It unwinds the DNA helix*
b. **False.** *Replication occurs in both directions*
c. **True.** *These fragments are joined by DNA ligase to form the lagging strand*
d. **False.** *DNA replication is semi-conservative as only one strand is newly synthesized*
e. **False.** *Uracil is incorporated in mRNA; thymine in DNA*

## CHAPTER 3: CHROMOSOMES AND CELL DIVISION

1. **Meiosis differs from mitosis in the following ways:**
a. **True.** *During human meiosis the number of chromosomes is reduced from 46 to 23*
b. **False.** *Early cell divisions in gametogenesis are mitotic; meiosis occurs only at the final division*
c. **True.** *In meiosis the two divisions are known as meiosis I and II*
d. **True.** *The bivalents separate independently during meiosis I and cross-overs (chiasmata) occur between homologous chromosomes*
e. **False.** *The 5 stages of meiosis I prophase are leptotene, zygotene, pachytene, diplotene and diakinesis*

2. **Chromosome abnormalities reliably detected by light microscopy include:**
a. **True.** *An extra chromosome (e.g. chromosome 21 in Down syndrome) is easily seen*
b. **True.** *A missing chromosome (e.g. Turner syndrome in females with a single X) is easily seen*
c. **False.** *A subtle translocation may not be visible*
d. **False.** *A small deletion may not be visible*
e. **True.** *Centric fusion of the long arms of two acrocentric chromosomes is readily detected*

3. **Fluorescence in situ hybridization using whole chromosome (painting) or specific locus probes enables routine detection of:**
a. **False.** *Changes in gene dosage may be identified by comparative genomic hybridization (CGH)*
b. **True.** *Subtelomeric probes are useful in the investigation of non-specific learning difficulties*
c. **True.** *Trisomies can be detected in interphase cells*
d. **True.** *The origin of marker chromosomes can be determined by chromosome painting*
e. **True.** *Subtle rearrangements can be detected by chromosome painting*

**4. Chemicals used in the preparation of metaphase chromosomes for analysis by light microscopy include:**

*a.* **True.** *Colchicine inhibits spindle formation, thus arresting cells at metaphase*

*b.* **True.** *Phytohemagglutinin stimulates cell division of T lymphocytes*

*c.* **True.** *Giemsa is used to stain chromosomes a pink/purple color*

*d.* **False.** *Quinacrine is a fluorescent stain not visible by light microscopy*

*e.* **True.** *Hypotonic saline swells the cells, causing cell lysis and spreading of chromosomes*

## CHAPTER 4: DNA TECHNOLOGY AND APPLICATIONS

**1. The following statements apply to restriction enzymes:**

*a.* **True.** *Double-stranded DNA can be digested to give overhanging (sticky) ends or blunt ends*

*b.* **False.** *Over 300 restriction enzymes have been isolated from various bacteria*

*c.* **True.** *If the mutation creates or destroys a recognition site*

*d.* **True.** *DNA digestion by a restriction enzyme is the first step in Southern blotting*

*e.* **False.** *They are endonucleases as they digest DNA fragments internally, as opposed to exonuclease digestion from the 5′ or 3′ ends of DNA fragments*

**2. The following describe the polymerase chain reaction (PCR):**

*a.* **True.** *Millions of copies of DNA can be produced from one template without using cloning vectors*

*b.* **False.** *PCR uses the heat-stable Taq polymerase, as a high denaturing temperature (around 95°C) is required to separate double-stranded products at the start of each cycle*

*c.* **True.** *PCR may be used to amplify DNA from single cells (e.g. in preimplantation genetic diagnosis), hence appropriate control measures are important to avoid contamination*

*d.* **False.** *PCR routinely amplifies targets up to 1 kb and long-range PCR is limited to around 40 kb*

*e.* **False.** *Knowledge of the sequence is required to design primers to flank the region of interest*

**3. Types of nucleic acid hybridization include:**

*a.* **True.** *Southern blotting describes the hybridization of a radioactively labeled probe with DNA fragments separated by electrophoresis*

*b.* **True.** *Hybridization between the target and probe DNA takes place on a glass slide*

*c.* **False.** *Western blotting is used to analyze protein expression using antibody detection methods*

*d.* **True.** *Northern blotting is used to examine RNA expression*

*e.* **True** *DNA fingerprinting employs a minisatellite DNA probe to hybridize to hypervariable DNA fragments*

**4. The following techniques can be used to screen genes for unknown mutations:**

*a.* **True.** *Sequencing can be used to detect known or unknown mutations and will characterize an unknown mutation*

*b.* **True.** *SSCP is a cheap method for mutation screening although its sensitivity is limited*

*c.* **True.** *DHPLC is an efficient method for detecting heterozygous mutations*

*d.* **False.** *OLA is used to detect known mutations as the probe design is mutation specific*

*e.* **False.** *Real-time PCR is also used to detect known mutations as the probe design is mutation specific*

## CHAPTER 5: MAPPING AND IDENTIFYING GENES

**1. Genes can be mapped to subchromosomal regions using:**

*a.* **False.** *Somatic cell hybridization permits assignment of genes to chromosomes but not the subchromosomal region*

*b.* **True.** *FISH using a gene probe can map the chromosomal location*

*c.* **False.** *PFGE is used to map DNA fragments to a physical map rather than a subchromosomal region*

*d.* **True.** *Radiation hybrids contain chromosome fragments*

*e.* **False.** *Flow cytometry separates chromosomes that can be used as whole chromosome probes*

**2. Methods of high-resolution physical mapping include:**

*a.* **True.** *DNA sequencing is the ultimate method of high-resolution physical mapping*

*b.* **True.** *PFGE is used to map DNA fragments up to 20 kb*

*c.* **True.** *Chromosome walking is used to isolate sequences adjacent on the chromosome to a characterized clone*

*d.* **True.** *Fibre FISH allows mapping of DNA sequences which are between 2 and 700 kb apart*

*e.* **False.** *DNA fingerprinting is used to compare the identity of samples, not for mapping*

**3. Positional cloning utilizes:**

*a.* **True.** *Now the human genome sequence is complete it is possible to identify a disease-associated gene in silico*

*b.* **True.** *Once a gene has been mapped to a region it can be helpful to check for syntenic regions in animal models*

*c.* **True.** *Many genes have been identified through mapping of translocation or deletion break-points*

*d.* **False.** *Positional cloning describes the search for genes based on their chromosomal location*

*e.* **True.** *A genome-wide scan uses microsatellite markers located throughout the genome for linkage mapping*

**4. A candidate gene is likely to be a disease associated gene if:**

*a.* **True.** *This implies causality*

*b.* **True.** *This is strong evidence*

*c.* **True.** *This excludes the possibility that a single variant is a marker in linkage disequilibrium rather than a pathogenic mutation*

*d.* **True.** *For example a gene associated with blindness might be expected to be expressed in the eye*

*e.* **False.** *A pseudogene does not encode a functional protein and mutations are therefore unlikely to be pathogenic*

## CHAPTER 6: DEVELOPMENTAL GENETICS

**1. In development, *HOX* genes:**

*a.* **True.** *They are important in spatial determination and patterning*

*b.* **False.** *Only a few malformation syndromes can be directly attributed to HOX gene mutations at present, probably because of paralogous compensation*

*c.* **False.** *They contain an important conserved homeobox of 180 bp*

*d.* **True.** *They are probably only important in early development*

*e.* **True.** *Where malformation-causing mutations have been identified, different organ system may be involved, e.g. the hand–foot–genital syndrome (HOXA13)*

**2.**

*a.* **False.** *This occurs later and is the process of laying down the primary body axis in the second and third weeks*

*b.* **False.** *Organogenesis takes places mainly between 4 and 18 weeks gestation*

*c.* **True.** *The genes in these pathways are widely expressed throughout the body*

*d.* **False.** *Somites form in a rostro-caudal direction*

*e.* **True.** *When mutated these genes lead to ulnar–mammary syndrome and Holt–Oram syndrome*

**3.**

*a.* **False.** *It is formed from the first pharyngeal (branchial) arch*

*b.* **True.** *Remodeling occurs so that these vessels become the great arteries*

*c.* **True.** *This has been established in animals and is proving to be highly likely in man*

*d.* **False.** *Achondroplasia is associated with very specific FGFR3 mutations affecting the membrane-bound part of the protein*

*e.* **False.** *These different types of mutation usually cause widely differing phenotypes, e.g. the RET gene*

**4.**

*a.* **True.** *Sometimes the SRY gene is involved in recombination with the pseudoautosomal regions of X and Y*

*b.* **False.** *Not all regions of the X are switched off, otherwise there would presumably be no phenotypic effects in Turner syndrome*

*c.* **True.** *However, only when there is a mutated gene on one X chromosome does this have any consequences*

*d.* **False.** *SRY has an important initiating function, but other genes are very important*

*e.* **True.** *Some unusual phenomena occur in twins which lead to the conclusion that these processes are linked*

**5. Transcription factors:**

*a.* **False.** *They are usually proteins that bind to specific regulatory DNA sequences*

*b.* **False.** *They also switch genes on*

*c.* **True.** *For example, a leg might develop in place of an antenna*

*d.* **False.** *Transcription factors are crucial to normal laterality*

*e.* **True.** *The zinc finger motif encodes a finger-like projection of amino acids that forms a complex with a zinc ion*

## CHAPTER 7: PATTERNS OF INHERITANCE

**1. Concerning autosomal recessive inheritance:**

*a.* **False.** *Sex ratio is equal*

*b.* **False.** *The risk at the time of conception is* $\frac{1}{2}$

*c.* **True.** *All people carry mutated genes; cousins are more likely to share a mutated gene inherited from a common grandparent*

*d.* **True.** *Affected individuals would have to partner a carrier or another affected person for their offspring to be affected as well*

*e.* **False.** *The mechanisms causing Angelman syndrome are varied but autosomal recessive inheritance is not one of them*

**2. Concerning X-linked inheritance:**

*a.* **True.** *A father passes his Y chromosome to his son*
*b.* **True.** *He might have affected grandsons through his daughters who are carriers*
*c.* **False.** *Although the condition affects females, the males are more severely affected because the female has a normal copy of the gene on her other X, and X-inactivation means that the normal copy is expressed in about half of her tissues*
*d.* **True.** *All daughters of an affected man will be affected, but none of his sons*
*e.* **False.** *Germ-line mosaicism always needs to be considered when an isolated case of an X-linked condition occurs*

**3.**

*a.* **False.** *This refers to two populations of mitochondrial DNA, one normal, one mutated*
*b.* **False.** *The opposite, probably because they replicate more frequently*
*c.* **False.** *Any tissue with mitochondria can be affected*
*d.* **True.** *If the affected woman's oocytes contain only mutated mitochondria*
*e.* **False.** *Many mitochondrial proteins are encoded by nuclear genes*

**4.**

*a.* **False.** *The same disease caused by different genes – but not necessarily on different chromosomes*
*b.* **False.** *The basic pattern of inheritance in pseudodominance is autosomal recessive*
*c.* **True.** *A proportion of individuals with the mutated gene show no signs or symptoms*
*d.* **True.** *Diseases showing anticipation show increased severity, and earlier age of onset, with succeeding generations*
*e.* **False.** *Not a variation in severity (variable expression) but two or more apparently unrelated effects from the same gene*

**5.**

*a.* **True.** *Both copies of a mutated gene can be passed to a child this way*
*b.* **True.** *This explains a proportion of cases of Prader-Willi and Angelman syndromes*
*c.* **False.** *Digenic inheritance refers to heterozygosity for two different genes causing a phenotype*
*d.* **True.** *This explains presenile baldness and gout*
*e.* **False.** *Only a small proportion*

## CHAPTER 8: MATHEMATICAL AND POPULATION GENETICS

**1. In applying the Hardy-Weinberg equilibrium the following assumptions are made:**

*a.* **False.** *The population should be large to increase the likelihood of non-random mating*
*b.* **True.** *Consanguinity is a form of non-random mating*
*c.* **True.** *The introduction of new alleles introduces variables*
*d.* **True.** *In theory, if the population is small and donors are used many times this would introduce a form of non-random mating*
*e.* **True.** *Migration introduces new alleles*

**2. If the population incidence of a recessive disease is 1:10 000, the carrier frequency in the population is:**

*a.* **False.**
*b.* **False.**
*c.* **False.**
*d.* **True.** *The carrier frequency is double the square root of the incidence*
*e.* **False.**

**3. Heterozygote advantage:**

*a.* **False.** *It refers to conditions following autosomal recessive inheritance*
*b.* **True.** *The homozygote may show markedly reduced biological fitness, e.g. cystic fibrosis*
*c.* **True.** *People with sickle-cell trait are more able to remove parasitized cells from the circulation*
*d.* **True.** *A process of selective advantage may be at work*
*e.* **False.** *The presence of the allele in a population may indeed be a founder effect*

**4. Polymorphic loci:**

*a.* **False.** *The alleles need have frequencies of only 1%*
*b.* **True.** *They are crucial to gene mapping by virtue of their co-segregation with disease*
*c.* **True.** *Linkage analysis using polymorphic loci may be the only way to determine genetic status in presymptomatic diagnosis and prenatal testing*
*d.* **False.** *The association of polymorphic loci with disease segregation is key to calculating a LOD score*
*e.* **False.** *They may be important, e.g. blood groups*

**5. In population genetics:**

*a.* **False.** *The incidence of the disease must also be known*
*b.* **True.** *In autosomal recessive disease most of the genes in the population are present in unaffected heterozygotes*
*c.* **True.** *In recessive conditions unaffected sibships will not be ascertained*
*d.* **True.** *Basically, only males are affected and they always manifest the condition*
*e.* **False.** *It is only useful when there is a common ancestor from both sides of the family, i.e. inbreeding*

## CHAPTER 9: POLYGENIC AND MULTIFACTORIAL GENETICS

### 1. Concerning autism:

a. **False.** *It is a neurodevelopmental disorder and no metabolic abnormalities are found*
b. **False.** *This would imply autosomal dominant inheritance. The figure is about 20%.*
c. **False.** *Although autism occurs in Fragile-X syndrome the vast majority of affected individuals do not have this condition*
d. **True.** *The figure is nearly 3% for full-blown autism and a further 3% for milder features – autistic spectrum disorder*
e. **False.** *The male:female ratio is approximately 4:1*

### 2. Linkage analysis is more difficult in multifactorial conditions than in single-gene disorders because:

a. **True.** *Detection of polygenes with small effects is very difficult*
b. **True.** *In a fully penetrant single-gene disorder it is easier to find families with sufficient informative meioses*
c. **True.** *Parametric linkage analysis requires that the mode of inheritance is known*
d. **True.** *Different genetic and environmental factors may be involved*
e. **True.** *The late age of onset means that affection status may be uncertain*

### 3. Association studies:

a. **True.** *The disease and variant tested may be common in a population subset but there is no causal relationship*
b. **True.** *The TDT test uses family controls and thus avoids population stratification effects*
c. **True.** *Replication of positive studies in different populations will increase the evidence for an association*
d. **False.** *Association studies are used to test variants identified by gene mapping techniques, including affected sibling pair analysis*
e. **True.** *Variants with small effects may be missed if the patients and controls are not closely matched*

### 4. Variants in genes which confer susceptibility to type 2 diabetes (T2DM) have been found:

a. **True.** *The calpain-10 gene was identified by positional cloning in Mexican-American sibling pairs*
b. **False.** *No confirmed T2DM susceptibility genes have been identified by this approach*
c. **True.** *Examples include two subtypes of maturity-onset diabetes of the young (MODY)*
d. **True.** *The genes encoding the potassium channel subunits in the pancreatic $\beta$-cell were biological candidates*
e. **True.** *For example the HNF-1$\alpha$ variant G319S has only been reported in the Oji Cree population*

### 5. Variants in the *NOD2/CARD15* gene:

a. **False.** *Evidence to date supports a role in Crohn disease but not ulcerative colitis*
b. **True.** *Increased risk is estimated at 40-fold for homozygotes and 2.5x for heterozygotes*
c. **True.** *A genome-wide scan for inflammatory bowel disease (IBD) initially identified the 16p12 region*
d. **False.** *The NOD2/CARD15 gene activates NF-κB, but this complex is already targeted by the most effective drugs used to treat Crohn disease*
e. **False.** *The three reported variants are found at a frequency of 5% in the general population, compared to 15% in patients with Crohn disease*

## CHAPTER 10: HEMOGLOBIN AND THE HEMOGLOBINOPATHIES

### 1.

a. **True.** *The population should be large to increase the likelihood of non-random mating*
b. **False.** *This true for the $\alpha$ and $\gamma$ chains only; the $\beta$ chain appears towards the end of fetal life*
c. **False.** *There are too few $\alpha$ chains, which are replaced by $\beta$ chains*
d. **False.** *It is a form of $\alpha$-thalassemia*
e. **False.** *They have a mild anemia and clinical symptoms are rare*

### 2. Regarding sickle-cell disease:

a. **False.** *The effect is due to reduced solubility and polymerization*
b. **True.** *Obstruction of arteries can be the result of sickling crises*
c. **True.** *A valine residue is substituted for a glutamic acid residue*
d. **False.** *Life-threatening sepsis can result from splenic infarction*
e. **True.** *These mutations give rise to an amino-acid substitution*

### 3.

a. **True.** *This applies to the majority of those known*
b. **False.** *All types of mutation are known*
c. **False.** *Bone marrow hyperplasia occurs, which leads to physical changes such as a thickened calvarium*
d. **True.** *Oxygen is not released so readily to tissues*
e. **True.** *Hb H, for example, is unstable*

**4.**

*a.* **False.** *It is a hereditary condition*

*b.* **False.** *This is true only between about 2 and 7 months gestation*

*c.* **False.** *The bone marrow starts producing Hb from 6-7 months of fetal life*

*d.* **False.** *Production ceases from 2-3 months of postnatal life*

*e.* **True.** *It gives rise to no symptoms - the Hb chains produced are normal*

## CHAPTER 11: BIOCHEMICAL GENETICS

**1. In congenital adrenal hyperplasia (CAH):**

*a.* **True.** *The most common enzyme defect is 21-hydroxylase deficiency*

*b.* **True.** *This occurs in the rare forms - 3β-dehydrogenase, 5α-reductase, and desmolase deficiencies*

*c.* **True.** *Hyponatremia and hyperkalemia may be severe and lead to circulatory collapse*

*d.* **False.** *Cortisol and fludrocortisone are required lifelong in salt-losing CAH*

*e.* **False.** *Fertility is reduced in the salt-losing form*

**2. Phenylketonuria:**

*a.* **False.** *There is a benign form as well as abnormalities of cofactor synthesis*

*b.* **False.** *Dietary restriction of phenylalanine is only necessary during childhood and pregnancy*

*c.* **True.** *These are features if untreated*

*d.* **True.** *Affected individuals have reduced pigment and are fair*

*e.* **False.** *A different pathway*

**3. Hepatomegaly is an important feature of:**

*a.* **True.** *Hepatomegaly is a feature of most of the mucopolysaccharidoses*

*b.* **True.** *Hepatomegaly is a feature of most of the glycogen storage disorders, though not all*

*c.* **False.** *This is not a feature, even in the so-called hepatic porphyrias*

*d.* **True.** *This is one of the sphingolipidoses, lipid storage diseases*

*e.* **False.** *Cirrhosis can occur in the untreated*

**4. Concerning mitochondrial disorders:**

*a.* **False.** *The main patterns of inheritance also apply where mitochondrial proteins are encoded by nuclear genes*

*b.* **True.** *Especially in NARP and MIDD, respectively*

*c.* **True.** *There are 37 gene products*

*d.* **False.** *Leigh disease is genetically heterogeneous*

*e.* **True.** *The G4.5 gene is mutated, urinary 3-methyglutaconic acid is raised, but the link remains to be elucidated*

**5.**

*a.* **True.** *The carnitine cycle is important for long-chain fatty acid transport into mitochondria*

*b.* **True.** *90% of alleles are due to the same mutation and neonatal population screening has been suggested*

*c.* **False.** *These are inborn errors of copper transport metabolism*

*d.* **True.** *These features should prompt investigation for organic acidurias and mitochondrial disorders, among others*

*e.* **False.** *Important radiological features may be seen in peroxisomal and storage disorders*

## CHAPTER 12: PHARMACOGENETICS

**1. Thiopurine drugs used to treat leukemia:**

*a.* **True.**

*b.* **True.** *They are used to treat autoimmune disorders and to prevent rejection of organ transplants*

*c.* **False.** *They can be toxic in 10–15% of patients*

*d.* **True.** *These include leukopenia and severe liver damage*

*e.* **True.** *Variants in the TPMT gene are associated with thiopurine toxicity*

**2. Liver enzymes which show genetic variation of expression and hence influence the response to drugs include:**

*a.* **True.** *Complete deficiency of this enzyme causes type 1 Crigler–Najjar disease*

*b.* **False.** N-*acetyltransferase (NAT2) variation influences metabolism of isoniazid*

*c.* **False.** *Absence of ALDH2 (acetaldehyde dehydrogenase) is associated with an acute flushing response to alcohol*

*d.* **True.** *Approximately 5–10% of the European population are poor metabolizers of debrisoquine owing to a homozygous variant in the CYP2D6 gene*

*e.* **True.** *CYP2C9 variants are associated with decreased metabolism of warfarin*

**3. The following have an increased risk of complications from anesthesia:**

*a.* **True.** *Malignant hyperthermia is dominantly inherited*

*b.* **True.** *RYR1 mutations are associated with malignant hyperthermia*

*c.* **False.** *G6DP deficiency results in sensitivity to certain drugs and fava beans*

*d.* **True.** *Homozygous CHE1 mutations cause suxamethonium sensitivity*

*e.* **False.** *Pseudocholinesterase metabolizes suxamethonium, hence decreased levels are associated with suxamethonium sensitivity*

**4. Examples of diseases where treatment maybe influenced by pharmacogenetics include:**

*a.* **False.** *Patients with glucokinase mutations are usually treated with diet alone*
*b.* **True.** *Patients with HNF-1$\alpha$ mutations are sensitive to sulphonylureas*
c. **True.** *Abacavir is an effective drug but approximately 5% of patients show potentially fatal hypersensitivity*
*d.* **True.** *Some patients show adverse reactions to the drug felbamate*
e. **True.** *Slow inactivators of isoniazid are more likely to suffer side-effects*

## CHAPTER 13: IMMUNOGENETICS

**1.**

*a.* **False.** *The cascade can also be activated by the alternative pathway*
*b.* **True.** *C4 levels are reduced and production of C2b is uncontrolled*
c. **False.** *C3 levels are normal, C4 are reduced*
*d.* **True.** *C3b adheres to the surface of microorganisms*
e. **False.** *Complement is a series of at least 20 interacting plasma proteins*

**2.**

*a.* **False.** *It is made up of four polypeptide chains - 2 'light' and 2 'heavy'*
*b.* **False.** *They are distributed around different chromosomes*
c. **False.** *Donors are likely to share HLA haplotypes, which are crucial to tissue compatibility*
*d.* **True.** *These are variable, diversity, junctional and constant regions*
e. **True.** *Antigen receptors contain two immunoglobulin-like domains*

**3.**

*a.* **False.** *They are protected for 3–6 months only*
*b.* **False.** *X-linked SCID is 50–60% of the total*
c. **True.** *B-cell positive SCID due to JAK3 deficiency can be subclinical*
*d.* **True.** *A defect in either T-cell function or development*
e. **False.** *CGD is an X-linked disorder of cell-mediated immunity*

**4.**

*a.* **False.** *It is classed as a secondary or associated immunodeficiency*
*b.* **True.** *Immunodeficiency is usually mild and the immune system improves with age as the thymus grows; there is a proneness to viral infections in childhood*
c. **False.** *The causes of CVID are not known and it is often a disorder of adult life*
*d.* **False.** *The risk to first-degree relatives is increased but the pedigree pattern is more suggestive of multifactorial conditions*
e. **True.** *FTT may be the only clue to an immunodeficiency disorder*

## CHAPTER 14: CANCER GENETICS

**1.**

*a.* **True.** *The best-known example is chronic myeloid leukemia and the Philadelphia chromosome*
*b.* **False.** *Tumor suppressor genes are more common than oncogenes*
c. **True.** *Apoptosis is normal, programmed cell death*
*d.* **False.** *LOH refers to the presence of two defective alleles in a tumor suppressor gene*
e. **False.** *Although important, APC mutations are part of a sequence of genetic changes leading to colon cancer*

**2.**

*a.* **True.** *The paradigm was retinoblastoma and the hypothesis was subsequently proved to be correct*
*b.* **False.** *Mutations in TP53 are found in many cancers, but are germline in Li–Fraumeni syndrome*
c. **False.** *It is implicated in MEN 2 but not MEN 1*
*d.* **True.** *There is a significant risk of small bowel polyps and duodenal cancer*
e. **True.** *Women with this condition have a lifetime risk of up to 50%*

**3.**

*a.* **True.** *This syndrome is allelic with Cowden disease, in which papillary thyroid cancer can occur*
*b.* **True.** *The lifetime risk may be in the region of 16%*
c. **False.** *The* BRCA1 *and* BRCA2 *genes do not account for all familial breast cancer*
*d.* **False.** *The lifetime risk of breast cancer for female* BRCA1 *or* BRCA2 *carriers is 60–85%*
e. **False.** *The figure is approximately 15%*

**4.**
- *a.* **False.** *Cerebellar hemangioblastoma is a common tumor in VHL*
- *b.* **False.** *This tumor is seen in MEN 2 and VHL disease*
- *c.* **True.** *There is also an increased risk in familial breast cancer*
- *d.* **True.** *Melanin spots in PJS, BCCs in Gorlin syndrome, and skin tumors in the Muir–Torre form of HNPCC*
- *e.* **False.** *The figure is approximately one-third*

**5.**
- *a.* **True.** *Clear cell renal carcinoma is a significant risk in VHL*
- *b.* **False.** *It is easier to detect breast cancer by mammography in postmenopausal women*
- *c.* **False.** *It should begin at birth*
- *d.* **False.** *This does not meet the Amsterdam criteria for HNPCC*
- *e.* **False.** *It is strongly indicated in FAP but not women positive for* BRCA1 *mutations*

## CHAPTER 15: GENETIC FACTORS IN COMMON DISEASES

**1.**
- *a.* **False.** *The figure is approximately 40%*
- *b.* **True.** *One form of epilepsy is autosomal dominant benign familial neonatal convulsions*
- *c.* **False.** *This epilepsy is non-Mendelian*
- *d.* **True.** *A large proportion of cases have epilepsy of different kinds, including infantile spasms*
- *e.* **False.** *It is Mendelian (autosomal recessive) but is progressive with neurodegeneration*

**2.**
- *a.* **False.** *The high risk is for schizophrenia*
- *b.* **False.** *The risk lies between 40 and 50%*
- *c.* **True.** *This is the case despite many studies suggesting significant linkage*
- *d.* **True.** *The concordance rates in monozygotic and dizygotic twins are 67% and 20%, respectively*
- *e.* **False.** *Although present in about 40% of Alzheimer's disease it is not discriminatory enough for screening*

**3.**
- *a.* **True.** *Conversion of the prion protein to the abnormal isoform, $PrP^{Sc}$, is more likely*
- *b.* **True.** *The genes are APP, Presenilin-1 and Presenilin-2*
- *c.* **False.** *The penetrance is very high for all Mendelian Alzheimer's disease so far reported*
- *d.* **False.** *Epidemiological studies using twins have proved more important so far in answering this question*
- *e.* **True.** *However, the reasons are not entirely clear, despite the APP gene being located on chromosome 21*

**4. Hemochromatosis:**
- *a.* **True.** *Mutations in at least five genes can cause hemochromatosis*
- *b.* **False.** *Males are five times more likely to be affected*
- *c.* **True.** *Regular phlebotomy is an effective treatment*
- *d.* **False.** *Penetrance may be as low as 1%*
- *e.* **False.** *The most common cause is homozygosity for the C282Y HFE mutation*

**5. The following statements about venous thrombosis are true:**
- *a.* **True.** *They account for more than 50% of cases*
- *b.* **False.** *Unlikely, but their first-degree relatives can be offered testing and prophylactic treatment if necessary*
- *c.* **False.** *The factor V Leiden mutation renders the factor V protein resistant to cleavage by activated protein C*
- *d.* **True.** *Elevated serum prothrombin levels result from the G20210A variant*
- *e.* **True.** *The risks are multiplicative*

## CHAPTER 16: CONGENITAL ABNORMALITIES AND DYSMORPHIC SYNDROMES

**1.**
- *a.* **False.** *The figure is approximately 25%*
- *b.* **True.** *This is the figure from chromosome studies. The figure might be much higher if all lethal single-gene abnormalities could be included*
- *c.* **False.** *The figure is 2–3%*
- *d.* **False.** *This is an example of deformation*
- *e.* **True.** *'Sequence' implies a cascade of events traced to a single abnormality*

**2.**
- *a.* **False.** *Syndrome is correct because of the highly recognizable nature of the condition*
- *b.* **False.** *It has been found to be due to mutations in a single gene*
- *c.* **True.** *The figure varies between populations and is lowered by periconceptional folic acid*
- *d.* **False.** *This well-defined entity is an autosomal recessive condition*
- *e.* **True.** *It may be chromosomal, autosomal dominant, and autosomal recessive*

**3.**
- *a.* **True.** *A teratogen represents a chemical or toxic disruption*
- *b.* **True.** *Renal agenesis causes oligohydramnios, which leads to talipes through deformation*
- *c.* **False.** *A variety of limb defects can occur*
- *d.* **True.** *There is a generalized effect on a particular tissue, such as bone or skin*
- *e.* **False.** *The figure is much higher, at around 50%*

**4.**

*a.* **True.** *Deafness and various visual defects are features*

*b.* **False.** *The first trimester is much more dangerous*

*c.* **True.** *Vertebral defects at any level are possible, including sacral agenesis*

*d.* **False.** *This is true for some populations, not all*

*e.* **True.** *Peripheral pulmonary artery stenosis in the case of congenital rubella*

**5.**

*a.* **True.** *The incidence is between 1:500 and 1:1000*

*b.* **False.** *Low recurrence risk because they are thought not to be genetic*

*c.* **False.** *Large studies of many families are required*

*d.* **True.** *Smith-Lemli-Opitz syndrome is a defect of cholesterol metabolism, affecting the sonic hedgehog pathway*

*e.* **False.** *The figure is much nearer 1:100*

## CHAPTER 17: GENETIC COUNSELING

**1.**

*a.* **False.** *This is the consultand; the proband is the affected individual*

*b.* **False.** *Retinitis pigmentosa can follow all the main patterns of inheritance*

*c.* **False.** *It is far more – transfer of relevant information, presentation of options and facilitating decision making in the face of difficult choices*

*d.* **False.** *Non-directive counseling is the aim because patients/clients should be making their own decisions*

*e.* **True.** *Patients do not remember risk information accurately and there are other important measures of patient satisfaction*

**2.**

*a.* **False.** *The risk is approximately twice the background risk*

*b.* **True.** *This is a second-degree relationship*

*c.* **False.** *The risk is roughly 25%*

*d.* **False.** *It is perfectly normal in many societies*

*e.* **False.** *It refers to anything from, e.g. uncle–niece partnerships (second degree) to third cousins (seventh degree)*

**3.**

*a.* **False.** *Guilt feelings from parents and grandparents are common when a genetic disease is first diagnosed in a child*

*b.* **False.** *Many patients make the choice they would have made before genetic counseling – but after the counseling they should be much better informed*

*c.* **True.** *The risk from each grandparent is 1:64*

*d.* **False.** *Such a practice is strongly discouraged and the indications for genetic testing should be the same*

*e.* **False.** *Good patient support groups have a huge role, and the patients/families themselves become the experts for their condition*

## CHAPTER 18: CHROMOSOME DISORDERS

**1.**

*a.* **True.** *Chromosome number was identified in 1956; DNA structure in 1953*

*b.* **True.** *A wide variety of abnormal karyotypes occur in spontaneous abortuses but 45,X is the single most common one*

*c.* **False.** *It is estimated that 80% of all Down syndrome fetuses are lost spontaneously*

*d.* **True.** *Although the risk of Down syndrome increases with maternal age the large proportion of babies born to younger mothers means that most Down syndrome babies are born to this group*

*e.* **False.** *A small proportion have an IQ at the lower end of the normal range*

**2.**

*a.* **False.** *Such cases usually die within days or weeks of birth*

*b.* **True.** *Males with Klinefelter syndrome (47,XXY) are usually infertile*

*c.* **True.** *This accounts for a substantial proportion of cases*

*d.* **False.** *This is not seen in either uniparental disomy or imprinting center defect cases*

*e.* **True.** *The deletion on 22q11.2 is a 3 Mb region flanked by very similar DNA sequences*

**3.**

*a.* **True.** *Probably due to haploinsufficiency for elastin*

*b.* **False.** *Congenital heart disease is not a recognized feature of Prader–Willi syndrome*

*c.* **False.** *Chromosome 11p13, and may be a feature of WAGR and Beckwith–Wiedemann syndrome*

*d.* **True.** *A mutation in PAX6 or a deletion encompassing this locus at 11p15*

*e.* **True.** *Behavioral phenotypes can be very informative, e.g. Smith–Magenis syndrome*

**4.**

*a.* **False.** *The figure is approximately 1 in 1000*

*b.* **False.** *IQ is reduced by 10-20 points but learning difficulties are not a feature*

*c.* **True.** *The other cell line may be normal but could also contain Y chromosome material*

*d.* **False.** *They have normal fertility*

*e.* **True.** *This occurs because of DNA instability*

**5.**

*a.* **True.** *The mutation passes from a normal transmitting male to his daughters essentially unchanged*

*b.* **False.** *In addition to FRAXA there is also FRAXE and FRAXF*

*c.* **True.** *Androgen insensitivity syndrome can present this way*

*d.* **False.** *This is unreliable. DNA analysis is necessary*

*e.* **False.** *The figure is around 5%*

## CHAPTER 19: SINGLE-GENE DISORDERS

**1.**

*a.* **False.** *Meiotic instability is greater in spermatogenesis than in oogenesis*

*b.* **True.** *This has been shown from studies in Venezuela*

*c.* **False.** *The duration is approximately 10–15 years*

*d.* **True.** *This is so for the reduced penetrance alleles of 36–39 repeats*

*e.* **True.** *The condition is due to a very large triplet repeat expansion, as in Fragile-X syndrome*

**2.**

*a.* **False.** *Somnolence is common*

*b.* **False.** *Neonatal hypotonia*

*c.* **True.** *Through a CUG RNA-binding protein, which interferes with a variety of genes*

*d.* **True.** *An important feature of myotonic dystrophy and the defining abnormality of many channelopathies*

*e.* **True.** *Males with mild or subclinical CF have congenital bilateral absence of the vas deferens*

**3.**

*a.* **False.** *The ΔF508 mutation is the most common*

*b.* **True.** *The polythymidine tract – 5T, 7T and 9T – can be crudely correlated with different CF phenotypes*

*c.* **False.** *This is true for most of the inherited cardiac arrhythmias; cardiomyopathies are often due to defects in cardiac muscle proteins*

*d.* **True.** *This glycoprotein complex in the muscle membrane contains a variety of units; defects in these cause various limb girdle dystrophies*

*e.* **False.** *These patients have normal intelligence*

**4.**

*a.* **False.** *They are good candidates according to current thinking*

*b.* **False.** *It is only a component of the skeletal system criteria*

*c.* **False.** *It is believed to be a fully penetrant disorder*

*d.* **True.** *This is not usually severe but is a recognized feature*

*e.* **False.** *The opposite is the case*

**5.**

*a.* **False.** *This is a neurophysiological classification*

*b.* **True.** *Autosomal dominant, autosomal recessive and X-linked*

*c.* **True.** *Mutations in the peripheral myelin protein affect Schwann cells*

*d.* **False.** *They are not good discriminatory tests and DNA analysis is much preferred*

*e.* **False.** *It is an inherited cardiac arrhythmia*

## CHAPTER 20: SCREENING FOR GENETIC DISEASE

**1.**

*a.* **True.** *By looking for evidence of two populations of cells*

*b.* **True.** *Firm clinical signs are the exception rather than the rule*

*c.* **False.** *DNA sequence variants must be polymorphic to be useful*

*d.* **False.** *There is far too much locus heretogeneity in this condition*

*e.* **True.** *As a general rule this may be vital, but should be undertaken with informed consent*

**2.**

*a.* **False.** *The facial rash of angiokeratoma (adenoma sebaceum) is often not present*

*b.* **False.** *There may not be sufficient numbers of café-au-lait spots until 5–6 years*

*c.* **False.** *They may be fully in formative of an individual's genetic status*

*d.* **True.** *Dural ectasia of the lumbar spine is one of the major criteria*

*e.* **False.** *Linked DNA markers, and sometimes biochemical tests, may be the best modality available*

**3.**

*a.* **False.** *Participation should, in principle, be voluntary*

*b.* **True.** *The outcome of population screening programs should be an improvement in health benefit*

*c.* **False.** *This is the specificity of a test*

*d.* **True.** *This is different from the sensitivity, which refers to the proportion of affected cases that are detected (i.e. there may be some false negatives)*

*e.* **True.** *Adequate expert counseling should be part of the predictive test program*

4.
a. **True.** *Recall of the result itself, or the interpretation, is frequently inaccurate*
b. **False.** *The highest incidence for a serious disease is β thalassemia – 1 in 8 are carriers*
c. **False.** *This has happened before and should be a major concern*
d. **False.** *The benefit lies in informing the family for subsequent reproductive decisions*
e. **False.** *The first assay is biochemical, a measure of immuno-reactive trypsin*

5.
a. **False.** *Although the carrier frequency is about 1:10, no population screening is undertaken in the UK*
b. **False.** *In general, unless a beneficial medical intervention can be offered, such testing should be deferred until the child is old enough to make the decision*
c. **True.** *They have been operational for about 30 years*
d. **False.** *This is only at the research stage*
e. **False.** *Their prime function in a service department is for clinical management of patients and families*

## CHAPTER 21: PRENATAL TESTING AND REPRODUCTIVE GENETICS

1.
a. **False.** *It is still mainly performed around 16 weeks gestation*
b. **False.** *They also derive from the amnion and fetal urinary tract epithelium*
c. **True.** *The risk is 1–2% compared to 0.5–1%*
d. **False.** *There is a small risk of causing limb abnormalities; CVS should not be performed before 11 weeks gestation*
e. **False.** *Fetoscopy would be required for this if a DNA test is not available*

2.
a. **True.** *This forms part of the triple test*
b. **True.** *This forms part of the triple test*
c. **False.** *In trisomy 18 all maternal serum markers are low*
d. **False.** *The best figure achieved is around 86%*
e. **True.** *There are two fetuses rather than one*

3.
a. **False.** *The figure is about 1%*
b. **True.** *Especially aneuploidies*
c. **True.** *Probably due to the presence of inspissated meconium*
d. **True.** *Most Down syndrome is due to meiotic non-disjunction*
e. **True.** *They are unlikely to have different clinical effects in different members of the same family*

4.
a. **False.** *A licence from the HFEA is required*
b. **False.** *It is not illegal but does require an HFEA licence*
c. **True.** *This is undertaken to avoid the presence of extraneous sperm*
d. **False.** *The figure is about 25%*
e. **False.** *Chromosome disorders are the largest group*

5.
a. **True.** *Chromosome abnormalities are present in10–12% of men with azoospermia or severe oligospermia, some of them heritable*
b. **False.** *Currently, the rule is that no more than 10 pregnancies may result from one donor*
c. **False.** *They are not currently entitled to know the identity of their biological parents*
d. **True.** *Analyzing fetal cells in the maternal circulation only removes the miscarriage risk*
e. **False.** *The figure is approximately 1 in 7*

## CHAPTER 22: RISK CALCULATION

1.
a. **True.** *These are two ways of expressing the same likelihood*
b. **True.** *A probability of one means that the event will happen 100% of the time*
c. **True.** *The probability that both will be boys is* $\frac{1}{2}\times\frac{1}{2}=\frac{1}{4}$*; for girls the same; therefore the chance of being the same sex is* $\frac{1}{4}+\frac{1}{4}=\frac{1}{2}$ *(0.5)*
d. **True.** *These two approaches to a probability calculation are essential*
e. **True.** *70% of heterozygotes will manifest the condition*

2. **For an autosomal recessive condition the chance that the first cousin of an affected individual is a carrier is:**
a. **False.**
b. **False.**
c. **True.** *The affected individual's parents are obligates carriers, aunts and uncles have a 1 in 2 risk, cousins a 1 in 4 risk*
d. **False.**
e. **False.**

3. **In X-linked recessive inheritance:**
a. **False.** *The risk is 1 in 2 if the sex of the fetus is known to be male*
b. **False.** *The male might be affected because a new mutation has occurred*
c. **True.** *This is significant and has to be allowed for in risk calculation and counseling*
d. **True.** *This is conditional information that can be built into a Bayes' calculation*
e. **False.** *This is a key individual whose risk must be calculated before the consultand's risk*

**4. In autosomal recessive inheritance the risk that the nephew of an affected individual, born to the affected individual's healthy sibling, is a carrier is:**

*a.* **False.**
*b.* **False.**
*c.* **False.**
*d.* **True.** *The healthy sibling of the affected individual has a 2 in 3 chance of being a carrier; this person's son has a risk which is half that*
*e.* **False.**

**5.**

*a.* **True.** *For example, negative mutation findings when testing for cystic fibrosis*
*b.* **True.** *Age of onset (clinical expression) data must be derived from large family studies*
*c.* **False.** *Without this information huge errors will be made*
*d.* **True.** *An empiric risk is really a compromise figure*
*e.* **False.** *It may matter a lot because it is a measure of the likelihood that a meiotic recombination event will take place between the marker and the gene mutation causing the disease*

## CHAPTER 23: THE HUMAN GENOME PROJECT, TREATMENT OF GENETIC DISEASE AND GENE THERAPY

**1. Achievements of the Human Genome Project include:**

*a.* **False.** *The draft sequence was completed in 2000, but its publication date was February 2001*
*b.* **True.** *Sequencing was finished two years ahead of the original schedule*
*c.* **True.** *Annotation tools such as Ensembl were developed to assist users*
*d.* **False.** *Nearly 1500 have been identified to date*
*e.* **True.** *Around 5% of the US budget for the Human Genome Project was devoted to studying these issues*

**2. Methods currently used to treat genetic disease include:**

*a.* **False.** *Germ-cell gene therapy is considered unacceptable because of the risk of transmitting genetic changes to future generations*
*b.* **True.** *For example bone marrow transplantation is used to treat various inherited immunodeficiencies*
*c.* **True.** *Examples include the replacement of factor VIII or IX in patients with hemophilia*
*d.* **True.** *For example, restricted phenylalanine in patients with phenylketonuria*
*e.* **False.** *This potential treatment has been tested in animal models*

**3. Gene therapy may be delivered by:**

*a.* **True.** *Liposomes are widely used as they are safe and can facilitate transfer of large genes*
*b.* **True.** *CFTR gene therapy trials have used adeno-associated viral vectors*
*c.* **False.** *Antisense oligonucleotides need to be delivered to the target cells*
*d.* **True.** *Lentiviruses may be useful for delivery of genes to non-dividing cells*
*e.* **True.** *An example is the injection of plasmid-borne factor IX into fibroblasts from patients with hemophilia B*

**4. Gene therapy has been used to successfully treat patients with the following diseases:**

*a.* **False.** *Trials have shown safe delivery of the CFTR gene to the nasal passages but effective treatment of cystic fibrosis is not possible at present*
*b.* **True.** *A number of patients have been successfully treated, although concern was raised when two boys developed leukemia*
*c.* **False.** *This will be difficult because the number of $\alpha$- and $\beta$-globin chains must be equal or a thalassemia phenotype might result*
*d.* **True.** *Some patients have been able to reduce their exogenous clotting factors*
*e.* **True.** *Although early attempts were unsuccessful, two patients have now been successfully treated by ex vivo gene transfer*

**5. Potential gene therapy methods for cancer include:**

*a.* **True.** *An example is the protein kinase inhibitor used to treat chronic myeloid leukemia*
*b.* **True.** *Perhaps through overexpression of interleukins*
*c.* **False.** *Anti-angiogenic factors might be used to reduce blood supply to tumors*
*d.* **True.** *RNA interference is a promising new technique which can used to target overexpressed genes associated with cancers*
*e.* **True.** *A number of trials are ongoing to determine the utility of this technique*

# Case-based answers

## CHAPTER 6: DEVELOPMENTAL GENETICS

**Case 1**

1. The combination of macrocephaly, odontogenic keratocysts, and basal cell carcinomas occurs in Gorlin (basal cell nevoid carcinoma) syndrome. This condition should be in the differential diagnosis of a child with macrocephaly, with appropriate exploration of the family history. It is understandable that hydrocephalus would be the main concern, but true hydrocephalus is unusual in Gorlin syndrome.
2. The child's father is an obligate carrier for the *PTCH* gene mutation causing Gorlin syndrome in the family. He should be regularly screened (at least annually) by X-ray for odontogenic keratocysts and come under regular surveillance by a dermatologist for basal cell carcinomas. *PTCH* gene mutation analysis is possible for any affected family member.

**Case 2**

1. The two most likely causes of sex reversal in a young 'girl' are androgen insensitivity syndrome (AIS), which is X-linked and due to mutations in the androgen receptor gene, and mutations in the *SRY* gene on the Y chromosome.
2. Mutation analysis in both the androgen receptor and *SRY* genes can be performed to determine the genetic basis of the sex reversal. It is very important to investigate and locate, if present, remnants of gonadal tissue because this will have to be removed to avoid the risk of malignant change. Because of this the parents should be given a full explanation but the phenotypic sex of the child should be affirmed as female.

## CHAPTER 7: PATTERNS OF INHERITANCE

**Case 1**

1. It is possible that the problems described in family members are unrelated but this is unlikely. If the condition has passed from the grandfather then mitochondrial inheritance is very unlikely. The condition is either autosomal dominant with variability, or X-linked.
2. The spinocerebellar ataxias are a genetically heterogeneous group of conditions that usually follow autosomal dominant inheritance and could present in this way. A form of hereditary spastic paraparesis is possible, also genetically heterogeneous and usually following autosomal dominant inheritance, though recessive and X-linked forms are described. Apart from these, X-linked adrenoleukodystrophy must be considered, especially as the man has signs of cognitive and behavioral problems. This is very important, not only because it can present early in life but also because of the potential for adrenal insufficiency.

**Case 2**

1. The information *may* be correct but is probably not and other possibilities must be explained to them.
2. Most forms of osteogenesis imperfecta (brittle bone disease) follow autosomal dominant inheritance. Sibling recurrence, when neither parent has signs or symptoms, can be explained by somatic and/or germline mosaicism in one of the parents. The risk to the offspring of those affected would then be 50%, i.e. high. In this case history the possibility of a non-genetic diagnosis must be considered, namely non-accidental injury. It is therefore important to try and confirm the diagnosis.

## CHAPTER 8: MATHEMATICAL AND POPULATION GENETICS

**Case 1**

1. Clearly, it is essential to know whether the condition in question has ever knowingly occurred in the families of either of the two consultands. If this had occurred it would potentially modify the carrier risk for one of the consultands regardless of the frequency of the disease in the population.
2. Assuming the disorder in question has not previously occurred in the family, the carrier frequency in the population A is 1:50, and 1:15 in the population B. The risk in the first pregnancy is therefore $\frac{1}{50} \times \frac{1}{15} \times \frac{1}{4} = \frac{1}{3000}$.

**Case 2**

1. From the figures given four cases in the town appear to be new mutations, i.e. four new mutations per 100 000 genes inherited. The mutation rate is therefore 1 per 25 000 gametes.
2. The population sample is small and may not therefore be representative of the larger, wider population. For example, if there is a bias towards an older, retired population, the reproducing sub-population may be smaller and the figures

distorted by the migration of younger people away from the town. Also, the four 'new mutation' cases should be verified by proper examination of the parents.

## CHAPTER 9: POLYGENIC AND MULTIFACTORIAL INHERITANCE

### Case 1

1. Testing for the factor V Leiden and prothrombin 20210A variant is appropriate. A positive result would provide a more accurate risk of her developing thromboembolism and would inform her choice of contraception. Heterozygosity for factor V Leiden or the prothrombin 29219A variant would increase her risk by 4–5-fold. Homozygosity or compound heterozygosity would increase her risk by up to 80-fold.
2. Negative results for FVL and the prothrombin 20210A variant in the consultand should be interpreted with caution since up to 50% of cases of venous thrombosis are not associated with these genetic risk factors.

### Case 2

1. The proband might have type 1 diabetes (T1DM), type 2 diabetes (T2DM) or maturity-onset diabetes of the young (MODY). Since both have normal hearing a diagnosis of maternally inherited diabetes and deafness (MIDD) is unlikely. T1DM and T2DM show multifactorial inheritance with environmental factors playing a role in addition to predisposing genetic susceptibility factors. MODY shows autosomal dominant inheritance.
2. The brother's risk of developing diabetes is 6%, 35% or 50%, respectively. If his sister is found to have a mutation in one of the genes causing MODY then he could have predictive genetic testing. A negative test would reduce his risk to that of the population. A positive test would allow regular monitoring in order to make an early diagnosis of diabetes and avoid diabetic complications due to longstanding undiagnosed diabetes.

## CHAPTER 10: HEMOGLOBIN AND THE HEMOGLOBINOPATHIES

1. The ethnic origin of the couple and the limited information should suggest the possibility of a hematological disorder. α-Thalasssemia is the likely cause of stillbirth, hydrops being secondary to heart failure, which in turn is secondary to anemia. Rhesus isoimmunization and glucose-6-phosphate dehydrogenase deficiency are other possibilities. Severe forms of congenital heart disease are frequently associated with hydrops, but the chance of a sibling recurrence (which occurred in the case history) is low. However, there are many other causes of hydrops and these would need to be considered. Among those that are genetic with a chance of recurrence are lethal forms of rare skeletal dysplasias and a wide range of metabolic disease.
2. A full blood count, blood groups, Hb electrophoresis, and maternal autoantibody and glucose-6-phosphate dehydrogenase deficiency screens should be performed for the couple. DNA analysis may detect the common mutation seen in SE Asia, which would then make it possible to offer genetic prenatal diagnosis by chorionic villus sampling. If no disorder is identified by these investigations it is unlikely that further diagnostic progress will be made unless the couple have another affected pregnancy that can be fully investigated by examination of the fetus.

### Case 2

1. This presentation is consistent with acute intermittent porphyria and hemolytic uremic syndrome. However, the ethnic origin should suggest the possibility of sickle-cell disease. The contents of the dark urine, and specific tests for porphyria, will help to differentiate these and a sickle-cell test should be performed.
2. If the diagnosis is sickle-cell disease there are various agents that can be tried to reduce the frequency of sickling crises – hydroxyurea in particular. Prophylactic penicillin is important for reducing the risk of serious pneumococcal infections, and the family should be offered genetic counseling and cascade screening of relatives.

## CHAPTER 11: BIOCHEMICAL GENETICS

### Case 1

1. Hypoglycemia can be part of severe illness in young children but in this case the intercurrent problem appears relatively minor, suggesting that the child's metabolic capacity to cope with stress is compromised. This history should prompt investigations for a possible inborn error of metabolism and, if a diagnosis is made, the younger sibling should be tested.
2. Hypoglycemia is a common consequence of a number of inborn errors of amino acid and organic acid metabolism. Investigation should begin with analysis of urinary organic acids, and plasma amino acids, ammonia and liver function tests.

### Case 2

1. If there is a family history of similar symptoms it might demonstrate matrilinear inheritance with all the offspring of affected males being normal. If this person is the only affected individual a family history will not be informative with respect to the diagnosis.
2. All causes of myopathy need to be considered but the combination of features is suggestive of a mitochondrial cytopathy. This would explain the muscular symptoms, ptosis, and hearing impairment – and there might also be evidence of a cardiomyopathy, neurological disturbance, retinitis pigmentosa and diabetes mellitus. Mitochondrial DNA analysis on peripheral lymphocytes might identify a mutation but a negative result would not rule out the diagnosis. A muscle biopsy might show ragged red fibers and DNA analysis on this tissue might be more informative than lymphocytes.

## CHAPTER 13: IMMUNOGENETICS

### Case 1

1. The nature of his grandfather's symptoms are rather non-specific – back pain and arthritis are both very common in

the general population. However, it is certainly possible that he also had ankylosing spondylitis, a form of enthesitis (inflammation at the site of insertion of a ligament or tendon into bone) with involvement of synovial joints, as the heritability is greater than 90%.
2. About 95% of patients with ankylosing spondylitis are positive for the HLA-B27 antigen; however, in the general population this test has only a low positive predictive value. His children have a 50% chance of being HLA-B27 positive; if positive, the risk of developing clinical ankylosing spondylitis is about 9%; if negative, the risk is less than 1%.

**Case 2**

1. This history points very strongly towards a diagnosis of deletion 22q11 (DiGeorge/Sedláčková) syndrome, which can easily be confirmed by specific FISH testing. Immunity is impaired but usually only mildly, and gradual improvement occurs through childhood and adolescence.
2. Deletion 22q11 syndrome can be familial and does not always give rise to congenital heart disease. If confirmed in the child, both parents should be offered FISH testing, and other family members as appropriate. Genetic counseling for the child will be important when she is older.

## CHAPTER 14: CANCER GENETICS

**Case 1**

1. The family history should first of all be confirmed with the consent of the affected individuals. If the thyroid cancer in the cousin was papillary in type, and the polyps in her father hamartomatous, the pattern would be very suspicious for Cowden disease. This is also known as multiple hamartoma syndrome, which is autosomal dominant and often due to mutations in *PTEN*, and the risk of breast cancer is approximately 50% in females.
2. Macrocephaly, a cobblestone appearance of the oral mucosa, and generalized lipomas are other features to look for in patients with this unusual history.

**Case 2**

1. If the *BRCA2* mutation has not been confirmed in another family member or by testing another sample from the deceased cousin (e.g. a tissue section embedded in paraffin), the possibility of a sample mix-up in the research laboratory cannot be excluded. If, however, the uncle tests positive for the mutation, then the consultand's mother is a phenocopy. Alternatively the mutation may have been inherited from the cousin's mother.
2. If the uncle tests positive for the *BRCA2* mutation then his lifetime risk of developing breast cancer is approximately 6%, more than 100-fold higher than that of the general population.

## CHAPTER 15: GENETIC FACTORS IN COMMON DISEASES

**Case 1**

1. Generally, the risk of epilepsy to first-degree relatives is around 4%. However, mother and daughter are affected here, which suggests the possibility of a Mendelian form of epilepsy. Furthermore, it seems that both have an abnormal finding on brain imaging and the mother's CT films should be located and reviewed. At this stage an explanation of both autosomal dominant and X-linked inheritance should be given, as well as the possibility that the two cases of epilepsy are coincidental.
2. The condition that the mother's doctors mentioned would almost certainly have been tuberous sclerosis (TS), which follows autosomal dominant inheritance. Further evaluation of both mother and daughter looking for clinical features of TS might be indicated and genetic testing is available. However, the nodules on the lateral ventricle walls may be pathognomonic of bilateral periventricular nodular heterotopia (BPVNH) and the images should be reviewed by someone who can recognize this. BPVNH is an abnormality of neuronal migration and inherited as an X-linked dominant, caused by mutations in the filamin-1 (*FLNA*) gene. Testing is available. In general, Mendelian forms of epilepsy are rare.

**Case 2**

1. Not necessarily. Many people with glucokinase gene mutations are asymptomatic and their mild hyperglycemia is only detected upon screening (routine medicals, during pregnancy or intercurrent illness). Gestational diabetes in the father's sister suggests that the mutation could have been inherited from his side of the family.
2. Identifying a glucokinase gene is 'good news' as the mild hyperglycemia is likely to be stable throughout life, treated by diet alone (except during pregnancy) and unlikely to result in diabetic complications. Cascade testing can be offered to other relatives. If the mutation has been inherited from the father, his sister and her child may be tested. The sister might avoid the anxiety of having a young child diagnosed with unexplained hyperglycemia.

## CHAPTER 16: CONGENITAL ABNORMALITIES AND DYSMORPHIC SYNDROMES

**Case 1**

1. This is not an unusual scenario. The karyotype on amniocentesis was normal and polyhydramnios suggests the possibility of a gastrointestinal obstruction such as esophageal atresia. The abnormalities are more likely to represent an 'association' rather than a syndrome or Mendelian condition. The empiric recurrence risk is low, and all that can be offered is ultrasound examination in subsequent pregnancies.
2. A fetal postmortem is highly desirable in this situation to know the full extent of internal organ anomalies. A repeat karyotype on fetal skin might have shown something that was not detected on amniocentesis, and DNA should be stored for possible future use. Maternal diabetes should be excluded. As a last resort the parents' chromosomes could be tested, including telomere screens to look for the possibility of a cryptic translocation.

**Case 2**

1. Isolated, non-syndromic cleft palate is statistically the most likely diagnosis but the mild short stature might be significant. Syndromic possibilities include spondyloepiphyseal dysplasia congenita (SEDC) – though there are many rare syndromes with more severe short stature and other features.
2. The short stature appears mild; it is therefore important to try and determine whether this might be familial – the parents need to be assessed. Follow-up of the baby is indicated, including a radiological skeletal survey to see if there is an identifiable skeletal dysplasia. SEDC may be accompanied by myopia and sensorineural hearing impairment, therefore hearing and vision assessment is important. However, the child has cleft palate and is at risk of conductive hearing problems as a result. The cleft palate team need to be involved from the beginning.

## CHAPTER 17: GENETIC COUNSELING

**Case 1**

1. The couple are at risk of having further affected children and prenatal diagnosis can be offered. The father may have inherited the balanced translocation from one of his parents and his sister may also be a carrier. Carrier testing should be offered to his family, especially as his sister is trying to get pregnant.
2. The father's wider family need to be made aware of the child's diagnosis, but they have their own fixed misconceptions and it might be very difficult to accept that the child's problems have their origin on their side of the family. There is a severe communication problem but a way needs to be found to inform the father's wider family of the genetic risk. It might be necessary to involve their GPs.

**Case 2**

1. There is now no need for the woman to undergo an invasive prenatal test in future pregnancies, which would be a waste of resources and place the pregnancy at a small but unnecessary risk of a miscarriage.
2. There is the difficulty of communicating the fact that a prenatal test is not necessary, but disclosure of non-paternity may have far reaching consequences or the marriage. The counselors do not know if the 'father' suspects non-paternity, and the mother may think he is the biological father of the child.

## CHAPTER 18: CHROMOSOME DISORDERS

**Case 1**

1. Head-banging is not rare in early childhood, especially in children with developmental delay, and it is not necessarily a helpful feature in making a diagnosis. However, combined with the persistently disturbed sleep pattern the diagnosis of Smith–Magenis syndrome should be considered. These children can be quiet as babies and have congenital heart disease.
2. Smith–Magenis syndrome is usually due to a microdeletion at 17p11.2, for which a FISH probe test is available. They can also exhibit self-hugging behavior and develop scoliosis. Melatonin has proved a very effective treatment for sleep disturbance.

**Case 2**

1. The previous counseling given naturally assumed the girl was *pure* 47,XXX. However, the subsequent course raises the possibility that she has chromosome mosaicism, and in particular she might be mosaic for Turner syndrome (45,X). A buccal smear and/or skin biopsy should be offered to look at chromosomes in a tissue other than blood. If this is normal, other causes of short stature would need to be considered.
2. If the child is indeed found to be a 45,X:47,XXX mosaic, she needs to be investigated for the complications of Turner syndrome – congenital heart disease and horseshoe kidney. In addition, her fertility is in question and she would need to be referred to a pediatric endocrinologist, who would also assess her for possible growth hormone treatment.

## CHAPTER 19: SINGLE-GENE DISORDERS

**Case 1**

1. The history in the brother is consistent with his having Becker muscular dystrophy (BMD) but is also consistent with other diagnostic possibilities, e.g. limb–girdle muscular dystrophy (LGMD). These two conditions have sometimes been difficult to distinguish and the inheritance is different, with quite different implications for the woman who wishes to start a family.
2. The medical records of the affected brother should be reviewed and he should be reassessed. Thirty years ago the tests for BMD were very basic but now dystrophin gene mutation analysis is available. A muscle biopsy subjected to specific dystrophin staining may be diagnostic, but if this is negative staining techniques for different forms of LGMD are available. If one of the LGMD group, the woman can be reassured because these follow autosomal recessive inheritance. If BMD, carrier testing for the consultand would only be straightforward if a specific mutation is found in her brother.

**Case 2**

1. The sudden, unexpected death of young adults, especially when no cause can be identified, is extremely shocking for a family. The focus of attention becomes the inherited arrhythmias and cardiomyopathies – sometimes the latter show no obvious features at postmortem. All close family members are eligible for cardiac evaluation by echocardiogram, ECG and provocation tests, looking for evidence of the long QT and Brugada syndromes. Genetic testing is available but not guaranteed to identify a pathogenic mutation. Some forms of inherited arrhythmia/cardiomyopathy are amenable to prophylactic treatment; for others very little is currently available.
2. Management will depend on the outcome of investigations and genetic testing. However, if no specific findings are made it is very difficult to know how to advise families like this. High-intensity sports and swimming should probably be avoided in case such activity is a precipitating factor for a life-threatening arrhythmia.

## CHAPTER 20: SCREENING FOR GENETIC DISEASE

### Case 1

1. Mutation analysis in the fibrillin-1 gene is possible on the consultand but not guaranteed to identify a mutation even if the clinical diagnosis is confident. Linkage analysis at the fibrillin-1 locus on chromosome 15 would be possible using DNA from the consultand's mother and inferring the haplotype of the father, whose affected status would have to be assumed. In a small family, however, linkage may be consistent with segregation of the condition by chance. Furthermore, in unusual cases Marfan syndrome is due to a mutated gene at a separate locus on chromosome 3. There are serious pitfalls to genetic testing in this situation.
2. The important life-threatening complication of Marfan syndrome is progressive aortic root dilatation carrying a risk of dissection. Those with a firm diagnosis must be followed until at least age 30. If there is doubt about the diagnosis, regular cardiac screening is probably a sensible precaution for all those at risk until their mid-twenties.

### Case 2

1. The sensitivity is the proportion of true positives detected by the test, i.e $\frac{45}{45+5}$ = 90%. The specificity is the proportion of true negatives detected by the test, i.e. 99 190 (the unaffected cases who test negative) / 99,190 + 760 (the unaffected cases who test positive) = 99.2%.
2. The positive predictive value is the proportion of cases with a positive test who truly have the disease, i.e. $\frac{45}{805}$ = 5.6%.

## CHAPTER 21: PRENATAL TESTING AND REPRODUCTIVE GENETICS

### Case 1

1. The finding of mosaicism for trisomy 20 in CV tissue might have been a case of confined placental mosaicism. The latter is not a rare event for a wide variety of chromosome aberrations but, as long as it is confined, there are no serious consequences for the pregnancy. The problem with going on to perform an amniocentesis is in interpretation of the result. If no abnormal cells are found this does not completely rule out chromosome mosaicism in the fetus. If abnormal cells are found, the clinical implications are very difficult, if not impossible, to predict.
2. This case illustrates the rollercoaster of emotions and experiences that some women and couples have to cope with as a result of different forms of prenatal test and their interpretation. In fact, trisomy 20 mosaicism is unlikely to be of great clinical significance – but it is very difficult to be sure. Renal abnormalities have been reported and detailed fetal anomaly scanning can be offered for the remainder of the pregnancy. However, what might have been an enjoyable pregnancy will probably continue to be an anxious one.

### Case 2

1. In the large majority of autism cases no specific diagnosis is reached. Chromosome analysis including a multi-telomere screen, fragile-X syndrome, a metabolic screen, and examination for neurocutaneous disorders, should all be performed.
2. This is a very difficult situation. However, there is no proof in this case that autism is X-linked, and therefore no guarantee that any daughter will be unaffected. It would, therefore, be very difficult to support this request in the UK where PGD is regulated by the Human Fertilisation and Embryology Authority and sex selection for anything other than clearly X-linked conditions is not licenced. In other countries, where these techniques are not regulated, the couple might find clinicians who acquiesce to their request.

## CHAPTER 22: RISK CALCULATION

### Case 1

1. The siblings of the affected aunt each have a $\frac{2}{3}$ chance of being carriers; therefore each of the couple have a $\frac{1}{3}$ chance of being carriers. The chance of their first baby being affected is $\frac{1}{3} \times \frac{1}{3} \times \frac{1}{4} = \frac{1}{36}$.
2. Even though genetic studies cannot be performed, biochemical prenatal testing can be offered for their pregnancies, but biochemical tests will not reliably determine whether they are carriers. If they elect for prenatal testing it would also be worth testing for Hunter syndrome, which can easily be confused with Hurler syndrome clinically, and is X-linked.

### Case 2

1. A simple Bayes' calculation can be performed, taking into account that she has had two normal sons (Table 1). She therefore has a $\frac{1}{5}$, or 20%, chance of being a carrier.
2. There is a good chance of identifying the factor VIII gene mutation in either her brother or uncle if either of them is still alive. If so, it should then be possible to determine her carrier status definitively. If not, tests of factor VIII levels and factor VIII related antigen may give a result that can modify her risk but this is not necessarily discriminatory. DNA linkage analysis would be much more reliable, provided DNA samples are available.

Table 1

| Probability | Is a carrier | Is not a carrier |
|---|---|---|
| Prior<br>Conditional<br>(2 normal sons) | $\frac{1}{2}$<br><br>$\frac{1}{2} \times \frac{1}{2}$ | $\frac{1}{2}$<br><br>1 |
| Joint | $\frac{1}{8}$ | $\frac{1}{2}$ |
| Posterior | $\frac{1}{8} / \frac{1}{8} + \frac{1}{2} = \frac{1}{5}$ | |

# Index